HUSZAR'S
ECG AND 12-LEAD INTERPRETATION

HUSZAR'S

ECG AND 12-LEAD INTERPRETATION

SIXTH EDITION

KEITH WESLEY, MD, FACEP, FAEMS

Medical Director
United Emergency Medical Response
Wisconsin Rapids, Wisconsin

ELSEVIER

Elsevier
3251 Riverport Lane
St. Louis, Missouri 63043

HUSZAR'S ECG AND 12-LEAD INTERPRETATION, SIXTH EDITION   ISBN: 978-0-323-71195-1

Notices

Knowledge and best practice in this field are constantly changing. As new research and experience broaden our understanding, changes in research methods, professional practices, or medical treatment may become necessary. Practitioners and researchers must always rely on their own experience and knowledge in evaluating and using any information, methods, compounds or experiments described herein. Because of rapid advances in the medical sciences, in particular, independent verification of diagnoses and drug dosages should be made. To the fullest extent of the law, no responsibility is assumed by Elsevier, authors, editors or contributors for any injury and/or damage to persons or property as a matter of products liability, negligence or otherwise, or from any use or operation of any methods, products, instructions, or ideas contained in the material herein.

Library of Congress Control Number: 2021938409

Senior Content Strategist: Sandra Clark
Senior Content Development Manager: Laura Schmidt
Content Development Specialist: Laura Fisher
Publishing Services Manager: Deepthi Unni
Project Manager: Janish Ashwin Paul
Design Direction: Renee Duenow

Printed in India

Last digit is the print number: 9 8 7 6 5 4 3 2

To all the emergency medical technicians, paramedics, physicians,
and nurses I've had the honor to work with during my career.
You are the tireless heroes of medicine.

To my wife, Karen.
You are the light of my life.

To my three sons: JT, Austin, and Camden.
Thank you for being such incredible men.

And to their wives: Nikki, Jen, and Brenna.
Thank you for loving them as much as I do.

To all you: without your love, confidence, and patience,
I could not have pursued my dream.

I love you.

Keith Wesley, MD, FACEP, FAEMS

ABOUT THE AUTHOR

Keith Wesley is board certified in emergency medicine and holds subspecialty certification in emergency medical service (EMS) medicine. Originally from Tyler, Texas, he graduated from Brigham Young University in 1982 and Baylor College of Medicine in Houston, Texas, in 1986. He completed an emergency medicine residency at Methodist Hospital in Indianapolis, Indiana, where he gained his first exposure to EMS flying air medical missions.

Dr. Wesley has been involved in EMS since 1989, working with many services in Wisconsin. In 1992, he was selected by the governor as a founding member of the Wisconsin State Physician Advisory Committee and served for 12 years, the last 4 years as chair.

From 1992 to 2004, Dr. Wesley was a clinical assistant professor at the University of Wisconsin Family Practice Residency in Eau Claire, Wisconsin. There he was responsible for the training and education of family practice residents rotating through the emergency department.

In 2006, Dr. Wesley was selected as the Wisconsin State EMS medical director. He held that position until 2008, when he moved his practice to Minnesota and accepted the position of Minnesota State EMS medical director, which he held until 2010. From 2008 to 2020, he worked for M Health Fairview EMS, formally HealthEast Medical Transportation, in St. Paul, Minnesota, as the EMS medical director for Emergency Medical Services. From 2007 to the present, he has been the medical director for United Emergency Medical Response in Wisconsin Rapids, Wisconsin.

Dr. Wesley is a former chair of the National Council of State EMS Medical Directors and is active in the National Association of EMS Physicians. He has coauthored four textbooks and numerous articles and papers and is a frequent speaker at state and national conferences. He is currently on the editorial board of *JEMS* magazine.

An active member of the American College of Emergency Physicians and the National Association of EMS Physicians, Dr. Wesley has been actively involved in creating educational programs for medical and nursing students, emergency medical technicians (EMTs), and physicians.

When not engaged in EMS duties, Dr. Wesley enjoys spending time with his wife, Karen, who is a retired police officer and tactical paramedic. They live in Eau Claire, Wisconsin, with their golden retriever, Charly, and shih tzu, Sammie.

FOREWORD TO THE SIXTH EDITION

Dr. Keith Wesley's *Huszar's ECG and 12-Lead Interpretation* has been a mainstay of emergency medical services (EMS) and allied health education for decades. It has always provided a pragmatic approach to the interpretation and utilization of the electrocardiogram (ECG) in the clinical setting. The sixth edition is an important update for this essential textbook and reflects the evolving science and practice of acute cardiac care.

I had the honor of meeting Dr. Robert J. Huszar many years ago when this book was released by a different publisher. He was passionate about cardiology from an emergency standpoint. He was witty and knowledgeable and had a great amount of respect for those learning ECGs and ECG monitoring. When I was instructing paramedics in the late 1970s in Texas, we always required Dr. Huszar's book (then called *Emergency Cardiac Care*) for our students for ECG interpretation instruction. Dr. Keith Wesley is a fellow emergency physician and longtime friend and colleague. He has taken Dr. Huszar's book to a new level, which is why it remains popular decades later. He has continued the great tradition of Dr. Huszar.

The Centers for Disease Control and Prevention reports that one person dies every 37 seconds in the United States from cardiovascular disease. As with many medical conditions, early diagnosis and treatment of certain cardiovascular conditions are essential. Electrocardiography, the science of the ECG, is one of the most sensitive tools was have for rapidly detecting heart attacks and other life-threatening conditions. Because of this, EMS providers and other healthcare practitioners must be adept at ECG recognition and interpretation. Drs. Huszar and Wesley have recognized this, and using the book you are holding, they will help you understand ECGs and help ensure that your patients with acute cardiac conditions receive the prompt and efficient emergency care they need.

The sixth edition of *Huszar's ECG and 12-Lead Interpretation* has been extensively updated and provides a concise and comprehensive discussion of the science of electrocardiography. It is an excellent educational tool and reference for any provider who deals with ECG monitoring and interpretation.

Bryan E. Bledsoe, DO, FACEP, FAEMS
Professor, Emergency Medicine and Trauma
University of Nevada, Las Vegas, School of Medicine
Las Vegas, Nevada

PUBLISHER'S NOTE

The author and publisher have made every attempt to check dosages and advanced life support content for accuracy. The care procedures presented here represent accepted practices in the United States. They are not offered as a standard of care. Advanced life support–level emergency care is performed under the authority of a licensed physician. It is the student's responsibility to know and follow local care protocols as provided by his or her medical advisors. It is also the student's responsibility to stay informed of changes in emergency care procedures, including the most recent guidelines set forth by the American Heart Association and printed in their textbooks.

PREFACE

This text was written to teach medical, nursing, and emergency medical service (EMS) providers basic skills in cardiac rhythm interpretation. It also provides a wealth of advanced instruction in the clinical signs, symptoms, and management of patients presenting with cardiac dysrhythmias.

With the advent of electrocardiogram (ECG) monitoring has come readily accessible 12-lead electrocardiography, an essential tool in the detection and management of acute coronary syndromes. Accordingly, this edition has several chapters dedicated to 12-lead ECG interpretation. The book also offers in-depth coverage of the pathophysiology, clinical signs and symptoms, and management of acute coronary syndromes.

Each rhythm is first presented in its classic form, with a quick-reference box outlining its unique characteristics. The accompanying text contains a detailed explanation of these features and a discussion of the range of variability and the possible exceptions to each pattern. Many of the rhythm strips are from real patients. Thus they do not necessarily have all of the classic characteristics described in the text. That's the challenge of ECG rhythm interpretation.

The treatment algorithms are based on the latest resuscitation guidelines issued by the American Heart Association and the American College of Cardiology. However, because the science continues to evolve and local policy and protocol may vary, it's important to stay abreast of new treatments as they evolve.

This edition of the text offers information in a more visual format that allows quick reference and review.

ECG KEYS BOXES

Skillful diagnosis and treatment of rhythm disorders are based on mastery of a body of foundational knowledge. ECG Keys boxes highlight this core information, such as clinical indications and end points for the administration of certain agents.

AUTHOR'S NOTES

It's critical to be aware of the broad range of variables that might make a patient's rhythm look less than classic. In Author's Notes, I point out some of these considerations. Many of the notes pertain to diagnosis or treatment and not strictly interpretation. For example, I advise asking patients about discomfort, not just pain, when taking a history. Author's Notes also point out ways in which my recommendations may differ from the course of action suggested in other texts or required by local protocols.

KEY DEFINITIONS

This text contains a full glossary. Key Definitions call attention to the most relevant terms, making them easily accessible while you're reviewing the surrounding topics. These on-page definitions often elaborate on the information given in the glossary.

TAKE-HOME POINTS

When you don't have time to read or reread an entire chapter, Take-Home Points hit the highlights. This bulleted summary gives you need-to-know information about the most important topics covered.

CHAPTER REVIEW QUESTIONS

Appendix A provides answers to the Chapter Review Questions sections to check your knowledge of the main points presented. Appendix B contains 290 ECG rhythms for interpretation, along with case scenarios, with answers provided in Appendix C.

Each chapter in this book builds on the skills and principles explored earlier. By moving sequentially through the chapters, you'll have all the tools you need for accurate rhythm interpretation, diagnosis, and clinical management. If you're a seasoned veteran, you already know how rewarding such competence can be. If you're a student, welcome to this exciting, critical, and sometimes challenging subject.

Keith Wesley, MD, FACEP, FAEMS

ACKNOWLEDGMENTS

First, I would like to thank the dedicated men and women of M Health Fairview EMS, formally HealthEast Medical Transportation, and United Emergency Medical Response, who provided me encouragement, criticism, and reams of rhythm strips and 12 leads.

Next, I must acknowledge the successful foundation upon which this book is based. Dr. Huszar expertly crafted this text in its first three editions. To be given the opportunity to carry on where this great man left off is an honor.

Keith Wesley, MD, FACEP, FAEMS

PUBLISHER'S ACKNOWLEDGMENTS

The editors wish to acknowledge the reviewers of the fifth edition of this book for their invaluable assistance in developing and fine-tuning this manuscript.

Vincent M. DiGiulio Jr., BS, EMT-CC
EMT–Critical Care
Binghamton, New York

Hugh Grantham, ASM, MBBS, FRACGP
Professor of Paramedics
Flinders University
South Australia

Brent M. Lopez, MSN, RN
LPN Instructor
Applied Tech
St. Louis, Missouri

Lane Miller, MBA/HCM, BS/BM
Adjunct Faculty
Community College of Baltimore County
Baltimore, Maryland

Brooks Walsh, MD
Attending Physician
Department of Emergency Medicine
Bridgeport, Hospital–Yale–New Haven
Bridgeport, Connecticut

Our continued thanks also go out to the previous edition reviewers, whose hard work continues to contribute to the ongoing success of this book:

Robert Carter, Kevin T. Collopy, Robert Cook, Robert Elling, Janet Fitts, Timothy Frank, Mark Goldstein, Glen A. Hoffman, Robert L. Jackson, Kevin B. Kraus, Lynn Pierzchalski-Goldstein, Ronald N. Roth, Mikel Rothenburg, Judith Ruple, Ronald D. Taylor, Glen Treankler, Andrew W. Stern, David L. Sullivan, and Gilbert N. Taylor.

CONTENTS

HUSZAR'S

ECG AND 12-LEAD INTERPRETATION

1 Anatomy and Physiology of the Heart

CARDIAC ANATOMY AND PHYSIOLOGY

The primary purpose of the heart is to pump blood through the circulatory system. The heart is a muscle made up of four chambers (Fig. 1.1) arranged in pairs: the upper chambers are called *atria,* and the lower chambers are called *ventricles.* The two upper chambers, the *right and left atria,* have thin walls. The two lower chambers, the *right and left ventricles,* have thick, muscular walls. The point at which the two atria connect to the vascular system is referred to as the *base of the heart.* The ventricles form a rounded cone attached at the *apex of the heart.* This arrangement may seem a bit backward when you look at a diagram of the heart because the base is at the top and the apex at the bottom (see Fig. 1.1).

> **AUTHOR'S NOTE** The heart is also part of the endocrine system. It secretes hormones that help regulate blood pressure and kidney function. In this text, we will limit our discussion to the heart's role in pumping blood.

Composition

The walls of the atria and ventricles are composed of three layers of tissue (Fig. 1.2):
1. **Endocardium.** The innermost layer, called the *endocardium,* is thin and smooth. The endocardium reduces friction between the blood and the inner walls of the atria and ventricles.
2. **Myocardium.** The middle layer is called the *myocardium.* It contains the muscle cells that contract and relax. In the

ventricles, where the muscular walls are much thicker than in the atria, the myocardium is divided into the *subendocardial area,* which is the inner half of the myocardium, and the *subepicardial area,* the outer half of the myocardium.
3. **Epicardium.** The outermost tissue layer, the *epicardium,* is a thin layer of smooth connective tissue similar to the endocardium. The epicardium reduces friction between the heart and the pericardial sac that envelops it.

The walls of the left ventricle are more muscular and about three times thicker than the walls of the right ventricle. The atrial walls, like those of the ventricles, are also composed of three layers of tissue, but the middle muscular layer of the atrial walls is much thinner than that of the ventricles.

> **AUTHOR'S NOTE** The epicardium is also referred to as the *visceral pericardium.*

Protection

The heart is enclosed in a protective dual-layered membrane called the *pericardium,* or *pericardial sac.* Its tough outer layer, the parietal pericardium (see Fig. 1.2), comes into direct contact with the lungs and the diaphragm. The inner layer of the pericardium is called the *visceral pericardium.* It is in contact with the outer surface of the heart. The space between the visceral pericardium and the parietal pericardium contains a small amount of pericardial fluid. This fluid reduces friction between the beating heart and the pericardial sac.

Inferiorly (at the bottom), the pericardium is attached to the center of the diaphragm. Anteriorly (at the front), it's attached to the sternum; posteriorly (at the back), to the esophagus,

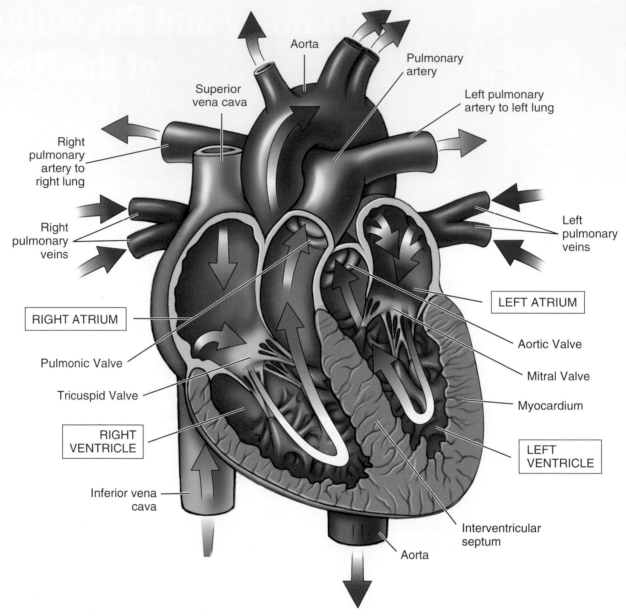

FIG. 1.1 Anatomy and circulation of blood through the heart. (Modified from Herlihy, B. [2011]. *The human body in health and illness* [4th ed.]. Saunders.)

trachea, and main bronchi; and at the base (top) of the heart, to the aorta, the superior and inferior vena cava (collectively referred to as the *venae cavae*), and the right and left pulmonary veins. In this way, the pericardium anchors the heart to the chest and limits its movement within the mediastinum.

Two Pumps

The interatrial septum (a thin, membranous wall) separates the two atria. A thicker, more muscular wall, the interventricular septum, separates the two ventricles. These two septa, in effect, divide the heart lengthwise into two pumping systems: the right heart and the left heart. Each consists of an atrium and a ventricle.

RIGHT HEART

The right heart pumps blood into the pulmonary circulation. The left heart pumps blood into the systemic circulation. The systemic circulation includes the arteries that supply blood to the body and the arteries of the coronary circulation, which supply blood to the heart.

The right atrium receives deoxygenated blood from the body from two sources:

1. Two of the body's largest veins, the superior vena cava and inferior vena cava (together called the *venae cavae*).
2. The coronary sinus, a large vein located on the back side of the heart. This vein receives venous blood from the coronary circulation.

The blood in the right atrium is then delivered to the right ventricle through the tricuspid valve. Next, the right ventricle pumps the deoxygenated blood through the pulmonary valve and into the lungs through the right and left pulmonary arteries. In the lungs, the blood picks up oxygen and releases carbon dioxide.

- Next, the ventricles contract vigorously (ventricular systole). This causes a sharp spike in ventricular pressure. As the tricuspid and mitral valves close completely, the aortic and pulmonary valves snap open. This allows the forceful ejection of blood into the pulmonary and systemic circulation.
- Meanwhile, the atria have again relaxed and begun filling with blood. As soon as the ventricles empty and begin to relax (ventricular diastole), the ventricular pressure falls, the aortic and pulmonary valves shut tightly, the tricuspid and mitral valves open, and the rhythmic cardiac sequence begins anew.

> **AUTHOR'S NOTE** Coronary perfusion occurs during ventricular diastole, when the aortic valve is closed.

The sequence of one ventricular systole followed by ventricular diastole is called a *cardiac cycle*. The cardiac cycle extends from the initiation of atrial contraction to ventricular relaxation.

ELECTRICAL CONDUCTION SYSTEM OF THE HEART

The conduction system of the heart (Fig. 1.4) is composed of the following structures:
- The sinoatrial (SA) node
- The conduction tracts between the SA and AV nodes and the conduction tract between the atria (Bachmann's bundle)
- The atrioventricular (AV) junction, consisting of the AV node and bundle of His
- The right bundle branch and the left bundle branch and its anterior and posterior small conduction tracts, called *fascicles*
- The Purkinje network

The SA node lies in the wall of the right atrium near the inlet of the superior vena cava. It consists of pacemaker cells that generate electrical impulses automatically and regularly. These impulses travel to the atria and ventricles, causing them to contract (Fig. 1.5).

Three conduction tracts run through the walls of the right atrium between the SA node and the AV node: the anterior, middle, and posterior internodal tracts. These tracts conduct the electrical impulse from the SA node to the AV node in 0.03 seconds. The interatrial conduction tract (Bachmann's bundle), a branch of the anterior internodal tract, extends across the atria, conducting the electrical impulses from the SA node to the left atrium.

The AV node, the proximal part of the AV junction, lies partly in the right side of the interatrial septum in front of the opening of the coronary sinus and partly in the upper part of the interventricular septum above the base of the tricuspid valve.

The AV node consists of three regions:
1. **Atrionodal region.** The small upper region, located between the lower part of the atria and the nodal region, is called the *atrionodal region.*

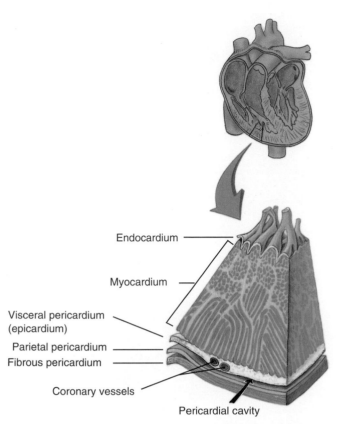

Endocardium

Myocardium

Visceral pericardium (epicardium)

Parietal pericardium

Fibrous pericardium

Coronary vessels

Pericardial cavity

FIG. 1.2 Pericardium and pleura. (Applegate, E. [2011]. *The anatomy and physiology learning system* [4th ed.]. Saunders.)

LEFT HEART

The left atrium receives the newly oxygenated blood from the lungs via the right and left pulmonary veins and delivers it to the left ventricle through the mitral valve. The left ventricle then pumps the oxygenated blood out through the aortic valve and into the aorta, the largest artery in the body. From there, the blood is distributed throughout the body, including the heart, where the blood supplies oxygen to the cells.

ATRIAL AND VENTRICULAR DIASTOLE AND SYSTOLE

The heart performs its pumping action repeatedly in a rhythmic sequence, as follows (Fig. 1.3):
- First, the atria relax (atrial diastole), allowing the blood to pour in from the venae cavae and pulmonary veins. The pressure of blood in the venae cavae and pulmonary veins is referred to as *preload.*
- As the atria fill with blood, the ventricles begin to relax. As the atrial pressure rises above that in the ventricles, the tricuspid and mitral valves (collectively called the *atrioventricular valves*) open. Blood empties rapidly through the open valves into the relaxed ventricles.
- Then the atria contract (atrial systole) to maintain the preload pressure required to keep the atrioventricular valves open. Blood continues to fill the ventricles to capacity. Toward the end of atrial contraction, the pressure in the atria and ventricles equalizes, and the tricuspid and mitral valves begin to close.

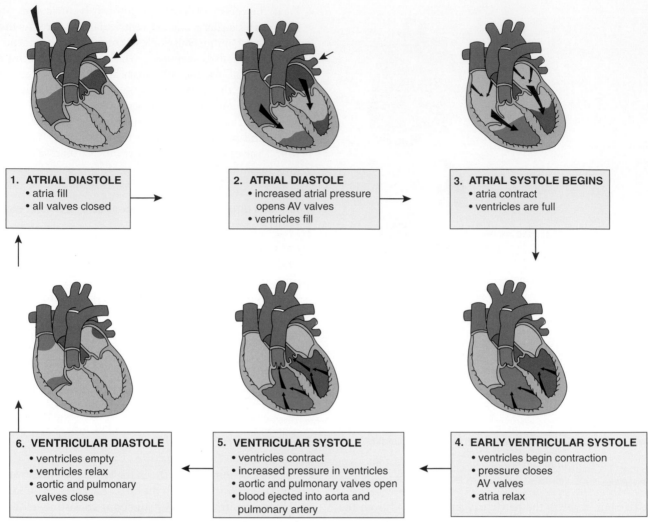

FIG. 1.3 Ventricular diastole and systole. (VanMeter, K. C., & Hubert, R. J. [2014]. *Gould's pathophysiology for the health professions* [5th ed.]. Saunders.)

2. **Middle nodal region.** The large, central area of the AV node is called the *middle nodal region*. In this area, the progression of electrical impulses from the atria to the ventricles is slowed.
3. **Nodal-His region.** The small, lower nodal-His region is located between the nodal region and the bundle of His. The atrionodal and nodal-His regions contain pacemaker cells (described later in the chapter), whereas the nodal region does not.

The primary function of the AV node is to ensure that electrical impulses from the atria to the bundle of His follow the most efficient pathway and to slow their progression so that they arrive at the ventricles after the ventricles have filled with blood. A ring of fibrous tissue insulates the remainder of the atria from the ventricles, preventing electrical impulses from entering the ventricles except through the AV node, unless there are accessory conduction pathways, as described later.

The electrical impulses slow as they travel through the AV node, taking about 0.06 to 0.12 seconds to reach the bundle of His. This delay allows the atria time to contract and empty and the ventricles to fill completely before they (the ventricles) are stimulated to contract.

The bundle of His, the distal part of the AV junction, lies in the upper part of the interventricular septum. It connects the AV node to the two bundle branches. Once the electrical impulses enter the bundle of His, they travel rapidly through the fibrous tissue that electrically separates the atria from the ventricles and enter the bundle branches.

The right and left bundle branches arise from the bundle of His. The bundle of His, the right and left bundle branches, and the Purkinje network are also known as the *His–Purkinje system of the ventricles*. Pacemaker cells are located throughout the His–Purkinje system.

The bundle branches and their fascicles subdivide into smaller and smaller branches, with the smallest ones connecting with the Purkinje network. This intricate web of tiny fibers, distributed widely throughout the ventricles beneath the endocardium, conducts the electrical impulses. The ends of the Purkinje fibers terminate at the myocardial cells.

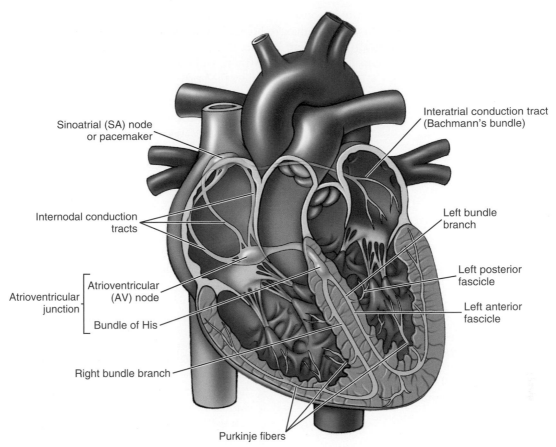

FIG. 1.4 Electrical conduction system. (Modified from Herlihy, B. [2011]. *The human body in health and illness* [4th ed.]. Saunders.)

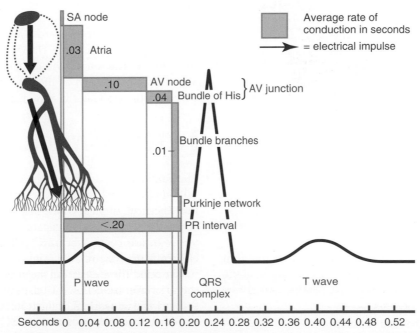

FIG. 1.5 The average rate of conduction of the electrical impulse through various parts of the electrical conduction system.

The electrical impulses travel very rapidly (in less than 0.01 second) through the bundle branches to the Purkinje network. Overall, it normally takes an electrical impulse less than 0.02 seconds to travel from the SA node to the Purkinje network in the ventricles.

CARDIAC CELLS

There are two basic kinds of cardiac cells—the myocardial, or "working," cells and the pacemaker cells of the electrical conduction system (Fig. 1.6 and Table 1.1).

Myocardial Cells

Myocardial cells are cylindrical. At their ends, they partially divide into two or more branches. These branches connect to the ends of adjacent cells, forming a network of cells called a *syncytium* (pronounced *syn-SIE-shee-um,* from *syn-,* meaning "together," and *cyto-,* meaning "cell"). At the junctions where the branches intersect, there are specialized cell membranes not found in any other cells. These membranes are called the *intercalated disks.* They contain areas of low electrical resistance called *gap junctions.* They permit very rapid conduction of electrical impulses from one cell to another. The ability of cardiac cells to conduct electrical impulses is called the *property of conductivity.*

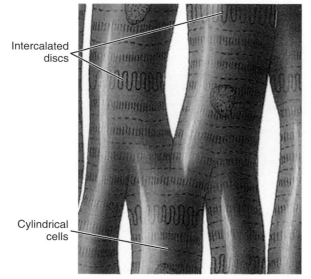

Intercalated discs

Cylindrical cells

FIG. 1.6 Cardiac cells. (Modified from McCance, K. L., & Huether, S. E. [2015]. *Pathophysiology: The biologic basis for disease in adults and children* (5th ed.). Mosby.)

TABLE **1.1**	Cardiac Cells and Their Function
Type	**Primary Function**
Myocardial cells	Contraction and relaxation
Pacemaker cells	Generation and conduction of electrical impulses

Each myocardial cell is enclosed in a semipermeable membrane. This membrane allows charged chemical particles, called *ions,* to flow in and out of the cells. The ability of sodium, potassium, and calcium ions to enter and leave myocardial cells allows the heart to contract and relax.

> **AUTHOR'S NOTE** Recall that a permeable cell membrane allows ions to flow freely through the cell wall. A cell membrane that is impermeable, on the other hand, does not permit the flow of ions across it. A semipermeable cell membrane is selective, allowing only certain ions to enter and leave the cell.

The myocardial cells form the thin muscular layer of the atrial wall and the much thicker muscular layer of the ventricular wall (myocardium). These cells contain many thin muscle fibers, or *myofibrils,* made up of protein filaments called *actin* and *myosin.* Myofibrils give myocardial cells the property of contractility, that is, the unique ability to shorten when stimulated by an electrical impulse and then return to their original length.

> **AUTHOR'S NOTE** The force of myocardial contractility increases in response to certain drugs (for example, digitalis and stimulants) and physiologic conditions such as increased venous return to the heart, exercise, emotion, hypovolemia, and anemia. In contrast, drugs such as procainamide, quinidine, beta blockers, and potassium, as well as conditions such as hypocalcemia and hypothyroidism, decrease the force of myocardial contractility.

Pacemaker Cells

The pacemaker cells of the heart's electrical conduction system contain no myofibrils and therefore cannot contract. They do, however, contain more gap junctions than do myocardial cells. Thus they can conduct electrical impulses very rapidly—at least six times faster than myocardial cells. The pacemaker cells are also capable of generating electrical impulses spontaneously. Myocardial cells, on the other hand, cannot normally do so. This capability, known as the *property of automaticity,* will be discussed in detail later in this chapter.

ELECTROPHYSIOLOGY OF THE HEART

The human heart is regulated by electrical impulses. Pacemaker cells in the heart are capable of generating and conducting the electrical impulses. The myocardial cells are capable of contracting but are also capable of conducting electrical impulses to adjacent myocardial cells, although they do so less efficiently and at a slower rate than do the specialized pacemaker cells. These electrical impulses are conducted because of the brief but rapid flow of positively charged ions (primarily sodium and potassium and, to a lesser extent, calcium) back and forth across the pacemaker cell membrane. The difference in the concentration of these ions inside compared with outside the cell membrane at any given instant produces an electrical potential. This potential energy, or charge, is measured in millivolts (mV).

Resting State of the Cardiac Cell

At rest, a cardiac cell has a layer of positive ions surrounding its cell membrane. It has an equal number of negative ions lining the inside of the cell membrane directly opposite each positive ion. When the positive and negative ions are aligned this way, like rival football teams at the 50-yard line, the resting cell is said to be *polarized* (Fig. 1.7).

When a cardiac cell is in the resting state, there is a high concentration of positively charged sodium (Na^+) ions called *cations* outside the cell. At the same time, inside the cell, there is a high concentration of negatively charged ions called *anions* (especially organic phosphate, organic sulfate, and proteins), mixed with a lower concentration of potassium cations (K^+). Cations carry a positive charge, whereas anions carry a negative charge. This makes the interior of the cell electrically negative compared with the outside of the cell. Under these conditions, a negative electrical potential exists across the cell membrane. This is possible because the cell membrane is not permeable to either the positively charged sodium cations outside the cell

membrane or the negatively charged phosphate, sulfate, and protein anions inside the cell.

The electrical potential maintained across the membrane of a resting cardiac cell is called the *resting membrane potential.* The resting membrane potential in atrial and ventricular cardiac cells and in the pacemaker cells of the electrical conduction system is normally −90 mV. Remember, a negative (−) membrane potential indicates that the concentration of positive ions, or cations, outside the cell is greater than the concentration inside the cell. A positive (+) membrane potential indicates the opposite—that there are more cations inside the cell than outside.

Depolarization and Repolarization

When stimulated by an electrical impulse, the membrane of a polarized cardiac cell becomes permeable to sodium cations, allowing sodium to flow into the cell. This causes the interior of the cell to become less negative compared with its exterior.

The process by which the cell's resting, polarized state is reversed is called *depolarization* (Fig. 1.8). When the membrane potential drops from its resting potential of −90 mV to about −65 mV, large pores in the membrane momentarily open. These pores are called *fast sodium channels.* They facilitate the rapid, free flow of sodium across the cell membrane, resulting in a sudden large influx of positively charged sodium cations into the cell. This quickly causes the interior of the cell to become more positively charged. The moment the concentration of sodium cations within the cell reaches the concentration outside the cell, the membrane potential drops to zero, and the cardiac cell is depolarized. The influx of sodium cations continues, however, causing a temporary rise in the membrane potential to about +20 to +30 mV—the so-called *overshoot.*

The fast sodium channels are found in the myocardial cells but not in the pacemaker cells. The pacemaker cells have slow calcium–sodium channels that open when the membrane potential drops to about −50 mV. During depolarization, these channels permit calcium and sodium cations to enter the cardiac cells at a slow and gradual rate. The result is a slower rate of depolarization compared with the depolarization rate of myocardial cells that contain fast sodium channels.

As soon as a cardiac cell depolarizes, potassium cations flow out of the cell. This movement across the cell membrane initiates a process by which the cell returns to its resting polarized state. This process, called *repolarization* (see Fig. 1.8), involves a complex exchange of sodium, calcium, and potassium ions across the cell membrane.

Depolarization of one cardiac cell acts as an electrical impulse that stimulates and depolarizes adjacent cells. Depolarization of the myocardial cells results in contraction of the muscle

Polarized resting cardiac cell

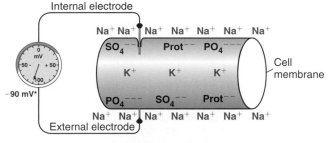

Depolarizing cardiac cell

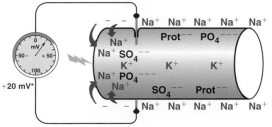

*Resting membrane potential   ⚡ = Electrical impulse

Na^+	sodium ion
K^+	potassium ion
PO_4^{---}	phosphate ion
SO_4^{--}	sulfate ion
$Prot^{--}$	protein ion

FIG. 1.7 Membrane potentials of polarized and depolarized cardiac cells.

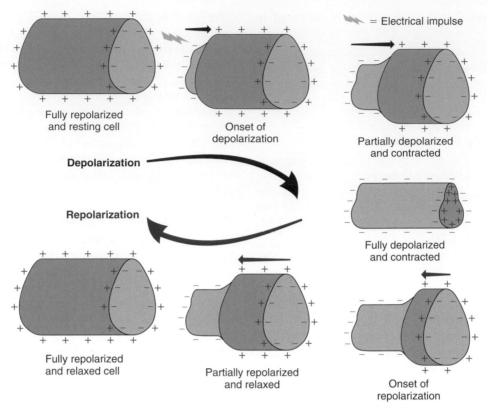

FIG. 1.8 Depolarization and repolarization of a myocardial cell.

and propagation (generation) of an impulse. Depolarization of the pacemaker cells propagates an impulse to adjacent pacemaker cells. This wave of depolarization from cell to cell produces a wave of electrical energy that can be measured as an electrical current flowing through the heart.

> **AUTHOR'S NOTE** The electrocardiogram (ECG) machine detects only the electrical current of the myocardial cells because their size and number far exceed the size and number of the pacemaker cells.

Threshold Potential

A cardiac cell need not be repolarized completely to its resting polarized state (−90 mV) before it can be stimulated to depolarize again. The cells of the SA and AV nodes can be depolarized when they have been repolarized to about −30 to −40 mV. The remaining cells within the electrical conduction system of the heart and the myocardial cells can be depolarized when they have been repolarized to about −60 to −70 mV. The level to which a cell must be repolarized before it can be depolarized again is known as its *threshold potential.*

> **AUTHOR'S NOTE** The fact that the myocardial cells have a higher (more negative) threshold potential than the pacemaker cells helps to ensure that the dedicated electrical pathways are the primary and most efficient means of electrical conduction through the heart.

Action Potential

The *action potential* refers to the change in membrane potential (from a positive to a negative state) during depolarization and repolarization. This change can be represented by a diagram in which the action potential is divided into five phases: phase 0 to phase 4 (Fig. 1.9):

- **Phase 0.** Phase 0 (depolarization phase) is the sharp, tall upstroke of the action potential, during which the cell membrane reaches its threshold potential. This triggers the fast sodium channels to open momentarily, permitting the rapid entry of sodium into the cell. As the cations flow into the cell, the interior of the cell becomes electrically positive. During the upstroke, the cell depolarizes and begins to contract.
- **Phase 1.** During phase 1 (early rapid repolarization phase), the fast sodium channels close, terminating the rapid flow of sodium into the cell, followed by a loss of potassium from the cell. The net result is a decrease in the number of positive electrical charges within the cell and a drop in the membrane potential to zero.
- **Phase 2.** Phase 2 is the prolonged plateau phase, during which the myocardial cell is slowly repolarized. The gradual completion of this phase allows the myocardial cell to finish contracting and begin relaxing. During phase 2, the membrane potential remains near zero. In a complicated exchange of ions across the cell membrane, calcium gradually enters the cell through the slow calcium channels. Sodium enters gradually as well, whereas potassium continues to leave the cell.

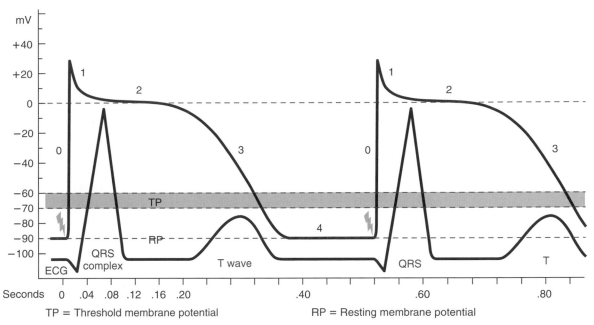

FIG. 1.9   Action potential of myocardial cells.

- **Phase 3.** Phase 3 is the final or terminal phase of rapid repolarization. During this phase, the inside of the cell becomes markedly negative, and the membrane potential once again returns to its resting level of about −90 mV. This change is caused primarily by the flow of potassium from the cell. Repolarization is complete by the end of phase 3.

- **Phase 4.** At the onset of phase 4 (the period between action potentials), the membrane has returned to its resting potential, and the inside of the cell is once again maximally negative (−90 mV) compared with the outside. But there is still an excess of sodium in the cell and an excess of potassium outside. At this point, a physiologic mechanism known as the *sodium–potassium pump* is activated, transporting the excess sodium out of the cell and ushering potassium back in. Because of this mechanism and the impermeability of the cell membrane to sodium during this phase, the myocardial cell normally maintains a stable membrane potential between action potentials.

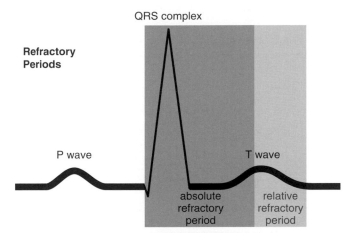

FIG. 1.10   Refractory periods.

REFRACTORY PERIODS

The refractory period of a cardiac cell begins with the onset of phase 0 of the cardiac action potential and ends just before the end of phase 3. On the ECG, this period extends from the onset of the QRS complex to about the end of the T wave.

The refractory period is divided into absolute and relative refractory periods (Fig. 1.10). The absolute refractory period (ARP) constitutes the first two-thirds of the refractory period. It begins with the onset of phase 0 and ends midway through phase 3, at about the peak of the T wave. During this period, the cardiac cells—having completely depolarized—are in the process of repolarizing. Because they have not repolarized to their threshold potential, the cardiac cells cannot be stimulated to depolarize. In other words, the myocardial cells cannot contract, and

the cells of the electrical conduction system cannot depolarize during the ARP.

The relative refractory period (RRP) occupies the remaining one-third of the refractory period. The RRP extends through most of the second half of phase 3, corresponding to the downslope of the T wave. During this period, the cardiac cells can be stimulated to depolarize if the stimulus is strong enough because they have been repolarized to their threshold potential. This period is also called the *vulnerable period of repolarization.*

refractory period
The period between the onset of depolarization and the end of repolarization of a cardiac cell, during which it cannot be stimulated to repolarize.

AUTOMATICITY

The ability of a cardiac cell to depolarize spontaneously during phase 4 is called the *property of automaticity*. To depolarize spontaneously, the cell membrane must become permeable to sodium during phase 4, thus allowing a steady leakage of sodium ions into the cell. This causes the resting membrane potential to become progressively less negative. As soon as its threshold potential is reached, the cell rapidly depolarizes (phase 0). The rate of spontaneous depolarization depends on the slope of phase 4 depolarization (Fig. 1.11). The steeper the slope of phase 4 depolarization, the faster the rate of spontaneous depolarization and impulse formation (the firing rate). The flatter the slope is, the slower the firing rate.

> ### automaticity (auto-ma-TISS-ity)
>
> A property of cardiac cells that allows them to reach threshold potential and then depolarize spontaneously and completely, without external stimulation.

> **AUTHOR'S NOTE** Increased sympathetic activity and administration of catecholamines increase the slope of phase 4 depolarization, which increases the automaticity of the pacemaker cells and their firing rate. On the other hand, increased parasympathetic activity or administration of drugs that decrease the slope of phase 4 depolarization reduces the automaticity and firing rate of the pacemaker cells.

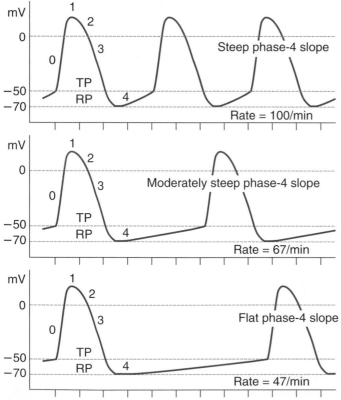

FIG. 1.11 Action potential of pacemaker cells. Rate of spontaneous depolarization is dependent on the slope of phase 4 depolarization. *RP,* Resting membrane potential; *TP,* threshold potential.

Dominant and Escape Pacemakers of the Heart

As we have described, pacemaker cells are specialized cells in the electrical conduction system that normally have the property of automaticity. These cells are located in the SA node; in some areas of the internodal atrial conduction tracts and AV node; and throughout the bundle of His, bundle branches, and Purkinje network. The pacemaker cells of the SA node have the fastest spontaneous firing rate (60–100 times per minute). As a result, they are normally the dominant (or primary) pacemaker cells of the heart (Fig. 1.12). The pacemaker cells in the rest of the electrical conduction system have a lower rate of automaticity and are normally called on to depolarize only if the SA node fails to function properly or if electrical impulses fail to reach them. For this reason, these pacemaker cells are called *escape pacemaker cells.*

Normally, the heart rate is controlled by the pacemaker cells with the highest level of automaticity. Each time these pacemaker cells generate an electrical impulse, the more slowly firing escape pacemaker cells are depolarized before they can do so spontaneously. This phenomenon is called *overdrive suppression.*

The SA node is normally the dominant and primary pacemaker of the heart (see Fig. 1.11) because it possesses the highest level of automaticity; that is, its spontaneous rate of automatic firing (60–100 times per minute) is normally greater than that of the other pacemaker cells.

If the SA node fails to depolarize at its normal rate or stops functioning entirely, or if the conduction of the electrical impulse is blocked for any reason (for example, in the AV node), escape pacemaker cells in the AV junction will usually assume the role of pacemaker of the heart but at a slower rate (40–60 times per minute). If the AV junction is unable to take over as the pacemaker, an escape pacemaker in the electrical conduction system below the AV junction or in the ventricles (in the bundle branches or Purkinje network) may take over at an even slower rate (fewer than 40 times per minute).

The rate at which the SA node or an escape pacemaker normally generates electrical impulses is called the *pacemaker's inherent firing rate.* A beat or a series of beats arising from an escape pacemaker is called an *escape beat* or *rhythm* and is identified according to its origin (for example, junctional, ventricular).

Mechanisms of Ectopic Electrical Impulse Formation

Under certain circumstances, cardiac cells in any part of the heart, whether they are escape pacemaker cells or myocardial cells, are capable of generating additional electrical impulses. Such activity within the heart is referred to as *ectopic* because it originates outside the normal conduction pathway. The result can be ectopic rhythms. These rhythms are identified according to the location of the ectopic pacemaker (for example, atrial, junctional, or ventricular). The three basic mechanisms that are responsible for ectopic beats and rhythms are (1) enhanced automaticity, (2) reentry, and (3) triggered activity.

> ### ectopy
>
> Origination of electrical impulses in a site outside the heart's normal conduction pathway, resulting in abnormal (ectopic) rhythms or beats.

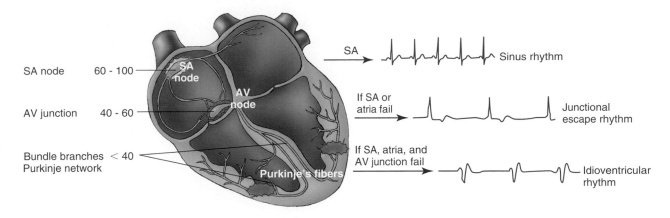

FIG. 1.12 Dominant and escape pacemakers.

ENHANCED AUTOMATICITY

Enhanced automaticity is a condition in which the cell's firing rate is increased beyond its inherent rate. This occurs when the cell membrane becomes abnormally permeable to sodium during phase 4. The result is an abnormally high leakage of sodium ions into the cells and, consequently, a sharp rise in the phase 4 slope of spontaneous depolarization. Even myocardial cells that do not ordinarily possess automaticity may acquire this property and depolarize spontaneously. Enhanced automaticity can cause atrial, junctional, and ventricular ectopic rhythms.

Common causes of enhanced automaticity include elevated levels of catecholamines (stimulants), digitalis toxicity, and administration of atropine. In addition, hypoxia, hypercapnia, myocardial ischemia or infarction, stretching of the heart muscle, hypokalemia, hypocalcemia, and heating or cooling of the heart may also cause enhanced automaticity.

REENTRY

Reentry is a condition in which the progression of a wave of depolarization is delayed or blocked (or both) (Fig. 1.13, *A* and *B*) in one or more segments of the electrical conduction system while being conducted normally through the rest of the conduction system. This delays antegrade (forward) or retrograde (backward) conduction of electrical impulses into adjacent cardiac cells that have just been depolarized by the normally conducted electrical impulse. If these cardiac cells have repolarized sufficiently, the delayed electrical impulse depolarizes them prematurely, producing ectopic rhythms. Myocardial ischemia and hyperkalemia are the two most common causes of a delay or block in the conduction of an electrical impulse through the electrical conduction system responsible for the reentry mechanism. Another cause of the reentry mechanism is the presence of an accessory conduction pathway (see Fig. 1.13, *C* and *D*), such as the accessory AV pathways located between the atria and ventricles described earlier in this chapter.

After normal antegrade progression of a wave of depolarization through the electrical conduction system and depolarization of the cardiac cells, the electrical impulse enters the accessory conduction pathway and progresses in a retrograde fashion to reenter the proximal end of the electrical conduction system much sooner than the next expected normal electrical impulse. The electrical impulse is then conducted antegrade as before, causing depolarization of the cardiac cells prematurely. Thus a reentry circuit is a condition that can result in the conduction of a rapid series of electrical impulses through the electrical conduction system. The electrical impulse can also progress in an antegrade direction through the accessory conduction pathway and retrogradely through the electrical conduction system.

This reentry mechanism can result in the abnormal generation of single or repetitive electrical impulses in the atria, AV junction, bundle branches, and Purkinje network. It produces atrial, junctional, or ventricular ectopic rhythms, such as atrial, junctional, and ventricular tachycardias. Such reentry tachycardias typically start and stop abruptly.

TRIGGERED ACTIVITY

Triggered activity is an abnormal condition of myocardial cells in which the cells may depolarize more than once after stimulation by a single electrical impulse. The cellular membrane action potential spontaneously increases after the first depolarization until it reaches threshold potential, causing the cells to depolarize, once or repeatedly. This phenomenon, called *afterdepolarization*, can occur almost immediately after depolarization in phase 3 or later in phase 4. Triggered activity can result in atrial or ventricular ectopic complexes occurring singly, in groups of two (paired or coupled), or in bursts of three or more complexes (paroxysms of tachycardia).

AUTHOR'S NOTE Common causes of triggered activity, like those of enhanced automaticity, include an increase in catecholamines, digitalis toxicity, hypoxia, myocardial ischemia or injury, and stretching or cooling of the heart.

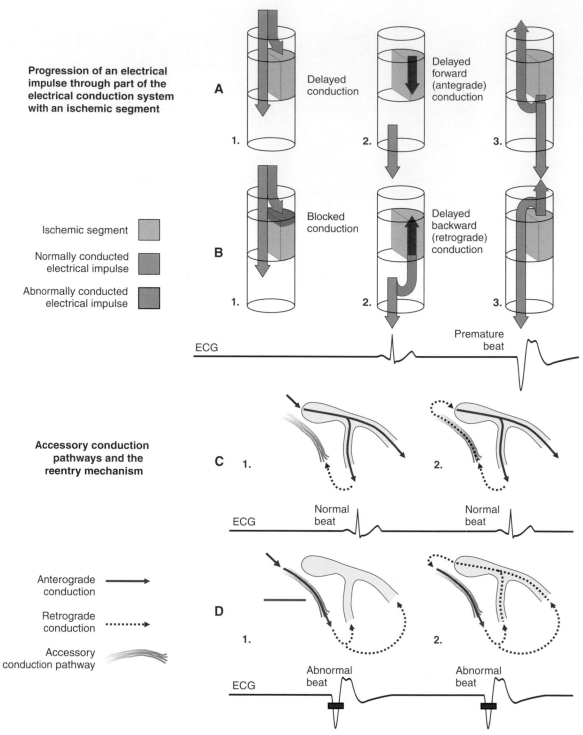

Progression of an electrical impulse through part of the electrical conduction system with an ischemic segment

Ischemic segment

Normally conducted electrical impulse

Abnormally conducted electrical impulse

A 1. Delayed conduction

2. Delayed forward (antegrade) conduction

3.

B 1. Blocked conduction

2. Delayed backward (retrograde) conduction

3.

ECG Premature beat

Accessory conduction pathways and the reentry mechanism

C 1. 2.

ECG Normal beat Normal beat

Anterograde conduction

Retrograde conduction

Accessory conduction pathway

D 1. 2.

ECG Abnormal beat Abnormal beat

FIG. 1.13 Examples of reentry mechanisms. (A) Delayed conduction. (B) Blocked and delayed conduction. (C) Antegrade conduction through the conduction system. (D) Retrograde conduction through the conduction system.

AUTONOMIC NERVOUS SYSTEM CONTROL OF THE HEART

The heart is under constant control of the autonomic nervous system (ANS), which includes the sympathetic and parasympathetic divisions (Fig. 1.14). By producing opposite effects, these divisions work together to regulate cardiac output and blood pressure.

ANS control of the heart originates in two separate nerve centers in the medulla oblongata, a part of the brainstem:

1. **Cardioaccelerator center.** This center is part of the sympathetic nervous system. Impulses from the cardioaccelerator center reach the electrical conduction system of the

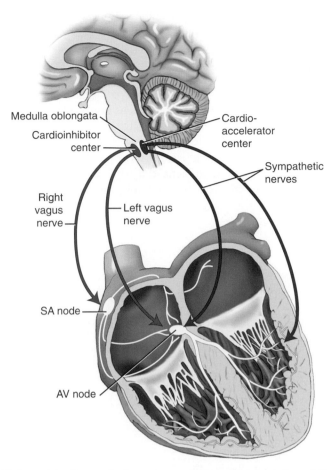

FIG. 1.14 Sympathetic and parasympathetic regulation of the heart.

heart and the atria and ventricles by way of the sympathetic nerves.

Stimulation of the sympathetic nervous system produces the following effects:

- An increase in the firing rate of the SA node and escape and ectopic pacemakers throughout the heart
- An increase in the conductivity of electrical impulses through the atria and ventricles, especially through the AV node
- An increase in the force of atrial and ventricular contractions
- The result is an increase in heart rate, cardiac output, and blood pressure.

2. **Cardioinhibitor center.** This center is part of the parasympathetic nervous system. Impulses from the cardioinhibitor center travel to the SA node, atria, and AV junction and, to a small extent, the ventricles by way of the right and left vagus nerves. When the vagus nerve fires, the heart rate slows. When it fires less, the effects of the sympathetic nervous system dominate, and the heart rate increases. The rate at which the vagus nerve fires is referred to as *vagal tone*. Another important cardioinhibitor (parasympathetic) nerve center is the carotid sinus. The carotid sinus is a slight dilation of the common carotid artery, located at the point where it branches into the internal and external carotid arteries. Sensory nerve endings in the carotid sinus help regulate blood pressure and heart rate.

Stimulation of the parasympathetic nervous system produces the following effects:

- A decrease in the firing rate of the SA node and escape and ectopic pacemakers in the atria and AV junction
- A slowing of conduction of electrical impulses through the AV node

The result is a decrease in heart rate, cardiac output, and blood pressure and, sometimes, a complete block of the electrical impulse through the AV node.

As the blood pressure requirements of the body change, multiple sensors in the body relay impulses to the cardioinhibitor and cardioaccelerator centers for analysis. From there, the sympathetic and parasympathetic nerves transmit the appropriate impulses to the electrical conduction system of the heart and to the atrial and ventricular myocardium, where they influence the automaticity, conductivity, and contractility of the cardiac cells.

> **AUTHOR'S NOTE** The parasympathetic nervous system can be stimulated by putting pressure on the carotid sinus, performing the Valsalva maneuver (the action of straining against a closed glottis [airway]), straining to move the bowels, or distention of the urinary bladder. Nausea, vomiting, bronchial spasm, sweating, faintness, and hypersalivation are manifestations of excessive parasympathetic activity. The drug atropine effectively blocks the parasympathetic nervous system.

TAKE-HOME POINTS

- The heart lies in the center of the chest, with its base at the atria and its apex at the ventricles. It is surrounded by the pericardium, enveloped by the epicardium, and lined by the endocardium.
- The walls of the ventricles are composed of three layers: the innermost layer is the smooth tissue of the endocardium, the middle layer is the muscular myocardium, and the outermost is a thin layer of connective tissue called the *epicardium*.
- Blood from the venae cavae and lungs enters the atria and then moves into the ventricles, where it is pumped to the lungs and body during the cardiac cycle.
- The cardiac cycle has two phases: Diastole is the phase during which the atria and ventricles relax and fill with blood. Systole is the phase during which the atria and ventricles contract to pump blood out.
- The heart has specific pathways that allow electrical impulses to be transmitted in order to stimulate contraction of the atria and ventricles. The primary pathway consists of the SA node, the internodal/interatrial tract, the AV junction, the right and left bundle branches, and the Purkinje network. Signals may also travel along accessory pathways, causing various rhythm disturbances.
- The specific properties of conductivity, automaticity, and contractility allow the cardiac muscle to perform its unique duty to ensure coordinated contraction and relaxation

of the heart in order to generate blood flow through the body.

- The heart has three layers. The innermost layer is the smooth tissue of the endocardium. The middle layer is the muscular myocardium. The outermost layer is a thin layer of connective tissue.
- The electrophysiology of the heart is regulated by the movement of positive and negative ions across cell membranes. The unique properties of these ions change the permeability of the membrane.
- This process of ion movement charges the cell with an action potential that allows it to cause adjacent cells to depolarize and transmit the electrical impulse forward.

- The action potential has five phases: phase 0, depolarization; phase 1, early rapid repolarization; phase 2, the prolonged plateau phase; phase 3, the terminal phase of rapid repolarization; and phase 4, the period between action potentials.
- The presence of dominant and escape pacemakers ensures that the heart has backup mechanisms in place to generate a pulse in the event that one of the higher pacemakers fails.
- The process of depolarization and repolarization causes electrical impulses to move down the conduction pathway. This process can be influenced by the autonomic nervous system and other environmental stimuli and pathologic conditions.

CHAPTER REVIEW QUESTIONS

1. Which term is commonly used to describe the inner layer of the pericardium, which covers the heart itself?
   A. Endocardium
   B. Epicardium
   C. Myocardium
   D. Pericardium

2. The _____ side of the heart pumps blood into the _____ circulation, and the _____ side of the heart pumps blood into the _____ circulation.
   A. left; pulmonary; right; systemic
   B. left; ventricular; right; atrial
   C. right; pulmonary; left; systemic
   D. right; systemic; left; pulmonary

3. The right ventricle pumps deoxygenated blood through the _____ valve and into the lungs through the _____ artery.
   A. aortic; mitral
   B. mitral; tricuspid
   C. pulmonary; pulmonary
   D. tricuspid; pulmonary

4. Which term best describes the period during which the heart relaxes and the ventricles fill with blood?
   A. Atrial diastole
   B. Atrial systole
   C. Ventricular diastole
   D. Ventricular systole

5. Which structure is a normal component of the heart's electrical conduction system?
   A. Atrial septa
   B. Coronary sinus
   C. Right bundle branch
   D. Vagus nerve

6. Which term best describes the ability of cardiac cells to depolarize spontaneously?
   A. Automaticity
   B. Conductivity
   C. Contractility
   D. Self-excitation

7. In the resting state, a myocardial cell has a high concentration of the _____ charged _____ ions present outside the cell.
   A. negatively; potassium
   B. negatively; sodium
   C. positively; potassium
   D. positively; sodium

8. Cardiac cells cannot be stimulated to depolarize during which part of the cardiac cycle?
   A. Absolute refractory period
   B. Ectopic period
   C. Relative refractory period
   D. Resting state

9. Which term best describes the normal and dominant pacemaker of the heart?
   A. AV node
   B. Bundle of His
   C. Purkinje fibers
   D. SA node

10. Under what conditions does the vagus nerve, part of the parasympathetic nervous system, slow the heart?
    A. When the vagus nerve fires
    B. When the vagus nerve is blocked by atropine
    C. When the vagus nerve is severed
    D. When the patient is given a stimulant

11. Label the figure.

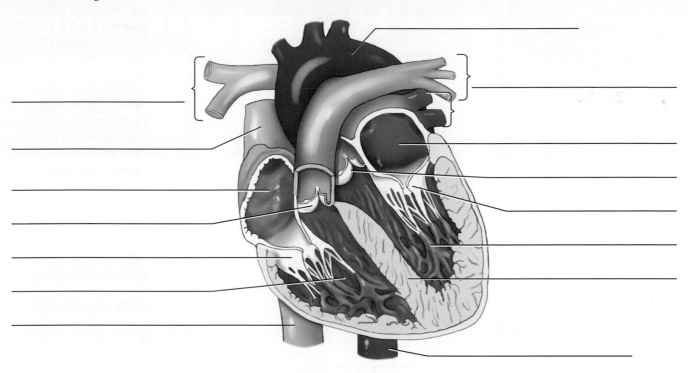

2 ECG Leads and Cardiac Monitoring

BASIC ECG CONCEPTS

AUTHOR'S NOTE Throughout this text, we will use the term *ECG* for *electrocardiogram*. Some texts use the abbreviation *EKG*, which is derived from the German word *Elektrokardiogramm*. Also, *EKG* is often the abbreviation used verbally because *ECG* can be confused with *EEG*, which refers to an electroencephalogram that measures electrical activity in the brain.

Electrical Basis of the ECG

The ECG is a graphic record of changes in the magnitude and direction of the heart's electrical activity. The ECG does not detect the depolarization of individual cells. In fact, it does not detect the combined depolarization of the pacemaker cells because the resulting impulse is too small to detect with standard electrodes. What the ECG does detect is the combined electrical impulse generated by the wave of depolarization and repolarization that progresses through the myocardial cells of the atria and ventricles during each cardiac cycle. This electrical activity is sufficient enough to be detected by electrodes attached to the skin.

ECG Paper

ECGs are printed on grid paper that shows time in seconds (sec) along the horizontal axis. Voltage or strength (amplitude) in millimeters (mm) appears along the vertical axis (Fig. 2.1).

These intersecting dark and light vertical and horizontal lines form a grid of large and small squares. The distance between the vertical lines depends on the rate of paper output when the ECG is recorded. For example, the grid will look different at an output rate of 25 millimeters per second (mm/sec) compared with 50 mm/sec. The standard recording speed is 25 mm/sec. Other speeds are used only for specialized purposes.

AUTHOR'S NOTE All ECGs in this text will be based on the standard recording speed of 25 mm/sec unless otherwise noted.

When the ECG is recorded at the standard speed of 25 mm/sec, the measurements between the vertical lines are as follows:
- The dark vertical lines are 5 mm apart.
- If 1 second = 25 mm, then 5 mm = ⅕ of a second, or 0.20 second.
- The light vertical lines are 1 mm apart.
- If 5 mm = ⅕ of a second, then 1 mm = ¹⁄₂₅ of a second, or 0.04 second.

Regardless of the speed of the recording, the measurements between the horizontal lines are as follows:
- The dark horizontal lines are 5 mm apart.
- The light horizontal lines are 1 mm apart.

Therefore at the standard paper speed of 25 mm/sec, the large and small squares have the following characteristics:
- One large square is 5 mm tall and 0.2 second long.
- One small square is 1 mm tall and 0.04 second long.

The sensitivity of an ECG machine must be calibrated. Conventionally, a 1-millivolt (mV) electrical signal should produce a 10-mm (2 large squares or 10 small squares) deflection on the ECG.

Short vertical lines (or small arrowheads) are printed along the top or bottom edge of the ECG paper at regular intervals. These lines denote intervals of time and thus are called *time lines*. They are spaced 15 large squares apart (75 mm, or about 3 inches apart). When the ECG is recorded at the standard paper speed of 25 mm/sec, the distance between the time lines represents 3 seconds. Every third vertical line, then, represents the passage of 6 seconds.

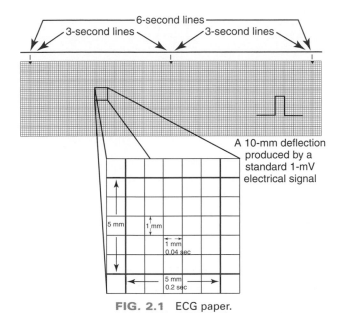

FIG. 2.1 ECG paper.

Short vertical lines (or small arrowheads) that denote intervals of time on an ECG. At the standard paper speed, the distance between the lines represents a period of 3 seconds.

BASIC COMPONENTS OF A NORMAL ECG

It is vital to understand the relationship between the various components of the ECG and the electrical activity occurring in the heart. The current generated by depolarization and repolarization of the atria and ventricles is detected by electrodes. It is then amplified and displayed on a screen. It is also recorded on the ECG paper as a series of waves and complexes. This combination of waves and complexes is referred to as the

ECG waveform (Fig. 2.2). Between the ECG waveforms, the ECG tracing returns to a nearly flat line, called the *baseline* or *isoelectric line*. During this period, no electrical activity occurs. Generally speaking, when we examine the ECG waveform, we will be evaluating the waves and complexes based on their shape, duration, and timing; the intervals based on their length; and the segments based on their relationship to the baseline.

| baseline |

A nearly flat line on the ECG that reflects a period during which no electrical activity occurs in the heart. The baseline serves as a point of reference for measuring and interpreting waves, complexes, intervals, and segments.

The next chapter will discuss each component in greater detail, but let's take a look at the basics:
- The electric impulse generated by atrial depolarization is recorded as the P wave.
- The impulse generated by ventricular depolarization is recorded as the Q, R, and S waves. Together they are called the *QRS complex*.
- Ventricular repolarization is manifested by the *T wave*. Because atrial repolarization normally occurs during ventricular depolarization, it is hidden in the QRS complex.

In a normal ECG waveform, the P wave occurs first. It is followed by the QRS complex and then the T wave. The sections of the ECG between waves and complexes are called *segments* and *intervals*. Their shape and length reveal the speed of electrical conduction through the heart:
- The PR segment starts at the beginning of the P wave and ends at the start of the QRS complex.
- The ST segment starts at the end of the QRS complex and ends at the start of the T wave.
- The start of the ST segment, where the QRS complex ends, is the J point.
- The TP segment starts at the end of the T wave and stops at the start of the next P wave.

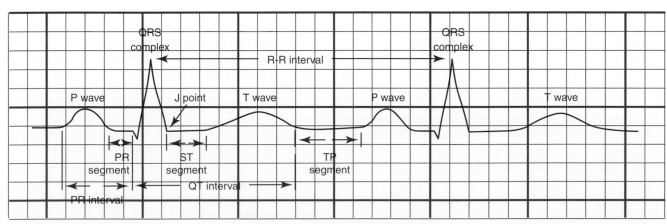

FIG. 2.2 Components of the ECG.

- The PR interval starts at the beginning of the P wave and ends at the beginning of the QRS complex.
- The QT interval starts at the beginning of the QRS complex and stops at the end of the T wave.
- And finally, the R-R, or "R to R," interval is measured from the tips of two consecutive QRS complexes.

ECG LEADS

Lead Basics

Electrodes, attached to the skin, detect the electrical impulse generated by the depolarization and repolarization of the myocardial cells. Each electrode is designated as either negative or positive and is placed on a specified area of the body, such as the right or left arm, the left leg, or one of several locations on the chest wall. The positive and corresponding negative electrodes are referred to as *leads*.

electrode
A sensing device attached to the skin that detects positive or negative electrical activity in the heart.

The ECG represents the movement of the negatively charged electrical impulse toward and away from the positive electrode. Therefore the orientation of the lead around the heart determines its "view" of the heart's electrical activity.

lead
The view of the heart's electrical activity from the perspective of the positive electrode.

To obtain an ECG, self-adhesive electrodes are affixed to the patient's skin and then connected to the ECG machine with wires. The machine then designates each electrode as positive or negative and changes its polarity depending on the lead selected. Two types of leads are used in ECG analysis: bipolar and unipolar.

Bipolar Leads

A lead with both a positive and negative electrode is a bipolar lead. Bipolar leads are referred to as *standard limb leads* because the electrodes are usually attached to the arms and legs of the patient. The standard limb leads are leads I, II, and III.

bipolar lead
A view of the electrical impulse between a positive and negative electrode from the positive electrode's perspective.

When monitoring the heart solely for rhythms, a single bipolar ECG lead, such as lead II (Fig. 2.3), is usually used. MCL$_1$

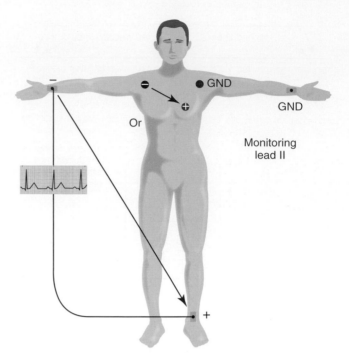

FIG. 2.3 Monitoring lead II.

is another bipolar monitoring lead that's often used. *MCL* stands for *modified chest lead*. This lead is especially useful in monitoring heart rhythms in the hospital. Bipolar leads used less often for monitoring include leads I, III, and MCL.

MONITORING LEAD II

Lead II is usually obtained by attaching the negative electrode to the right arm and the positive electrode to the left leg. Electrodes sometimes detect respiratory chest movement rather than electrical activity of the heart. This electrical interference, or noise, can move the baseline or leave other traces on the ECG. To reduce this distortion when using lead II for monitoring, we attach a third, electrically neutral electrode, or ground electrode. It can be attached to the upper left chest; to an extremity (the left arm or right leg); or, for that matter, to any part of the body.

When an electrical impulse flows toward the positive electrode of a lead, a positive (upward) deflection is recorded on the ECG. Conversely, a negative (downward) deflection is recorded when the electrical impulse flows away from the positive electrode. If the positive electrode is attached to the left leg, all of the electric impulses generated in the heart that flow toward the left leg will be recorded as positive (upward) deflections. Those that flow away from the left leg will be recorded as negative (downward) deflections (Fig. 2.4).

Normal depolarization of the atria and ventricles progresses from the right upper chest downward toward the left leg. As a result, the electrical impulses generated during depolarization will also flow toward the left leg. They will be recorded as two positive (upward) deflections—a positive P wave (atrial depolarization) and a large positive R wave (ventricular depolarization)—in lead II.

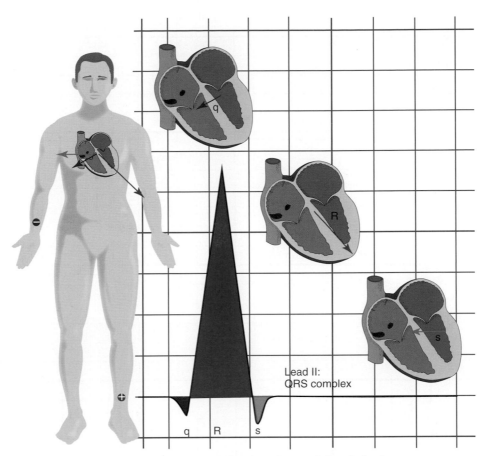

FIG. 2.4 Sequence and direction of normal depolarization.

Depolarization and repolarization of the atria and ventricles appear in the P wave, QRS complex, and T wave (Fig. 2.5) in predictable ways:

- **P wave.** Depolarization of the atria normally begins near the sinoatrial (SA) node and proceeds downward and to the left, producing a positive P wave.
- **QRS complex.** Depolarization of the ventricles usually starts with the depolarization of the relatively thin interventricular septum from left to right, resulting in a small negative deflection—the Q wave. This is immediately followed by the depolarization of the large left ventricle from right to left, which overshadows the almost simultaneous left-to-right depolarization of the smaller right ventricle, resulting in a large R wave. In addition, depending on the position of the heart in the chest, the size of the ventricles, and the rotation of the heart, depolarization of the base of the left ventricle from left to right usually produces a small negative (inverted) deflection after the R wave—the S wave.
- **T wave.** Finally, the T wave is produced as the ventricles repolarize from left to right.

AUTHOR'S NOTE The ECG components and strips shown in this book are depicted as they would appear in lead II unless otherwise noted.

MONITORING LEADS I AND III

The two other bipolar leads, leads I and III, are also used for ECG monitoring (Fig. 2.6):

- **Lead I.** Lead I is obtained by attaching the negative electrode to the right arm, the positive electrode to the left arm, and the ground electrode to the right leg. Lead I can also be obtained by attaching the negative electrode to the upper right anterior chest wall below the right clavicle and the positive electrode to the upper left anterior chest wall below the left clavicle. The ground electrode is attached to the right or left lower chest wall.
- **Lead III.** Lead III is obtained by attaching the negative electrode to the left arm, the positive electrode to the left leg, and the ground electrode to the right leg. Lead III can also be obtained by attaching the negative electrode to the upper left anterior chest wall below the left clavicle and the positive electrode to the lower-left anterior chest wall at the intersection of the fifth intercostal space and the midclavicular line. The ground electrode is attached to the right lower chest wall.

MODIFIED CHEST LEADS

MCLs are similar to the unipolar chest leads used in 12-lead ECGs but have less sensitivity. They can, however, be used to monitor certain rhythms.

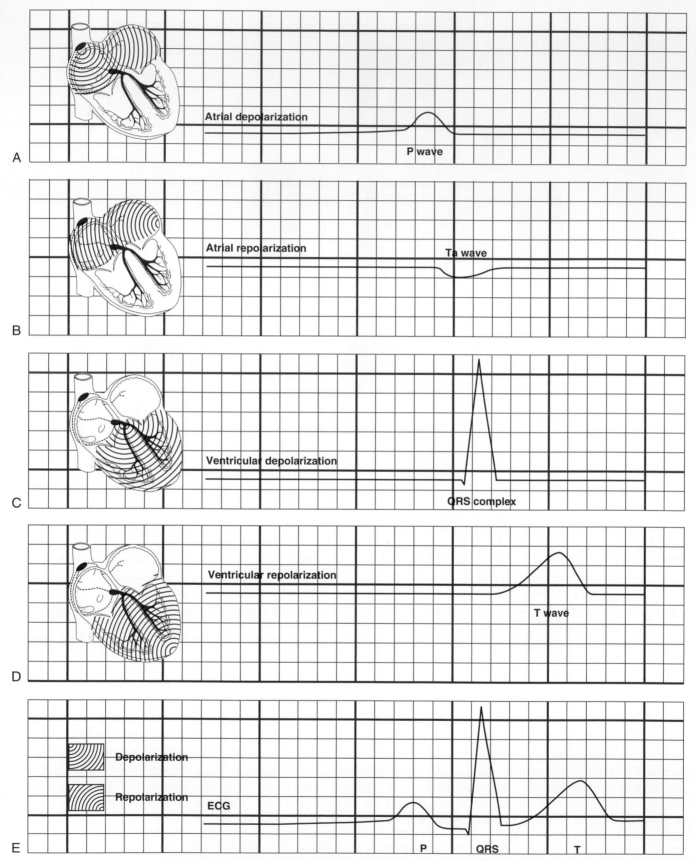

FIG. 2.5 Depolarization and repolarization of the atria and ventricles and the ECG. (A) P wave. (B) T$_a$ wave. (C) QRS complex. (D) T wave. (E) ECG in lead II.

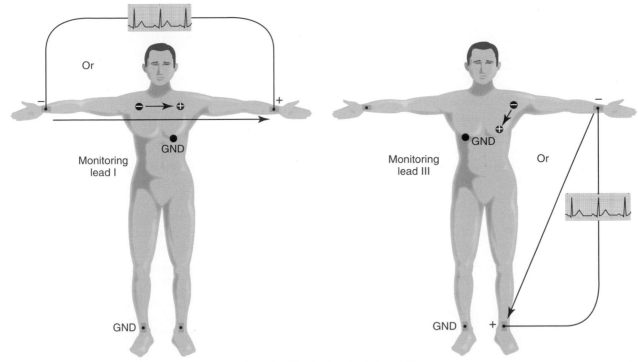

FIG. 2.6 Monitoring leads I and III.

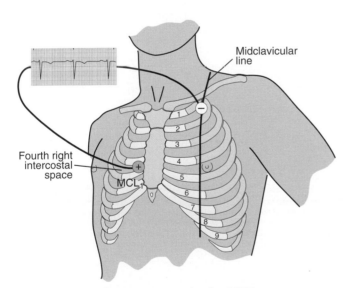

FIG. 2.7 Monitoring lead MCL₁.

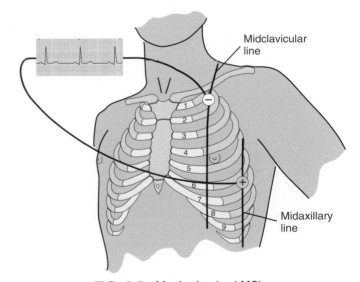

FIG. 2.8 Monitoring lead MCL₆.

- **Monitoring lead MCL₁.** Lead MCL₁ is a bipolar lead similar to lead V_1 of the 12-lead ECG (Fig. 2.7). It is obtained by attaching the positive electrode from lead III to the right side of the anterior chest in the fourth intercostal space just right of the sternum and the negative electrode to the left chest in the midclavicular line below the clavicle. Lead MCL₁ is helpful in identifying the origin of certain rhythms with wide QRS complexes, particularly when a full 12-lead ECG can't be obtained.
- **Monitoring lead MCL₆.** Lead MCL₆, a bipolar lead that resembles the unipolar lead V_6 of the 12-lead ECG, is obtained by attaching the positive electrode of lead III to the left chest in the fifth intercostal space in the midaxillary line and the

negative electrode in the midclavicular line below the clavicle on the same side (Fig. 2.8). The P waves, QRS complexes, and T waves are similar to those in lead II. MCL₆, like MCL₁, is often used when a full 12-lead ECG can't be obtained.

Unipolar Leads

A lead that has only one electrode (which is positive) is called a *unipolar lead*. It does not have a corresponding negative lead. Instead, a theoretical electrode is created by the ECG machine to represent the center of the heart's electrical field. Unipolar leads are used extensively in 12-lead ECGs. As with bipolar leads, the view of the heart is from the perspective of the positive electrode.

unipolar lead

A view of the heart's electrical impulses from a single positive electrode.

There are 12 different leads in a standard ECG (Fig. 2.9), providing a detailed analysis of the heart's electrical activity. We will discuss 12-lead ECGs in detail in later chapters, but let's take a quick look now.

A 12-lead ECG consists of the following:
- Three standard (bipolar) limb leads (leads I, II, and III)
- Three augmented (unipolar) leads (leads aVR, aVL, and aVF)
- Six precordial (unipolar) leads (V$_1$, V$_2$, V$_3$, V$_4$, V$_5$, and V$_6$)

Augmented and precordial leads will be fully explained in Chapter 12.

The 12-lead ECG is used to diagnose changes associated with acute coronary syndrome (ACS), or "heart attack," and bundle-branch block. It also helps us differentiate between certain kinds of tachycardias (for instance, supraventricular versus ventricular). Clinicians frequently rely on the 12-lead ECG in the hospital, and it is the standard of care in prehospital medicine because of its accuracy in identifying patients with ACS so that they can be delivered efficiently to the most appropriate facility for definitive care.

ACQUIRING A QUALITY ECG

Artifacts

Artifacts are abnormal waves and spikes in an ECG that come from sources other than the heart's electrical activity. These traces of other activity or movement can interfere with or distort the components of the ECG, making interpretation difficult. The causes of artifacts include muscle tremor, alternating current (AC) interference, poor electrode contact with the skin, and external chest compression.

artifacts

Traces of activity or movement other than the heart's electrical activity that can distort the components of the ECG.

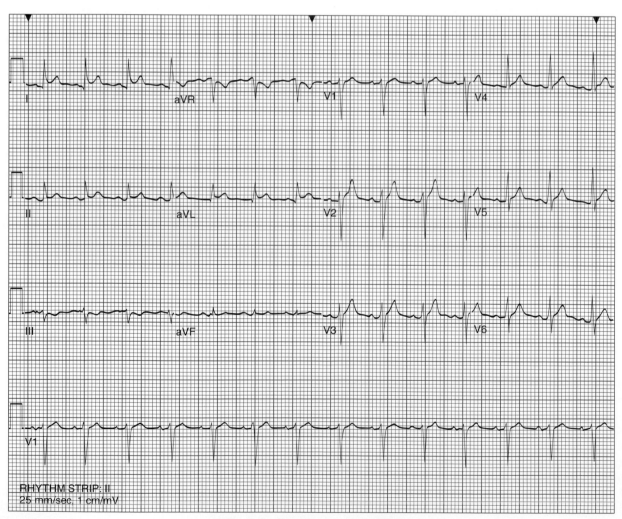

FIG. 2.9 Sample of a 12-lead ECG.

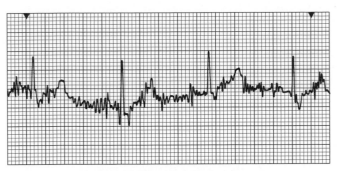

FIG. 2.10 Muscle tremor.

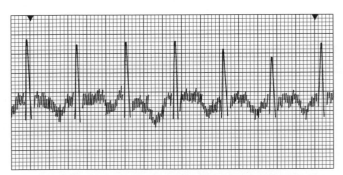

FIG. 2.11 Alternating current interference.

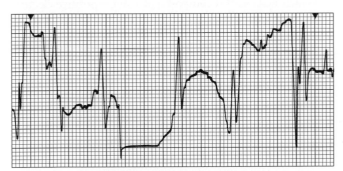

FIG. 2.12 Loose electrodes.

Muscle tremor (Fig. 2.10), for example, can occur in tense, nervous, or shivering patients, giving the ECG a jagged appearance that can be either fine or coarse. An artifact can also occur as a result of the patient breathing. This can cause the baseline of the ECG rhythm to wander up and down, making the determination of various abnormalities difficult.

AC electrical interference (Fig. 2.11) can occur when an improperly grounded AC-operated ECG machine is used or when an ECG is obtained near high-tension wires, transformers, or electrical appliances. This results in a thick baseline composed of 60-cycle waves.

Loose electrodes, or electrodes that are in poor contact with the skin (Fig. 2.12) (because of insufficient or dried electrode paste or jelly) can cause multiple sharp spikes and waves in the ECG. This is the most common cause of artifacts. Loose connecting wires can cause similar artifacts. In addition, any extraneous matter on the skin, such as blood, vomit, sweat, or hair, can result in poor electrode contact and the appearance of artifacts.

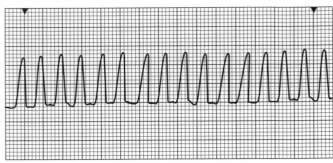

FIG. 2.13 External chest compression.

External chest compression (Fig. 2.13) during cardiopulmonary resuscitation (CPR) causes regularly spaced, wide, upright waves. The waves occur in sync with the rhythmic downward compressions.

> **AUTHOR'S NOTE** Unfortunately, the appearance of waves on the ECG during CPR does not necessarily indicate that the chest compression is producing adequate cardiac output and circulation.

QRS Size and Wandering Baseline

The ECG machine can amplify the signal it receives and display it on the monitor. If the signal strength is low, most machines have a control that allows you to increase the amplitude. This control is called the *gain*. Increasing the gain will increase the size of the ECG waveform printed on the ECG graph paper and can be very helpful when you are using only the monitor to interpret the rhythm.

> **gain**
>
> An adjustable control on an ECG machine that allows the operator to amplify its electrical signal.

Dense tissue increases resistance to the signal as it passes through the chest. Causes of low-amplitude waveforms on the ECG include large barrel chests and/or obesity.

TAKE-HOME POINTS

- An electrocardiogram or ECG is a graphical representation of the electrical impulses generated during the depolarization and repolarization of the atria and ventricles. This signal is detected by electrodes attached to the body.
- The resulting ECG waveform is displayed on the monitor and printed on ECG graph paper for analysis.
- The ECG graph paper is designed to allow accurate measurement of both the strength (amplitude) and duration or timing of the various components of the waveform.
- The ECG waveform is detected by multiple leads, each of which provides a different view of the electrical activity of the heart.
- Waves and complexes are evaluated by shape and duration, intervals are analyzed by length, and segments are measured in relation to the baseline.

- The basic components of the ECG are the P wave; Q, R, and S waves; the T wave; the PR, ST, and TP segments; the PR, QT, and R-R intervals; and the J point.
- There are bipolar and unipolar leads. The bipolar leads (leads I, II, and III) have two electrodes attached to the body, whereas the unipolar leads have one. Lead II is the most common lead used in ECG rhythm interpretation.
- MCL1 and MCL6 are bipolar leads that can be used when a full 12-lead ECG cannot be obtained. They mimic the unipolar leads V1 and V6.
- Unipolar leads have only one electrode attached to the body and are used only in 12-lead ECGs.

- Rhythm interpretation generally relies on bipolar leads, whereas unipolar leads are commonly used to identify various ACSs.
- Artifacts on an ECG are traces of activity or movement other than the heart's electrical activity that can distort the components of the ECG. Artifacts can be caused by muscle tremors, AC interference, poor electrode contact with the skin, or external chest compression.
- Adjusting the gain on an ECG machine to amplify the signal can be helpful when using only the monitor for rhythm interpretation.

CHAPTER REVIEW QUESTIONS

1. What kind of electrical activity does an ECG record?
   A. The depolarization and repolarization of the atria and ventricles
   B. The flow of blood through the heart
   C. The mechanical contraction and relaxation of the atria and ventricles
   D. The transmission of electrical impulses responsible for initiating depolarization of the atria and ventricles

2. When an ECG is recorded at the standard paper speed of 25 mm/sec, how many seconds apart are the dark vertical lines and the light vertical lines?
   A. 5 sec and 1 sec
   B. 20 sec and 4 sec
   C. 0.20 sec and 0.4 sec
   D. 0.20 sec and 0.04 sec

3. The sensitivity of the ECG machine is calibrated so that a(n) _____ electrical signal produces a(n) _____ deflection on the ECG.
   A. 0.5-mV; 1-mm
   B. 1-mV; 10-mm
   C. 5-mV; 10-mm
   D. 10-mV; 5-mm

4. Which part of the waveform shows the electrical impulses generated by ventricular depolarization?
   A. P wave
   B. QRS complex
   C. Atrial T wave (T_a)
   D. T wave

5. Which part of the waveform shows the electrical impulses generated by ventricular repolarization?
   A. P wave
   B. QRS complex
   C. Atrial T wave (T_a)
   D. T wave

6. Which of the following is the most common cause of an ECG artifact?
   A. External chest compression
   B. Muscle tremor
   C. Poor electrode contact with the skin
   D. Turning up the gain

7. Which ECG lead is composed of a single positive electrode and a reference point located at the center of the heart?
   A. Bipolar lead
   B. MCL_1 lead
   C. Multifocal lead
   D. Unipolar lead

8. Monitoring lead II is obtained by attaching the negative electrode and positive electrode to what?
   A. Left arm and left leg
   B. Right arm and left arm
   C. Right arm and left leg
   D. Right arm and left upper chest

9. If the positive electrode is attached to the left leg or lower left anterior chest, in which direction will the electrical impulses that flow toward the positive electrode be deflected on the ECG?
   A. Negative (downward)
   B. Negative (upward)
   C. Positive (downward)
   D. Positive (upward)

10. Monitoring lead MCL_1 is obtained by attaching the positive electrode from lead III to which part of the body?
    A. Left chest below the clavicle
    B. Middle of the sternum at the level of the fourth intercostal space
    C. Left side of the sternum in the fourth intercostal space
    D. Right side of the anterior chest in the fourth intercostal space next to the sternum

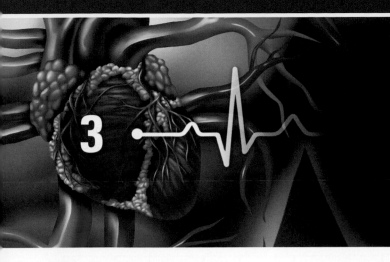

3   Components of the ECG Waveform

In 1887, Professor A. D. Waller was the first to record the electrical activity of the human heart. Using a device called the *Lippmann capillary electrometer,* Waller initially detected only two waves. He labeled them V_1 and V_2, to indicate ventricular events in the heart. Using the same device, Dr. William Einthoven detected four waves, which he initially labeled A, B, C, and D. Further refinement of the device revealed more wave patterns. Einthoven chose to relabel these waveforms P, Q, R, S, and T, in recognition of the letters used by the analytical mathematician René Descartes to describe points along a curve. In 1903, Einthoven invented a more sophisticated ECG machine that could record a detailed tracing of the heart's electrical activity. For that accomplishment, he was awarded the Nobel Prize in Medicine in 1924. As a result, Einthoven is sometimes called "the father of modern electrocardiography."

> **AUTHOR'S NOTE** Lead II is the most common lead used to analyze the heart's electrical activity. For that reason, the shape (morphology) of the ECG waveforms presented in this and subsequent chapters will be described as they are seen in lead II unless other leads provide a better "view."

As noted in Chapter 2, the ECG waveform is composed of waves, intervals, and segments (see Fig. 2.2).

WAVES

P WAVE

P wave

A P wave represents depolarization of the right and left atria.

Normal Sinus P Wave
CHARACTERISTICS

Origin	Sinoatrial (SA) node
Physiology	Atrial depolarization
Onset/End	TP segment/ PR segment
Direction	Upward
Duration	0.08–0.10 sec
Amplitude	0.5–2.5 mm
Shape	Smooth and rounded
Sequence	Precedes QRS complex unless a block is present

Origin
The normal P wave originates in the SA node and is called a *sinus P wave.*

Relationship to Cardiac Anatomy and Physiology
A normal sinus P wave (Fig. 3.1) represents normal depolarization of the myocardial cells of the atrial wall. Depolarization of the atria begins near the SA node and progresses from right to left and downward. The first part of the sinus P wave represents depolarization of the right atrium; the second part represents depolarization of the left atrium. During the P wave, the electrical impulse progresses from the SA node through the internodal atrial conduction tracts and most of the atrioventricular (AV) node.

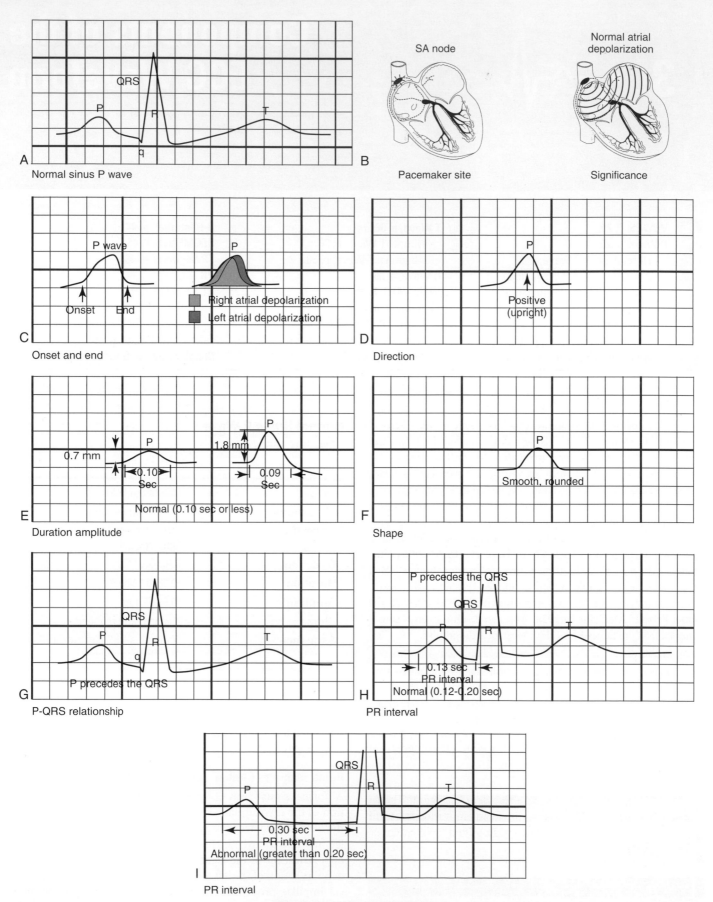

A Normal sinus P wave

B Pacemaker site   Significance

SA node

Normal atrial depolarization

C Onset and end

P wave

Onset   End

Right atrial depolarization

Left atrial depolarization

D Direction

P

Positive (upright)

E Duration amplitude

0.7 mm

P

0.10 Sec

1.8 mm

P

0.09 Sec

Normal (0.10 sec or less)

F Shape

P

Smooth, rounded

G P-QRS relationship

QRS

P   R

q

T

P precedes the QRS

H PR interval

P precedes the QRS

QRS

P   R

T

0.13 sec

PR interval

Normal (0.12-0.20 sec)

I PR interval

QRS

P

R

T

0.30 sec

PR interval

Abnormal (greater than 0.20 sec)

FIG. 3.1 Normal sinus P wave.

DESCRIPTION

Onset and End

The onset of the normal P wave is identified as the first gradual deviation from the baseline. The point at which the wave flattens out to return to the baseline, joining with the PR segment, marks the end of the P wave.

Direction

The direction is positive (upward). This is because most of the impulse is directed toward the positive electrode of lead II, which is on the right upper chest or right arm.

Duration

From 0.08 and 0.10 second.

Amplitude

Ranges from 0.5 to 2.5 mm, although it rarely exceeds 2 mm in height.

Shape

Smooth and rounded.

Sequence

A QRS complex follows each sinus P wave except in certain rhythms, such as AV blocks (see Chapter 9).

SIGNIFICANCE

A normal sinus P wave indicates that the electrical impulse responsible for the P wave originated in the SA node and that normal depolarization of the right and left atria has occurred.

Abnormal Sinus P Wave

CHARACTERISTICS

Origin

The abnormal sinus P wave originates in the SA node.

Relationship to Cardiac Anatomy and Physiology

An abnormal sinus P wave (Fig. 3.2) represents depolarization of damaged or abnormal atria. Increased right atrial pressure and right atrial dilatation and hypertrophy may result in P waves that are abnormally tall or wide or that deflect in abnormal directions.

P waves that occur in two phases are called *biphasic P waves.* This pattern occurs in both right and left atrial dilation and hypertrophy. Biphasic P waves are best detected in leads V_1 and V_2 because these two unipolar leads have direct views of the SA node from the front of the chest. They will show an initial positive deflection during right atrial depolarization. Then a negative deflection will appear as the left atrium is depolarized. Conditions with biphasic P waves are described in Chapter 14.

DESCRIPTION

Onset and End

Same as for those of a normal P wave.

Direction

Positive (upright) in lead II; may be biphasic (initially positive, then negative) in leads V_1 and V_2.

Duration

Usually normal (0.08–0.10 sec) and rarely greater than 0.16 second.

Amplitude

Either normal (0.5–2.5 mm) or greater than normal. When the amplitude of the P wave is greater than 2.5 mm, it is referred to as *P pulmonale.*

Shape

Tall and symmetrically peaked or wide and notched. By definition, notched P waves equal to or greater than 0.12 second with the top of each mound greater than 0.04 second apart is called *P mitrale* and may be biphasic in leads V_1 and V_2.

Sequence

Same as that of a normal sinus P wave.

SIGNIFICANCE

The presence of an abnormal sinus P wave indicates that although the electrical impulse responsible for the P wave originated in the SA node, changes in the atrial walls altered depolarization of the atrial muscle.

Ectopic P Wave: P Prime, or P′

ectopic P wave

A P wave produced by depolarization of the atria in an abnormal direction.

CHARACTERISTICS

Origin

An ectopic P wave is called *P prime,* denoted as P′. It can originate in the AV junction or anywhere in the atrium other than the SA node.

> **AUTHOR'S NOTE** The word *ectopic* comes from the Greek *ek-,* meaning "outside of," and *topos,* meaning "place or location." An ectopic P wave is one that originates outside the SA node.

Relationship to Cardiac Anatomy and Physiology

An ectopic P wave (P′) (Fig. 3.3) represents atrial depolarization originating somewhere in the atrium other than the SA node and proceeding in an abnormal direction, sequence, or both, depending on where the impulse originates. We call this location an *ectopic pacemaker* because the site sets the pace of the rhythm.

- If the ectopic pacemaker is in the upper or middle right atrium, depolarization of the atria occurs in a normal, antegrade direction (right to left and downward).

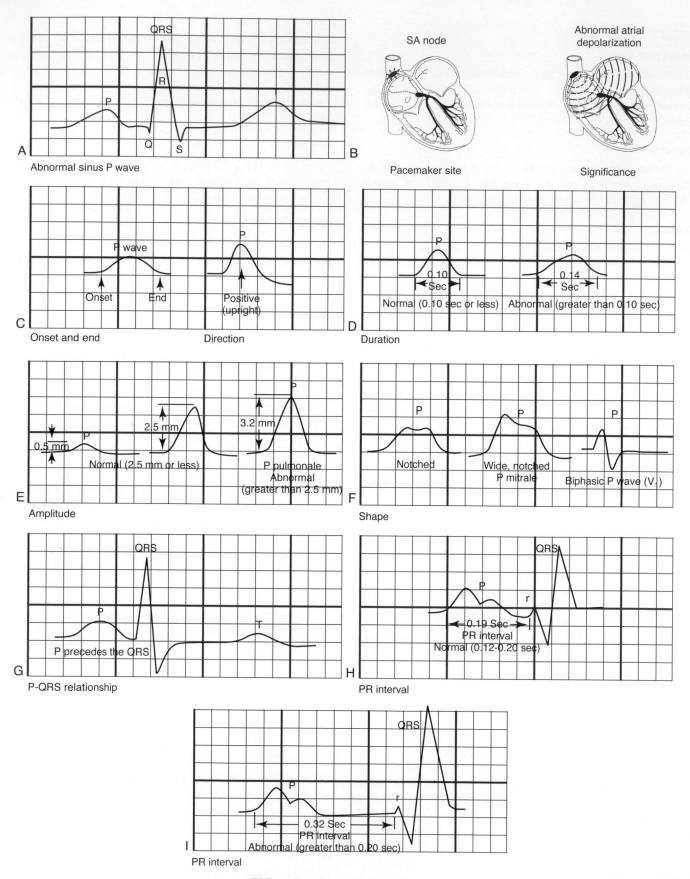

A — Abnormal sinus P wave

B — Pacemaker site — SA node; Significance — Abnormal atrial depolarization

C — Onset and end; Direction

D — Duration

E — Amplitude

F — Shape

G — P-QRS relationship

H — PR interval

I — PR interval

FIG. 3.2 Abnormal sinus P wave.

- If the ectopic pacemaker is in the lower right atrium near the AV node or in the left atrium, depolarization of the atria occurs in a retrograde direction (left to right and upward).
- If the ectopic pacemaker is in the AV junction, the electrical impulse travels upward through the AV junction into the atria (retrograde conduction), causing retrograde atrial depolarization. Ectopic P waves occur in the following ECG rhythms:
  - Wandering atrial pacemaker
  - Premature atrial complexes
  - Atrial tachycardia

DESCRIPTION

Onset and End

Same as those of a normal P wave.

Direction

Either positive (upright) or negative (inverted) if the ectopic pacemaker is in the atria. Generally, if the ectopic pacemaker is in the upper part of the right atrium, the P′ wave is positive, resembling a normal sinus P wave.

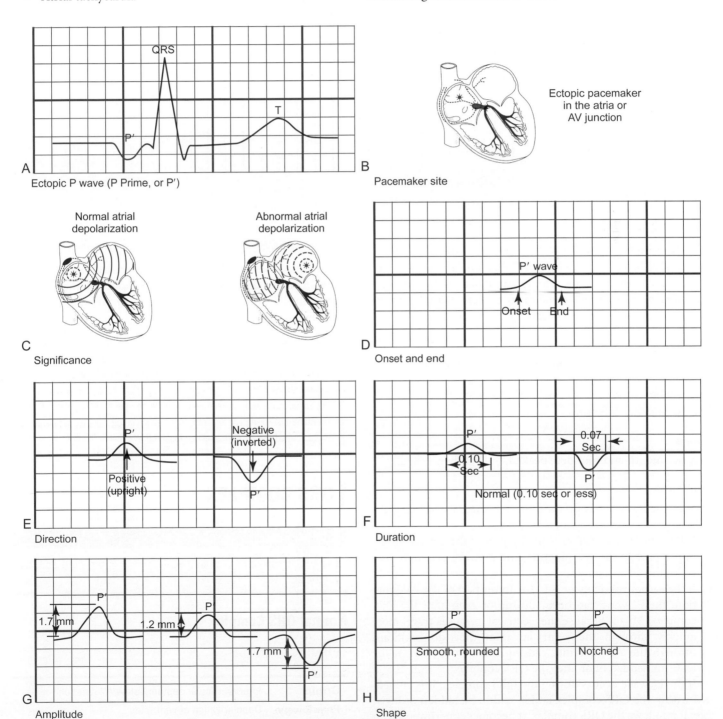

FIG. 3.3 Ectopic P wave (P prime, or P′).

Continued

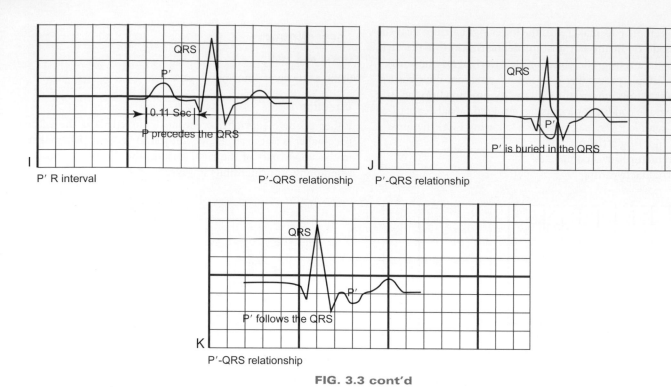

FIG. 3.3 cont'd

If the ectopic pacemaker is in the middle of the right atrium, the P′ wave is less positive (upright) than one arising from the upper right atrium. If the ectopic pacemaker is in the lower right atrium near the AV node or in the left atrium or in the AV junction, the P′ wave is negative (inverted).

Duration
Normal or prolonged, depending on the site of origin.

Amplitude
Usually less than 2.5 mm.

Shape
May be smooth and rounded, peaked, or slightly notched.

Sequence
The ectopic P wave may precede, be embedded in, or follow the QRS complex with which it is associated.
- If the ectopic pacemaker is in any part of the atria or in the upper part of the AV junction, the P′ wave generally precedes the QRS complex.
- If the ectopic pacemaker is in the lower part of the AV junction, the P′ wave can occur during or even after the QRS complex. This is because the electrical impulses travel more quickly through the ventricles than they do backward through the AV junction, causing them to appear on the ECG embedded in or after the QRS complex.

If the P′ wave occurs during the QRS complex, it is embedded within the QRS complex and is said to be hidden or invisible. If it follows the QRS complex, it becomes superimposed on (laid on top of) the ST segment and/or T wave, distorting them.

SIGNIFICANCE

An ectopic P wave indicates that the electrical impulse originated in part of the atria outside the SA node and that depolarization of the right and left atria has occurred in an abnormal direction, sequence, or both.

> **AUTHOR'S NOTE** Another type of ectopic atrial depolarization is seen in atrial fibrillation and atrial flutter. In atrial fibrillation, multiple randomly located ectopic impulses result in the absence of a single P wave. These are called *f waves*. In atrial flutter, a single ectopic atrial depolarization is spontaneously firing at a high rate. This results in regular sawtooth-shaped waves called *F waves*. This will be explored in detail in Chapters 4 and 6.

QRS COMPLEX

QRS complex

The QRS complex represents depolarization of the right and left ventricles.

Normal QRS Complex

CHARACTERISTICS

Origin	Interventricular septum below AV junction
Physiology	Depolarization of ventricles
Onset/End	Deviation from PR interval/beginning of ST segment

Duration	0.06–0.12 sec
Direction	
Q wave	First negative deflection
R wave	First positive deflection
S wave	First negative deflection after an R wave
QS wave	Single negative deflection
RS wave	Single positive deflection
Amplitude	2–15 mm
Shape	Narrow and sharply pointed
Sequence	Follows the P wave and precedes the T wave

Origin

Interventricular septum just below the AV junction.

Relationship to Cardiac Anatomy and Physiology

A normal QRS complex (Fig. 3.4) represents normal depolarization of the ventricles. Depolarization begins in the left side of the interventricular septum near the AV junction and progresses across the interventricular septum from left to right. Then, beginning at the endocardial surface of the ventricles, depolarization progresses through the ventricular walls to the epicardial surface.

The first short part of the QRS complex, usually the Q wave, represents depolarization of the interventricular septum; the rest of the QRS complex represents the simultaneous depolarization of the right and left ventricles. Because the left ventricle is larger than the right ventricle and has more muscle mass, the QRS complex represents, for the most part, depolarization of the left ventricle.

DESCRIPTION

Onset and End

The onset of the QRS complex is identified as the point where the first wave of the complex just begins to deviate, usually abruptly, from the baseline of the PR interval following the end of the P wave. The end of the QRS complex is the point where the last wave of the complex sharply flattens to meet the ST segment. This point, the junction between the QRS complex and the ST segment, is called the *junction* or *J point*.

Components

The QRS complex consists of one or more of the following: positive (upright) deflections called *R waves* and negative (inverted) deflections called *Q, S,* and *QS waves*. The characteristics of the waves that make up the QRS complex are as follows:
- **Q wave:** The Q wave is the first negative deflection in the QRS complex not preceded by an R wave.
- **R wave:** The R wave is the first positive deflection in the QRS complex. Subsequent positive deflections are called *R prime (R′), R double prime (R″),* and so forth.
- **S wave:** The S wave is the first negative deflection in the QRS complex after an R wave. Subsequent negative deflections are called *S prime (S′), S double prime (S″),* and so forth.

- **QS wave:** A QS wave is a QRS complex that consists entirely of a single, large negative deflection without an intervening positive deflection.

Whereas there is only one Q wave, there can be more than one R and S wave in the QRS complex.

The waves comprising the QRS complex are usually identified by uppercase (capital) or lowercase (small) letters, depending on the relative size of the waves. In other words, the major deflections—the large waves—are identified by the letters Q, R, and S. The smaller waves, which are less than half the amplitude of the major deflections, are identified by the letters q, r, and s. Thus the ventricular depolarization complex can be described more accurately by using the specific letters assigned to the waves (for example, qR, Rs, or qRs). However, we still refer to it as a QRS complex when discussing this complex in general.

Direction

The QRS complex is described as being mostly positive (upright), mostly negative (inverted or downward), or biphasic (positive and negative). In a mostly positive QRS complex, for example, the R wave—the major deflection—covers more area than the Q and S waves do. Usually this is easy to see simply by looking at the QRS complex; however, if you are unsure, place a ruler at the baseline and estimate the number of small squares covered by the height and depth of the QRS complex above and below the baseline.

Duration

The duration of the QRS complex is measured from the onset of the Q or R wave to the end of the last wave of the complex, called the *J point,* and is normally 0.06 to 0.12 second in adults and 0.08 second or less in children. The duration of the Q wave is normally 0.04 second or less.

> **AUTHOR'S NOTE** The time between the onset of the Q wave and the peak of the R wave is the ventricular activation time (VAT). The VAT is the time it takes for depolarization of the interventricular septum and depolarization of the ventricle from the endocardium to the epicardium under the facing lead. The upper limit of the normal VAT is 0.05 second. Some texts refer to the VAT as the *intrinsicoid deflection.*

Amplitude

The amplitude of the R or S wave in the QRS complex varies from 2 to 15 mm or more. The normal Q wave is less than 25% of the height of the R wave that follows it.

Shape

The normal QRS complex is generally narrow and sharply pointed.

Sequence

The normal QRS complex follows the P wave and precedes the T wave.

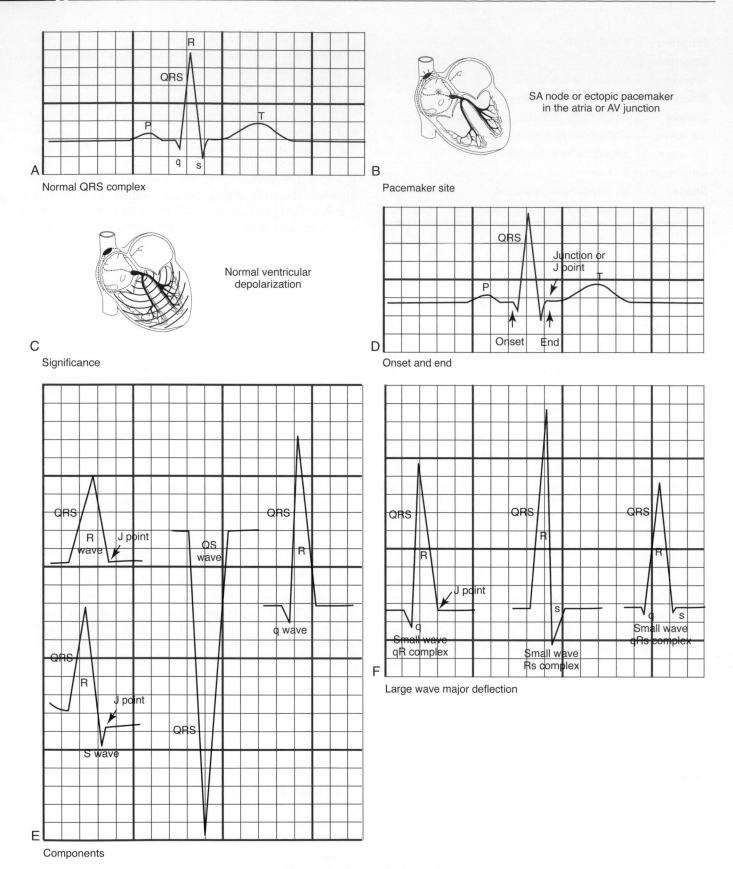

A Normal QRS complex

B Pacemaker site
SA node or ectopic pacemaker in the atria or AV junction

C Significance
Normal ventricular depolarization

D Onset and end

E Components

F Large wave major deflection

FIG. 3.4 Normal QRS complex.

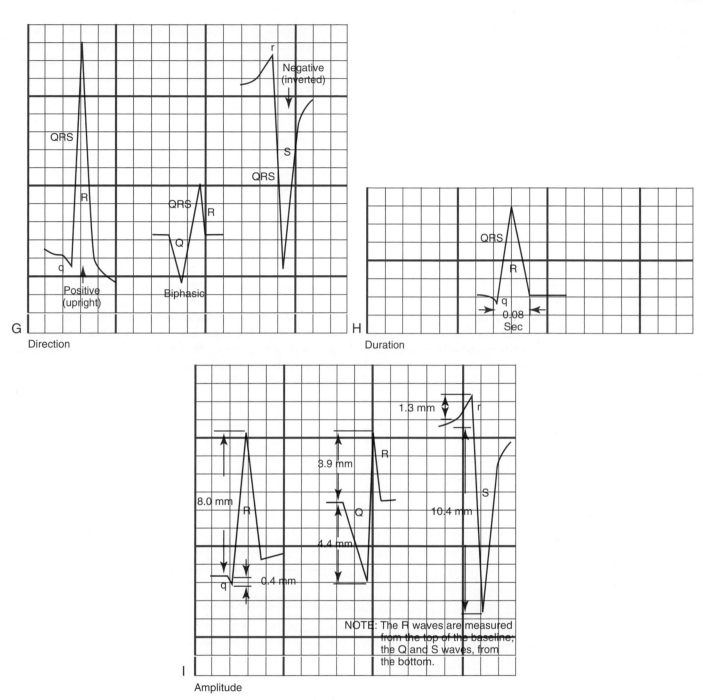

FIG. 3.4 cont'd

SIGNIFICANCE

A normal QRS complex indicates that the electrical impulse has progressed normally from the AV junction down the bundle of His to the Purkinje network and through the right and left bundle branches to depolarize the right and left ventricles normally.

Abnormal QRS Complex

CHARACTERISTICS

Origin

Within or below the AV junction or from the bundle branches, Purkinje network, or ventricular myocardium.

Relationship to Cardiac Anatomy and Physiology

An abnormal QRS complex (Fig. 3.5) represents abnormal depolarization of the ventricles. It is referred to as *aberrant (abnormal) ventricular conduction.* The cause may be any of the following:

- Intraventricular conduction disturbance (such as a bundle-branch block)
- Ventricular preexcitation
- An ectopic electrical impulse
- Ventricular pacing by an implanted cardiac pacemaker
  Intraventricular conduction disturbance is most often caused by right or left bundle-branch block. It can also be caused by a nonspecific, widespread electrical conduction defect associated

with specific types of heart diseases, electrolyte imbalances, or excessive administration of certain cardiac drugs. Bundle-branch block is caused by the blockage or partial blockage of electrical impulses from the bundle of His to the Purkinje network through the right or left bundle branch. Conduction through the unaffected bundle branch is unimpeded (see Chapter 13). A block in one bundle branch causes depolarization of the ventricle on that side to occur later than on the unaffected side because the affected ventricle must wait until the electrical impulse travels through a longer and less efficient route to depolarize the myocardial cells. This delay results in a widened QRS that exceeds 0.12 seconds in duration.

In partial or incomplete bundle-branch block, conduction of the electrical impulse is only partially blocked, resulting in less of a delay in depolarization of the ventricle on the side of the block than in complete bundle-branch block. Consequently, the QRS complex is greater than 0.10 but less than 0.12 seconds in duration and often appears normal.

Complete and incomplete bundle-branch block may be present in normal sinus rhythm and in any supraventricular arrhythmia (that is, any arrhythmia arising above the ventricles in the SA node, atria, or AV junction).

Ventricular preexcitation is a transient inability of the right or left bundle branch to conduct an electrical impulse normally. This may occur when an electrical impulse arrives at the bundle branch that has just conducted an electrical impulse while it is still refractory to conducting another. This occurs with premature atrial complexes and some tachycardias. It results in an abnormal QRS complex that often resembles an incomplete or complete bundle-branch block.

Abnormal ventricular conduction may occur in the following supraventricular rhythms that mimic ventricular rhythms (see Chapter 8):
- Premature atrial and junctional complexes
- Atrial tachycardia
- Atrial flutter and fibrillation
- Nonparoxysmal junctional tachycardia
- Paroxysmal supraventricular tachycardia

An electrical impulse originating in an ectopic or escape pacemaker in the bundle branches, Purkinje network, or myocardium of one of the ventricles depolarizes that ventricle earlier than the other. The result is an abnormal QRS complex that is greater than 0.12 second in duration and appears bizarre. Such QRS complexes typically occur in ventricular rhythms such as

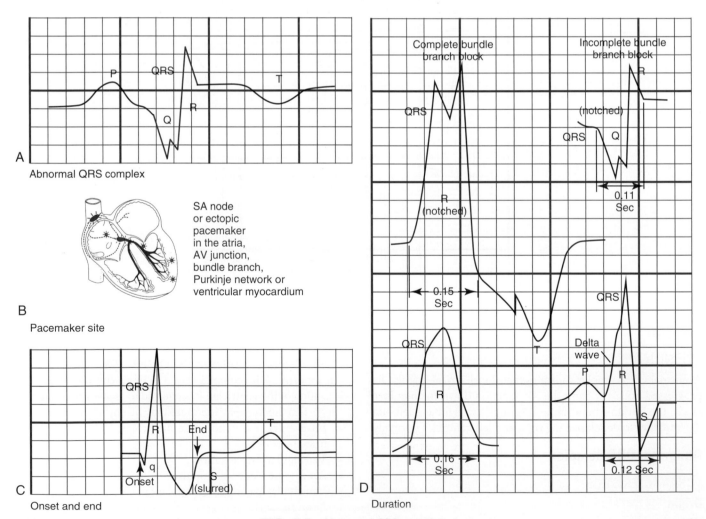

FIG. 3.5 Abnormal QRS complex.

1. Blockage of conduction of the electrical impulse through a bundle branch

Block in right bundle branch

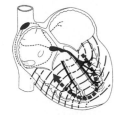

Right bundle branch block

Block in left bundle branch

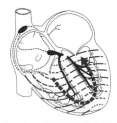

Left bundle branch block

Direction of ventricular depolarization

Bundle branch block and aberrant ventricular conduction

2. Conduction of the electrical impulse through accessory conduction pathways

Ventricular preexcitation

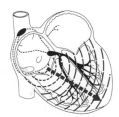

3. Ventricular ectopic or artificial cardiac pacemaker

Abnormal ventricular depolarization

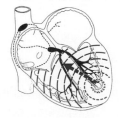

Ventricular pacemaker

E

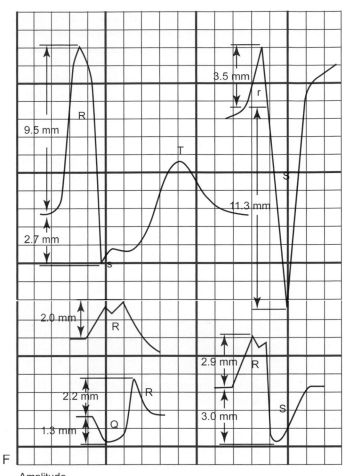

F

Amplitude

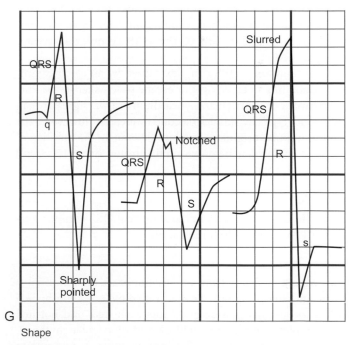

G

Shape

FIG. 3.5 cont'd

accelerated idioventricular rhythm, ventricular escape rhythm, ventricular tachycardia, and premature ventricular complexes (see Chapter 8). The occurrence of ventricular ectopic beats or rhythms is often referred to as *ventricular ectopy.*

Implanted cardiac pacemaker–induced QRS complexes are generated by the electrical stimulation from a wire embedded in the inner wall of the right ventricle. The resulting QRS complexes are generally 0.12 second or greater in width, similar to a left bundle-branch block because the impulse must travel through a slower pathway from the right to the left ventricle. However, because the depolarization occurs in the endocardium of the ventricle, the cardiac pacemaker–induced QRS complex has a similar shape as a ventricular ectopic complex. A common indicator of a pacemaker-induced QRS complex is a narrow deflection, often biphasic, preceding the QRS complex called the *pacemaker spike,* which is the electrical stimulus from the pacemaker wire. (see Chapter 10).

DESCRIPTION

Onset and End

Same as those of a normal QRS complex.

Direction

Mostly positive (upright), mostly negative (inverted), or biphasic (positive and negative).

Duration

Greater than 0.12 second. If a bundle-branch block is present and the duration of the QRS complex is between 0.10 and 0.12 second, the bundle-branch block is called *incomplete.* If the duration of the QRS complex is greater than 0.12 second, the bundle-branch block is called *complete.* In ventricular preexcitation, the duration of the QRS complex is greater than 0.12 second.

The duration of a QRS complex caused by an electrical impulse originating in an ectopic or escape pacemaker in the Purkinje network or ventricular myocardium is always greater than 0.12 second; typically, it is 0.16 second or greater. However, if the electrical impulse originates in a bundle branch, the duration of the QRS complex may be only slightly greater than 0.10 second and appear normal.

Amplitude

The amplitude of the waves in the abnormal QRS complex varies from 1 to 2 mm to 20 mm or more.

Shape

Varies widely in shape, from one that appears quite normal—narrow and sharply pointed (as in incomplete bundle-branch block)—to one that is wide and bizarre, slurred, and notched (as in complete bundle-branch block and ventricular rhythms). In ventricular preexcitation, the QRS complex is wider than normal at the base because of an initial slurring or bulging of the upstroke of the R wave (or of the downstroke of the S wave, as the case may be) known as the *delta wave.*

Sequence

The abnormal QRS may or may not follow a P wave but will be preceded by a T wave.

SIGNIFICANCE

Indicates that abnormal depolarization of the ventricles has occurred because of one of the following:

- A block in the progression of the electrical impulse from the bundle of His to the Purkinje network through the right or left bundle branch (bundle-branch block and aberrant ventricular conduction)
- The progression of the electrical impulse from the atria to the ventricles through an abnormal accessory conduction pathway (ventricular preexcitation)
- The origination of the electrical impulse responsible for the ventricular depolarization in a ventricular ectopic or escape pacemaker
- The depolarization of the ventricles initiated by an implanted cardiac pacemaker

T WAVE

T wave
A T wave represents ventricular repolarization. T waves are characterized as normal or abnormal.

Normal T Wave

CHARACTERISTICS

Origin	Epicardial surface of the ventricles
Physiology	Repolarization of ventricles
Onset/End	Deviation from ST segment/TP segment
Direction	Positive
Duration	0.10–0.25 sec
Amplitude	Less than 5 mm
Shape	Bluntly rounded and asymmetrical
Sequence	Always follows a QRS

Origin

Epicardial surface of the ventricles.

Relationship to Cardiac Anatomy and Physiology

A normal T wave (Fig. 3.6) represents normal repolarization of the ventricles. Normal repolarization begins at the epicardial surface of the ventricles and progresses inwardly through the ventricular walls to the endocardial surface. The T wave occurs during the last part of ventricular systole.

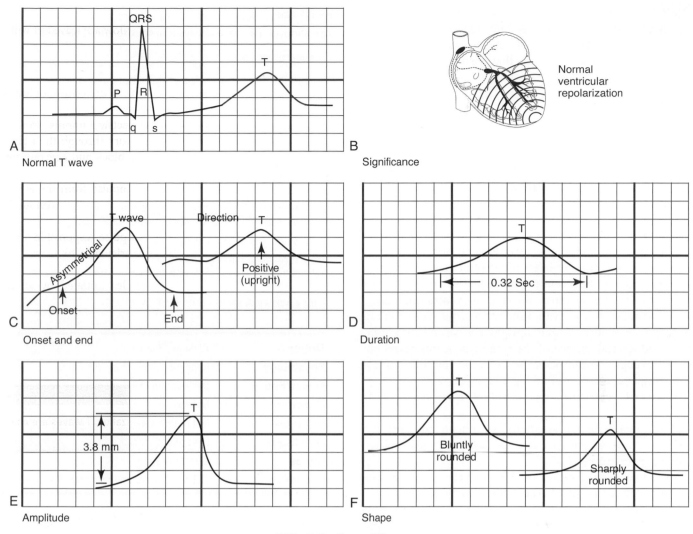

FIG. 3.6 Normal T wave.

DESCRIPTION

Onset and End

Begins at the first deviation from the ST segment (or the point at which the slope of the ST segment appears to become steeper). If the T wave begins at the end of the QRS complex (the J point), the ST segment is absent. The point at which the T wave returns to the baseline marks the end of the T wave. In the absence of an ST segment, the T wave is sometimes called the *ST-T wave*. Occasionally the onset and end of the T wave are difficult to pinpoint.

Direction

Positive (upright).

Duration

Ranges from 0.10 to 0.25 second or greater. The duration of the T wave alone is less important than the QT interval.

Amplitude

Normally less than 5 mm.

Shape

Bluntly rounded and asymmetrical. The first upward part of the T wave is longer than the second downward part. It is asymmetrical, with the majority of the wave occurring before the peak of the T wave.

Sequence

Always follows the QRS complex.

> **AUTHOR'S NOTE** The normal T wave is usually in the same direction as the QRS complex and is never more than two-thirds the height of the R wave. Symmetrical T waves usually indicate some pathology, such as ischemia or electrolyte imbalance.

SIGNIFICANCE

Examination of T waves must also include examination of the ST segment (to be discussed later). A normal T wave preceded by a normal ST segment indicates that normal repolarization of the right and left ventricles has occurred.

Abnormal T Wave

CHARACTERISTICS

Origin

The impulse responsible for the abnormal T wave originates in either the epicardial or endocardial surface of the ventricles.

Relationship to Cardiac Anatomy and Physiology

An abnormal T wave (Fig. 3.7) represents abnormal ventricular repolarization. Abnormal repolarization may begin at either the epicardial or endocardial surface of the ventricles. When abnormal repolarization begins at the epicardial surface of the ventricles, it progresses inwardly through the ventricular walls to the endocardial surface, as it normally does, but at a slower rate, producing an abnormally tall, upright T wave. When it begins at the endocardial surface of the ventricles, it progresses outwardly through the ventricular walls to the epicardial surface, producing a negative, inverted, or "flipped" T wave.

Abnormal ventricular repolarization may occur in the following:

- Myocardial ischemia, associated with acute coronary syndromes, myocarditis, pericarditis, and ventricular enlargement (hypertrophy)
- Abnormal depolarization of the ventricles (as in bundle-branch block and ectopic ventricular rhythms)
- Electrolyte imbalance, such as hyperkalemia and administration of certain cardiac drugs, such as quinidine or procainamide

DESCRIPTION

Onset and End

Same as those of a normal T wave.

Direction

Positive (upright) and abnormally tall, low, and negative (inverted), or biphasic (partially positive and partially negative). The abnormal T wave may or may not be deflected in the same direction as the QRS complex.

Duration

From 0.10 to 0.25 seconds or more.

Amplitude

Variable.

Shape

Rounded, blunt, sharply peaked, wide, or notched. The most common abnormal shape is a symmetrical T wave or one with reverse asymmetry, in which the first portion of the T wave is steep and short, whereas the second portion is more gradual and long.

Sequence

The abnormal T wave always follows the QRS complex.

SIGNIFICANCE

An abnormal T wave indicates that abnormal repolarization of the ventricles has occurred. An examination of the ST segment must also be taken into consideration to fully understand the clinical significance of the abnormal T wave.

U WAVE

U wave
A U wave follows the T wave and probably represents delayed repolarization of Purkinje fibers.

CHARACTERISTICS

Origin	Purkinje fibers
Physiology	Repolarization of Purkinje fibers
Onset/End	Deviation from TP segment/TP segment
Direction	Positive
Duration	Not determined
Amplitude	Less than 5 mm
Shape	Less than 2 mm
Sequence	Follows T wave and precedes P wave

Origin

Arises from the Purkinje fibers.

Relationship to Cardiac Anatomy and Physiology

A U wave (Fig. 3.8) probably represents repolarization of the Purkinje fibers or delayed repolarization of some small portion of the ventricle. Although uncommon and not easily identified, the U wave can best be seen when the heart rate is slow.

DESCRIPTION

Onset and End

The onset of the U wave is identified as the first gradual deviation from the baseline or the downward slope of the T wave. It should not be mistaken for a P wave. The point where the U wave returns to the baseline or downward slope of the T wave marks the end of the U wave.

Direction

Positive (upright), the same as that of the preceding normal T wave.

Duration

The duration is not routinely determined.

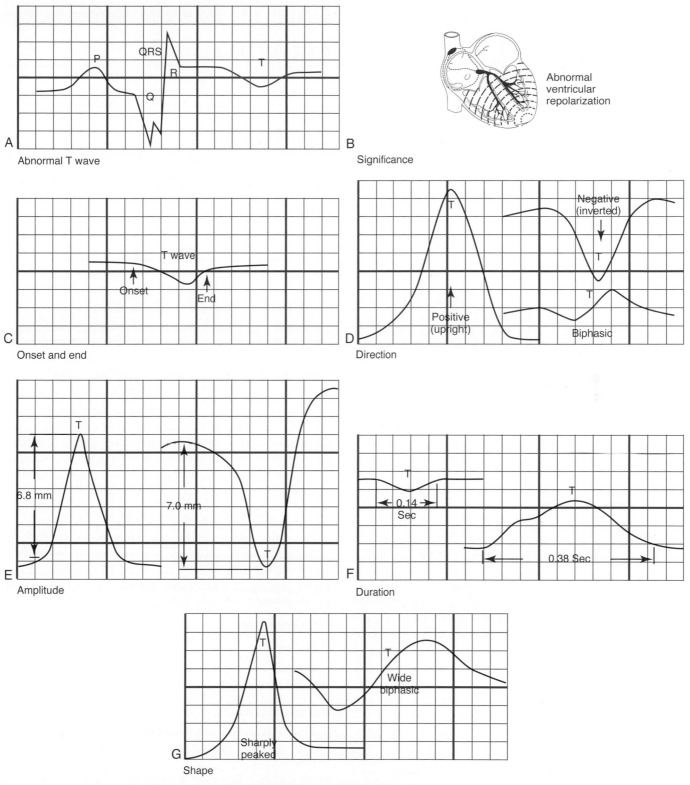

FIG. 3.7 Abnormal T wave.

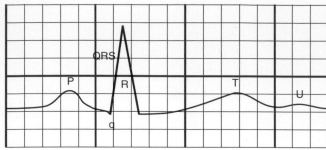

U wave

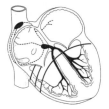

Repolarization of part
of the ventricles

Significance

FIG. 3.8 U wave.

Amplitude

Usually less than 2 mm and always smaller than that of the preceding T wave. A U wave taller than 2 mm is considered abnormal.

Shape

Rounded and symmetrical.

Sequence

If present, it follows the peak of the T wave and occurs before the next P wave.

SIGNIFICANCE

A U wave indicates that repolarization of the ventricles has occurred. Small U waves of less than 2 mm are a normal finding. Abnormally tall U waves of more than 2 mm in height may be present in the following:

- Hypokalemia
- Cardiomyopathy
- Left ventricular hypertrophy
- Excessive administration of digitalis, quinidine, and procainamide

> **AUTHOR'S NOTE** A large U wave may sometimes be mistaken for a P wave. If a P wave is absent, as in a junctional rhythm, and a large U wave is present, a sinus rhythm with a first-degree AV block may be mistakenly diagnosed. If both a large P wave and a large U wave are present, a 2:1 AV block may be diagnosed incorrectly. The fact that a U wave bears a constant relationship to the T wave and not to the P wave or QRS complex helps identify the U wave and differentiate it from a P wave.

INTERVALS

PR INTERVAL

> **PR interval**
>
> A PR interval (Fig. 3.9) represents the time it takes for the electrical impulse to travel from the atria to the bundle of His below the AV junction. It starts at the beginning of the P wave and ends at the start of the QRS complex. PR intervals are either normal or abnormal.

Normal PR Interval
CHARACTERISTICS

Physiology	Represents the normal time delay between atrial and ventricular depolarization
Onset/End	Onset of P wave/onset of QRS complex
Duration	From 0.12 to 0.20 sec, depending on heart rate

Relationship to Cardiac Anatomy and Physiology

Before atrial depolarization, blood fills the ventricles passively because the pressure in the ventricles is lower than that in the atria. As the pressure equalizes, the flow stops. During atrial depolarization (the P wave), the atria contract and maintain an equal pressure between the filling ventricles and the vessels supplying blood to the atria. This ensures that the AV valves remain open so that the ventricles can fill completely. This "atrial kick" can promote up to 25% more volume to the ventricles.

As we discussed previously, the P wave represents atrial depolarization. After atrial depolarization, the electrical impulse passes through to the AV node, where it slows momentarily before being transmitted to the ventricles. This period of slowing, represented by the PR segment, provides the time necessary for the mechanical activity of atrial contraction to occur.

DESCRIPTION
Onset and End

Begins with the onset of the P wave and ends with the onset of the QRS complex.

Direction

Isoelectric (flat) running along the baseline of the ECG.

Duration

From 0.12 to 0.20 second, depending on heart rate. When the heart rate is fast, the PR interval is normally shorter than when the heart rate is slow (example: heart rate = 120, PR interval = 0.16 second; heart rate = 60, PR interval = 0.20 second).

Sequence

A QRS follows every P wave if conduction between the atria and the ventricles is normal.

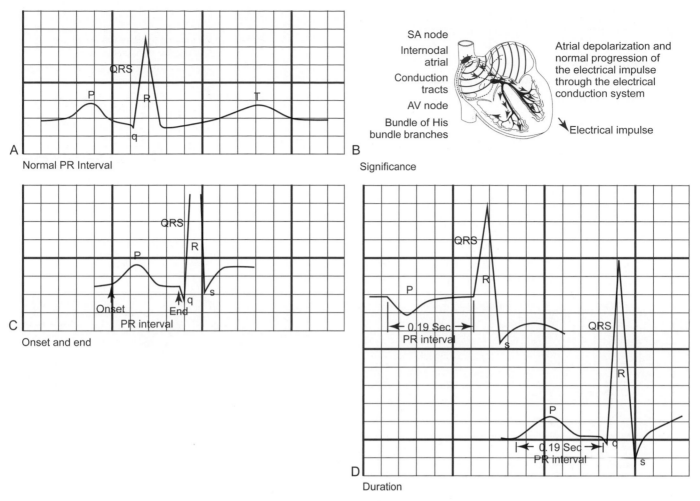

FIG. 3.9 Normal PR interval.

SIGNIFICANCE

A normal PR interval indicates that the electrical impulse originated in the SA node or an ectopic pacemaker in the atria and has progressed normally through the AV node to the bundle of His without delay.

Abnormal PR Interval

CHARACTERISTICS

Relationship to Cardiac Anatomy and Physiology

A PR interval of greater than 0.20 second (Fig. 3.10) represents delayed progression of the electrical impulse through the AV node of the bundle of His. A PR interval of less than 0.12 second is usually present when the electrical impulse originates in an ectopic pacemaker in the atria close to the AV node or in an ectopic or escape pacemaker in the AV junction. The short PR interval reflects the shorter distance the impulse traveled to reach the AV node.

A negative (inverted) P wave is often associated with abnormally short PR intervals because the impulse is conducted in a retrograde fashion (from left to right or upward) away from the AV node.

A positive and normal-appearing P wave with a PR interval of less than 0.12 second also occurs when the electrical impulse progresses from the atria to the ventricles through one of several accessory conduction pathways, which bypass the entire AV junction or just the AV node itself, depolarizing the ventricles earlier than usual.

DESCRIPTION

Onset and End

Same as those of a normal PR interval.

Direction

May be either isoelectric or gently sloping or slurring into the QRS complex.

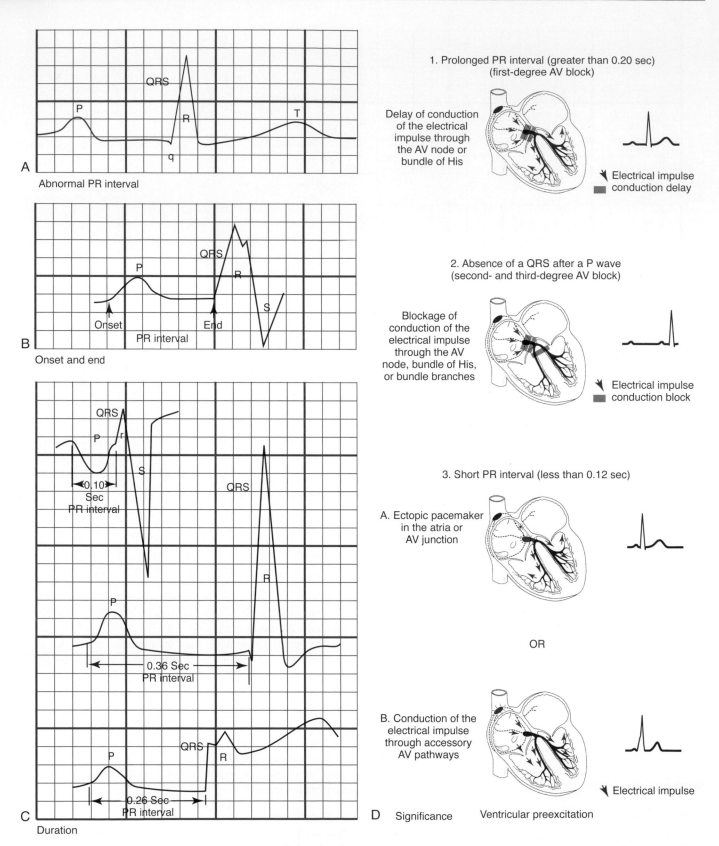

A Abnormal PR interval

B Onset and end

C Duration

1. Prolonged PR interval (greater than 0.20 sec) (first-degree AV block)

Delay of conduction of the electrical impulse through the AV node or bundle of His

Electrical impulse
conduction delay

2. Absence of a QRS after a P wave (second- and third-degree AV block)

Blockage of conduction of the electrical impulse through the AV node, bundle of His, or bundle branches

Electrical impulse
conduction block

3. Short PR interval (less than 0.12 sec)

A. Ectopic pacemaker in the atria or AV junction

OR

B. Conduction of the electrical impulse through accessory AV pathways

Electrical impulse

D Significance   Ventricular preexcitation

FIG. 3.10 Abnormal PR interval.

Duration

Rarely exceeds 0.48 second. The interval may vary from beat to beat or may be normal at times and then progressively lengthen until the impulse does not reach the bundle of His, resulting in no associated QRS complex.

Sequence

If a QRS complex is present after each P wave and prolonged PR interval, it can be assumed that the QRS complex resulted from the P wave.

SIGNIFICANCE

An abnormally prolonged PR interval indicates a delay in the progression of the electrical impulse through the AV node or bundle of His. If the prolongation is constant, then the conduction delay is not changing. If the PR interval is constantly lengthening, then the conduction delay is progressively worsening with each beat.

An abnormally short PR interval indicates one of the following:

- That the electrical impulse originated in an ectopic pacemaker in the atria near the AV node or in an ectopic or escape pacemaker in the AV junction
- That the electrical impulse originated in the SA node or atria and progressed through one of several abnormal accessory conduction pathways that bypass the entire AV junction or just the AV node

QT INTERVAL

QT interval

The QT interval represents the time between the onset of ventricular depolarization and the end of ventricular repolarization.

CHARACTERISTICS

Physiology	Total time for ventricles to depolarize and repolarize
Onset/End	First wave of QRS complex/T wave returns to baseline
Duration	Less than 0.45 sec, depending on rate

Relationship to Cardiac Anatomy and Physiology

The QT interval (Fig. 3.11) represents the total time for the ventricles to depolarize and repolarize. It encompasses the QRS complex, the ST segment, and the T wave. An abnormally prolonged QT interval, one that exceeds the average QT interval for any given heart rate by 10%, represents a slowing in the repolarization of the ventricles. Abnormally prolonged QT intervals may occur in the following:

- Pericarditis, acute myocarditis, acute myocardial ischemia and infarction, left ventricular hypertrophy, and hypothermia

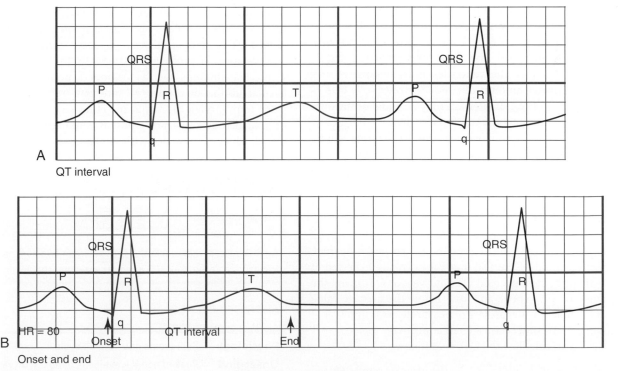

FIG. 3.11 QT interval.

- Slow rhythms (for instance, marked sinus bradycardia, third-degree AV block with slow ventricular escape rhythm)
- Electrolyte imbalance (hypokalemia and hypocalcemia) and liquid-protein diets
- Medication effects (sotalol, procainamide, amiodarone, phenothiazines, and tricyclic antidepressants; some antibiotics, such as ciprofloxacin and erythromycin)
- Central nervous system disorders (for example, cerebrovascular accident, subarachnoid hemorrhage, and intracranial trauma)
- Congenital prolonged QT syndrome

An abnormally short QT interval, one that is less than the average QT interval for any given heart rate by 10%, represents an increase in the rate of repolarization of the ventricles. This occurs in digitalis therapy and hypercalcemia.

DESCRIPTION

Onset and End

Begins at the point where the first wave of the QRS complex begins to deviate, whether abruptly or gradually, from the baseline. Ends at the point where the T wave returns to the baseline.

> **AUTHOR'S NOTE** The determination of the QT interval should be made in the lead where the T wave is most prominent and not deformed by a U wave and should not include the U wave.

Duration

Depends on heart rate. In general, a QT interval of less than half of the R-R interval is normal, one that is greater than half is abnormal, and one that is about half is "borderline." When the heart rate is fast, the QT interval is shorter than when the heart rate is slow (for example, heart rate 120, QT interval about 0.29 second; heart rate 60, QT interval about 0.39 second). As the heart rate increases, the time for ventricular systole decreases, and therefore the ventricles must depolarize and repolarize in a shorter amount of time. The reverse is true as the heart rate slows. The QT intervals may be equal or unequal in duration, depending on the underlying rhythm. For example, if portions of the rhythm are fast, the QT interval will be shorter than those portions of the rhythm that are slower. In these instances, it will be impossible to obtain an accurate measurement of the QT interval, but you can estimate an average interval.

Because the QT interval is dependent on heart rate, "normal" is therefore dependent on heart rate and must be "corrected." This new value is termed the *QTc*, or the *QT corrected interval*. The average duration of the QT interval normally expected at a given heart rate, the corrected QT interval (or QTc), and the normal range of 10% above and 10% below the average value are shown in Table 3.1. Regardless of heart rate, a QT interval of greater than 0.45 second is considered abnormal.

An easy way to calculate the QTc is as follows:

$$QTc = QT \text{ (milliseconds)} + 1.75 \text{ (ventricular rate } - 60)$$

$$\text{Example}: HR = 100, QT = 330$$

TABLE 3.1	QTc Intervals	
Heart Rate/min	**R-R Interval (sec)**	**QT$_c$ (sec) and Normal Range**
40	1.5	0.46 (0.41–0.51)
50	1.2	0.42 (0.38–0.46)
60	1.0	0.39 (0.35–0.43)
70	0.86	0.37 (0.33–0.41)
80	0.75	0.35 (0.32–0.39)
90	0.67	0.33 (0.30–0.36)
100	0.60	0.31 (0.28–0.34)
120	0.50	0.29 (0.26–0.32)
150	0.40	0.25 (0.23–0.28)
180	0.33	0.23 (0.21–0.25)
200	0.30	0.22 (0.20–0.24)

$$1.75 (100 - 60) = 1.75 \times 40 = 70$$

$$330 + 70 = 400, \text{ or } 0.400 \text{ second, which is normal}$$

SIGNIFICANCE

A QT interval represents the time between the onset of ventricular depolarization and the end of ventricular repolarization. Throughout the majority of the QRS complex, when the ventricles are depolarizing, the myocardial cells cannot be stimulated to further depolarize and contract. This is called the *absolute refractory period*. This period lasts for a portion of the initial period of repolarization, but at some point during the T wave, the cells are vulnerable to repolarization by a sufficient impulse. This is called the *relative refractory period*. A prolonged QT interval increases the relative refractory period.

Therefore QT prolongation increases the potential for lethal ventricular rhythms, such as torsades de pointes, a form of ventricular fibrillation. Short QT intervals are relatively rare, but when found (often in infants and children), they are a result of genetic disorders that predispose the individual to sudden cardiac death and are treated with implantable defibrillators.

R-R INTERVAL

> **R-R interval**
>
> An R-R interval represents the time between two successive ventricular depolarizations. R-R intervals are either regular or irregular.

CHARACTERISTICS

Physiology	Represents one cardiac cycle
Onset/End	Peak of one R wave/peak of next R wave
Duration	Depends on rate

Relationship to Cardiac Anatomy and Physiology

An R-R interval (Fig. 3.12) normally represents one cardiac cycle, during which the atria and ventricles contract and relax once.

> **AUTHOR'S NOTE** It is possible for there to be more than one atrial depolarization (P wave) between consecutive R waves. Noting the P waves and measuring the P-P interval will further assist your rhythm interpretation.

DESCRIPTION

Onset and End

Generally considered to begin at the peak of one R wave. Ends at the peak of the next R wave.

Duration

Depends on heart rate. When the heart rate is fast, the R-R interval is shorter than when the heart rate is slow (for example, heart rate 120, R-R interval, 0.50 second; heart rate 60, R-R interval, 1 second). The R-R intervals may be equal or unequal in duration, depending on the underlying rhythm.

We refer to this equality as *regularity*. If the R-R intervals are equal, the ventricular rate is regular. If they are unequal, the rate is irregular. Examples of irregular rhythms include the following:

- A regular rhythm interspersed with premature atrial, junctional, and ventricular premature beats
- Atrial fibrillation
- Atrial flutter with variable conduction ratio
- Second-degree AV blocks

SIGNIFICANCE

An R-R interval represents the time between two successive ventricular depolarizations. Measuring the R-R interval and correlating it with the presence and timing of the P waves and other intervals is a crucial step in rhythm interpretation that you should master.

> **AUTHOR'S NOTE** When measuring the R-R interval, it is important to measure from the same point on each consecutive QRS complex. This is particularly true when the QRS complex is wide.

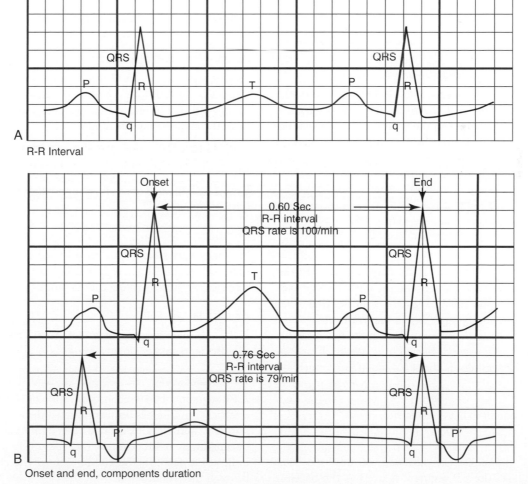

A R-R Interval

B Onset and end, components duration

FIG. 3.12 R-R interval.

SEGMENTS

TP SEGMENT

> **TP segment**
>
> The interval between two successive P-QRST complexes, during which electrical activity of the heart is absent. This is referred to as the *baseline* or *isoelectric line*.

> **AUTHOR'S NOTE** Segments are referred to as "elevated" or "depressed" relative to the baseline. Think of the baseline as neutral or zero, at which time there is no electrical activity occurring in the heart. Anything above the baseline is positive (elevated), and anything below it is negative (depressed). One method of determining the baseline of an ECG is to place a ruler or straight edge across successive TP segments.

CHARACTERISTICS

Physiology	Represents the time between ventricular repolarization and atrial depolarization
Onset/End	End of T wave/onset of next P wave
Duration	Depends on rate
Amplitude	Isoelectric (flat)

Relationship to Cardiac Anatomy and Physiology

A TP segment represents the time from the end of ventricular repolarization to the onset of the next atrial depolarization, during which electrical activity of the heart is absent. A TP segment may include a U wave after the T wave.

DESCRIPTION

Onset and End

Begins with the end of the T wave and ends with the onset of the following wave.

Duration

From 0.0 to 0.40 second or greater and depends on heart rate and the configuration of the P waves and the QRS-T complexes. When the heart rate is fast, the TP segment is shorter than when the heart rate is slow. For example, when the heart rate is about 120 or greater, the TP segment is absent, with the P wave either immediately after the T wave or buried in it. With a heart rate of 60 or less, the TP segment is about 0.4 second or longer.

Amplitude

Usually, the TP segment is flat (isoelectric).

SIGNIFICANCE

A TP segment indicates the absence of any electrical activity of the heart. The TP segment is used as the baseline reference for the determination of ST-segment elevation or depression.

> **AUTHOR'S NOTE** Be sure to avoid confusing a U wave with the P wave when evaluating the TP segment.

PR SEGMENT

> **PR segment**
>
> Represents the time it takes after atrial depolarization for the electrical impulse to progress from the AV node through the bundle of His, bundle branches, and Purkinje network to the ventricular myocardium.

CHARACTERISTICS

Physiology	Represents the time between the end of atrial depolarization and the start of ventricular depolarization
Onset/End	End of P wave/onset of QRS complex
Duration	0.02–0.10 sec
Amplitude	Isoelectric (flat)

Relationship to Cardiac Anatomy and Physiology

The PR segment (Fig. 3.13) represents the time from the end of atrial depolarization to the onset of ventricular depolarization, during which the electrical impulse progresses from the AV node through the bundle of His.

DESCRIPTION

Onset and End

Begins with the end of the P wave and ends with the onset of the QRS complex.

Duration

Normally varies from 0.02 to 0.10 second. It may be greater than 0.10 second if there is a delay in the progression of the electrical impulse through the AV node or bundle of His.

Amplitude

Normally the PR segment is flat (isoelectric), but it may be slightly depressed or downsloping.

SIGNIFICANCE

A PR segment of 0.10 second's duration or less indicates that the electrical impulse has been conducted through the AV junction normally and without delay or through an accessory conduction pathway. A PR segment exceeding 0.10 second's duration indicates a delay in the conduction of the electrical impulse through the AV junction.

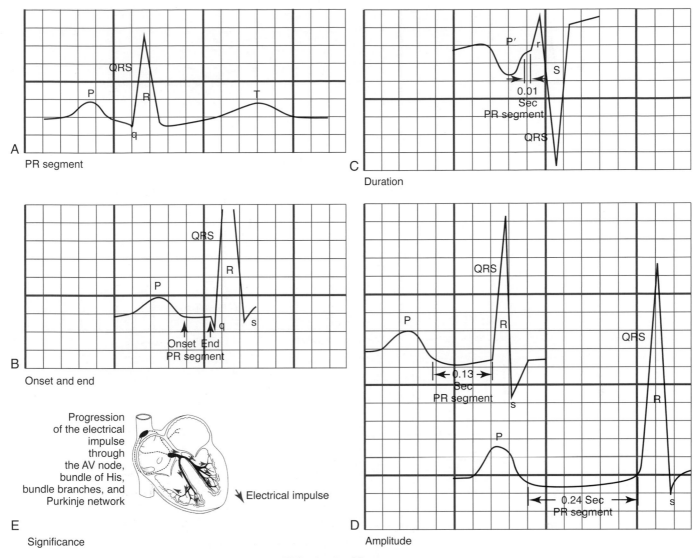

FIG. 3.13   PR segment.

ST SEGMENT

ST segment

Represents the period between the completion of ventricular depolarization and repolarization.

Normal ST Segment

CHARACTERISTICS

Physiology	Early portion of ventricular repolarization
Onset/End	End of QRS complex/onset of T wave
Duration	0.20 sec or less, depending on rate
Amplitude	Isoelectric (flat)

Relationship to Cardiac Anatomy and Physiology

The ST segment (Fig. 3.14) is the period between the completion of ventricular depolarization and repolarization. This is a period of electrical silence of the heart, during which the mechanical contraction of the ventricles (ventricular systole) is reaching completion.

DESCRIPTION

Onset and End

Begins with the end of the QRS complex and ends with the onset of the T wave. The junction between the QRS complex and the ST segment is called the *junction* or *J point*.

Duration

From 0.20 second or less and depends on heart rate. When the heart rate is fast, the ST segment is shorter than when the heart rate is slow.

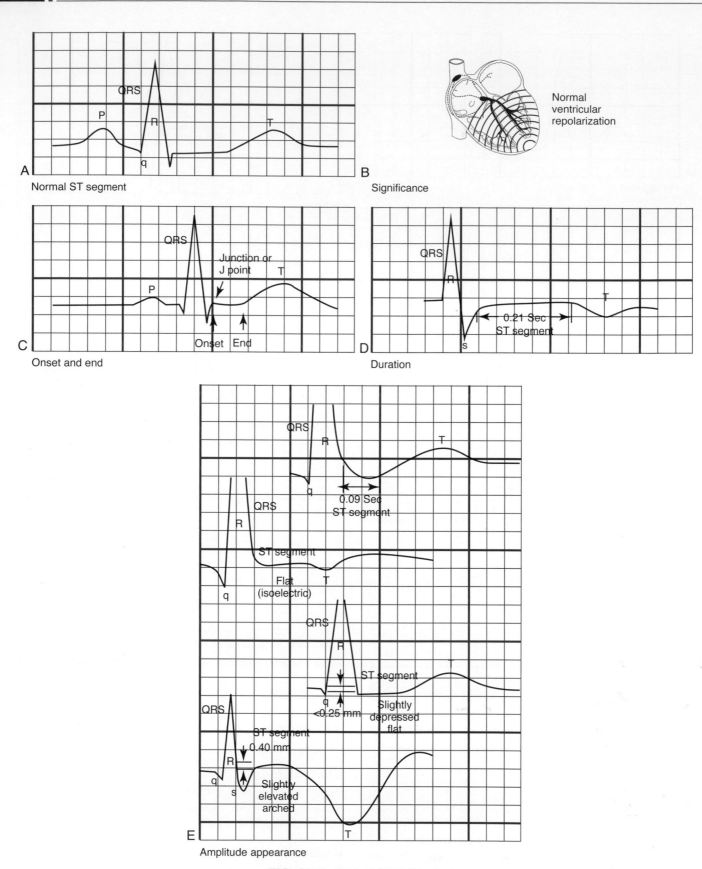

FIG. 3.14 Normal ST segment.

Amplitude

Normally flat (isoelectric). Slight elevation or depression of less than 1.0 mm during the first 0.04 second (1 small square) after the J point of the QRS complex is considered normal. The TP segment is normally used as a baseline reference for the determination of the amplitude of the ST segment. However, if the TP segment is absent because of a very rapid heart rate, the PR segment is used instead.

Appearance

If slightly elevated, the ST segment may be flat, concave, or arched. If slightly depressed, the ST segment may be flat, upsloping, or downsloping.

SIGNIFICANCE

A normal ST segment followed by a normal T wave indicates that repolarization of the right and left ventricles has occurred normally. Examination of the ST segment and its relationship with the T wave is critical when assessing for evidence of myocardial ischemia and/or infarction and will be explored in greater detail in Chapter 15.

Abnormal ST Segment

CHARACTERISTICS

Relationship to Cardiac Anatomy and Physiology

An abnormal ST segment (Fig. 3.15) signifies abnormal ventricular repolarization, a common consequence of myocardial ischemia and injury. It occurs because the damaged myocardium begins to repolarize earlier than the normal myocardium, and this electrical activity causes the ST segment to merge into the T wave. This can result in either ST-segment elevation or depression, depending on the area of the heart affected and the lead examined.

DESCRIPTION

Onset and End

Same as those of a normal ST segment.

Duration

Lasts 0.20 second or less.

Amplitude

An ST segment is abnormal when it is elevated or depressed more than 1.0 mm.

Appearance

If elevated, the ST segment may be flat, concave, or arched. If depressed, the ST segment may be flat, upsloping, or downsloping.

SIGNIFICANCE

Indicates that abnormal ventricular repolarization has occurred. Common causes of ST-segment elevation include the following:
- Acute myocardial infarction (cell death)
- Myocardial ischemia (hypoxia)

- Prinzmetal angina (severe transmural myocardial ischemia from coronary artery spasm)
- Ventricular aneurysm
- Acute pericarditis
- Early repolarization pattern (a form of myocardial repolarization seen in normal healthy people that produces ST-segment elevation closely mimicking that associated with myocardial ischemia)
- Left ventricular hypertrophy and left bundle-branch block (leads V1 to V3)
- Hyperkalemia (leads V1, V2)
- Hypothermia (along with the J wave and Osborn wave)

Common causes of ST-segment depression include the following:
- Subendocardial myocardial infarction (non–ST-elevation myocardial infarction)
- Angina pectoris (subendocardial myocardial ischemia)
- Reciprocal ECG changes in acute myocardial infarction
- Right and left ventricular hypertrophy ("strain" pattern)
- Right and left bundle-branch block
- Digitalis effect
- Hypokalemia

> **AUTHOR'S NOTE** Examination of the ST segment must take into consideration any changes in the T wave because both relate to repolarization of the ventricles. Therefore changes in either one can affect the other.

TAKE-HOME POINTS

- The ECG waveform consists of waves, intervals, and segments. Each has normal characteristics associated with the function of the underlying area of the heart from which it originates and through which it passes.
- The P wave is associated with the electrical activity of the atria, whereas the QRS complex and T wave are associated with the ventricles.
- The P wave and QRS complex are the result of depolarization of the atria and ventricles, respectively. The T wave represents repolarization of the ventricles.
- The size and width of each wave are a reflection of the speed and strength of the electrical impulses responsible for them.
- The PR interval is the period during which the electrical impulse is transmitted between the atria and the AV node.
- The QT interval represents the amount of time from the beginning of ventricular depolarization to repolarization.
- Abnormalities in either the PR interval or the QT interval indicate delays in the progression of the electrical impulse through the heart.
- The R-R interval represents the time between successive ventricular depolarizations. It is the best indicator of the rate of a rhythm.
- The TP segment represents the period of no electrical activity between the P-QRS-T cycle. This segment defines the

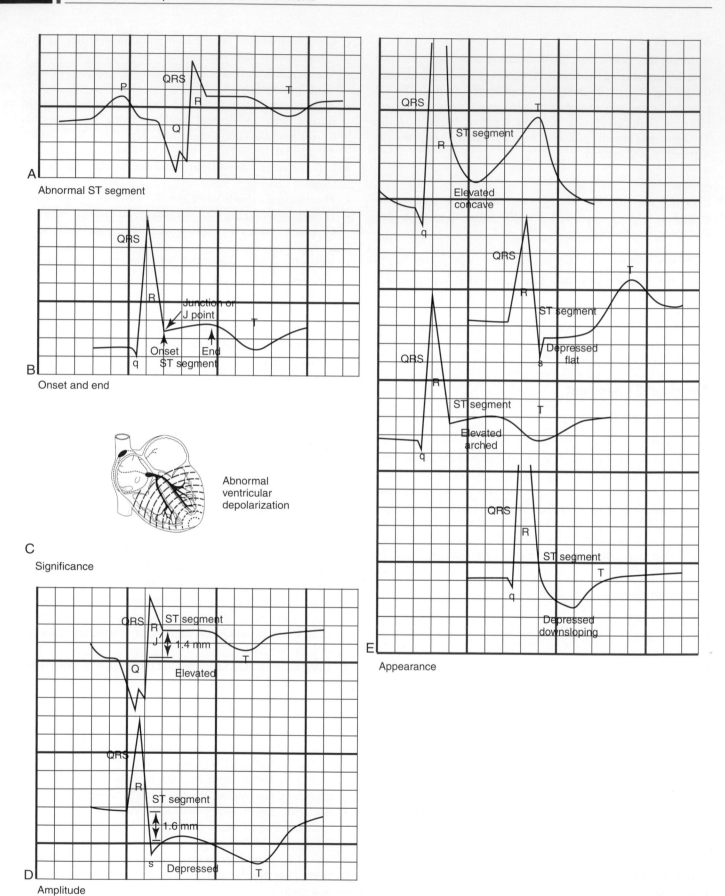

A
Abnormal ST segment

B
Onset and end

C
Significance

Abnormal ventricular depolarization

D
Amplitude

E
Appearance

FIG. 3.15 Abnormal ST segment.

isoelectric line (the baseline) against which other segments are compared.
- The PR segment is incorporated into the PR interval. It provides additional information about the passage of the electrical impulse from the atria to the AV node.
- The ST segment indicates the process leading to repolarization of the ventricles.

- Abnormality in the ST segment may indicate myocardial ischemia.
- Various conditions can affect the appearance of the waves, intervals, and segments of the ECG. Understanding what is normal and which conditions cause abnormalities is the key to successful ECG rhythm interpretation.

CHAPTER REVIEW QUESTIONS

1. Wide, notched P waves are most often caused by which condition or circumstance?
   A. Orthostatic hypotension
   B. Mitral and aortic valvular disease
   C. Pericarditis
   D. Faster ECG recording speeds

2. The normal PR interval lasts how long?
   A. 0.08 and 0.24 second
   B. 0.08 and 0.16 second
   C. 0.10 and 0.24 second
   D. 0.12 and 0.20 second

3. An ectopic P wave represents which kind of atrial depolarization?
   A. Arising from an implanted cardiac pacemaker
   B. Arising from the SA node
   C. Arising from the ventricle
   D. Occurring in an abnormal direction, sequence, or both

4. A normal QRS complex represents that what has occurred normally?
   A. Depolarization of the atria
   B. Depolarization of the ventricles
   C. Repolarization of the atria
   D. Repolarization of the ventricles

5. The time taken for the depolarization of the interventricular septum plus depolarization of the ventricle from the endocardium to the epicardium under the facing lead is called what?
   A. Atrial repolarization phase
   B. QT interval
   C. Septal excitation time
   D. Ventricular activation time

6. Which one of the following accessory conduction pathways is *not* involved in causing ventricular preexcitation with associated delta waves?
   A. Accessory AV pathways
   B. Atrio-His fibers
   C. Bundles of Kent
   D. Nodoventricular/fasciculoventricular fibers

7. Myocardial ischemia, acute myocardial infarction, excess serum potassium, and administration of procainamide can cause abnormality of what component of the ECG?
   A. P wave
   B. QRS complex
   C. T wave
   D. U wave

8. A U wave indicates that repolarization of the ventricles has occurred. An abnormally tall U wave may be present in which conditions?
   A. Cardiac tamponade, diabetes
   B. Cerebrovascular accident, syncope
   C. Hypokalemia, cardiomyopathy
   D. Hypothermia, vertigo

9. Delayed progression of the electrical impulse through the AV node or bundle of His would appear on an ECG as what?
   A. Elevated ST segment
   B. Peaked T wave
   C. Prolonged PR interval
   D. Prolonged QRS complex

10. What does an abnormal ST segment indicate?
    A. Abnormal atrial repolarization
    B. Abnormal ventricular contraction
    C. Abnormal ventricular repolarization
    D. Conduction delay in the AV node

Step-by-Step ECG Interpretation

SYSTEMATIC APPROACH TO ECG ANALYSIS

Regardless of how much experience you have at ECG analysis, it is essential to approach the process systematically. Although many ECG rhythms are easily recognized by their patterns, even the most common ones have variations that can be confusing if they are not analyzed systematically. Using a systematic approach will also help you explain to or teach others how you arrived at your interpretation. Finally, using the same method each time allows you to create a mental flowchart to follow, giving you greater confidence in your interpretation.

> **AUTHOR'S NOTE** All ECG texts recommend using a systematic approach. The steps outlined in other books may vary from those outlined here, but if examined closely, they are only slight variations on a common theme. No single system works for everyone. As your knowledge grows, learn, adapt, and adopt the techniques that work best for you.

Box 4.1 outlines the steps used in interpreting ECG findings, but let's go over them one at a time.

STEP ONE: DETERMINE THE RATE

The rate of the rhythm and the rate of the beating heart are not always the same. The heart rate, also called the *pulse rate*, is the rate of muscular contraction that results in a detectable pulse.

In some instances, electrical impulses that appear as a waveform on an ECG may not generate a detectable pulse. Comparing the rate of the ECG rhythm with the physical heart rate can reveal important information about the clinical significance of the rhythm.

The P wave is associated with atrial contraction, and the QRS complex is associated with ventricular contraction under normal circumstances. Therefore an ECG rhythm will have both an atrial and ventricular rate. If every P wave is followed by a QRS complex, both rates will be the same. However, there are

---

BOX 4.1 | **Dysrhythmia Interpretation**

Step One: Determine the heart rate.
Step Two: Determine the regularity of the rhythm.
Step Three: Identify and analyze the P, P′, F, or f waves.
    1. Determine the atrial rate and regularity.
    2. Compare and associate the atrial rate to the ventricular rate.
Step Four: Determine the PR or RP′ intervals and AV conduction rate.
    1. Assess the equality of the PR intervals.
    2. Determine whether all P waves are followed by a QRS complex.
    3. Determine the AV conduction ratio.
Step Five: Identify and analyze the QRS complexes.
    1. Note the duration and shape of the QRS complexes.
    2. Assess the equality of the QRS complexes.
    3. Determine whether there is a P wave associated with each QRS complex.
Step Six: Determine the site of origin of the dysrhythmia.
Step Seven: Identify the dysrhythmia.
Step Eight: Evaluate the clinical significance of the dysrhythmia.

rhythms that have no P waves and some where the P wave is not followed by a QRS complex. In those instances, you will need to calculate the atrial and ventricular rates separately. Generally speaking, the rate of a rhythm is most commonly based on the rate of the QRS complexes.

You can calculate the rate of the rhythm by determining the number of P waves or QRS complexes that occur in the ECG in 1 minute. Because counting every wave and complex in a 1-minute ECG recording is not practical, you will use the 6-second method, a rate calculator ruler, the R-R interval method, or the Rule of 300.

AUTHOR'S NOTE It is vital to recognize that for our purposes, "rate" refers only to the rate of ECG waveforms. The physiologic heart rate may or may not be equal to the ECG rate because only by physically assessing the patient can you determine whether a given QRS complex is associated with a pulse. For the sake of conformity, we will refer to the rate of an ECG rhythm simply as rate in beats/minute, even though you are actually counting the number of complexes (usually the QRS) per minute.

Six-Second Method

The 6-second method is the simplest and most common way of determining the rate. It can be used when the rhythm is either regular or irregular. Except for the rate calculator method, which is more accurate but does require its availability, the 6-second method is generally considered the fastest method. The downside is that it is the least accurate. Nevertheless, the rate calculated by this method is a close approximation of the actual rate.

The top or bottom of most ECG papers is marked with short vertical lines that divide the strip into 3-second intervals (Fig. 4.1). When the paper is run at a standard speed of 25 mm per second, the distance between every third line is equal to a 6-second interval. Calculate the rate by determining the number of QRS complexes in the interval and multiplying that number by 10 (Fig. 4.2). The result is the rate in beats per minute.

If premature complexes (to be discussed in later chapters) are present in the 6-second interval, they should be included in your count of QRS complexes.

Example

You count eight QRS complexes in a 6-second interval. A minute can be divided into ten 6-second intervals, so we'll multiply by 10:

$$8 \times 10 = 80 \text{ beats/min}$$

To obtain a more accurate rate when the rate is extremely slow and/or the rhythm is irregular, determine the number of QRS complexes in a longer interval, such as a 12-second interval, and adjust the multiplication accordingly.

Example

Let's say you count six QRS complexes in a 12-second interval. Because 1 minute contains only five 12-second intervals, we will multiply by 5 instead of 10:

$$6 \times 5 = 30 \text{ beats/min}$$

Rate Calculator Ruler Method

A rate calculator ruler, such as the one shown in Fig. 4.3, is a device that can be used to determine the ECG rate rapidly and accurately. This method is most accurate if the rhythm is regular. Be sure to follow the instructions printed on the ruler (for example, "Third complex from arrow is rate per minute"). If possible, you should not include premature complexes in your count of QRS complexes when using this method. Instead, find a portion of the ECG rhythm without premature complexes and measure using those QRS complexes.

---

premature complex

A premature complex is a QRS complex that occurs unexpectedly at some point between the P-QRS-T cycles.

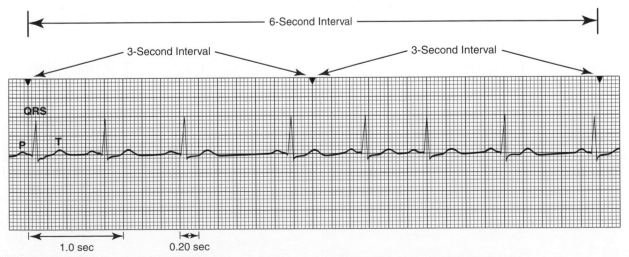

FIG. 4.1 Intervals of 3 and 6 seconds at an ECG recording speed of 25 mm/sec.

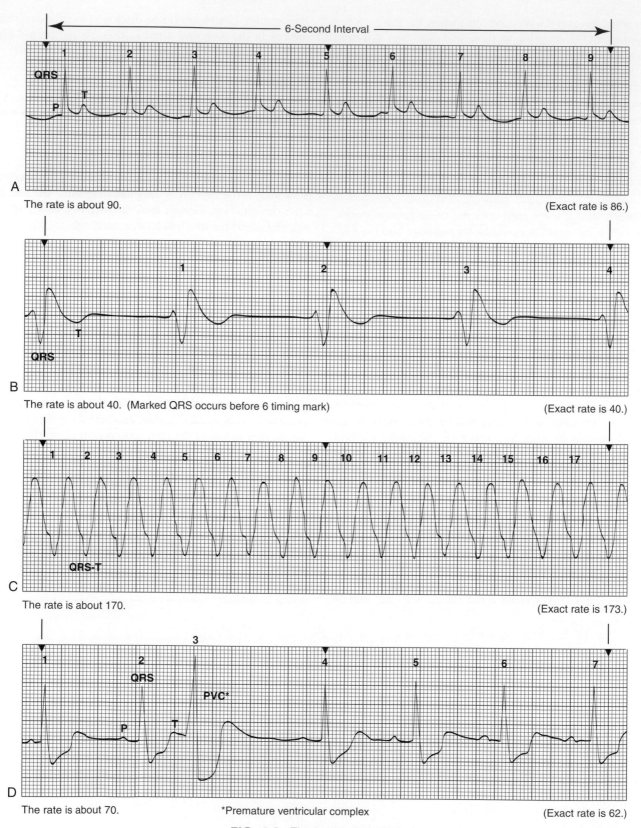

FIG. 4.2 The 6-second method.

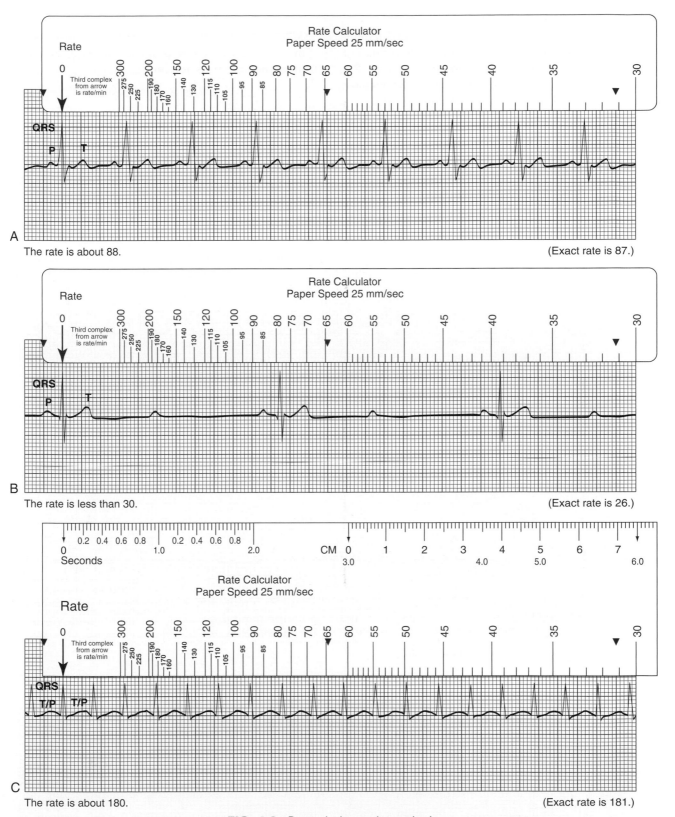

A The rate is about 88.   (Exact rate is 87.)

B The rate is less than 30.   (Exact rate is 26.)

C The rate is about 180.   (Exact rate is 181.)

FIG. 4.3   Rate calculator ruler method.

R-R Interval Method

The R-R interval may be used in four different ways to determine the rate. The rhythm must be regular if the calculation of the rate is to be accurate. The two R waves used for measuring the R-R interval should be those of the underlying rhythm and not those of premature complexes. The four methods are as follows.

METHOD 1

Measure the distance in seconds between the peaks of two consecutive R waves, remembering that each small box represents 0.04 second. Divide this number into 60, because there are 60 seconds in a minute, to obtain the rate (Fig. 4.4).

Example

If the distance between the peaks of two consecutive R waves is 0.56 second, the rate is as follows:

$$60 \div 0.56 = 107 \text{ beats/min}$$

METHOD 2

Count the large squares (0.20-second interval) between the peaks of two consecutive R waves. Divide this number into 300, because there are 300 large squares per minute, to obtain the heart rate (Fig. 4.5).

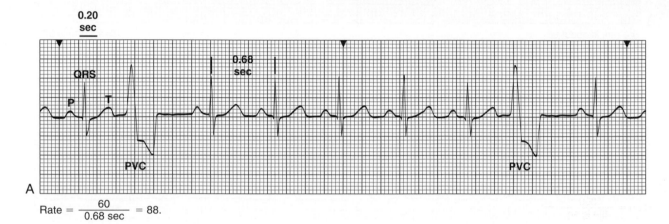

A

$$\text{Rate} = \frac{60}{0.68 \text{ sec}} = 88.$$

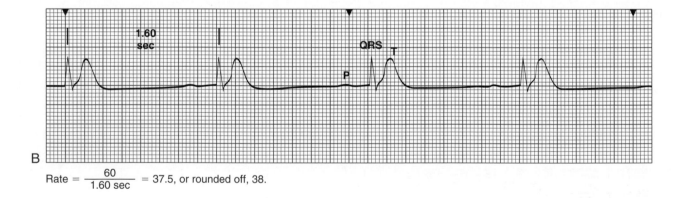

B

$$\text{Rate} = \frac{60}{1.60 \text{ sec}} = 37.5, \text{ or rounded off, } 38.$$

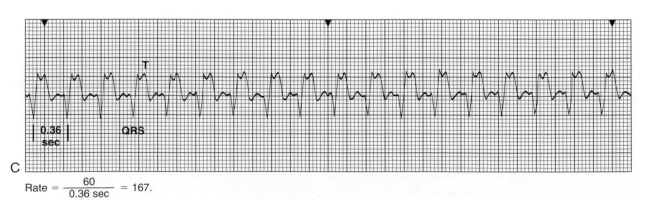

C

$$\text{Rate} = \frac{60}{0.36 \text{ sec}} = 167.$$

FIG. 4.4 R-R interval method 1.

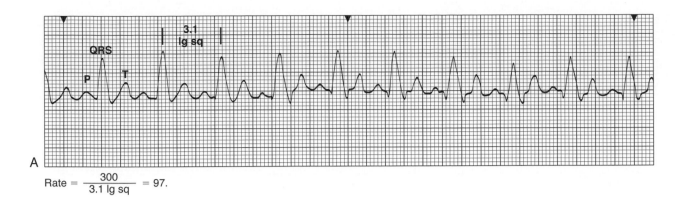

A

$$\text{Rate} = \frac{300}{3.1 \text{ lg sq}} = 97.$$

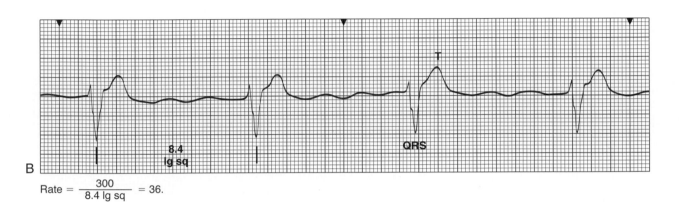

B

$$\text{Rate} = \frac{300}{8.4 \text{ lg sq}} = 36.$$

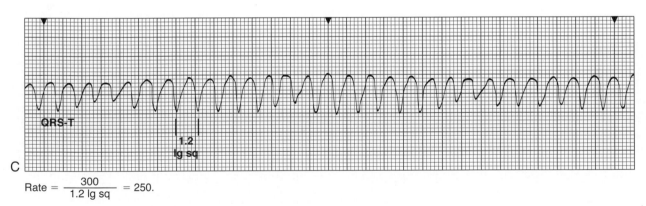

C

$$\text{Rate} = \frac{300}{1.2 \text{ lg sq}} = 250.$$

FIG. 4.5 R-R interval method 2.

Example

If there are 2.5 large squares between the peaks of two consecutive R waves, the rate is as follows:

$$300 \div 2.5 = 120 \text{ beats/min}$$

METHOD 3

Count the small squares (0.04-second interval) between the peaks of two consecutive R waves. Divide this number into 1500, because there are 1500 small squares per minute, to obtain the rate (Fig. 4.6).

Example

If there are 19 small squares between the peaks of two consecutive R waves, the rate is as follows:

$$1500 \div 19 = 78.9, \text{ or rounded off, } 79 \text{ beats/min}$$

METHOD 4

Count the small squares (0.04-second interval) between the peaks of two consecutive R waves. Using a rate-conversion table (Table 4.1), convert the number of small squares into the rate (Fig. 4.7).

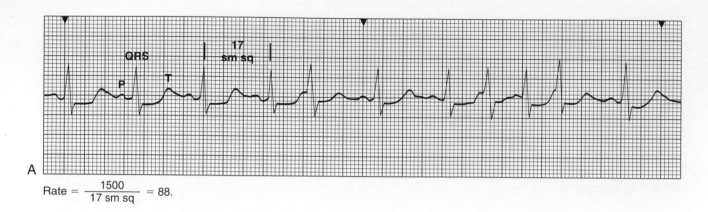

A

$$Rate = \frac{1500}{17 \text{ sm sq}} = 88.$$

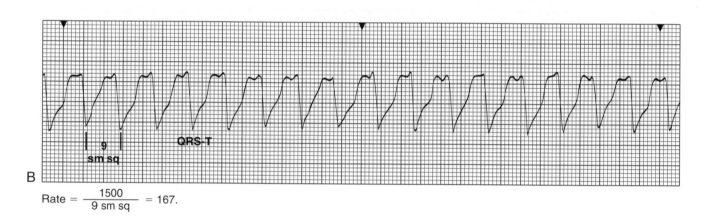

B

$$Rate = \frac{1500}{9 \text{ sm sq}} = 167.$$

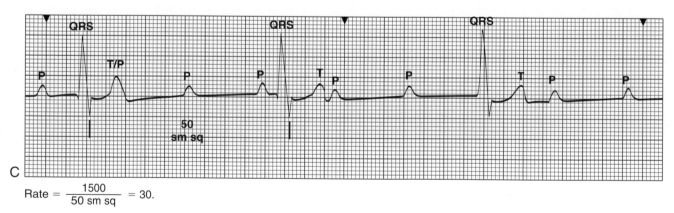

C

$$Rate = \frac{1500}{50 \text{ sm sq}} = 30.$$

FIG. 4.6 R-R interval method 3.

Example

There are 17 small squares between the peaks of two consecutive R waves. Therefore the rate is 88 beats/min.

> **AUTHOR'S NOTE** Methods 2 and 3 are more commonly used than the other two methods because they can be performed rapidly without difficult addition or the aid of tables.

Rule of 300

The Rule of 300 will be accurate in determining the rate only if the rhythm is regular (Fig. 4.8). It is a variation on method 2 of the previously described R-R interval method, where the rate is calculated by dividing 300 by the number of large red boxes between consecutive QRS complexes. Instead of performing the calculation, a number is assigned to each box. These boxes are numbered 300, 150, 100, 75, 60, 50, 43, 38, 33,

| TABLE 4.1 | Calculating ECG Rate From Space Between Consecutive R Waves | | |

To find the ECG rate, begin by counting the number of small squares (0.04-second spaces) between the peaks of two consecutive R waves. Then find the number in the following table:

Small Squares	ECG Rate/Min	Small Squares	ECG Rate/Min
5	300	27	56
6	250	28	54
7	214	29	52
8	188	30	50
9	167	31	48
10	150	32	47
11	136	33	45
12	125	34	44
13	115	35	43
14	107	36	42
15	100	37	41
16	94	38	40
17	88	39	39
18	84	40	38
19	79	41	37
20	75	42	36
21	72	43	35
22	68	44	34
23	65	45	33
24	63	47	32
25	60	48	31
26	58	50	30

and 30. Memorize this sequence, and when the need arises, write the numbers on a piece of graph paper. If the QRS complex falls between the dark lines of the large boxes, estimate the rate based on which dark line is closest to the QRS complex.

The rate per minute is determined as follows:

1. Select an R wave that lines up with a dark vertical line. Label it "A."
2. Place 300 above the next dark line to the right of A. Do the same for each of the remaining numbers in the progression above each of the dark lines to the right.
3. Identify the first R wave to the right of wave "A," and label it "B." If wave B lands on one of the dark vertical lines, the rate corresponds to the number above it.
4. If B does not land exactly on a dark vertical line, you can estimate the rate by checking the distance of B from the nearest dark line. This mark indicates the estimated beats per minute.

Example

If B is halfway between the dark lines labeled 150 and 100, the rate is about 125 beats/min.

Example

If B is one-third of the way between 75 and 60, the rate is about 70 beats/min.

> **AUTHOR'S NOTE** The same method of calculating rate can be used on the P waves. This is useful in determining whether the atrial rate and ventricular rate are the same.

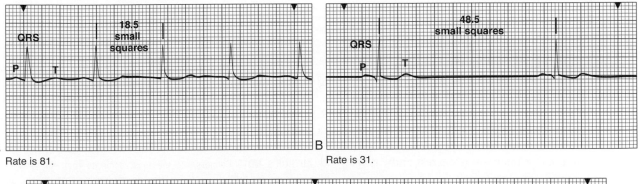

A   Rate is 81.

B   Rate is 31.

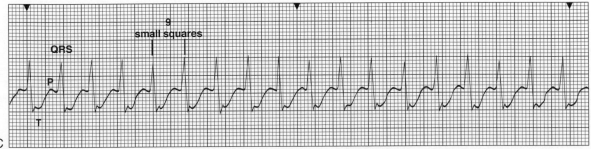

C   Rate is 167.

FIG. 4.7   R-R interval method 4.

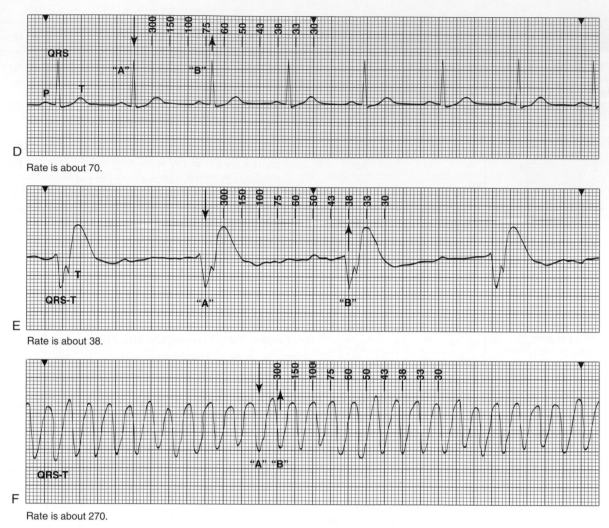

D
Rate is about 70.

E
Rate is about 38.

F
Rate is about 270.

FIG. 4.8 Rule of 300.

STEP TWO: DETERMINE REGULARITY

You can determine the regularity of the rhythm by comparing the R-R intervals to each other. The simplest way to determine regularity is to first estimate the length of one of the R-R intervals (Fig. 4.9). Choose an interval on the left side of the EGG strip and compare it to the R-R intervals in the rest of the strip, moving from left to right.

If you are using EGG calipers, place the first caliper tip on the peak of one R wave. Then adjust the calipers so that the other tip rests on the peak of the next R wave to the right. Then compare the other R-R intervals to the R-R interval measured by the calipers.

If you use pencil and paper, place the straight edge of the paper horizontally, near the peaks of the R waves, and mark off the distance between two consecutive R waves (the R-R interval). While moving the paper to the right along the ECG rhythm strip, compare this marked R-R interval with the following ones.

To determine the regularity of very fast rhythms, you can count the number of small squares. Each one represents 0.04 second. Count the number of small squares between the R waves. Then compare the width of the R-R intervals with each other.

> **AUTHOR'S NOTE** Calipers are the most accurate tool, not only for measuring the R-R interval but also for evaluating the width, height, and length of every component of the ECG waveform.

Regular

In general, if the difference between R-R intervals is less than 0.08 seconds (two small squares), the rhythm is considered to be regular (Fig. 4.10).

Irregular

If the shortest and longest R-R intervals vary by more than 0.08 second, the rhythm is considered to be irregular (Fig. 4.11).

The distances between the
R waves are determined:

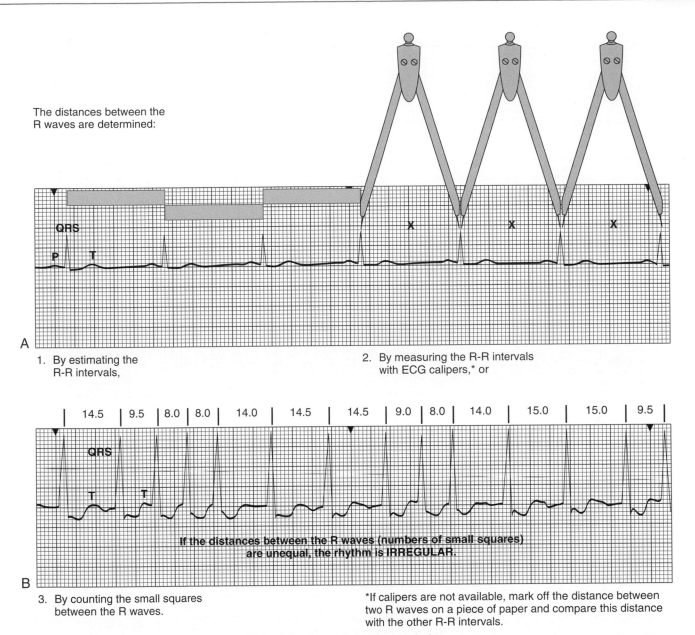

1. By estimating the
   R-R intervals,

2. By measuring the R-R intervals
   with ECG calipers,* or

3. By counting the small squares
   between the R waves.

*If calipers are not available, mark off the distance between
two R waves on a piece of paper and compare this distance
with the other R-R intervals.

FIG. 4.9 Determining the regularity.

The rhythm may be *slightly irregular*. This means that over the length of the ECG, the length of the R-R interval rarely varies more than 0.08 second, or 2 small boxes in length. This occurs in the rhythm called *sinus arrhythmia*.

> **AUTHOR'S NOTE** A good rule of thumb to remember: For the rhythm of any given rate to be considered regular, the R-R intervals should not vary more than 10%.

The degree of acceptable variability is related to the rate. The faster the rate, the less variability is acceptable for the rhythm to be considered regular. A regular rhythm may be *occasionally irregular* over a short segment. This occurs in certain conditions when premature atrial or ventricular complexes are present.

The rhythm may be *regularly irregular*. Another term for this type of regularity is *patterned irregularity*. This occurs when a pattern appears between the measured R-R intervals. For example, the R-R interval may progressively lengthen in a predictable manner, or there may be a pattern of short and long R-R intervals.

The rhythm may be *totally irregular*, also referred to as *irregularaly irregular*. When there is no fixed pattern or ratio of short to long R-R intervals, the rhythm is considered to be totally irregular. This is characteristic of the following:

- Atrial fibrillation
- Multifocal atrial tachycardia
- Ventricular fibrillation

> **AUTHOR'S NOTE** In this text we will use the term *totally irregular* because it is easier to pronounce, but just be aware that others will use the term *irregularly irregular*.

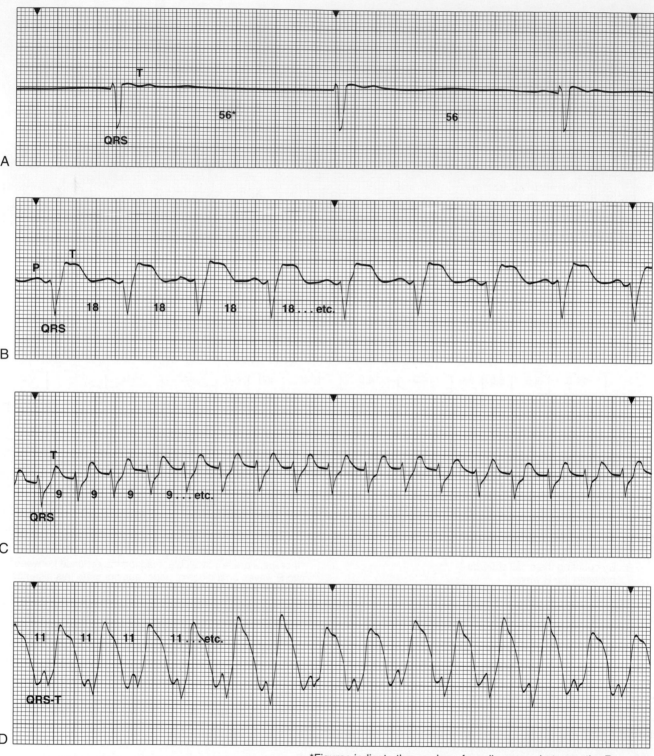

*Figures indicate the number of small squares between the R waves.

FIG. 4.10 Regular rhythms.

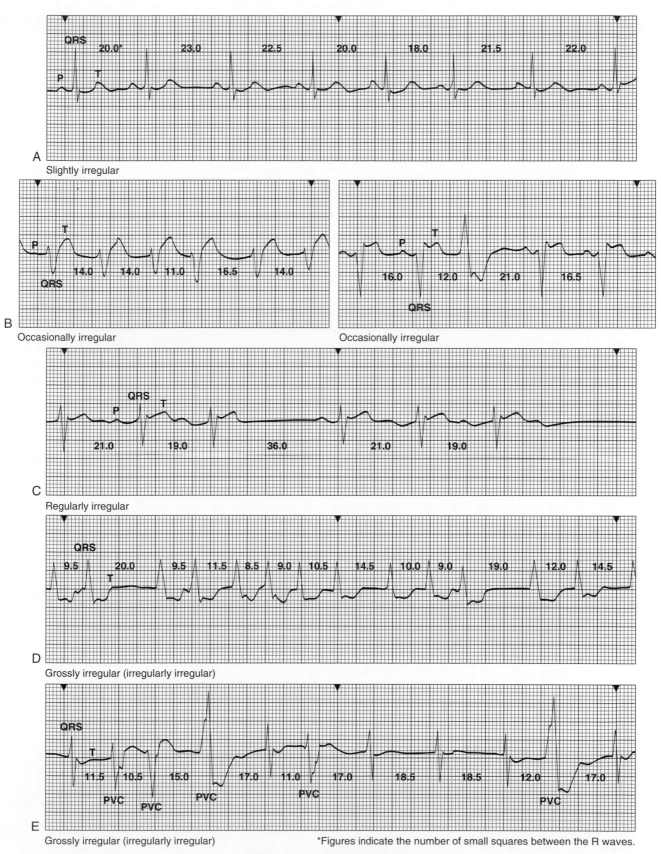

FIG. 4.11 Irregular rhythms.

STEP THREE: IDENTIFY AND ANALYZE THE P, P', F, OR f WAVES

A normal P wave is a positive, smoothly rounded wave in lead II (Fig. 4.12). It is 0.5 to 2.5 mm high and 0.10 second or less wide. It typically appears before each QRS complex. In conditions such as atrioventricular (AV) block, however, it may occur alone, without a QRS complex following it.

AV block

AV block is a condition in which there is a complete or incomplete (partial) blockage of electrical impulses from the atria to the ventricles through the AV junction or the bundle branches (see Chapter 9). This results in a rhythm with more P waves than QRS complexes.

An abnormal P wave is one that differs from any or all of the normal features just described. The P wave in lead II may

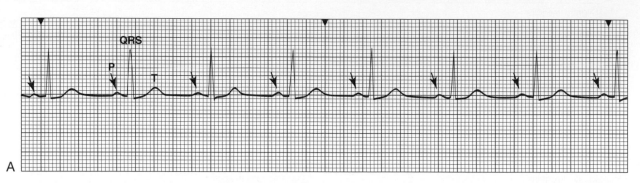

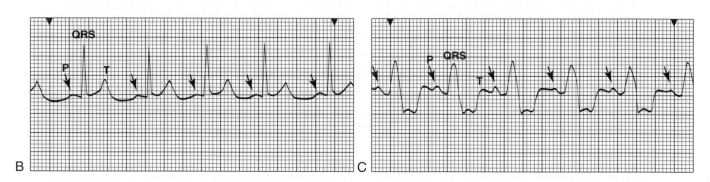

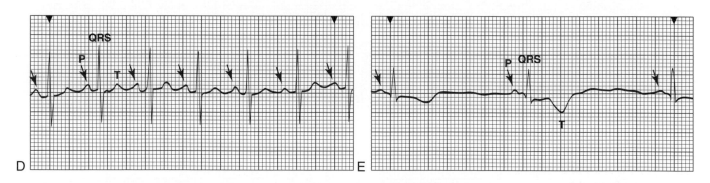

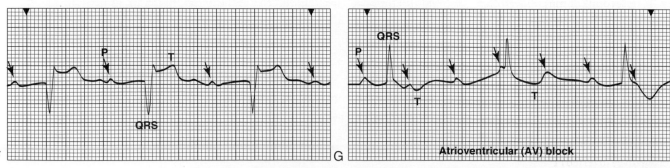

FIG. 4.12 Normal P waves.

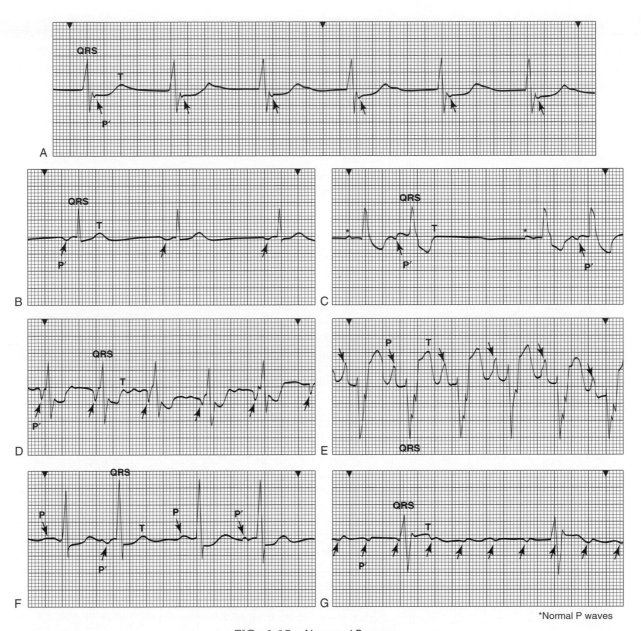

FIG. 4.13 Abnormal P waves.

be positive (upright), negative (inverted), or flat (Fig. 4.13). It may be smoothly rounded, peaked, or deformed (that is, wide and notched). Its height may be normal (0.5–2.5 mm) or abnormal (less than 0.5 mm or greater than 2.5 mm). Its duration may be normal (0.10 second or less) or abnormal (more than 0.10 second). It may appear before the QRS complex, like a normal P wave, or occur alone, without a QRS complex following it. Unlike a normal P wave, an abnormal P wave may appear after the QRS complex or be buried (hidden) within it.

You can determine the origin of the P wave by observing its positivity or negativity in lead II (Table 4.2):
- Positive (upright) P waves in lead II usually originate in the sinoatrial (SA) node or upper or middle right atrium. Although they are upright, they may have an abnormal (peaked or wide and notched) shape.
- Negative (inverted) P waves in lead II usually originate in the lower right atrium, left atrium, AV junction, or ventricles.

Any P wave that originates in the SA node, whether it appears normal or abnormal, is designated as a P wave and signified by *P* in the figures. A P wave that originates in the atria, AV junction, or ventricles, on the other hand, is designated as a *P'* wave, pronounced "P prime," and signified by *P'* in the figures.

If a P wave is present, first determine whether all the P waves look alike. Then determine the atrial rate using the same method you used to determine the heart rate. Finally, determine whether each QRS complex is accompanied by a P wave. The rate of the P wave and QRS complex will be the same if the electrical impulse is conducted normally from the atria to the ventricles. If the rates are different, either the conduction between the atria and ventricles is blocked or the rhythm is characterized by an ectopic QRS complex.

If P waves are absent, determine whether atrial flutter (F) or fibrillation (f) waves are present (Fig. 4.14). Atrial flutter, or F, waves are typically positive, sawtooth-shaped waves in lead II.

Origin of the P Wave	Appearance in Lead II	P Wave Location
TABLE 4.2	**Appearance of P Wave Relative to Its Site of Origin**	
SA node (P wave)	Positive (upright)	Precedes the QRS complex
Upper or middle right atrium (P′ wave)	Normal, peaked, or wide and notched	Precedes the QRS complex
Lower right atrium or left atrium (P′ wave)	Negative (inverted)	Precedes the QRS complex
AV junction (P′ wave)	Negative (inverted)	Buried in the QRS complex
Upper part	Negative (inverted)	Precedes the QRS complex
Middle or distal part	Absent	Buried in the QRS complex
Distal part	Negative (inverted)	Follows the QRS complex

AV, Atrioventricular; *SA,* sinoatrial.

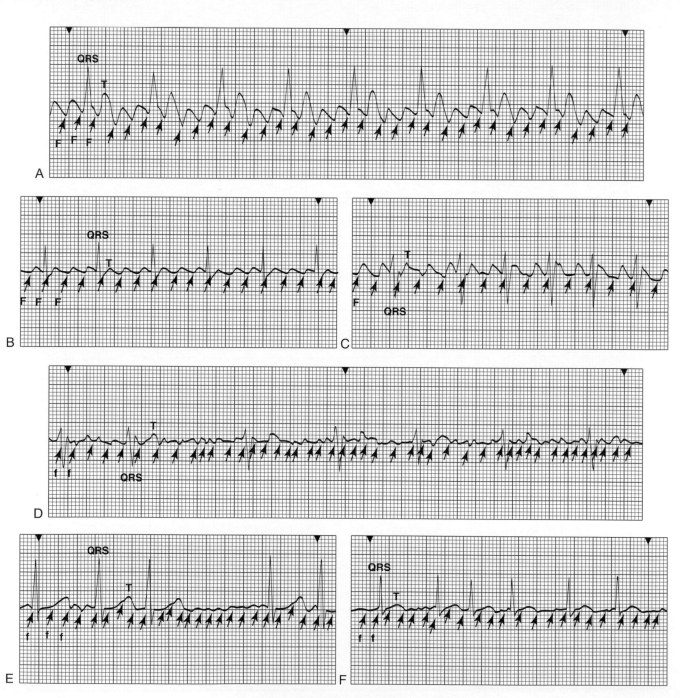

FIG. 4.14 F and f waves.

The rate of the F waves is usually between 240 and 360/min. Their rhythm is typically regular. QRS complexes usually occur regularly, after every second, third, or fourth F wave, but they may occur irregularly at varying F wave–to–QRS complex ratios if a *variable AV block* is present.

variable AV block

When the ratio of F waves to QRS complexes is constant, fixed AV block is present. When the ratio changes across the ECG strip, a variable AV block is present. A variable AV block is an AV block with varying conduction ratios of P, P′, F, or f waves to QRS complexes over the course of the ECG rhythm strip.

Atrial fibrillation, or f, waves are characterized by irregularly shaped, chaotic waves, each dissimilar in configuration and amplitude to the other. If the f waves are less than 1 mm high, they are called *fine* fibrillatory waves; if they are greater than 1 mm high, they are called *coarse* fibrillatory waves. If the f waves are extremely fine, they may not be identified as such, and the sections of the EGG between the T waves and QRS complexes may appear only slightly wavy or even flat (isoelectric).

The rate of the f waves is usually between 350 and 600 (average 400/min), and the rhythm is totally irregular. Typically, in atrial fibrillation, the QRS complexes occur irregularly, with no set pattern, reflecting the totally irregular atrial rhythm and variable rate of AV conduction. See Chapter 6 for a full description of ECG rhythms associated with F and f waves.

STEP FOUR: DETERMINE THE PR OR RP′ INTERVAL AND ATRIOVENTRICULAR CONDUCTION RATIO

Determine the PR interval by measuring the distance between the onset of the P wave and the onset of the first wave of the QRS complex. Neither F nor f waves have an interval to measure because there is no measurable time between them and the QRS complex. To complete this step, you will do the following:
- Compare the PR intervals to one another to determine whether they are equal in duration.
- Determine whether all of the P waves are followed by QRS complexes.
- Determine the AV conduction ratio by noting the number of P (or F) waves followed by QRS complexes in a given set of P (or F) waves.

AUTHOR'S NOTE Recall from math class that a ratio indicates the quantity of one thing in relation to another. In culinary school, for instance, students learn that the ideal ratio of oil to vinegar in a salad dressing is 3 to 1, or 3:1—that is, three parts oil for every one part vinegar. To make 1 quart (4 cups) of vinaigrette, a chef would need 3 cups olive oil and 1 cup balsamic vinegar. To make four quarts, the chef would use 12 cups oil and 4 cups vinegar. Although the quantity has been multiplied, the ratio of 3:1 is the same.

AV conduction ratio

The ratio of P, P′, F, or f waves to QRS complexes. For example, an AV conduction ratio of 4:3 indicates that for every four P waves, three are followed by QRS complexes.

A normal PR interval is 0.12 to 0.20 second in duration (Fig. 4.15). An interval within this range indicates that the electrical impulse causing the P wave originated in the SA node or in the upper or middle part of the atria. It also indicates normal conduction through the AV node and the bundle of His. When the heart rate is fast, the PR interval is shorter than when it is slow. It will remain within normal limits, however, unless there is abnormal conduction or the P wave did not originate from the SA node.

A PR interval of less than 0.12 second or more than 0.20 second is abnormal (Fig. 4.16).
- If the PR interval is less than 0.12 second, it indicates either (1) that the electrical impulse originated in the lower part of the atria or in the AV junction or (2) that the electrical impulse progressed from the atria to the ventricles through an abnormal conduction pathway.
- A PR interval of more than 0.20 second indicates a delay in conduction through the AV node or bundle of His. When this occurs and the PR intervals are all the same, a first-degree AV block is present (Table 4.3).

first-degree AV block

A dysrhythmia in which there is a constant delay in conduction through the AV node. It is characterized by abnormally prolonged PR intervals (longer than 0.20 second).

- If a P′ wave follows the QRS complex, an RP′ interval is present. In this case the electrical impulse responsible for the P′ wave and QRS complex originates in the lower part of the AV junction or in the ventricles. An RP′ interval is usually 0.12 second or less but can be as long as 0.20 second.
- If a QRS complex does not occur before the next P wave, the PR interval is absent for that beat. Such a pattern indicates a block of the electrical conduction through the AV node, bundle of His, or bundle branches into the ventricles. If QRS complexes follow some P waves and not others, an incomplete AV block is present. AV blocks will be presented in Chapter 9.

incomplete AV block (second-degree AV block)

A dysrhythmia in which one or more P waves are not conducted to the ventricles.

- If the PR intervals are unequal, check for an increase in their duration until you see a P wave that is not followed by a QRS complex following a nonconducted P wave as a dropped beat. The AV conduction ratio is the ratio of P waves and their associated QRS complexes.

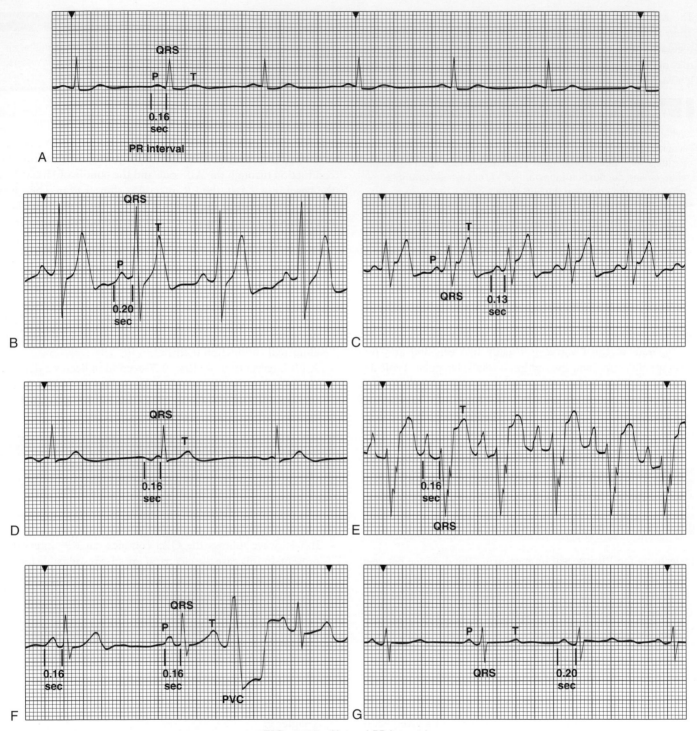

FIG. 4.15   Normal PR intervals.

- If the PR intervals are equal but some P waves are not associated with a QRS complex, a second-degree AV type II AV block is present. The type II AV block will have more

P waves than QRS complexes. This ratio of P wave to QRS complexes is the AV conduction ratio of the block. The following are examples of AV conduction ratios (Fig. 4.17):

- The AV conduction ratio is 1:1 if all P waves are followed by QRS complexes.
- The AV conduction ratio is 2:1 if, for every two P waves, one is followed by a QRS complex.

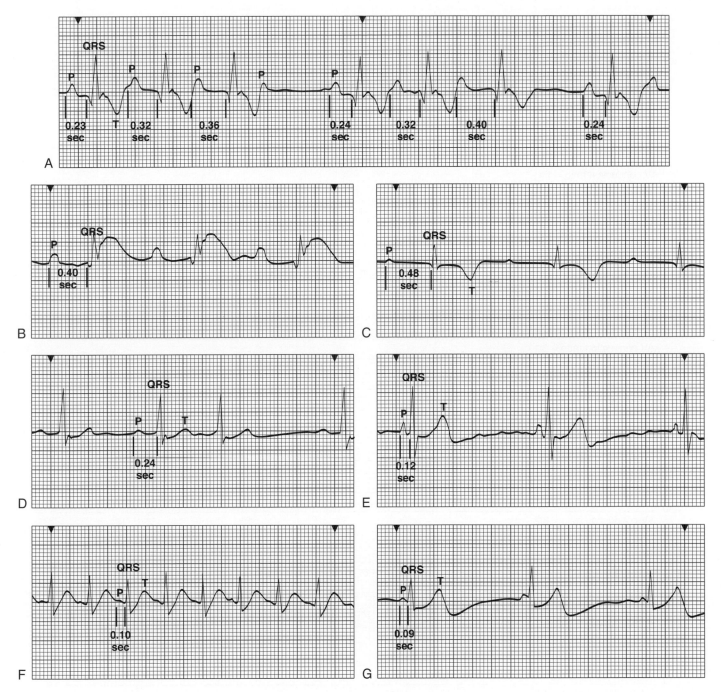

FIG. 4.16 Abnormal PR intervals.

TABLE **4.3**	PR Interval and AV Conduction Ratio in Relation to AV Block	
AV Block	**PR Intervals**	**AV Conduction Ratio**
First-degree AV block	Prolonged, equal	1:1
Second-degree type I AV block (Wenckebach)	Gradually lengthening	5:4, 4:3, 3:2 or 6:5, 7:6, etc.
Second-degree type II AV block	Equal	2:1, 3:1, 4:1, 5:1, etc.
Third-degree AV block	No relationship of P to R waves	None

AV, Atrioventricular.

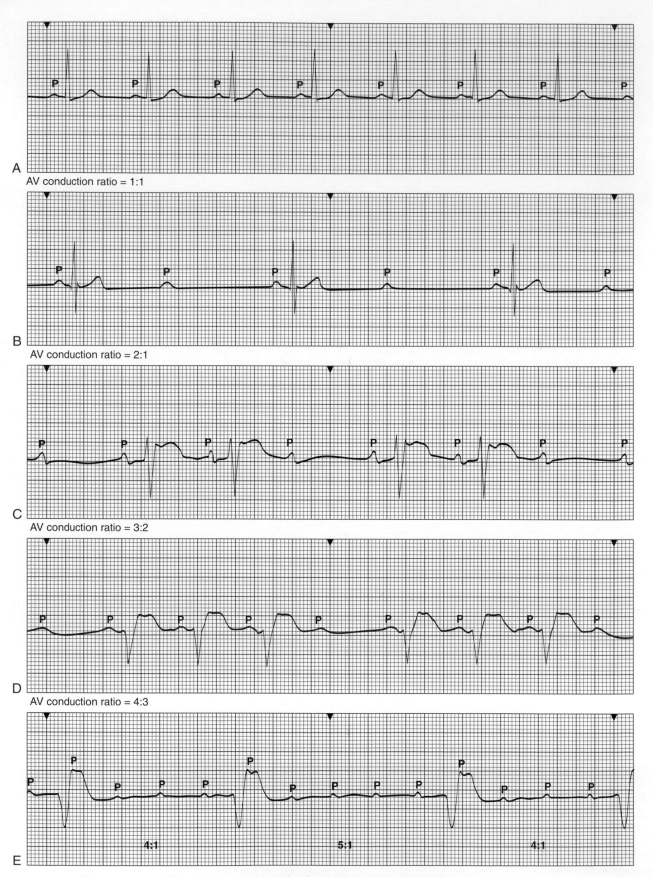

A
AV conduction ratio = 1:1

B
AV conduction ratio = 2:1

C
AV conduction ratio = 3:2

D
AV conduction ratio = 4:3

E
4:1   5:1   4:1

FIG. 4.17 Examples of atrioventricular (AV) conduction ratios.

- The AV conduction ratio is 3:2 if, for every three P waves, two are followed by QRS complexes.
- The AV conduction ratio is 4:3 if, for every four P waves, three are followed by QRS complexes and one is not.
- The AV conduction ratio is 5:1 if, for every five P waves, one is followed by a QRS complex.

If QRS complexes are present but do not regularly precede or follow the P waves, a complete AV block (third-degree AV block) is present. These QRS complexes tend to be abnormally wide.

---

complete (third-degree) AV block

A complete absence of electrical conduction from the atria to the ventricles through the AV junction. The condition may be temporary and reversible or permanent (chronic).

STEP FIVE: IDENTIFY AND ANALYZE THE QRS COMPLEXES

In this step you will analyze the QRS complexes in the following manner:

1. Identify the QRS complexes.
2. Note the duration of the QRS complexes. The duration of the QRS complexes may be normal (0.12 second or less) or long (more than 0.12 second).
3. Note the shape of the QRS complexes. The shape will be normal if conduction occurs through the normal pathway of the AV junction and bundle of His. The shape will be abnormal if there is a disturbance of the conduction pathway.
4. Compare the QRS complexes to determine whether all QRS complexes are equal in duration and shape or if one or more of the QRS complexes differ from the others.
5. Determine whether there is a P or P′ associated with the QRS.

A normal QRS complex, one that is 0.12 second or less in width (Fig. 4.18), indicates that the electrical impulse progressed normally through the ventricles.

An abnormal QRS complex, one that is greater than 0.12 second in width and/or bizarre in appearance, indicates that the electrical impulse responsible for it progressed through the ventricles abnormally.

Abnormally long and/or shaped QRS complexes occur with the following rhythms:

- **Ventricular rhythms.** Ectopic or escape complex and rhythms originating in the ventricles.
- **Bundle-branch block.** A block in the conduction of electrical impulses through the right or left bundle branch.
- **Intraventricular conduction defect (IVCD).** A delay in the conduction of electrical impulses through the myocardium caused by heart disease (myocardial infarction, fibrosis, and hypertrophy), electrolyte imbalance, and excessive administration of certain drugs.
- **Aberrant ventricular conduction (aberrancy).** A transient bundle-branch block caused by the arrival of electrical impulses at a bundle branch while it is still in the refractory stage.
- **Ventricular preexcitation.** Disfigurement (slurring and sometimes notching) of the initial upstroke (or downstroke) of the QRS complex caused by premature depolarization of the ventricles. This results when an electrical impulse in the atria bypasses the AV junction or bundle of His, entering the ventricles via an abnormal accessory conduction pathway.

---

accessory pathway

The word *accessory* in general refers to something extra or supplemental that aids or accelerates a process in some way. (An accessory road, for instance, might speed traffic on the main highway.) An accessory pathway, then, is one of several abnormal conduction pathways that bypass the AV node, the bundle of His, or both. These pathways allow electrical impulses to travel from the atria to the ventricles more rapidly than normal.

If the QRS complexes are identical and normal in duration and shape, they are most likely the result of an impulse that originated in the SA node, atria, or AV junction and was conducted through the bundle of His, bundle branches, and Purkinje network without delay.

If the QRS complexes are identical but abnormal in duration and shape, their origin may be either (1) ventricular or (2) supraventricular, combined with a bundle-branch block, intraventricular conduction defect, aberrancy, or ventricular preexcitation.

STEP SIX: DETERMINE THE ORIGIN OF THE RHYTHM

Determine the site of origin of the rhythm by analyzing the P waves, the QRS complexes, and their association to each other. Your goal is to determine the source of the electrical discharge that generated the rhythm because that usually defines the rhythm. Rhythms that originate in the SA node or anywhere in the atria are called *supraventricular rhythms,* whereas those that originate in the AV junction, AV node, or ventricles are called *ventricular rhythms.*

If the P wave is associated with a QRS complex, the rhythm originates from the source of the P wave (Fig. 4.19).

Table 4.4 summarizes the origin of rhythms with QRS complexes associated with P waves.

If the P′ waves are associated with QRS complexes, the rhythm originated in the lower part of the atria near the AV junction, in the AV junction itself, or in the ventricles. You can determine the exact origin of the negative P′ waves by analyzing their relationship to the QRS complexes in lead II as follows:

- If the negative P′ wave regularly precedes the QRS complex, the origin of the rhythm is either in the lower part of the atria near the AV junction or in the proximal part of the AV junction itself. Typically, the P′R interval is less than 0.12 second, but it may be longer if first-degree AV block is present.

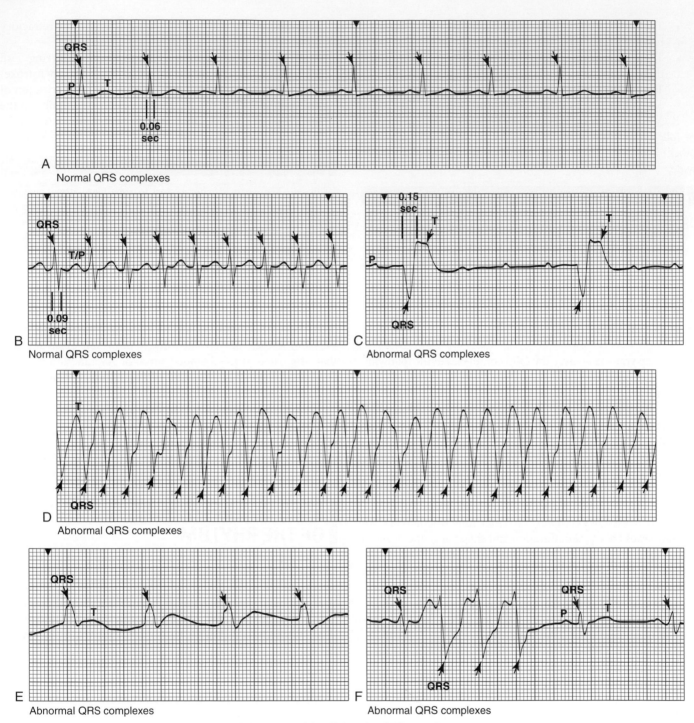

FIG. 4.18 Identifying the QRS complexes.

- If the negative P′ wave regularly follows the QRS complex, the origin of the rhythm is in the distal part of the AV junction. The RP′ interval is usually less than 0.20 second. If the QRS complex is longer than 0.12 second in duration and appears bizarre, it is likely that the rhythm originated in the ventricles.

If the QRS complexes have no set relationship to the P waves, you can still determine the origin of the electrical impulses responsible for them (Fig. 4.20). Note the duration and shape of the QRS complex and whether or not a bundle-branch block, an intraventricular conduction defect, or abnormal ventricular conduction is present. Often, the site of origin of wide and bizarre QRS complexes, occurring independently of the P waves or in their absence, cannot be determined accurately from monitoring only lead II. In such instances, a 12-lead ECG or lead MCL$_1$ is extremely helpful.

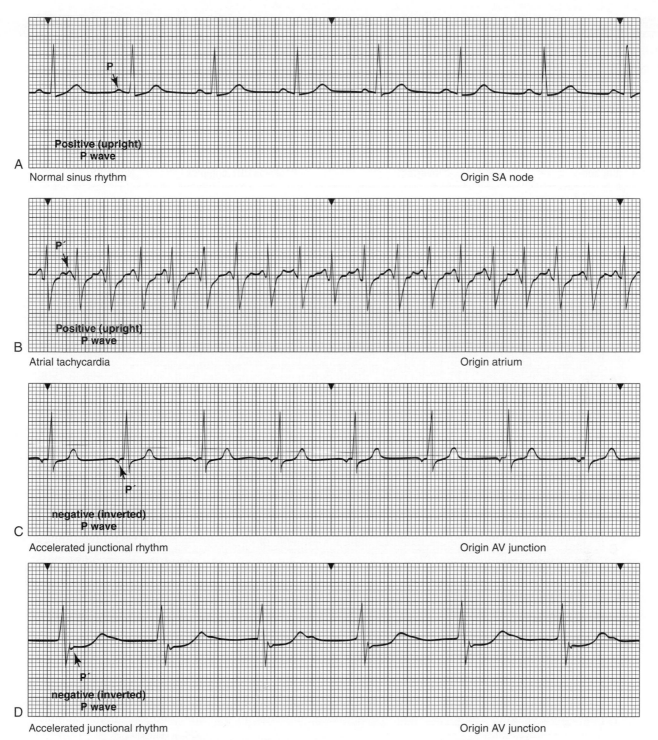

FIG. 4.19 Examples of rhythms with P waves associated with the QRS complexes.

Table 4.5 summarizes the origin of rhythms with QRS complexes not associated with P waves. Here are some key points to keep in mind:

- If the QRS complex is 0.12 seconds or less in duration and normal in appearance, the electrical impulse most likely originated in the AV junction or atrium.
- If the QRS complex is less than 0.12 seconds in duration and has a bizarre shape, the electrical impulse may have

originated in the AV junction or in the proximal part of a bundle branch in the ventricles near the bundle of His.

- If the QRS complex is longer than 0.12 second in duration and appears bizarre, the electrical impulse originated in the AV junction or in the distal part of a bundle branch, the Purkinje network, or ventricular myocardium.

TABLE **4.4**	Origin of Rhythms With P Wave Associated With the QRS Complex		
Origin	**Direction of P Waves in Lead II**	**P/QRS Relationship**	**PR Interval**
SA node or upper or middle right atrium	Positive (upright)	P precedes QRS complex	0.12–0.20 sec or greater or less than 0.12 sec[a]
Lower atria or proximal AV junction	Negative (inverted)	P precedes QRS complex	Less than 0.12 sec
Distal AV junction	Negative (inverted)	P follows QRS complex	None (RP′ interval, <0.20 sec)

AV, Atrioventricular; *SA,* sinoatrial.
[a]In association with an accessory conduction pathway.

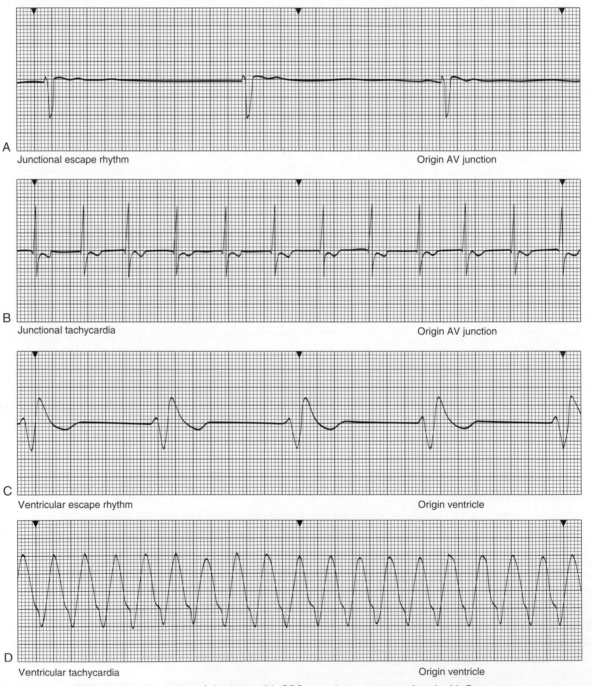

A Junctional escape rhythm   Origin AV junction

B Junctional tachycardia   Origin AV junction

C Ventricular escape rhythm   Origin ventricle

D Ventricular tachycardia   Origin ventricle

FIG. 4.20 Examples of rhythms with QRS complexes not associated with P waves.

TABLE 4.5	Origin of Rhythms With QRS Complex Not Associated With P Wave	
	QRS COMPLEX	
Origin	**Duration**	**Appearance**
AV junction	0.12 sec or less	Normal
AV junction[a] or	0.10–0.12 sec	Normal
Proximal bundle-branch AV junction[a] or	Longer than 0.12 sec	
Distal bundle branch, Purkinje network, or ventricular myocardium		Bizarre

AV, Atrioventricular.

[a]In association with a preexisting incomplete bundle-branch block, an intra-ventricular conduction defect, or aberrant ventricular conduction.

STEP SEVEN: IDENTIFY THE RHYTHM

Once you have performed each step, you will have enough information to interpret the rhythm. Most rhythms possess unique features that clearly identify them. However, in some cases, interpretation is based on a list of most probable rhythms. Figuring out which rhythm is actually present takes clinical experience with the clinical features that differentiate one rhythm from another. To draw a full clinical picture, you must also take into account which rhythms are more common than others. Chapters 5 through 9 will present the unique features of ECG rhythms and provide clues to distinguishing the common from the less common.

STEP EIGHT: ASSESS CLINICAL SIGNIFICANCE

Once the rhythm has been interpreted, you must determine its clinical significance. Rhythm interpretation concentrates on the electrical activity in the heart, whereas the clinical significance deals with the physiologic consequences of the rhythm on the ability of the heart to beat. Some rhythms significantly diminish the heart's ability to contract efficiently. Additionally, some rhythms provide clinically significant warning signs of a problem stemming from various causes, such as the following:

- Reduced blood flow to the body and shock
- The adverse effects of medications
- An electrolyte imbalance

We'll discuss the clinical significance of each rhythm in Chapters 5 through 9.

AUTHOR'S NOTE We apply the term *clinical* to any underlying problem that causes symptoms or observable signs of distress or illness in the patient. For example, atrial fibrillation often has no symptoms and generates no outward signs of a problem unless the rate is very fast, causing the blood pressure to drop and the patient to become symptomatic.

TAKE-HOME POINTS

- By using a systematic approach to the evaluation of an ECG rhythm, an interpretation can be made. This systematic approach consists of eight steps:
  1. Determining the rate: The most accurate method of determining the rate is using a rate calculator ruler; however, the 6-second method is a quick and easy estimate of the rhythm's rate.
  2. Determining the regularity: The regularity is assessed by comparing the R-R intervals. Rhythms are either regular or irregular. Irregular rhythms are either regularly (patterned) irregular or totally (irregularly) irregular.
  3. Identifying and analyzing the atrial activity: Atrial activity is assessed by noting the presence of P, P′, F, or f waves. P waves arise from the SA node, whereas P′ waves originate somewhere in the atrial walls or AV node. F and f waves arise from extremely fast firing sites in the atria and are associated with atrial flutter and atrial fibrillation, respectively.
  4. Determining the PR intervals and AV conduction ratio: The PR interval is measured from the start of the P wave to the first deflection of the QRS complex. It is normal, short, or long. If no QRS complex is associated with the P wave, a heart block is present.
  5. Identifying and analyzing the QRS complexes: QRS complexes are normally narrow (<0.12 seconds) but may be wide and bizarre if there is an intraventricular delay. If there are QRS complexes not associated with a P wave, then a premature complex is present. Premature QRS complexes may originate from either the AV node or the ventricles.
  6. Determining the origin of the electrical activity of the rhythm: The origin of any rhythm is the site in the heart that is primarily responsible for the P-QRS-T cycle.
  7. Identifying the rhythm: The combination of unique characteristics of any rhythm leads to its identification.
  8. Assessing the clinical significance of the rhythm: The ECG rhythm provides information related to the electrical activity in the heart. This activity may or may not be clinically significant. Clinical significance is based on the physiologic consequences of the rhythm.

CHAPTER REVIEW QUESTIONS

1. What is the most accurate regular ECG rate determined by?
   A. The 6-second count method
   B. A heart-rate calculator ruler
   C. The R-R interval method
   D. The Rule of 300

2. If the rhythm is irregular, which of the following is used to obtain an accurate calculation of the rate?
   A. The 6-second method
   B. Heart-rate calculator
   C. R-R interval
   D. Rule of 300

3. If there are four large squares between the peaks of two consecutive R waves, what is the rate?
   A. 50 beats/min
   B. 75 beats/min
   C. 100 beats/min
   D. 150 beats/min

4. Which of the following best describes the rate of the P wave in a normally conducted rhythm?
   A. It is unrelated to the rate of the QRS complex.
   B. It is sometimes less than the rate of the QRS complex.
   C. It is greater than the QRS rate in an AV block.
   D. It is the same as that of the QRS complexes.

5. If a wide, bizarre-shaped QRS complex is present but does not regularly precede or follow the P wave, which of the following is true?
   A. A complete AV block is present.
   B. The AV conduction ratio is fixed.
   C. The P waves will be abnormal.
   D. Aberrant conduction can be excluded.

6. When atrial flutter or fibrillation waves are present, what is the origin of the electrical impulses responsible for them?
   A. Ventricles
   B. Atria
   C. Septum
   D. Bundle of His

7. What is the electrical origin of inverted P waves in lead II?
   A. Ventricles
   B. Lower atria
   C. SA node
   D. Bundle of His

8. A PR interval of less than 0.12 second indicates that the origin of the P wave is in all of the following except where?
   A. AV junction
   B. Lower right atrium near the AV node
   C. Upper right atrium with an accessory AV pathway present
   D. SA node

9. If the QRS complex is 0.10 second or less in duration, the electrical impulse responsible for it most likely originated where?
   A. SA node
   B. Purkinje network
   C. AV junction in the presence of a right bundle-branch block
   D. Interventricular septum

10. A QRS that originates in the Purkinje network will have which of the following characteristics?
    A. Bizarre shape and duration between 0.10 and 0.12 second
    B. Normal shape and duration between 0.10 and 0.12 second
    C. Normal shape and duration of less than 0.12 second
    D. Wide, bizarre shape with duration longer than 0.12 second

5 Sinus Rhythms

NORMAL SINUS RHYTHM

normal sinus rhythm (NSR)

The most common rhythm found in the healthy human heart (Fig. 5.1). The electrical impulse originates in the sinoatrial (SA) node. The signal is then conducted through the atria to the atrioventricular (AV) node.

Characteristics

Rate	60–100
Regularity	Regular
P wave	Upright, rounded
PR interval	Normal, 0.12 to < 0.2 sec
P-P, R-R intervals	Equal
Conduction ratio	1:1
QRS complex	Normal; wide if conduction delay exists
Origin	Sinoatrial node

Rate

The rate is 60 to 100 beats/min. This is the normal resting rate in a healthy adult.

Regularity

Regular pattern with equal R-R and P-P intervals. There are no dropped or blocked QRS complexes.

P Wave

P waves are identical, precede each QRS complex, and are positive (upright) in lead II, indicating that they originated in the SA node and that depolarization of the atria has occurred normally.

PR Interval

Normal (less than 0.20 second) and constant but may vary slightly with the rate.

R-R and P-P Intervals

Equal but may vary slightly. The difference between the longest and shortest R-R (or P-P) interval, is usually to less than 0.04 second (one small box on an ECG strip).

Conduction Ratio

A P wave appears before every QRS complex, and a QRS complex follows each P wave. This 1:1 ratio indicates that the impulse is being conducted along the normal pathway and that no AV blocks are present.

QRS Complex

Follows each P wave. Duration is normally 0.12 second or less, but it may be prolonged (longer than 0.12 second) if the patient has an intraventricular conduction disturbance such as a bundle-branch block.

Origin

SA node.

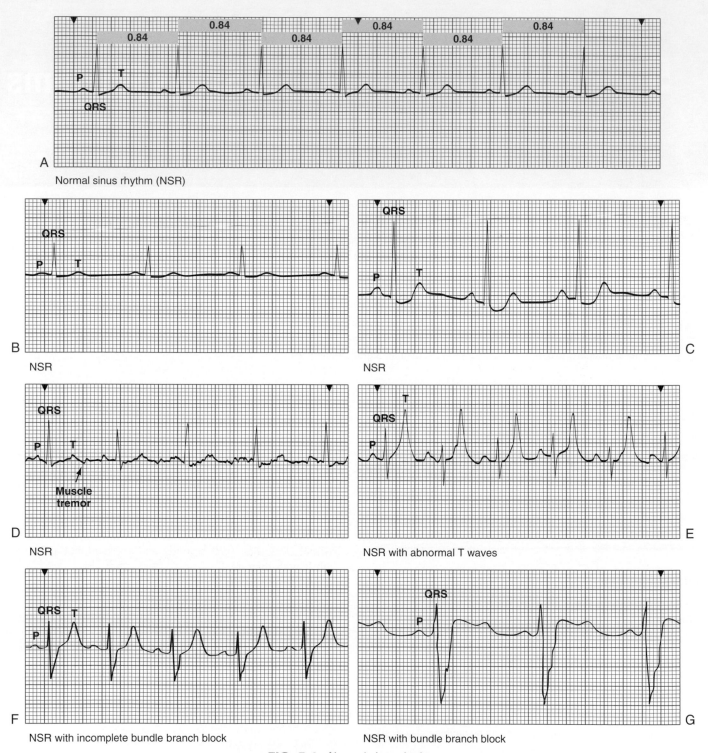

A Normal sinus rhythm (NSR)

B NSR

C NSR

D NSR

E NSR with abnormal T waves

F NSR with incomplete bundle branch block

G NSR with bundle branch block

FIG. 5.1 Normal sinus rhythm.

AUTHOR'S NOTE NSR is the standard against which all other rhythms are compared. In other words, we define abnormal ECG rhythms according to the ways in which they differ from NSR. These abnormal rhythms are more accurately called *dysrhythmia*, a term that quite literally means "disturbance of the rhythm." Going forward, you will find the terms *rhythm, rhythm disorder* or *disturbance*, and *dysrhythmia* used interchangeably.

Clinical Significance

NSR with a palpable pulse occurring simultaneously with the QRS indicates that the heart is ejecting blood with each P-QRST line cycle. However, the appearance of NSR on the cardiac monitor is no guarantee that a pulse has been generated, nor does it offer any indication of the quality of that pulse (blood pressure). If a pulse cannot be felt in a patient showing NSR on the ECG, he or she is probably in shock. If there is no pulse and the patient is not breathing, then a form of cardiac arrest called *pulseless electrical activity (PEA)* is occurring.

> **AUTHOR'S NOTE** The presence of a pulse and its correlation with the ECG rhythm should be one of the first tasks you perform when assessing a patient.

SINUS ARRHYTHMIA

> **sinus arrhythmia**
>
> An irregularity of the heartbeat caused by a cyclical change in the rate of sinus rhythm (Fig. 5.2). This rate change is usually associated with the patient's respiratory cycle.

> **AUTHOR'S NOTE** Sinus arrhythmia is technically a dysrhythmia. (Recall that arrhythmia means "without rhythm," and dysrhythmia refers to a disordered rhythm.) However, sinus arrhythmia is an old term with a long history of use. Therefore we will continue to use it in this book. Likewise, the term *dysrhythmia* is the most accurate way to describe a rhythm disturbance and will be commonly used in this text.

Characteristics

Rate	60–100
Regularity	Patterned irregularity

P wave	Upright, rounded
PR interval	Normal, 0.12 to < 0.2 sec
P-P, R-R intervals	Cyclically irregular
Conduction ratios	1:1
QRS complex	Normal; wide if conduction delay exists
Origin	Sinoatrial node

Rate

The rate is 60 to 100 beats/min. Occasionally, the rate may slow to slightly less than 60 or increase to slightly more than 100 beats/min. Typically, the rate increases when the patient breathes in (inhales) and decreases when the patient breathes out (exhales).

Regularity

Sinus arrhythmia is regularly irregular as the rate gradually rises and falls. These rate changes occur in cycles over the course of 15 to 30 seconds.

P Wave

P waves are identical, precede each QRS complex, and are positive (upright) in lead II, indicating normal depolarization of the atria.

PR Interval

Normal and constant.

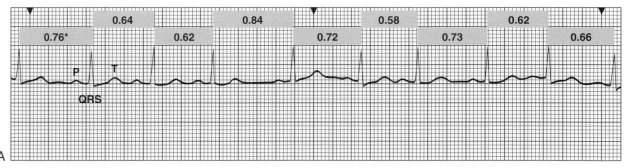

Sinus arrhythmia

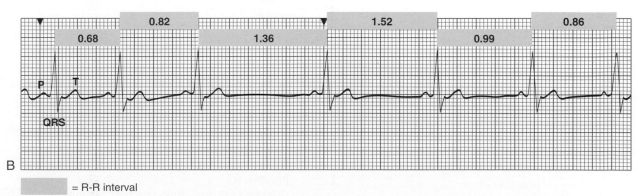

= R-R interval

*Seconds

FIG. 5.2   Sinus arrhythmia.

R-R Interval

Unequal. In sinus arrhythmia, the difference between the longest and shortest R-R intervals is greater than 0.04 second.

Conduction Ratio

A P wave appears before every QRS complex, and a QRS complex follows each P wave. This 1:1 ratio indicates that the impulse is being conducted along the normal pathway and that no AV blocks are present.

QRS Complex

Usually follows each P wave and has a normal duration unless an intraventricular conduction disturbance, such as a bundle-branch block, is present.

Origin

SA node.

Causes

The most common type of sinus arrhythmia is related to respiration. It is a normal phenomenon usually seen in children and young adults. It is caused by changes in the rate of impulse from the vagus nerve, which is part of the parasympathetic nervous system. During inhalation, the vagus nerve fires less frequently, resulting in an increased heart rate. During exhalation, the vagus nerve fires faster, resulting in a decreased heart rate.

The other, less common type of sinus arrhythmia is not related to respiration. It may occur in healthy individuals, but it is more often found in adult patients with heart disease, especially after an acute inferior wall myocardial infarction, or in patients receiving certain medications, such as digitalis. When this occurs in an elderly person, it may indicate a failing sinus node, or "sick sinus syndrome." In patients with this condition, the rate may alternate between being very slow (bradycardic) and very fast (tachycardic).

Clinical Significance

Usually, sinus arrhythmia is of no clinical significance and generally requires no treatment. In fact, this is evidence of a healthy heart that is appropriately responsive to the autonomic nervous system.

| SINUS BRADYCARDIA

sinus bradycardia
A rhythm originating in the SA node and characterized by a rate of less than 60 beats/min (Fig. 5.3).

Characteristics

Rate	Less than 60
Regularity	Regular
P wave	Upright, rounded
PR interval	Normal, 0.12 to < 0.2 sec
P-P, R-R intervals	Regular and equal
Conduction ratio	1:1
QRS complex	Usually normal; wide if conduction delay exists
Origin	Sinoatrial node

Rate

Less than 60 beats/min. The onset and termination of sinus bradycardia are typically gradual.

Regularity

Essentially regular, but it may be irregular if sinus arrhythmia is also present.

P Wave

Identical, precedes each QRS complex, and is positive (upright) in lead II, consistent with normal atrial depolarization.

PR Interval

Normal and constant; however, it tends to be near the upper limit of normal.

R-R Interval

Equal or may vary slightly.

Conduction Ratio

A P wave appears before every QRS complex, and a QRS complex follows each P wave. This 1:1 ratio indicates that the impulse is being conducted along the normal pathway and that no AV blocks are present.

QRS Complex

Follows each P wave. The duration of the complexes is normal unless an intraventricular conduction disturbance, such as a bundle-branch block, is present.

Origin

SA node.

Causes

Sinus bradycardia may be caused by any of the following:
- Hypokalemia (low potassium levels in the blood)
- Excessive influence of the parasympathetic nervous system on the SA node. This can occur from carotid sinus stimulation, vomiting, Valsalva maneuvers, or fainting caused by vagal nerve stimulation.
- Decreased influence of the sympathetic nervous system on the SA node. This can be caused by antihypertensive drugs—for example, beta blockers such as atenolol, metoprolol, and propranolol.
- Adverse effects of drugs, such as calcium-channel blockers (for example, diltiazem, verapamil, and nifedipine) and the cardiac glycoside drug digitalis

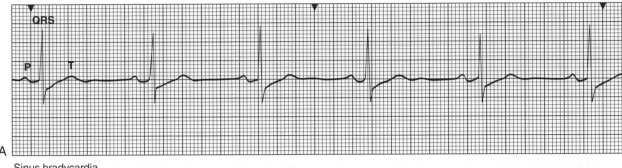

A

Sinus bradycardia

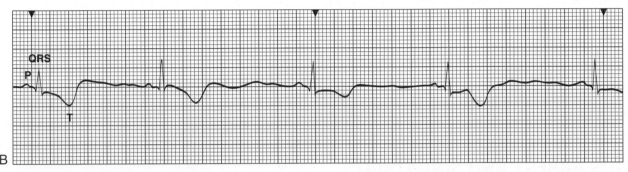

B

Sinus bradycardia with sinus arrhythmia

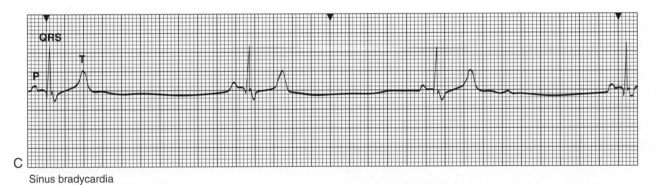

C

Sinus bradycardia

FIG. 5.3 Sinus bradycardia.

- Disease in the SA node, such as sick sinus syndrome
- Acute inferior wall or right ventricular myocardial infarction
- Hypothyroidism (myxedema)
- Hypothermia
- Hypoxia (especially in children)
- Sleep
- Decreased heart rate in a trained athlete

Valsalva maneuver

Any forced expiratory effort against a closed airway, such as when a person holds his or her breath and tightens the muscles in a concerted, strenuous effort to move a heavy object. It can also occur when straining during defecation. This causes a slowing of the heart rate as a result of increased firing of the vagus nerve.

Clinical Significance

In mild sinus bradycardia, the heart rate ranges from 50 to 59 beats/min. By itself, this condition usually does not produce symptoms, a condition referred to as *asymptomatic bradycardia*. In the presence of acute myocardial infarction, mild sinus bradycardia may actually be beneficial in some patients because it produces a decreased workload for the heart. With less work to do, the myocardium requires less oxygen, in turn minimizing the extension of the tissue damage and reducing the likelihood of other dysrhythmias that can worsen the patient's condition.

If the heart rate is 30 to 50 beats/min, cardiac output may drop, causing hypotension. However, many healthy athletes have resting heart rates between 40 and 60 beats/min and suffer no ill effect. In the older sedentary person, a heart rate of 30 to 50 beats/min will more commonly result in a drop in cardiac output. When the rate is less than 30 (marked sinus bradycardia), cardiac output is significantly reduced, causing hypotension. If blood pressure is too low, the brain and other vital organs may not receive adequate perfusion. Signs and symptoms of sinus bradycardia include the following:

- Dizziness, light-headedness, decreased level of consciousness, or fainting
- Shortness of breath
- Hypotension
- Shock
- Congestive heart failure
- Angina, myocardial ischemia, and/or myocardial infarction
- Predisposition to more serious dysrhythmias (for example, premature ventricular complexes, ventricular tachycardia, fibrillation, or asystole [absent heartbeat])

The well-conditioned athlete often has a resting heart rate of less than 50 and will be asymptomatic. However, when symptoms do occur, the dysrhythmia is called *symptomatic* bradycardia, regardless of the heart rate. Symptomatic sinus bradycardia, whatever the rate, must be treated promptly by addressing the underlying cause.

SINUS ARREST AND SINOATRIAL EXIT BLOCK

Sinus Arrest

sinus arrest

A rhythm caused by periodic failure of the SA node, resulting in bradycardia and/or asystole (Fig. 5.4).

Sinoatrial Exit Block

sinoatrial (SA) exit block

A rhythm caused by an interruption in the conduction of the electrical impulse from the SA node to the atria, resulting in bradycardia and/or no rhythm at all (asystole) (see Fig. 5.4).

Characteristics

Rate	60–100
Regularity	Irregular when the block is present
P wave	Upright, rounded, no P wave when arrest/block occurs
PR interval	That of the underlying rhythm. Duration may be normal or abnormal in duration.
P-P, R-R intervals	Sinus arrest: P wave following the pause is not a multiple of P-P interval.
	Sinoatrial block: P wave following the pause is a multiple of P-P interval
Conduction ratio	1:1 unless escape complexes are present
QRS complex	Normal; wide if conduction delay exists
Origin	SA node

Rate

Usually 60 to 100 beats/min but may be less.

Regularity

Irregular. The underlying rhythm will be seen, followed by a pause during which no QRS complex occurs. However, if the pause is sufficiently long, an escape complex may occur.

P Wave

P waves are identical, and a P wave precedes each QRS complex; however, when an electrical impulse is not generated by the SA node (known as *sinus arrest*), or if it is generated by the SA node but blocked from entering the atria (called *SA exit block*), atrial depolarization fails to occur. Consequently, no P wave will be seen. We call this a *dropped P wave*.

PR Interval

Reflects the underlying rhythm and thus may be normal or abnormal.

P-P and R-R Interval

It can be difficult to distinguish sinus arrest from SA block when a P wave does not occur in either condition. Normally, when the SA node fires, it resets itself and fires again at regular intervals. However, in sinus arrest and SA block, the SA node does not reset but instead fires at some random interval after the sinus arrest. This can be confirmed by measuring the P-P interval before and after the pause. When the SA node fails to fire, the next P wave (which represents SA-node firing) will not occur when expected. Therefore the P-P interval after the pause is totally different from any previous P-P interval.

With SA exit block, on the other hand, the SA node fires and *does* reset. But as with sinus arrest, the atria are not depolarized, and consequently, there is no P wave. However, the next P wave will occur at some predictable interval. The P-P interval after the SA exit block is a multiple of the P-P interval before the pause because the underlying rate of SA-node firing remains undisturbed.

Conduction Ratio

When sinus arrest or SA exit block occurs, there is no P wave. If a junctional escape complex occurs, there may be an inverted P′ or only a narrow QRS complex with a retrograde P wave. A ventricular escape complex will have a wide QRS complex and no P wave. If there is no escape complex, the next complex to occur will be the underlying rhythm P-QRS-T. The conduction ratio is thus said to be 1:1 except during the period of the pause.

QRS Complex

Follows each P wave. The duration is normal unless a preexisting intraventricular conduction disturbance (such as a bundle-branch block) is present. It is absent if there is no P wave unless an escape complex occurs.

Origin

SA node.

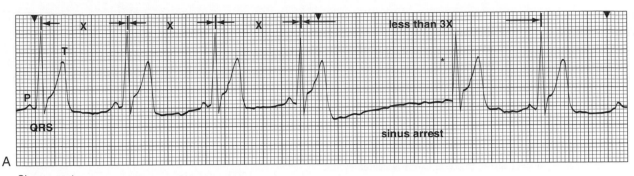

A

Sinus arrest

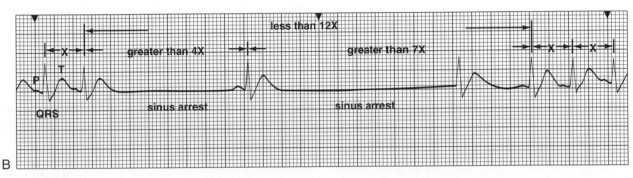

B

Sinus arrest

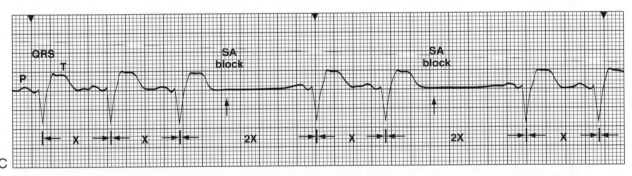

C

SA exit block

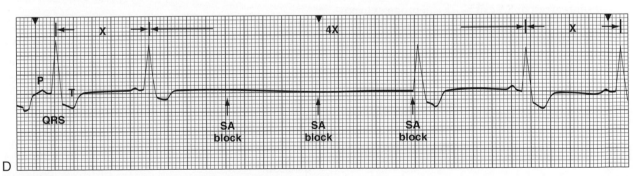

D

SA block

*Junctional Escape Complex. See Chapter 7, Junctional Rhythms.

FIG. 5.4 Sinus arrest and sinoatrial (SA) exit block.

Causes

Sinus arrest results from a marked decrease in the automaticity of the SA node. SA exit block occurs when conduction of the electrical impulse from the SA node into the atria is interrupted.

> **AUTHOR'S NOTE** Recall that automaticity is a unique property that allows certain cardiac cells to generate an electrical impulse spontaneously—that is, automatically. Increased automaticity is the most common cause of a rhythm disturbance. In sinus arrest, the disturbance is caused by decreased automaticity.

Sinus arrest or SA exit block may be brought on by any of the following:
- Increase in vagal (parasympathetic) influence on the SA node
- Hypoxia
- Hyperkalemia
- Sleep apnea
- Adverse effect of digitalis or beta blockers such as atenolol, metoprolol, propranolol, or quinidine
- Damage to the SA node or adjacent atrium from acute inferior wall and right ventricular myocardial infarction, acute myocarditis, or fibrosis (scarring) of the myocardium.

Clinical Significance

Sinus arrest and SA exit block may be unnoticeable to the patient or clinician if a junctional escape pacemaker takes over promptly. If, however, a ventricular escape pacemaker takes over and the patient's heart rate is slow, or if an escape pacemaker does not occur at all, the patient may have a transient (temporary) period of asystole during which there is no heartbeat. Light-headedness or fainting may occur. The signs and symptoms, clinical significance, and management of sinus arrest or SA exit block in a patient with an excessively slow heart rate are the same as for patients with symptomatic sinus bradycardia.

Intermittent sinus arrest or SA exit block can progress to prolonged sinus arrest accompanied by lack of electrical activity of the atria (atrial standstill). If a junctional or ventricular escape pacemaker does not take over, asystole occurs, requiring immediate life-saving treatment.

SINUS TACHYCARDIA

sinus tachycardia

A rhythm originating in the SA node, characterized by a rate of more than 100 beats/min (Fig. 5.5).

Characteristics

Rate	Greater than 100
Regularity	Regular
P wave	Upright, rounded
PR interval	Normal or short
P-P, R-R intervals	Regular and equal
Conduction ratio	1:1
QRS complex	Normal; wide if conduction delay exists
Origin	SA node

Rate

More than 100 beats/min. The rate may climb to 180 beats/min or more with extreme exertion. Onset and termination are typically gradual.

Regularity

Regular.

P Wave

Usually normal but may be slightly taller and more peaked. P waves are identical, precede each QRS complex, and are positive (upright) in lead II. When the heart rate is very rapid, the P wave may be hidden (buried) in the preceding T wave and therefore not easily identified. Such combined T and P waves are known as *T/P waves*.

PR Interval

Normal and constant. The higher the rate, the shorter the PR interval becomes.

P-P and R-R Intervals

Each is constant.

Conduction Ratio

A P wave appears before every QRS complex, and a QRS complex follows each P wave. This 1:1 ratio indicates that the impulse is being conducted along the normal pathway and that no AV blocks are present.

QRS Complex

Normal unless a preexisting intraventricular conduction disturbance (such as a bundle-branch block) or aberrant ventricular conduction is present. A QRS complex normally follows each P wave.

Origin

SA node.

Causes

Sinus tachycardia in adults is a normal response of the heart to the demand for increased blood flow, as occurs during exercise or other exertion. It may also be caused by any of the following:
- Ingestion of stimulants such as coffee or tea or from abuse of drugs such as cocaine or amphetamines
- Increase in the influence of the sympathetic nervous system, which can occur from excitement, anxiety, pain, or stress

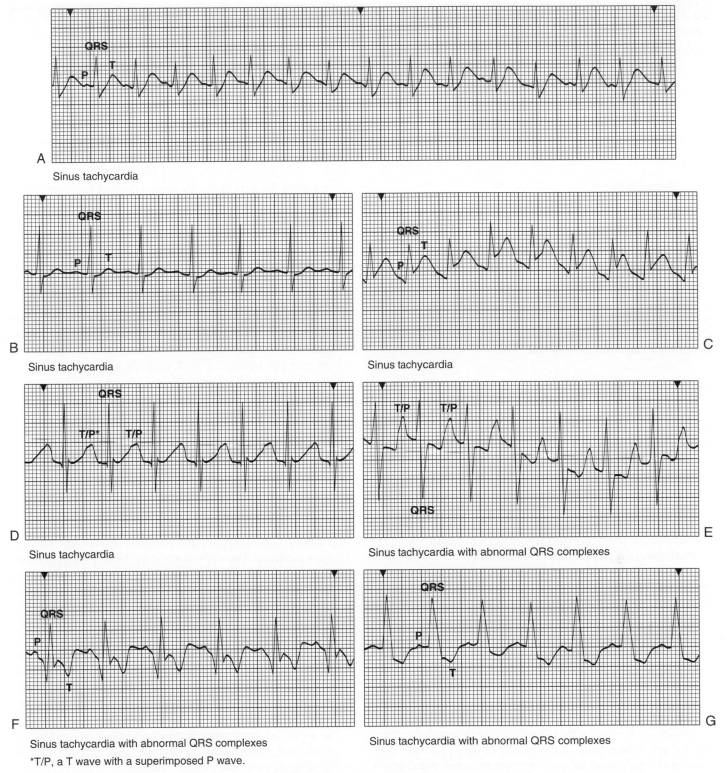

A Sinus tachycardia

B Sinus tachycardia

C Sinus tachycardia

D Sinus tachycardia

E Sinus tachycardia with abnormal QRS complexes

F Sinus tachycardia with abnormal QRS complexes

G Sinus tachycardia with abnormal QRS complexes

*T/P, a T wave with a superimposed P wave.

FIG. 5.5 Sinus tachycardia.

- As a response to conditions that increase the demands on the heart—in other words, when greater cardiac output is needed, as may occur in the following:
  - Severe bleeding or dehydration
  - Heart failure
  - Pulmonary embolism
  - Myocardial ischemia or acute myocardial infarction
  - Fever
  - Thyrotoxicosis
  - Anemia

TABLE 5.1	Typical Diagnostic ECG Features of Sinus Node Rhythms				
Rhythm	**Heart rate (beats/min)**	**Regularity**	**P Wave**	**PR Interval**	**QRS Complex**
Normal sinus rhythm	60–100	Regular	Normal	Normal	Normal
Sinus arrhythmia	60–100	Patterned irregularity	Normal	Normal	Normal
Sinus bradycardia	<60	Regular	Normal	Normal	Normal
Sinus arrest, SA exit block	60–100	Irregular	Normal	Normal	Normal
Sinus tachycardia	100–180	Regular	Normal; may be peaked	Normal	Normal

SA, Sinoatrial.

- Hypovolemia
- Hypoxia
- Shock
- Effects of sympathomimetic drugs, such as dopamine, epinephrine, isoproterenol, and norepinephrine, which affect the body's sympathetic nervous system

> **AUTHOR'S NOTE** As a general rule, the maximum rate for sinus tachycardia is often calculated as follows: 220 − age (years). Therefore a 50-year-old patient would generally not be expected to have a sinus tachycardia exceeding 170 beats/min.

Clinical Significance

Sinus tachycardia in healthy individuals is an abnormal but usually benign rhythm that requires no specific treatment. Instead, when its cause is removed or treated, sinus tachycardia resolves gradually and spontaneously. Because a rapid heart rate increases the workload of the heart, the heart's oxygen requirements increase. For this reason, sinus tachycardia in the setting of acute coronary syndrome may result in the following:

- Increase in myocardial ischemia (death of cardiac muscle tissue)
- Increase the frequency and severity of chest pain
- Predispose the patient to more serious dysrhythmias

The two most worrisome issues in addressing any tachycardia are the following:

1. What is the effect on oxygen demand in the heart? A heart with significant cardiovascular disease will not tolerate the increased oxygen demand of the tachycardia and will be prone to ischemia, infarction, and potentially lethal dysrhythmias.
2. The second and more common issue is that as the heart rate increases, there is less time for the heart to relax and fill completely during diastole. This can cause a significant decrease in cardiac output, leading to syncope and shock.

Treatment of sinus tachycardia should be directed at correcting the underlying cause of the dysrhythmia. For a brief summary of the various sinus node dysrhythmias discussed in this chapter, see Table 5.1.

TAKE-HOME POINTS

- NSR is the most common and physiologically normal rhythm of the human heart. It arises from the SA node, traverses the atria to the AV node, and then moves on to the ventricles via the bundle of His, bundle branches, and Purkinje network.
- All rhythm disturbances (dysrhythmias) are characterized according to how they differ from NSR.
- The SA node is the source of all sinus rhythms and is easily influenced by the sympathetic and parasympathetic nervous systems and external stimuli.
- With NSR, each heartbeat originates in the sinus node. The P wave is always positive in lead II. The PR interval is normal, and the heart rate is at its resting state, firing between 60 and 100 beats/min. NSR is characterized by upright P waves, a normal PR interval, and in most cases a narrow QRS complex.
- Sinus bradycardia and sinus tachycardia differ from NSR only by their rate, with bradycardia existing when the rate is less than 60 beats/min and tachycardia existing when the rate exceeds 100 beats/min.
- Both sinus bradycardia and sinus tachycardia may occur under normal conditions. However, a cause should be sought if your patient exhibits signs and symptoms related to a slow or fast rate.
- Although sinus rhythms are essentially regular, the rate can vary cyclically. This cyclical variation usually occurs in concert with inhalation and exhalation. This kind of variation constitutes sinus arrhythmia and is a normal finding, particularly in children and young adults.
- Disease may affect the SA node, either causing the node to fail to fire or blocking the impulse from reaching the atria. When this occurs, there is no P wave and consequently no QRS complex, and a pause is seen in the ECG rhythm strip.
- If the next P wave occurs at the expected time, sinus exit block exists. If the next P wave occurs later than expected, sinus arrest is present. Either condition can produce a prolonged period with no rhythm (asystole), resulting in inadequate perfusion or even death.
- The most important issue to address in any rhythm disturbance arising from the sinus node is the underlying cause. This is because, aside from sinus arrest and SA block, most sinus rhythm disorders are symptomatic of an underlying medical condition.
- Table 5.1 provides a summary of the ECG features of the sinus node dysrhythmias discussed in this chapter.

CHAPTER REVIEW QUESTIONS

1. Typically, in sinus arrhythmia, how does the heart rate change when the patient inhales and exhales?
   A. Decreases during inhalation and exhalation
   B. Decreases during inhalation and increases during exhalation
   C. Increases during inhalation and decreases during exhalation
   D. Increases during inhalation and increases during exhalation

2. Which description best applies to the most common type of sinus arrhythmia, the one related to respiration?
   A. It's a normal phenomenon commonly seen in middle-aged adults.
   B. It's caused by varying vagal activity.
   C. It's caused by the sympathetic effect on the SA node.
   D. It's extremely rare in children.

3. Another, less common type of sinus arrhythmia that is unrelated to respiration is sometimes associated with the use of which of the following?
   A. Cocaine
   B. Beta blockers
   C. Digitalis
   D. Calcium-channel blockers

4. Which of the following is a dysrhythmia originating in the SA node with a regular rate of less than 60 beats/min?
   A. Sinus arrest
   B. Sinus arrhythmia
   C. Sinus bradycardia
   D. Sinus tachycardia

5. Which of the following can cause sinus bradycardia?
   A. Increased firing of the vagus nerve
   B. Hyperthermia
   C. Increased influence of the sympathetic nervous system on the SA node
   D. Hyperthyroidism

6. What is the heart rate in mild sinus bradycardia?
   A. 30 to 39 beats/min
   B. 40 to 49 beats/min
   C. 50 to 59 beats/min
   D. 60 to 69 beats/min

7. A symptomatic patient with marked sinus bradycardia is likely to have which signs or symptoms?
   A. Hypertension and decreased cerebral perfusion
   B. Hypotension and decreased cerebral perfusion
   C. Hypothermia and chest pain
   D. Hypoxia and increased central venous pressure (CVP)

8. Symptomatic sinus tachycardia is best treated by doing what?
   A. Addressing the underlying cause
   B. Administering a beta blocker
   C. Administering oxygen
   D. Performing vagal maneuvers

9. Which term best describes a dysrhythmia caused by episodes of failure in the automaticity of the SA node resulting in bradycardia or asystole?
   A. Marked sinus arrhythmia
   B. Marked sinus bradycardia
   C. Sinus arrest
   D. Wenckebach phenomenon

10. SA exit block may result from the toxicity of which medication?
    A. Norepinephrine
    B. Digitalis
    C. Epinephrine
    D. Dopamine

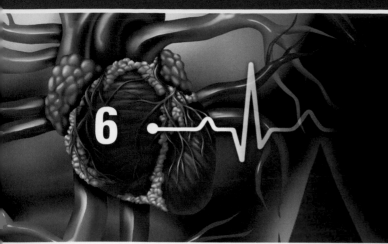

6

Atrial Rhythms

PREMATURE ATRIAL COMPLEXES

premature atrial complex (PAC)

A PAC (Fig. 6.1) is an extra P-QRS-T complex occurring earlier than the next expected beat of the underlying rhythm as a result of increased automaticity. A PAC is followed by a noncompensatory pause.

Characteristics

Rate	Underlying rhythm
Regularity	Irregular at point of PAC
P wave	P' wave is present. Shape of P' wave varies.
PR interval	Normal (0.12–0.20 sec) to very short (<0.12 sec)
P-P, R-R intervals	P-P' interval is unequal. Noncompensatory pause occurs. P-P and R-R intervals encompassing the PAC are less than 2 times the P-P and R-R intervals of the underlying rhythm.
Conduction ratio	1:1
QRS complex	Normal; wide if conduction delay exists
Origin	Multiple sites in the atria or high in the atrioventricular (AV) junction

Rate

Same as that of the underlying rhythm.

Regularity

Irregular at the period of time encompassing the PAC.

P Wave

A PAC is present when a P' wave accompanied by a QRS complex occurs earlier (prematurely) than the next expected sinus P wave. The premature P wave is called an *ectopic P'* (P prime) *wave*. Although the P' wave of a PAC may resemble a normal sinus P wave, it is usually different. The size, shape, and direction of the P' wave depend on the location of the ectopic atrial site that initiated the wave. For example, it may appear positive (upright) and quite normal in lead II if the ectopic site is near the sinoatrial (SA) node. It may appear negative (inverted) if the ectopic site is near the AV junction. P' waves originating in the same atrial ectopic site are usually identical. The P' waves precede the QRS complex and are sometimes buried in the preceding T waves (T/P wave), distorting them and often making the T wave more peaked and pointed than unaffected ones. A P' wave followed by a QRS complex is said to be a *conducted PAC* because the impulse originating in the ectopic site is conducted to the AV node and then on to the ventricles.

If the atrial ectopic site discharges too soon after the preceding QRS complex, the AV junction may not be sufficiently repolarized to accept another impulse. When this occurs, the AV node is said to be *refractory*, or unable to conduct the premature electrical impulse into the ventricles normally. In this case the AV junction or bundle branches may either slow the conduction of the premature impulse, resulting in a prolonged PR interval, or block its transmission completely, in which case the QRS complex will be absent. Such a PAC is called a *nonconducted* or *blocked PAC*.

PR Interval

May be normal but is usually different from that of the underlying rhythm. Their length will be as follows:

- 0.12 to less than 0.20 second when the ectopic site is near the SA node
- Less than 0.12 second when the ectopic site is near the AV junction

R-R Interval

The P-P′ interval of the PAC is shorter than the P-P interval of the underlying rhythm because the PAC occurs earlier than expected. The impulse from the ectopic P′ wave depolarizes the SA node, resetting its timing. Consequently, the next P-QRS-T cycle will appear earlier than it otherwise would have. The resulting R-R interval is called a *noncompensatory pause* because the rhythm did not compensate for the presence of the PAC. The interval between the R wave before the PAC and the R wave after the PAC will be less than twice the R-R interval of the underlying rhythm.

noncompensatory pause

A pause is termed *noncompensatory* if the normal beat after a premature complex occurs before it is expected, indicating that the SA node was reset. The R-R interval of the noncompensatory pause is less than twice the duration of the R-R interval before the pause.

QRS Complex

Usually resembles that of the underlying rhythm because conduction of the electrical impulse through the bundle branches is unchanged. If the atrial ectopic site discharges soon after the preceding QRS complex, the bundle branches may not repolarize sufficiently to conduct the PAC normally. If this occurs, the impulse may be conducted only down one bundle branch—usually the left one. It will be blocked in the other. The result is a wide and bizarre-looking QRS complex that resembles a right bundle-branch block. Such a PAC, called a *PAC with aberrancy* (or *with aberrant ventricular conduction*), can mimic a premature

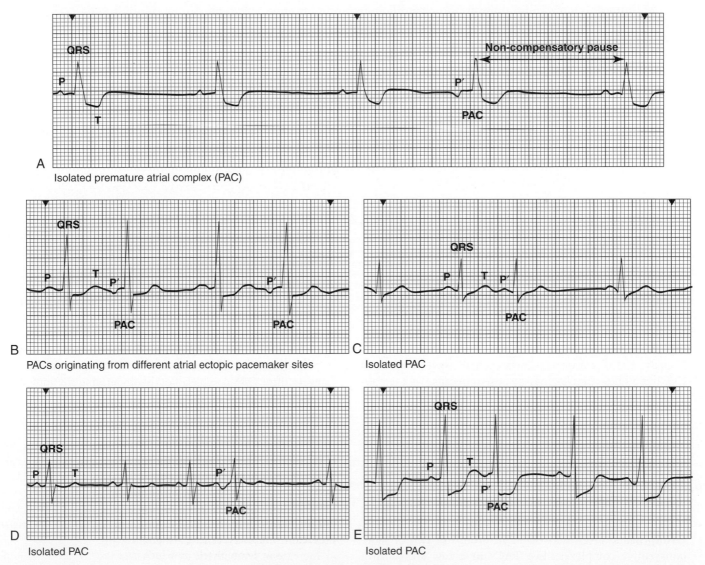

A Isolated premature atrial complex (PAC)

B PACs originating from different atrial ectopic pacemaker sites

C Isolated PAC

D Isolated PAC

E Isolated PAC

FIG. 6.1 Premature atrial complexes.   *Continued*

Lead II

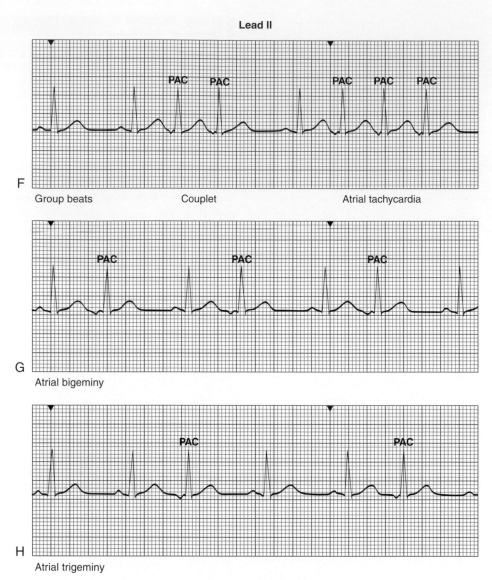

FIG. 6.1 cont'd

ventricular complex (PVC). You can differentiate it by the presence of a noncompensatory pause compared with the PVC, which has a compensatory pause (see Premature Ventricular Complexes).

Usually, a QRS complex follows each P′ wave (conducted PACs), but a QRS complex may be absent because of a temporary AV block resulting in a nonconducted PAC.

Conduction Ratio

The ratio is 1:1 when the PAC is conducted, and 1:0 when nonconducted or blocked.

Patterns

The following are the various forms in which PACs may appear:
- **Isolated:** PACs may occur singly (isolated events).
- **Group beats:** PACs may occur in groups of two or more consecutive complexes. Two PACs in a row are called a *couplet*. When three or more PACs occur in succession,

atrial tachycardia (discussed later in this chapter) is considered to be present.
- **Repetitive beats:** PACs may alternate with the QRS complexes of the underlying rhythm (atrial bigeminy) or occur after every two QRS complexes (atrial trigeminy) or after every three QRS complexes of the underlying rhythm (atrial quadrigeminy).

Origin

PACs originate at an ectopic site in the atria outside the SA node, such as the AV junction. They may originate from a single ectopic site or from multiple sites.

Causes

PACs are a result of increased automaticity of the ectopic atrial sites. Common causes include the following:
- Increase in sympathetic tone
- Infection

- Emotional stress
- Stimulants (such as caffeine or tobacco)
- Sympathomimetic drugs (such as epinephrine, albuterol, and norepinephrine)
- Hypoxia
- Digitalis toxicity
- Cardiovascular disease (especially acute coronary syndrome [ACS] or early heart failure)
- Dilated or hypertrophied atria caused by increased atrial pressure, usually as a result of mitral or tricuspid valve disease or atrial septal defect

In some patients, however, you may not be able to determine the cause.

Clinical Significance

Isolated PACs are not clinically significant and may occur in people with apparently healthy hearts. In those with heart disease, however, frequent PACs may indicate either enhanced automaticity of the atria or a reentry mechanism. The latter may have a variety of causes, such as heart failure or myocardial infarction. In addition, such PACs may initiate more serious supraventricular rhythms, such as atrial tachycardia, atrial flutter, atrial fibrillation, and paroxysmal supraventricular tachycardia (PSVT).

If nonconducted PACs are frequent and the heart rate is less than 50 beats/min, the signs and symptoms, clinical significance, and management are the same as those of symptomatic sinus bradycardia.

Because PACs with aberrancy often resemble PVCs (see Chapter 8), be sure to identify such PACs correctly so as to treat them appropriately.

WANDERING ATRIAL PACEMAKER

wandering atrial pacemaker (WAP)

A rhythm that is a result of increased automaticity, originates in multiple atrial sites, and shifts from one to the next (Fig. 6.2).

The rhythm may begin in and then shift from any of the following locations:
1. The SA node
2. Ectopic "pacemaker" sites in the walls of the atria
3. Upper portion of the AV junction
This rhythm is characterized by P waves of varying size, shape, and direction in any one lead.

AUTHOR'S NOTE The word *pacemaker* technically refers to sites of regular impulse generation within the heart. They include the SA node, the AV node, and the Purkinje fibers. Therefore WAP is not actually a pacemaker rhythm because the impulse may arise from an ectopic site in the atria. However, the impulse that generates WAP arises from the pacemaker cells in the conduction system.

Characteristics

Rate	60–100
Regularity	Irregular
P wave	P′ waves are present and vary in size and shape.
PR interval	Normal to very short
P-P, R-R intervals	Unequal
Conduction ratio	1:1
QRS complex	Normal; wide if conduction delay exists
Origin	SA node, ectopic atrial sites, AV junction (shifts randomly)

Rate

The rate is 60 to 100 beats/min but may be slower. Usually, the rate gradually slows as the pacemaker site shifts from the SA node to the atria or AV junction and increases as it shifts back to the SA node. This occurs because the SA node has greater automaticity (ability to depolarize spontaneously) than the other pacemaker sites.

Regularity

Slightly irregular.

P Wave

The P wave changes in size, shape, and direction over the course of several beats. It varies in lead II from positive (upright) to negative (inverted). It can even become buried in the QRS complex as the pacemaker site shifts. Ectopic atrial P waves (produced by signals generated outside the SA node or AV junction) do not always originate from the same site. Thus their progression from one point to another is unpredictable.

The shape of the P wave provides clues as to its source. A P wave arising from any site other than the SA node is referred to as a *P′ (P prime) wave*. The presence of varying P and P′ waves distinguishes a WAP from a normal sinus rhythm, in which the P wave remains constant in size, shape, and direction.

PR Interval

Varies between 0.12 and 0.20 seconds depending on whether the ectopic site is closer or farther away from the AV junction.

P-P and R-R Intervals

The P-P′ (or P′-P) and R-R intervals are usually unequal but may become nearly equal if the rate is fast.

Conduction Ratio

A P or P′ wave appears before every QRS complex, and a QRS complex occurs after each P wave. This 1:1 ratio indicates that the impulse is being conducted along the normal pathway and that no AV blocks are present.

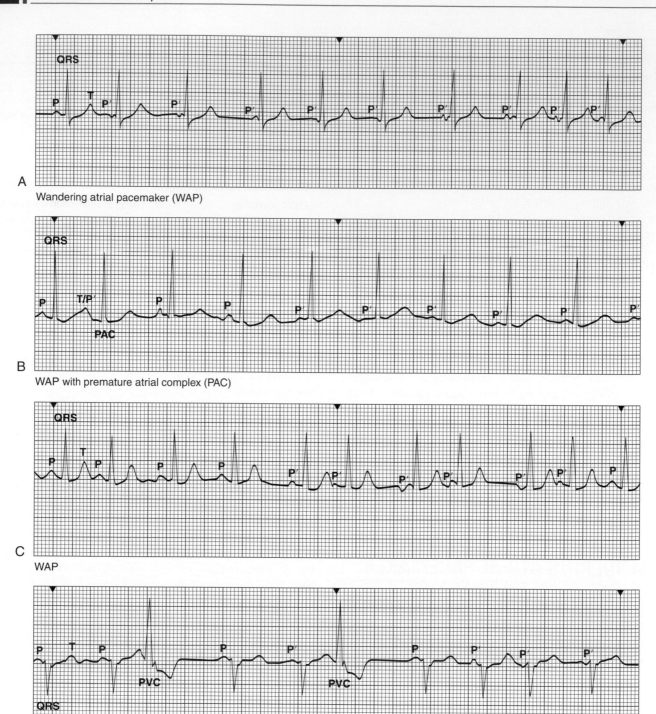

A
Wandering atrial pacemaker (WAP)

B
WAP with premature atrial complex (PAC)

C
WAP

D
WAP with premature ventricular complex (PVCs)*
*See Chapter 8, Ventricular Arrhythmias.

FIG. 6.2 Wandering atrial pacemaker.

QRS Complex

Normal unless a preexisting intraventricular conduction disturbance (such as a bundle-branch block) is present. A QRS complex follows each P or P′ wave.

Origin

The pacemaker site shifts back and forth between the SA node and one or more ectopic pacemaker sites in the atria.

Causes

A WAP may be a normal phenomenon seen in the very young, the elderly, or athletes. It most often occurs when respiration inhibits the effect of the vagal (parasympathetic) nerve on the SA node and AV junction. (A similar process occurs in sinus arrhythmia.) It may also be caused by administration of the drug digitalis.

Clinical Significance

A WAP is usually not clinically significant, and treatment is rarely indicated. When the heart rate slows excessively, the signs and symptoms, clinical significance, and management are the same as those in symptomatic sinus bradycardia.

ATRIAL TACHYCARDIA AND MULTI-FOCAL ATRIAL TACHYCARDIA

Rate	160–240 (half the rate if conduction ratio is 2:1); 100–150 for multifocal atrial tachycardia (MAT)
Regularity	Regular (usually); variable if conduction ratio changes
P wave	P′ waves are identical in atrial tachycardia. P′ waves vary in MAT.
PR interval	Normal in ectopic atrial tachycardia (0.12 to <0.20 sec); varies slightly in MAT
P-P, R-R intervals	Equal if AV conduction ratio is constant
Conduction ratio	1:1 (2:1 or higher if AV conduction block occurs)
QRS complex	Normal; wide if conduction delay exists
Origin	Atrial sites outside the SA node Called *MAT* when it originates in three or more ectopic sites

atrial tachycardia and multifocal atrial tachycardia (MAT)

Atrial tachycardia (Fig. 6.3) is a rhythm that originates in a single ectopic atrial site and has a rate of 160 to 240 beats/min. MAT is similar to WAP except that the rate is greater than 100. MAT differs from atrial tachycardia in that it originates in multiple ectopic sites in the atria. Both are caused by the increased automaticity of these ectopic atrial sites.

Characteristics

Rate

The rate is 160 to 240 beats/min for atrial tachycardia and 100 to 150 beats/min for MAT. The ventricular rate is usually the same as that of the atria, but if a 2:1 AV block is present, it will be half the atrial rate. Because atrial tachycardia usually starts and ends suddenly after a PAC, it is called *paroxysmal atrial tachycardia*. By definition, three or more consecutive PACs are considered to be atrial tachycardia.

Regularity

Regular if the AV conduction ratio is constant; variable if the AV conduction ratio changes.

P Wave

There are no normal P waves in atrial tachycardia because the ectopic P′ wave suppresses the normal automaticity of the SA node. The ectopic P′ wave in atrial tachycardia differs from normal sinus P waves. The P′ waves vary in size, shape, and direction, depending on the location of the pacemaker site. They may appear positive (upright) and quite normal in lead II if the pacemaker site is near the SA node but negative (inverted) if they originate near the AV junction. Regardless of their site of origin, the P′ waves in atrial tachycardia are all identical because the same site continues to generate the impulse at a high rate.

In ectopic atrial tachycardia, the P′ waves are usually identical and precede each QRS complex. In MAT, on the other hand, the P′ waves vary in size, shape, and direction because they arise from various ectopic sites. At least three different P′ waves must be present to classify the rhythm as MAT. They may be difficult to identify if they are buried in the preceding T wave or QRS complex.

> **AUTHOR'S NOTE** The distinguishing feature between atrial tachycardia and MAT is that the P′ waves are all identical in atrial tachycardia, whereas the P′ waves of MAT are not.

PR Interval

The PR interval is usually normal and constant in ectopic atrial tachycardia. In MAT, the PR interval usually varies slightly. It may vary from 0.20 second to less than 0.12 second, depending on the pacemaker site. If the impulse originating from the ectopic pacemaker reaches the AV node when it is refractory to depolarization, the impulse may be blocked. As a result, no QRS complex will follow. This pattern is referred to as *atrial tachycardia with block*.

P′-P′ and R-R Intervals

The P′-P′ and R-R intervals are equal if the AV conduction ratio is constant. But if the ratio varies (for example, 3:1, 2:1, 4:1, 3:1, and so forth), the R-R intervals will be unequal.

Conduction Ratio

In most patients with untreated atrial tachycardia not caused by digitalis intoxication, and in which the atrial rate is less than 200 beats/min, the AV conduction ratio is usually 1:1. When the atrial rate is greater than 200 beats/min, a 2:1 AV conduction ratio is common. When an AV block occurs during the tachycardia, the rhythm is called *atrial tachycardia with block*.

If the patient has a preexisting AV block because of cardiac disease or digitalis toxicity, or if drugs such as beta blockers or calcium-channel blockers have been administered, a 2:1 AV block may be present when the atrial rate is less than 200 beats/min. A higher-degree AV block (for example, 3:1, 4:1, and so forth) or a variable AV block may also occur, particularly in atrial tachycardia caused by digitalis toxicity.

QRS Complex

The QRS complex is normal unless a preexisting intraventricular conduction disturbance (such as a bundle-branch block), aberrant ventricular conduction, or ventricular preexcitation is

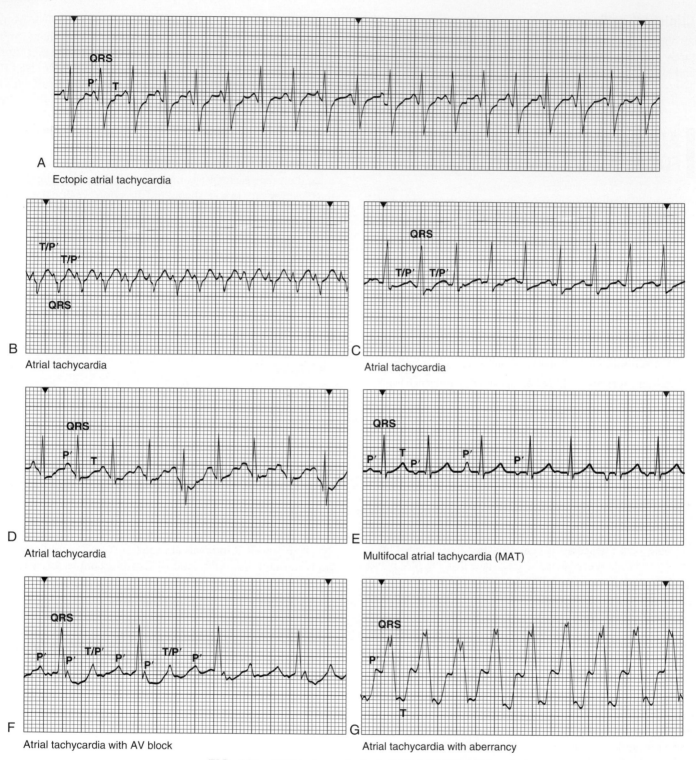

A   Ectopic atrial tachycardia

B   Atrial tachycardia

C   Atrial tachycardia

D   Atrial tachycardia

E   Multifocal atrial tachycardia (MAT)

F   Atrial tachycardia with AV block

G   Atrial tachycardia with aberrancy

FIG. 6.3   Atrial tachycardia (ectopic and multifocal).

present. If the QRS complex is abnormal only during the tachy-cardia, the arrhythmia is called *atrial tachycardia with aberrancy* (or *with aberrant ventricular conduction*). Atrial tachycardia with an abnormal QRS complex may resemble ventricular tachycardia (see Chapter 8).

Origin

Atrial tachycardia originates from an ectopic site in the atria—that is, any atrial site outside the SA node. When it originates in a single ectopic site, it is called *atrial tachycardia.* When it originates in three or more different ectopic atrial sites, it's called *MAT.* When atrial tachycardia occurs, the activity of the SA node is completely suppressed.

> **AUTHOR'S NOTE** Atrial tachycardia with aberrancy may mimic ventricular tachycardia.

Causes

Essentially the same as those of PACs. Like PACs, atrial tachycardia may occur in people with apparently healthy hearts or in those with diseased hearts.

Atrial tachycardia occurs in patients with the following conditions:

- Digitalis toxicity
- Acute alcohol toxicity
- Electrolyte disturbances
- Hypoxia
- Chronic lung disease
- Coronary artery disease (associated with ACS)
- Rheumatic heart disease

Atrial tachycardia caused by digitalis toxicity is often associated with either a 2:1 heart block or a varying AV block. Atrial tachycardia with AV block can also occur in patients with significant heart disease, such as coronary artery disease or lung disease, as a result of pathology in the atrial walls. MAT is most often associated with respiratory failure, as in decompensated chronic obstructive pulmonary disease (COPD).

Clinical Significance

The signs and symptoms of atrial tachycardia depend on the presence or absence of heart disease, the nature of the heart disease, the ventricular rate, and the duration of the rhythm disturbance. Atrial tachycardia is often accompanied by the perception of palpitations or feelings of nervousness or anxiety.

When the ventricular rate is very rapid, the ventricles are unable to fill completely during diastole, significantly reducing cardiac output and decreasing perfusion of the brain and other vital organs. Inadequate perfusion may cause confusion, dizziness, light-headedness, shortness of breath, near-syncope, or syncope.

In addition, because a rapid heart rate increases the workload of the heart, the oxygen requirements of the myocardium are usually increased in atrial tachycardia. As a result, in addition to the consequences of decreased cardiac output, atrial tachycardia in the setting of ACS may increase myocardial ischemia and the frequency and severity of chest pain, extend the size of the infarct, precipitate congestive heart failure, cause hypotension and cardiogenic shock, or predispose the patient to serious ventricular dysrhythmias.

Symptomatic atrial tachycardia must be treated promptly. Treatment is aimed at reversing the consequences of the reduced cardiac output and increased workload of the heart and preventing serious ventricular dysrhythmias. As noted earlier, atrial tachycardia with a wide QRS complex may resemble ventricular tachycardia. A 12-lead ECG may be useful in diagnosing this rhythm by detecting ectopic P waves in leads V_1, V_2, or MCL_1.

ATRIAL FLUTTER

> **atrial flutter**
>
> Atrial flutter (Figs. 6.4 and 6.5) is a rhythm arising in an ectopic atrial pacemaker as a result of increased automaticity or a rapid reentry circuit in the atria. It is characterized by rapid atrial flutter (F) waves, which have a sawtooth appearance and a slower, more regular ventricular response rate.

Characteristics

Rate	Atrial: 240–360 beats/min
	Ventricular: Half the atrial rate or less
Regularity	Regular if conduction ratio is constant
	Irregular if conduction ratio is variable
P wave	Normal P wave absent
	F waves (sawtooth) present
FR interval	FR interval is difficult to measure.
P-P, R-R intervals	No P-P intervals
	R-R intervals are equal unless the conduction ratio changes.
Conduction ratio	Usually 2:1, 3:1, or 4:1; rarely 1:1
QRS complex	Normal; wide if conduction delay exists

Rate

The rate of atrial flutter depends on the conduction ratio between the atria and ventricles. With a 1:1 conduction ratio, the resulting rate may be between 240 and 360 (average 300) beats/min. In uncontrolled (untreated) atrial flutter, the ventricular rate is usually about 150 beats/min (half the atrial rate) because of a 2:1 AV block. In controlled (treated) atrial flutter, or when this pattern occurs in a patient with a preexisting AV block, the ventricular rate is usually 60 to 75 beats/min. When the ventricular rate is greater than 100, the rhythm is referred to as *atrial flutter with rapid ventricular response (RVR).* When the ventricular rate is slower than 60, the rhythm is referred to as *atrial flutter with slow ventricular response (SVR).*

Regularity

Regular when the AV conduction is constant. Irregularly irregular when the AV conduction is variable.

P Wave

As discussed in Chapter 4, the P wave can assume many shapes. In atrial flutter, the ectopic atrial pacemaker fires rapidly, creating a waveform with a characteristic sawtooth pattern. This is called the *F wave,* which usually occurs at a rate of about 300 impulses per minute.

F Wave

The F wave represents depolarization of the atria in an abnormal direction, followed by atrial repolarization. Atrial depolarization

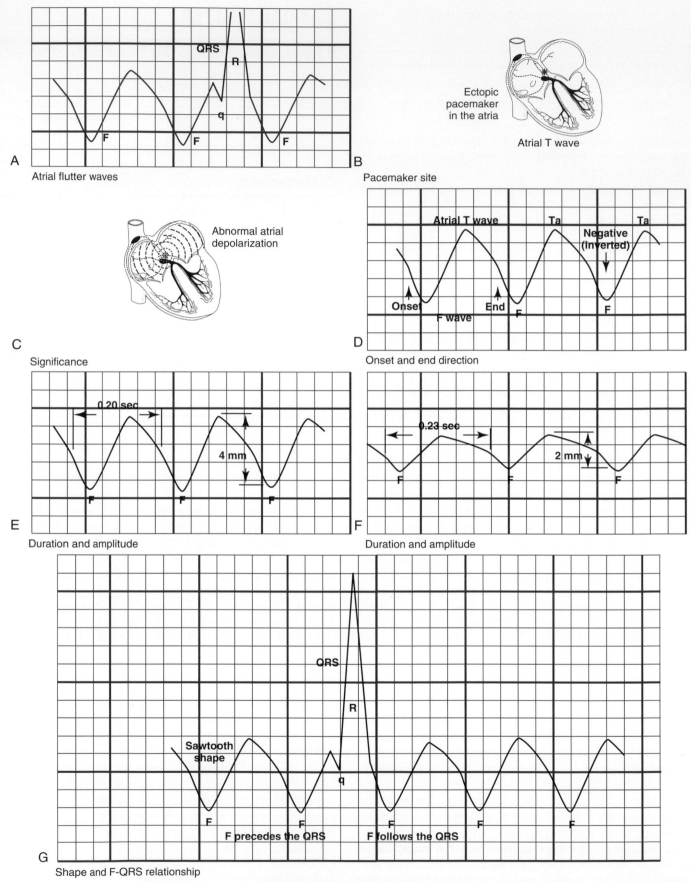

FIG. 6.4 Atrial flutter F waves.

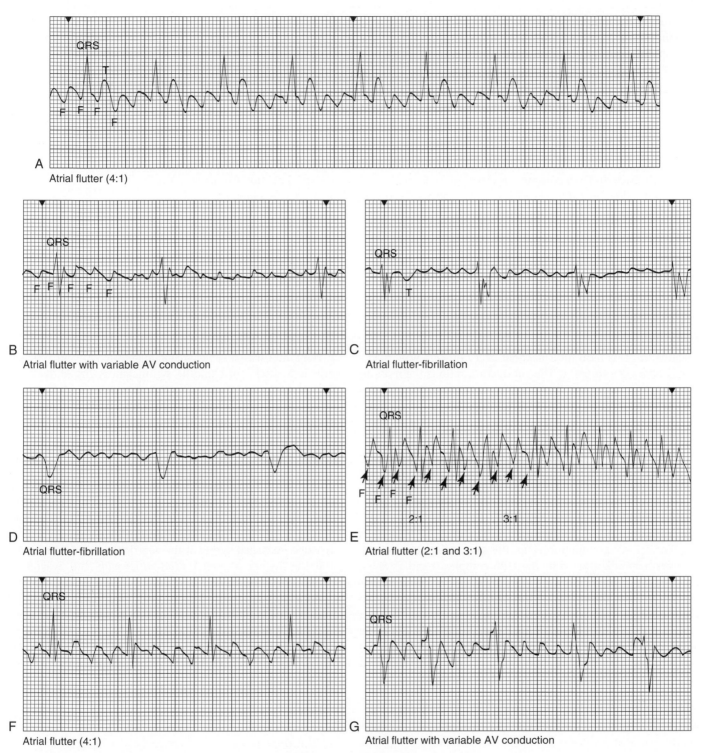

FIG. 6.5 Atrial flutter.

usually begins near the AV node and progresses across the atria in a retrograde direction. The following features are characteristic of F waves:

- **Onset and end:** Cannot be determined with certainty.
- **Shape:** The F wave has a jagged, zigzag appearance, like the edge of a serrated knife. A typical F wave viewed in lead II consists of a negative (inverted) deflection, representing an

abnormal wave of atrial depolarization, followed by a slower, positive (upright) deflection, representing atrial repolarization. An isoelectric line is seldom present between the waves. The first downward part of the F wave is typically shorter and more abrupt than the second upward part. F waves are generally identical in shape and size in any given lead but may vary slightly.

- **Duration:** Varies according to rate.
- **Amplitude:** Measured from peak to peak of the F wave, the amplitude can vary from less than 1 mm to more than 5 mm but is usually consistent in any given instance.

> **AUTHOR'S NOTE** Atrial fibrillation may occur during atrial flutter, and vice versa. Such a mixture of atrial fibrillation and flutter is called *atrial fib-flutter.*

- **Relationship to QRS complex.** F waves precede, are buried in, and follow the QRS complexes. They may also be superimposed on the T waves or ST segments.
- **FR interval.** Difficult to measure and irrelevant to interpretation.

R-R Interval

Equal if the AV conduction ratio is constant. Unequal if the AV conduction ratio varies.

Conduction Ratio

Usually 2:1. This ratio indicates that every other F wave is followed by a QRS complex. The conduction ratio is the result of the long refractory period of the AV junction, which prevents the conduction of all the rapid atrial impulses into the ventricles. This is an example of an *AV block.*

The AV block is either fixed at 2:1, 3:1, or 4:1 (or greater), or it may be variable, depending on the influence of the vagus nerve (parasympathetic tone) or if the patient is on medications such as digitalis, beta blockers, or calcium-channel blockers.

However, the AV conduction ratio is usually constant, producing a regular ventricular rhythm. If the AV conduction ratio varies, the ventricular rhythm will be irregular. When there is a 2:1 or 1:1 AV conduction ratio, the sawtooth pattern of the F waves may be distorted by the QRS complexes and T waves, making the F waves difficult to recognize. If a complete AV block is present, the atria and ventricles beat independently, and there is no set relationship between the F waves and the QRS complexes. This is referred to as *AV dissociation* because the atrial and ventricular rate are dissociated from (not related to) one another. The AV conduction ratio in new-onset untreated atrial flutter is usually 2:1.

QRS Complex

Normal except in the presence of a preexisting intraventricular conduction disturbance (such as a bundle-branch block), aberrant ventricular conduction, or ventricular preexcitation.

> **AUTHOR'S NOTE** Atrial flutter with rapid ventricular response and aberrant ventricular conduction may resemble ventricular tachycardia.

Origin

Atrial flutter originates in an atrial site outside the SA node, usually located low in the atria near the AV node. Atrial flutter completely suppresses the activity of the SA node.

Causes

Chronic (persistent) atrial flutter is seen most often in middle-aged and older adults with the following conditions:
- Mitral and/or tricuspid valvular stenosis
- Coronary heart disease
- High blood pressure

Transient (paroxysmal) atrial flutter usually indicates that the patient has heart disease; however, it can occur in healthy people. This rhythm is often associated with the following:
- Disease of the cardiac muscle
- Atrial dilation from any cause
- Hyperthyroidism
- Digitalis toxicity
- Low blood oxygen level
- Acute or chronic cor pulmonale
- Congestive heart failure
- Damage to the SA node or atria as a result of pericarditis or myocarditis
- Alcoholism

Clinical Significance

Atrial flutter with a ventricular rate between 60 and 100 beats/min is in itself not clinically significant. Atrial flutter at this ventricular rate is referred to as *controlled atrial flutter.* The signs, symptoms, and clinical significance of atrial flutter with a slow (less than 60 beats/min) ventricular response are related to the slow rate and possible effect on cardiac output, as seen with symptomatic bradycardia.

When the ventricular rate is very rapid, the ventricles are unable to fill completely during diastole, significantly reducing cardiac output and decreasing perfusion (blood flow) to the brain and other vital organs. Inadequate perfusion may cause confusion, dizziness, light-headedness, shortness of breath, near-syncope, or syncope. As stated earlier, if the ventricular rate is greater than 100, the rhythm is termed *atrial flutter with RVR,* whereas the clinical condition is referred to as *uncontrolled atrial flutter.*

In addition, because a rapid heart rate increases the workload of the heart, the oxygen requirements of the heart muscle are usually increased in atrial flutter with RVR. As a result, in addition to the consequences of decreased cardiac output, atrial flutter in the setting of ACS may further reduce blood flow to the heart muscle, with the following consequences:
- Episodes of angina (chest pain) may be more frequent and severe.
- A larger area of tissue may be damaged.
- This rhythm may precipitate congestive heart failure.
- The patient may have hypotension and experience cardiogenic shock, or he or she may be predisposed to developing serious ventricular dysrhythmias.

Regardless of the ventricular response rate, people with atrial flutter are at risk of developing thrombi (clots), which form on the walls of the atria. Small portions of these clots may break free and travel to the brain, causing a stroke.

Symptomatic atrial flutter must be treated promptly. Treatment is aimed at reducing the ventricular response by administering medications that decrease the conduction ratio to 3:1 or 4:1.

ATRIAL FIBRILLATION

> **atrial fibrillation**
>
> Atrial fibrillation (Figs. 6.6 and 6.7) is a rhythm arising in multiple ectopic atrial sites as a result of increased automaticity or rapid reentry circuits in the atria. It is characterized by very rapid atrial fibrillation (f) waves and an irregularly (totally) irregular ventricular response.

Characteristics

Rate	Atrial: 350–600 beats/min
	Ventricular:
	< 60 (slow ventricular response)
	<100 (controlled ventricular response)
	>100 (rapid or uncontrolled ventricular response)
Regularity	Totally (irregularly) irregular
P wave	Normal P waves absent
	f waves present
PR interval	Absent
P-P, R-R intervals	P-P absent
	R-R unequal
Conduction ratio	Random
QRS complex	Normal; wide if conduction delay exists
Pattern	Can be isolated or occur in group beats or repetitive beats
Origin	Atrial sites outside the SA node

Rate

Typically, the atrial rate is 350 to 600 (average 400) beats/min, but it can be as high as 700. However, because of this extremely fast rate, it is impossible to estimate from the ECG. The ventricular rate is usually greater than 100 beats/min and is often about 160 to 180 (or as high as 200) beats/min in an uncontrolled atrial fibrillation. The ventricular rate is less than 100 beats/min in a controlled one or when it occurs in a heart with a preexisting AV block. When the ventricular rate is greater than 100 beats/min, it is referred to as *atrial fibrillation with RVR* or, more simply, *a-fib with RVR*. When the rate is less than 60 beats/min, it is referred to as *atrial fibrillation with SVR*.

Regularity

Totally (irregularly) irregular.

P Wave

As discussed in Chapter 4, there are no normal P waves in atrial fibrillation. Instead, the chaotic rapid firing of the multiple ectopic atrial sites results in the characteristic f wave.

f Wave

The f waves seen in atrial fibrillation represent abnormal, chaotic (disorganized), incomplete depolarization of small individual groups of atrial muscle fibers called *islets*. Normal P waves are absent because impulses from the atrial sites suppress the SA node. Characteristics of f waves include the following:

- **Onset and end:** Cannot be determined with certainty.
- **Shape:** Irregular, rounded (or pointed), and dissimilar, varying randomly from positive (upright) to negative (inverted).
- **Duration:** Varies greatly and cannot be accurately determined.
- **Amplitude:** Usually 1 to 2 mm. If the f waves are small (less than 1 mm), they are called *fine fibrillatory waves;* if they are large (1 mm or greater), they are called *coarse fibrillatory waves.* If the f waves are so small or fine that they are not recorded, the sections of the ECG between the QRS complexes may appear as a wavy or flat (isoelectric) line.
- **Relationship to QRS complex.** The f waves precede, are buried in, and follow the QRS complexes and are superimposed on the ST segments and T waves.

R-R Interval

The R-R intervals are typically unequal. When no impulse is transmitted through the AV node, complete AV dissociation is present. Consequently, a junctional or ventricular escape rhythm may be present, resulting in a regular R-R interval.

Conduction Ratio

In atrial fibrillation, less than one-half, and often less than one-third, of the atrial electrical impulses are conducted through the AV junction into the ventricles. Conduction occurs randomly. This results in a totally or irregularly irregular ventricular rhythm. Remember, the AV junction has a long refractory period, which prevents the conduction of all the rapid atrial impulses into the ventricles. When more than 100 QRS complexes per minute are conducted, the rhythm is called *uncontrolled atrial fibrillation* or *atrial fibrillation with RVR.* When fewer than 100 QRS complexes per minute are conducted, the rhythm is termed *controlled atrial fibrillation.*

QRS Complex

The QRS complexes are normal unless a preexisting intraventricular conduction disturbance (such as a bundle-branch block), aberrant ventricular conduction, or ventricular preexcitation is present. Atrial fibrillation with RVR and abnormal QRS complexes may resemble ventricular tachycardia but can usually be differentiated by its total irregularity.

Origin

Atrial fibrillation originates from multiple ectopic sites in the atria, generating electrical impulses chaotically.

Causes

Atrial fibrillation is associated with the following:
- Mitral valve disease
- Coronary heart disease (with or without acute myocardial infarction)
- High blood pressure
- Hyperthyroidism

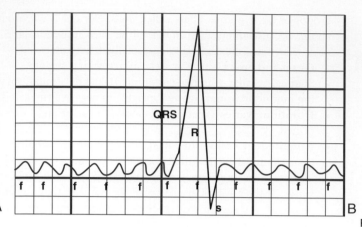

A

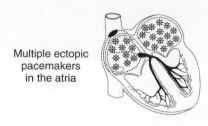

Multiple ectopic
pacemakers
in the atria

B Pacemaker site

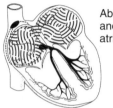

Abnormal chaotic
and incomplete
atrial depolarizations

C
Significance

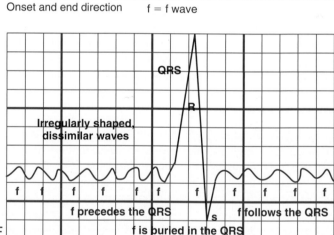

D
Onset and end direction   f = f wave

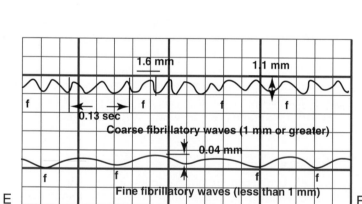

E
Duration and amplitude

F
Shape and f-QRS relationship

FIG. 6.6 Atrial fibrillation f waves.

Less often, atrial fibrillation may occur in the following:
- Disease of the cardiac muscle
- Acute myocarditis and pericarditis
- Chest trauma
- Lung disease
- Digitalis toxicity

Whatever the underlying form of heart disease, atrial fibrillation is often associated with congestive heart failure. In some cases, atrial fibrillation may occur in healthy people after excessive ingestion of alcohol or caffeine, during periods of emotional stress, and/or without any apparent cause.

> **AUTHOR'S NOTE** Atrial fibrillation may be intermittent, or it may be chronic (persistent). It can even occur in short bursts called *paroxysms*, similar to those that occur in PSVT.

Clinical Significance

The signs, symptoms, and clinical significance of atrial fibrillation with RVR are the same as those of atrial tachycardia and atrial flutter with RVR.

When the ventricular rate is very rapid, the ventricles are unable to fill completely during diastole. This significantly reduces

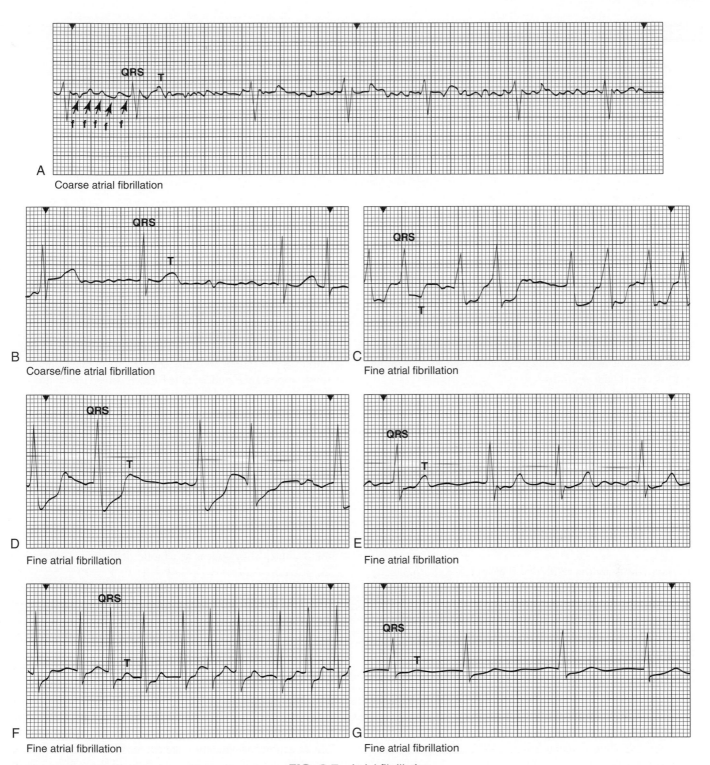

FIG. 6.7 Atrial fibrillation.

cardiac output and decreases perfusion of the brain and other vital organs. Inadequate perfusion may cause confusion, dizziness, light-headedness, shortness of breath, near-syncope, or syncope.

In addition, because a rapid heart rate increases the workload of the heart, the oxygen requirements of the myocardium are usually increased. As a result, in addition to the consequences of decreased cardiac output, uncontrolled atrial fibrillation in the setting of ACS may have the following effects:

- Episodes of chest pain may be more frequent and severe.
- A larger area of tissue may be damaged.
- This rhythm may precipitate heart failure.

TABLE 6.1	Typical ECG Features of Atrial Rhythms				
Rhythm	**Ventricular Rate (beats/min)**	**Rhythm**	**P Wave**	**P'R Interval**	**QRS Complex**[a]
Wandering atrial pacemaker	60–100	Slightly irregular	Varies from normal to inverted	Varies from 0.20 to 0.12 sec	Normal
Atrial tachycardia	160–240	Regular	Normal or abnormal At least three forms in MAT	Normal, constant (varying from 0.2 to ≤0.12 sec in MAT)	Normal
Atrial flutter	60–150	Usually regular; may be irregular if conduction ratio changes	Atrial flutter F waves	None	Normal
Atrial fibrillation	Atrial: 350–600 Ventricular: <100 (controlled) >100 (uncontrolled)	Totally irregular	Atrial fibrillation f waves (sawtooth appearance)	None	Normal

MAT, Multifocal atrial tachycardia.
[a]Unless a preexisting intraventricular conduction disturbance, such as a bundle-branch block, is present.

• The patient may have hypotension and experience cardiogenic shock, or he or she may be predisposed to developing serious ventricular rhythms.

Symptomatic atrial fibrillation must be treated promptly. Treatment is aimed at slowing the AV conduction to the ventricles and slowing the rate.

Patients with atrial fibrillation, regardless of ventricular response rate, are at significant risk of developing thrombi (clots), which form on the walls of the atria. Small portions of these clots may break free and travel to the brain, causing a stroke.

TAKE-HOME POINTS

• Atrial rhythms are the result of either increased automaticity or a reentry phenomenon that causes an ectopic pacemaker in the atria to fire. The result can be as benign as a single PAC or as malignant as atrial fibrillation with RVR.
• When the atrial site of the P wave fluctuates but the rate of the rhythm remains less than 100, the patient has a WAP rhythm.
• If the rate exceeds 100, the rhythm is termed *MAT.* If the atrial site of the P wave remains the same but is not in the SA node, atrial tachycardia exists.
• A PAC is an extra P-QRS-T complex occurring sooner than expected. It is differentiated from a PVC by a noncompensatory pause.
• A noncompensatory pause is present when the R-R interval of the premature beat and the subsequent beat is less than twice the R-R interval preceding the premature beat. A noncompensatory pause indicates that the SA node was reset by the premature beat.

• When an ectopic atrial site generates regularly occurring impulses at a rate of 300/min, the waveform takes on a sawtooth appearance and is called the *F wave.* This pattern is characteristic of atrial flutter.
• Because the AV node is unable to conduct every impulse that makes up an F wave, the resulting ventricular response rate is a ratio of the F waves to the QRS complexes. A ratio of 2:1 would result in a heart rate of 150 beats/min and could manifest with signs and symptoms of shock. This ratio is common with untreated, new-onset atrial flutter. The ratio can remain fixed or may vary.
• In atrial fibrillation, multiple ectopic atrial sites generate impulses at a rate as high as 700 but usually at a rate of about 400/minute. They appear as chaotic deflections, referred to as *f waves.*
• As in atrial flutter, in atrial fibrillation, the AV node is unable to conduct all the impulses it receives. However, unlike atrial flutter, the conduction ratio varies from beat to beat, resulting in a characteristic ventricular response that is totally (irregularly) irregular.
• When the ventricular response is greater than 100/minute, the rhythm is referred to as *uncontrolled atrial fibrillation* or *atrial fibrillation with RVR.*
• The primary concern when addressing a patient with an atrial rhythm is the resulting heart rate and cardiac output. Shock can occur when the rate exceeds 150 beats/minute or when the conduction ratio is so great that the resulting heart rate is too slow.
• Patients with atrial flutter and atrial fibrillation are at increased risk of stroke.
• Table 6.1 summarizes the characteristics of the various atrial rhythms discussed in this chapter.

CHAPTER REVIEW QUESTIONS

1. Which rhythm originates in multiple pacemaker sites and shifts back and forth among them?
   A. Alternating atrial flutter
   B. Atrial fibrillation
   C. Supraventricular tachycardia
   D. WAP

2. WAP may be a normal phenomenon seen in which patient population?
   A. Patients with acute myocardial infarction
   B. Patients with digitalis toxicity
   C. Smokers
   D. The very young

3. Which term describes an extra atrial complex consisting of a positive P wave in lead II followed by a normal or abnormal QRS complex that occurs before the next beat of the underlying rhythm?
   A. PAC
   B. Premature junctional contraction
   C. Premature ventricular contraction
   D. Intraventricular conduction delay

4. A nonconducted or blocked PAC often causes which artifact on the ECG?
   A. A distorted T wave
   B. The absence of a QRS complex after a P′ wave
   C. A short PR interval
   D. A bizarre-looking QRS complex

5. Which of the following best describes the QRS complex of a PAC?
   A. Resembles left bundle-branch block
   B. Can be mistaken for PVC
   C. Mimics right bundle-branch block
   D. Mirrors the underlying rhythm

6. Which term describes two PACs in a row?
   A. Atrial tachycardia
   B. A couplet
   C. A nonconducted PAC
   D. Bigeminy

7. Which term describes a rhythm originating in an ectopic atrial pacemaker and characterized by an atrial rate of between 160 and 240 beats/min and differing P waves?
   A. Atrial flutter
   B. Atrial tachycardia
   C. Junctional tachycardia
   D. Sinus tachycardia

8. Which of the following causes the symptoms associated with atrial tachycardia?
   A. Drug toxicity
   B. Increased vagal tone
   C. Palpitations
   D. Reduced cardiac output

9. Which of the following characterizes atrial flutter?
   A. An atrial rate of between 160 and 240 beats/min
   B. An atrial rate slower than the ventricular rate
   C. Varying and chaotic flutter waves
   D. Waves with a sawtooth appearance

10. Which rhythm is characterized by numerous dissimilar and chaotic atrial waves occurring at 350 or more beats/min?
    A. Atrial fibrillation
    B. Atrial flutter
    C. Ectopic atrial tachycardia
    D. Multifocal atrial tachycardia

7 — Junctional Rhythms

PREMATURE JUNCTIONAL COMPLEX

premature junctional complex (PJC)

A normal or abnormal QRS complex, with or without an inverted P wave, that originates from within the atrioventricular (AV) junction and occurs prematurely before the next expected beat of the underlying rhythm (Fig. 7.1). If a P wave is present, it may precede or follow the QRS complex. It is followed by a noncompensatory pause.

Characteristics

Rate	Underlying rhythm
Regularity	Irregular in the section encompassing the premature junctional complex (PJC)
P wave	P′ wave before or after QRS P′ may be absent.
PR interval	P′R interval less than 0.12 sec
P-P, R-R intervals	Compensatory pause present P-P′ and R-R interval encompassing the PJC is 2 times the R-R interval of the underlying rhythm.
Conduction ratio	1:1
QRS complex	Normal; wide if conduction delay exists
Origin	Ectopic pacemaker in AV junction

Rate

That of the underlying rhythm.

Regularity

Irregular over the segment encompassing the PJC.

P Wave

If present, it is a P′ wave, varying in size, shape, and direction from a normal P wave. The P′ wave may precede, be buried in, or follow the QRS complex of the PJC (Table 7.1).

A P′ wave that occurs before the QRS complex most likely originated in the proximal, upper part of the AV junction. A P′ wave that occurs during or after the QRS complex probably originated in the middle or distal part of the AV junction. If the PJC occurs very soon after the previous complex, the P′ may be buried in and distort the T wave, creating a T/P wave. If the P′ wave follows the QRS complex, it is usually buried in the ST segment.

Atrial depolarization occurs in a retrograde fashion. In other words, it moves backward through the conduction system from the AV node. The P′ wave that precedes or follows the QRS complex is therefore negative (inverted) in lead II. The P′ wave may be absent. The absence of a P′ wave indicates one of two circumstances:

1. Retrograde atrial depolarization occurred during the QRS complex.
2. Atrial depolarization did not occur because a retrograde AV block prevented the impulse from reaching the atria. This AV block would be located between the ectopic pacemaker site in the AV junction and the atria.

PR Interval

A P′R interval exists if the P′ precedes the QRS. An RP′ interval exists if the P′ follows the QRS. Both result in an interval of less than 0.12 second in duration.

104

R-R Interval

The R-R interval is unequal when PJCs are present. The interval between the PJC and the preceding QRS complex is shorter than the R-R interval of the underlying rhythm. A compensatory pause ordinarily follows a PJC. That's because the PJC does not depolarize the sinoatrial (SA) node and rest it. The beat following the PJC occurs when it normally should. Therefore the R-R interval encompassing the PJC is two times the R-R interval of the underlying rhythm. (See the discussion of compensatory and noncompensatory pauses under Premature Atrial Complexes.)

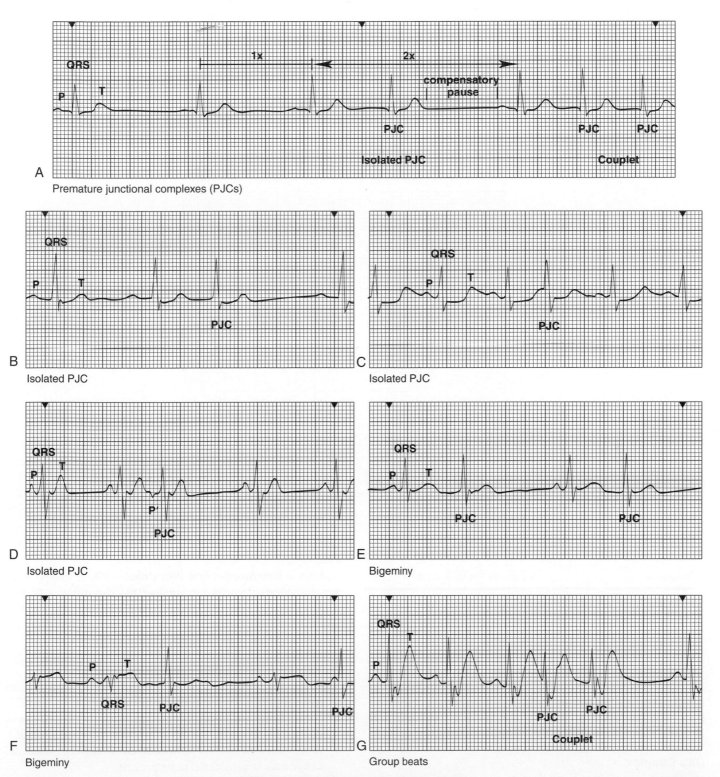

FIG. 7.1 Premature junctional complexes.

Continued

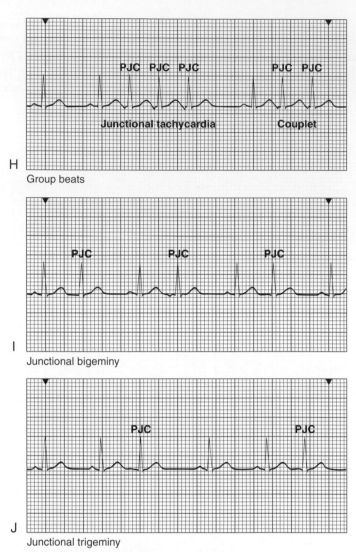

FIG. 7.1 cont'd

TABLE **7.1**	Relationship of P′ Wave to the QRS Complex[a]
Origin of the PJC Within the AV Junction	**Location of P′ Wave**
Upper part	Precedes the QRS complex
Middle or distal part	Is buried in the QRS complex
Distal part	Follows the QRS complex

AV, Atrioventricular; *PJC,* premature junctional complex.
[a]Depends on the PJC's site of origin.

Conduction Ratio

The impulse causing the PJC originates above the ventricles. It is conducted down the bundle of His, resulting in ventricular depolarization. This is a 1:1 ratio. A QRS complex usually follows each premature P′ wave (conducted PJC), but it may be absent if a complete AV block is present (nonconducted PJC).

QRS Complex

Usually resembles that of the underlying rhythm. If the site within the AV junction discharges too soon after the preceding QRS complex, the bundle branches may not respond to the electrical impulse of the PJC. As a result, the electrical impulse may be conducted down only one bundle branch—usually the left one. This produces a wide and bizarre-appearing QRS complex that resembles a right bundle-branch block (see Chapter 13).

Such a bizarre-appearing PJC, called a *PJC with aberrancy* (or *with aberrant ventricular conduction*), can mimic a premature ventricular complex (PVC). That's because both the PJC and the PVC are characterized by a compensatory pause (see Premature Ventricular Complex).

Frequency of Occurrence and Pattern

The following are the various forms in which PJCs may appear:
- **Isolated**: PJC occurs singly.
- **Group beats**: PJCs occur in groups of two or more beats in succession. A set of two PJCs in a row is called a *couplet.* When three or more PJCs occur consecutively, *junctional tachycardia* is considered to be present.
- **Repetitive beats**: PJCs may alternate with the QRS complexes of the underlying rhythm *(bigeminy)* or occur after

every two QRS complexes *(trigeminy)* or after every three QRS complexes *(quadrigeminy)*.

Origin

Within the AV junction.

Causes

Occasional PJCs may occur in a healthy person without apparent cause. Common causes of PJCs include the following:

- Digitalis toxicity (most common cause)
- Excessive dose of certain cardiac drugs, such as quinidine and procainamide
- Excessive dose of sympathomimetic drugs, such as epinephrine, isoproterenol, and norepinephrine
- Hypoxia
- Congestive heart failure
- Coronary artery disease (especially after a myocardial infarction [MI])

Clinical Significance

Isolated PJCs are not significant. However, if digitalis is being administered, PJCs may indicate digitalis toxicity and enhanced automaticity of the AV junction. Frequent PJCs—more than four to six per minute—may indicate an enhanced automaticity or a reentry mechanism in the AV junction. Such a condition warns of the potential for more serious dysrhythmias.

JUNCTIONAL ESCAPE RHYTHM

junctional escape rhythm

Originates from a pacemaker site within the AV junction and has a rate of 40 to 60 beats/min (Fig. 7.2). When fewer than three consecutive QRS complexes arising from the escape pacemaker are present, they are called *junctional escape beats* or *junctional escape complexes*.

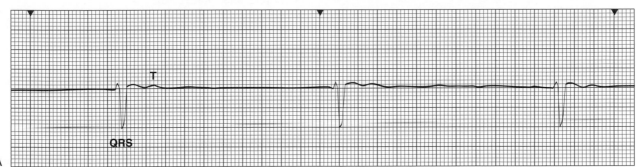

A Junctional escape rhythm

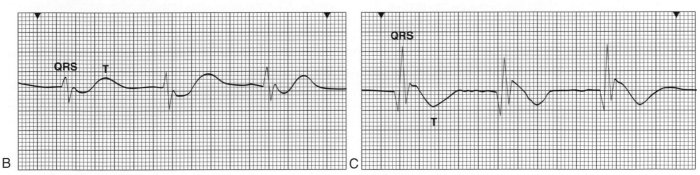

B Junctional escape rhythm

C Junctional escape rhythm with bundle branch block

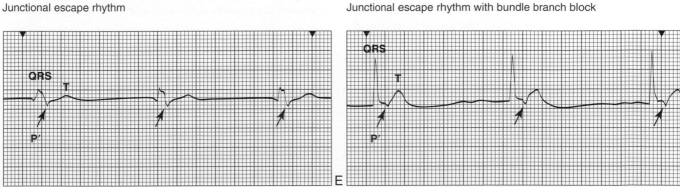

D Junctional escape rhythm with retrograde P wave

E Junctional escape rhythm

FIG. 7.2 Junctional escape rhythm.

Characteristics

Rate	40–60
Regularity	Regular
P wave	P′ waves before or after QRS P′ may be absent.
PR interval	P′R interval less than 0.12 sec
P-P, R-R intervals	R-R intervals equal
Conduction ratio	1:1
QRS complex	Normal; wide if conduction delay exists
Origin	Ectopic pacemaker in AV junction

Rate

Usually 40 to 60 beats/min, but it may be less.

Regularity

The ventricular rhythm is essentially regular.

P Wave

Normal P waves are absent. When the electrical impulses arise in the AV junction, the atria depolarize in a retrograde manner. The P′ wave is therefore negative (inverted) in lead II. If the P′ waves regularly precede or follow the QRS complex and are identical to one another, the electrical impulse originated in an ectopic pacemaker site of the AV junction.

The P′ wave may be buried in the QRS complex and therefore difficult to see. When a junctional escape rhythm is present with a complete AV block, normal sinus P waves (upright) may be present. When this occurs, the sinus P waves have no relationship to the QRS complexes. The rate of the P waves will typically be faster than the ventricular rate of the junctional escape rhythm. This constitutes a *complete (third-degree) heart block*. See Chapter 9.

PR Interval

Less than 0.12 second, regardless of whether the P′ wave precedes or follows the QRS complex.

R-R Interval

The R-R intervals are equal.

Conduction Ratio

The impulse causing the QRS originates above the ventricles and is conducted down the bundle of His, resulting in ventricular depolarization. This is a 1:1 ratio. The presence of a junctional escape rhythm indicates, however, that there is either a complete AV block or a failure of the SA node or any atrial pacemaker site to generate an impulse.

QRS Complex

Normal unless a preexisting intraventricular conduction disturbance (such as a bundle-branch block) is present. A junctional escape rhythm with abnormal QRS complexes may resemble a ventricular escape rhythm. Three or more consecutive junctional escape complexes must be present to constitute a junctional escape rhythm.

Origin

A pacemaker site within the AV junction.

Causes

Generally, when an electrical impulse fails to arrive at the AV junction within about 1 to 1.5 seconds, the escape pacemaker in the AV junction begins to generate electrical impulses. These signals fire at a rate of 40 to 60 beats/min. The result is one or more junctional escape beats or a junctional escape rhythm.

A junctional escape rhythm is a normal response of the AV junction under the following circumstances:

- The rate of impulse formation of the dominant SA node pacemaker drops below that of the escape pacemaker in the AV junction, which is typically 40 to 60 beats/min.
  OR
- The electrical impulses from the SA node or atria fail to reach the AV junction because of sinus arrest, SA exit block, or third-degree AV block.

A junctional escape rhythm often occurs in the following clinical conditions:

- Severe sinus bradycardia
- Sinus arrest
- SA exit block
- High-grade second-degree AV block
- Third-degree AV block
- High level of potassium in the blood (hyperkalemia)
- Drugs: beta blocker, calcium-channel blocker, or digoxin poisoning

Clinical Significance

The signs, symptoms, and clinical significance of a junctional escape rhythm are similar to those of symptomatic sinus bradycardia. A junctional escape rhythm is often seen after successful cardiac arrest resuscitation because it is one of the first pacemakers to "awaken" after a prolonged period without organized electrical activity in the heart. However, because of its relatively slow rate and the fact that the resulting rate would be even slower if it should fail, prompt therapy must be instituted to prevent cardiovascular collapse. Treatment is aimed at increasing the rate of the ectopic pacemaker and addressing any associated hypotension.

A junctional escape rhythm may also be seen with new-onset third-degree heart block. The patient may or may not have symptoms. Treatment will be guided by the underlying cause but often involves the placement of an internal electronic pacemaker.

NONPAROXYSMAL JUNCTIONAL TACHYCARDIA (ACCELERATED JUNCTIONAL RHYTHM, JUNCTIONAL TACHYCARDIA)

nonparoxysmal junctional tachycardia

A regular rhythm originating within the AV junction (Fig. 7.3) with a rate of 60 to 150 beats/min. It includes accelerated junctional rhythm and junctional tachycardia.

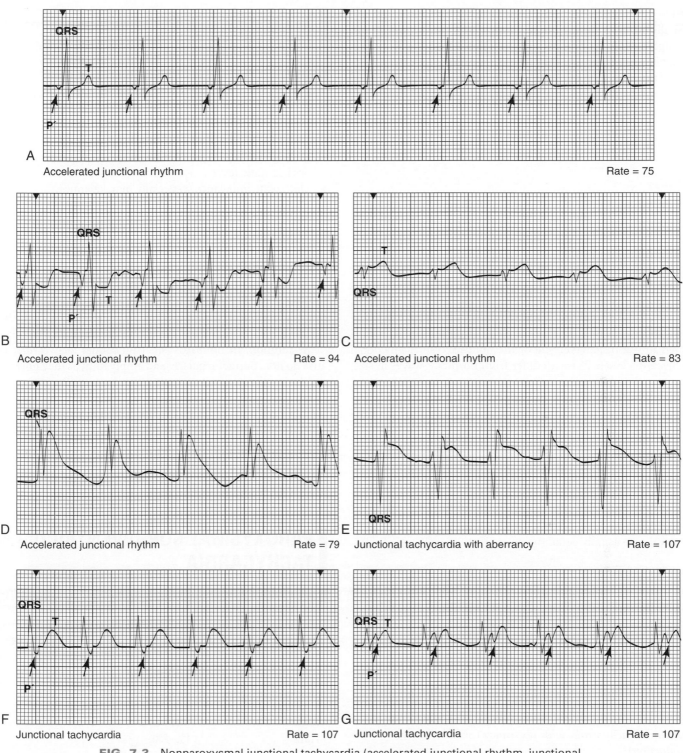

FIG. 7.3 Nonparoxysmal junctional tachycardia (accelerated junctional rhythm, junctional tachycardia).

Characteristics

Rate	60–100: accelerated junctional rhythm
	Greater than 100: junctional tachycardia
Regularity	Regular
P wave	P′ waves before or after QRS
	P′ may be absent.

PR interval	P′R intervals less than 0.12 sec
P-P, R-R intervals	R-R intervals equal
Conduction ratio	1:1
QRS complex	Normal; wide if conduction delay exists
Origin	Ectopic pacemaker in AV junction

Rate

Usually 60 to 130 beats/min, but it may be greater than 130 and as high as 150. Nonparoxysmal junctional tachycardia with a rate between 60 and 100 beats/min is called *accelerated junctional rhythm*. If the rate is greater than 100 beats/min, it's called *junctional tachycardia*. The onset and termination of nonparoxysmal junctional tachycardia are gradual.

Regularity

The rhythm is essentially regular.

P Wave

A normal sinus P wave is usually absent. If present, it may have no relation to the QRS complex, appearing independently at a rate (usually) faster than that of the QRS complex. This constitutes a *complete (third-degree) heart block*.

Instead, P′ waves are seen. When the electrical impulses arise in the AV junction, the atria depolarize in a retrograde manner. The P′ waves are therefore negative (inverted) in lead II. P′ waves that are identical and regularly precede or follow the QRS complexes indicate that the electrical impulses have originated in the pacemaker site of the nonparoxysmal junctional tachycardia. Such P′ waves differ from normal P waves in size, shape, and direction.

P′ waves are not seen in nonparoxysmal junctional tachycardia if they occur during (and thus are buried in) the QRS complexes.

PR Interval

Less than 0.12 second, regardless of whether the P′ wave precedes or follows the QRS complex.

R-R Interval

Intervals are usually equal to one another.

Conduction Ratio

The impulse causing the QRS complexes originates above the ventricles and is conducted down the bundle of His, depolarizing the ventricles. This is a 1:1 ratio.

QRS Complex

Normal unless a preexisting intraventricular conduction disturbance (such as a bundle-branch block) or aberrant ventricular conduction is present. If abnormal QRS complexes occur only when junctional tachycardia is present, the rhythm is called *junctional tachycardia with aberrancy* (or *aberrant ventricular conduction*).

If the rate is 60 to 100 beats/min (accelerated junctional rhythm), nonparoxysmal junctional tachycardia with abnormal QRS complexes may resemble accelerated idioventricular rhythm. If the rate is over 100 beats/min, it may resemble ventricular tachycardia. See Chapter 8.

Origin

An ectopic pacemaker in the AV junction.

> **AUTHOR'S NOTE** Junctional tachycardia with aberrancy may resemble ventricular tachycardia.

Causes

Common causes of nonparoxysmal junctional tachycardia include the following:

- Digitalis toxicity (most common cause)
- Excessive administration of catecholamines
- Damage to the AV junction from an acute inferior wall MI or rheumatic fever
- Electrolyte imbalance (especially hypokalemia)
- Hypoxia

The mechanism most often responsible for nonparoxysmal junctional tachycardia is enhanced automaticity of the AV node.

Clinical Significance

Nonparoxysmal junctional tachycardia is clinically significant because it usually indicates digitalis toxicity. The signs, symptoms, and clinical significance of rapid nonparoxysmal junctional tachycardia are the same as those of atrial tachycardia.

In addition, in nonparoxysmal junctional tachycardia, the atria do not contract regularly and empty fully, as they normally do, during the last part of ventricular diastole. The loss of this "atrial kick" may result in incomplete filling of the ventricles before they contract, reducing cardiac output by as much as 25%.

Accelerated junctional tachycardia is also common after successful cardiac arrest resuscitation and results from the catecholamines (epinephrine) administered. However, as the effects of these agents diminish, the rate of the rhythm slows, and a junctional escape rhythm results that may lead to significant hypotension.

PAROXYSMAL SUPRAVENTRICULAR TACHYCARDIA

paroxysmal supraventricular tachycardia (PSVT)

A rhythm originating paroxysmally (abruptly) at the site of a reentry circuit in the AV junction, with a rate between 150 and 250 beats/min (Fig. 7.4). PSVT may present as an AV nodal reentry tachycardia (AVNRT) or an AV reentry tachycardia (AVRT).

Characteristics

Rate	150–250
Regularity	Regular
P wave	Usually absent
PR interval	P′R interval less than 0.12 sec
P-P, R-R intervals	R-R intervals equal
Conduction ratio	1:1
QRS complex	Normal; wide if conduction delay exists
Origin	Reentry mechanism in the AV junction

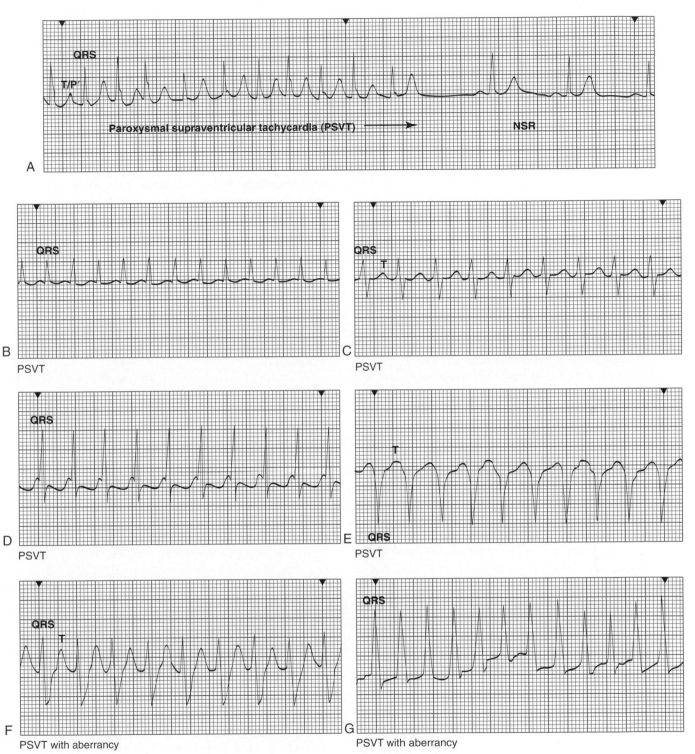

FIG. 7.4 Paroxysmal supraventricular tachycardia.

Rate

Usually 150 to 250 beats/min and constant but may exceed 250 beats/min. In the elderly or those on calcium-channel–blocking medications, the rate can be slower than 150 but is only rarely below 140 beats/min. The onset and termination of PSVT are abrupt. The onset is often initiated by a premature atrial complex.

A brief period of asystole (no electrical activity) may follow the termination of PSVT. The rate may be slower during the few beats after onset and before termination.

Regularity

Regular.

P Wave

Normal sinus P waves are absent. The P′ wave is usually absent because it is buried in the QRS complex. If P′ waves are present, they are identical and typically follow the QRS complexes. Because atrial depolarization occurs in a retrograde fashion, the P′ wave is negative (inverted) in lead II.

PR Interval

Less than 0.12 second, regardless of whether the P′ wave precedes or follows the QRS complex.

R-R Interval

The R-R intervals are equal.

Conduction Ratio

The impulse causing the QRS complex originates above the ventricles and is conducted down the bundle of His, resulting in ventricular depolarization. This is a 1:1 ratio.

QRS Complex

Normal unless a preexisting intraventricular conduction disturbance (such as a bundle-branch block) or aberrant ventricular conduction is present. If abnormal QRS complexes occur only with the tachycardia, the rhythm is called *PSVT with aberrancy* (or *aberrant ventricular conduction*). PSVT with aberrancy may resemble ventricular tachycardia.

Origin

A reentry mechanism in the AV junction that may involve the AV node alone or the AV node and an accessory conduction pathway between the atria and ventricles, as described in Chapter 1. When the reentry mechanism involves only the AV node, the rhythm is called *AVNRT*. When both the AV node and an accessory conduction pathway are involved in the reentry mechanism, the rhythm is called *AVRT*. A 12-lead ECG is required to differentiate them. See Chapter 14.

> **AUTHOR'S NOTE** Technically, any rhythm that originates above the ventricles and results in a rate greater than 100 beats/min is, by definition, a *supraventricular tachycardia* (SVT). Therefore atrial flutter with a 1:1 conduction ratio and multifocal atrial tachycardia are SVTs. Even sinus tachycardia can be considered an SVT. However, the treatment of each SVT is directed at the underlying cause, whether it is a result of increased automaticity or reentry. Although AVNRT and AVRT are both supraventricular in origin, they differ from other supraventricular rhythms in that they are a result of a reentry mechanism that precipitates their paroxysmal (abrupt) onset.

Causes

PSVT may occur without apparent cause in healthy people of any age with no apparent underlying heart disease. In those susceptible, this rhythm may be precipitated by any of the following:

- Increase in catecholamine level and sympathetic tone
- Overexertion
- Stimulants (for example, alcohol, coffee, and tobacco)
- Amphetamine and cocaine abuse
- Electrolyte or acid–base abnormalities
- Hyperventilation
- Emotional stress

The mechanism responsible for PSVT is a reentry mechanism involving either the AV node alone or the AV node in conjunction with an accessory conduction pathway, as described earlier.

Clinical Significance

The signs, symptoms, and clinical significance of PSVT are the same as those of atrial tachycardia. In addition, syncope may occur after the termination of PSVT if it is followed by a prolonged period of asystole.

PSVT is characterized by repeated, sudden episodes (paroxysms) of tachycardia that last from a few seconds to many hours or days. Vagal maneuvers, such as carotid sinus massage, usually terminate PSVT.

When PSVT with a wide QRS complex is encountered, it may be difficult to distinguish from ventricular tachycardia. A discussion of this topic will be presented in Chapter 8.

TAKE-HOME POINTS

- Junctional rhythms are characterized by the presence of a P′ wave, indicating that atrial depolarization occurred in a retrograde fashion. It may be buried in the QRS complex or ST segment and not easily identified.
- The PJC is a lone premature complex, whereas a junctional escape rhythm occurs when the atrial impulse fails to reach the AV node or when the SA node firing rate falls below that of the AV node, causing an AV junctional pacemaker to fire.
- Junctional rhythms may occur in a nonparoxysmal (gradual) or paroxysmal (abrupt) manner.
- Accelerated junctional rhythm and junctional tachycardia are examples of nonparoxysmal junctional tachycardia. This rhythm originates within the AV node and is the result of increased automaticity of the AV node.
- PSVT arises from a reentry pathway within the AV node or from an accessory pathway. PSVT also differs from other forms of supraventricular tachycardia in that its onset and termination are abrupt.
- The presence of a junctional rhythm should prompt investigation of the underlying cause. Distinguishing SVT from ventricular tachycardia may be difficult and usually requires the use of a 12-lead ECG.
- Table 7.2 summarizes the diagnostic characteristics of junctional rhythms.

TABLE **7.2**	Typical ECG Features of Junctional Rhythms				
Rhythm	**Heart Rate (beats/min)**	**Rhythm**	**P Wave**	**P′R/RP′ Interval**	**QRS Complex**
Junctional escape rhythm	40–60	Regular	Present or absent; if they precede or follow QRS complexes, negative; if no relation to QRS complexes, usually normal	• If P′R, less than 0.12 sec • If RP′ less than 0.20 sec	Normal
Nonparoxysmal junctional tachycardia	60–150	Regular	Present or absent; if they precede or follow QRS complexes, negative; if no relation to QRS complexes, usually normal	• If PR less than 0.12 sec • If RP′ less than 0.20 sec	Normal
Paroxysmal supraventricular tachycardia	160–240	Regular	Present or absent; if they precede or follow QRS complexes, negative; if no relation to QRS complexes, usually normal	• If PR less than 0.12 sec • If RP less than 0.20 sec	Normal

CHAPTER REVIEW QUESTIONS

1. Absent P′ waves in a junctional rhythm indicate what?
   A. Atrial depolarization has not occurred because of a retrograde AV block.
   B. Retrograde atrial depolarization occurred after the QRS complexes.
   C. Atrial depolarization was too weak to detect.
   D. Atrial depolarization occurred normally.

2. If the ectopic pacemaker (of a PJC) in the AV junction discharges too soon after the preceding QRS complex, what happens next?
   A. A premature atrial complex with aberrancy occurs.
   B. A PVC occurs.
   C. No QRS complex follows.
   D. A wide and bizarre QRS complex follows.

3. Which term best describes an extra QRS that originates from an ectopic pacemaker in the AV junction and occurs before the next expected beat of the underlying rhythm?
   A. Premature atrial complex
   B. PJC
   C. PVC
   D. Nonconducted PJC

4. Which of the following is true of the QRS complex of a PJC?
   A. It always follows the P′ wave associated with it.
   B. It is always narrow.
   C. It is present if the PJC is nonconducted.
   D. It resembles a PVC if aberrant ventricular conduction is present.

5. Why does a compensatory pause usually follow the PJC?
   A. The SA node was reset.
   B. The SA node was not reset.
   C. The P′ wave was premature.
   D. The impulse originated in the ventricles.

6. More than four to six PJCs per minute may indicate what?
   A. A normal variation
   B. An SA reentry mechanism
   C. Enhanced AV junction automaticity
   D. Risk of a more serious ventricular dysrhythmia

7. Which term best describes a rhythm originating within the AV junction with a rate greater than 100 beats/min?
   A. Junctional escape rhythm
   B. Junctional tachycardia
   C. Sinus bradycardia
   D. Ventricular rhythm

8. Which term best describes any rhythm that originates above the ventricles and results in a heartbeat of greater than 150 beats/min?
   A. AVT
   B. PSVT
   C. Ventricular tachycardia
   D. Ventricular fibrillation

9. Which of the following is a cardinal feature of PSVT?
   A. A heart rate between 60 and 130 beats/min
   B. A reentry mechanism in the bundle of His
   C. An abrupt onset and termination
   D. Increased automaticity of the SA node

10. Which rhythm is the most difficult to distinguish from SVT with aberrancy?
    A. Atrial flutter with 1:1 conduction
    B. Atrial tachycardia
    C. Ventricular fibrillation
    D. Ventricular tachycardia

8 — Ventricular Rhythms

PREMATURE VENTRICULAR COMPLEX

premature ventricular complex (PVC)

An unexpected QRS complex that is usually wide and bizarre because it originates in an ectopic site in the ventricles, bundle branches, Purkinje network, or ventricular myocardium. It occurs earlier than the next expected beat of the underlying rhythm and is followed by a compensatory pause (Fig. 8.1).

Characteristics

Rate	Underlying rhythm
Regularity	Irregular when PVC occurs
P wave	That of underlying rhythm
PR interval	That of underlying rhythm
P-P, R-R intervals	Unequal; compensatory pause
QRS complex	Wide (greater than 0.12 sec)
Origin	Ectopic site in ventricles, bundle branches, Purkinje network, or ventricular myocardium

Rate

The presence of a single PVC does not contribute noticeably to that of the underlying rhythm, so the rate is that of the underlying rhythm.

Regularity

The regularity of the underlying rhythm is not disturbed by the presence of the PVC.

P Wave

If present, it is generated by the underlying rhythm and has no relation to the PVC. Typically, a PVC does not disturb the P-P cycle of the underlying rhythm. As a result, the P waves occur without disruption at the expected time during and after the PVC.

PR Interval

Because the PVC does not depolarize the AV node or atria, there is not an associated PR interval.

R-R Interval

The R-R interval between the PVC and the preceding QRS complex of the underlying rhythm is shorter than the R-R interval of the underlying rhythm. This abbreviated segment is called the *coupling interval.* PVCs with the same coupling interval in a given ECG lead usually originate from the same ectopic site.

A compensatory pause occurs after a PVC because the SA node is not depolarized by the PVC. That is, the P wave of the underlying rhythm that follows the PVC appears at the expected time. Consequently, the interval between the R waves of the underlying rhythm immediately before and after the PVC is twice the duration of the R-R interval of the underlying rhythm.

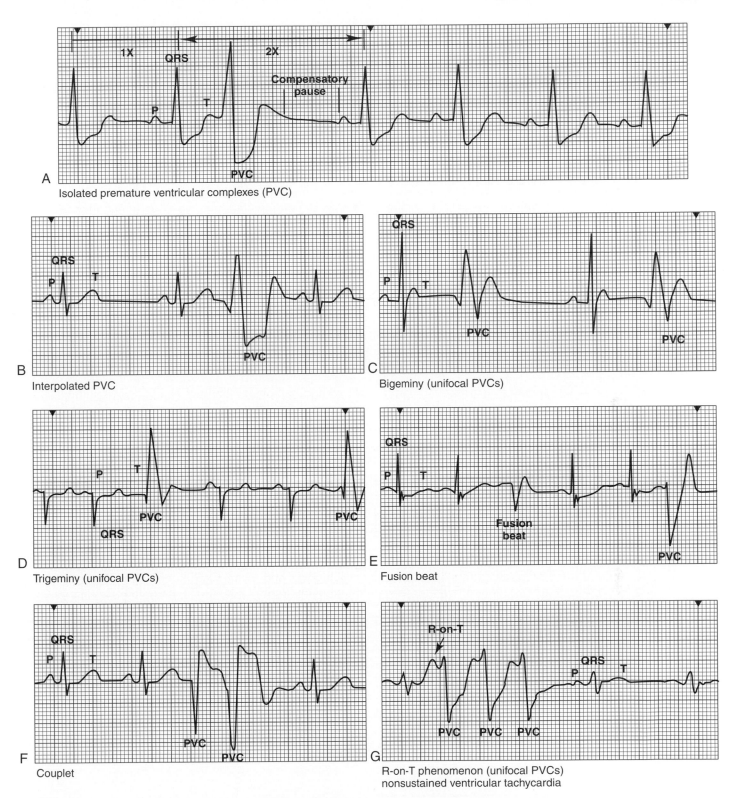

A Isolated premature ventricular complexes (PVC)

B Interpolated PVC

C Bigeminy (unifocal PVCs)

D Trigeminy (unifocal PVCs)

E Fusion beat

F Couplet

G R-on-T phenomenon (unifocal PVCs) nonsustained ventricular tachycardia

FIG. 8.1 Premature ventricular complexes.

Continued

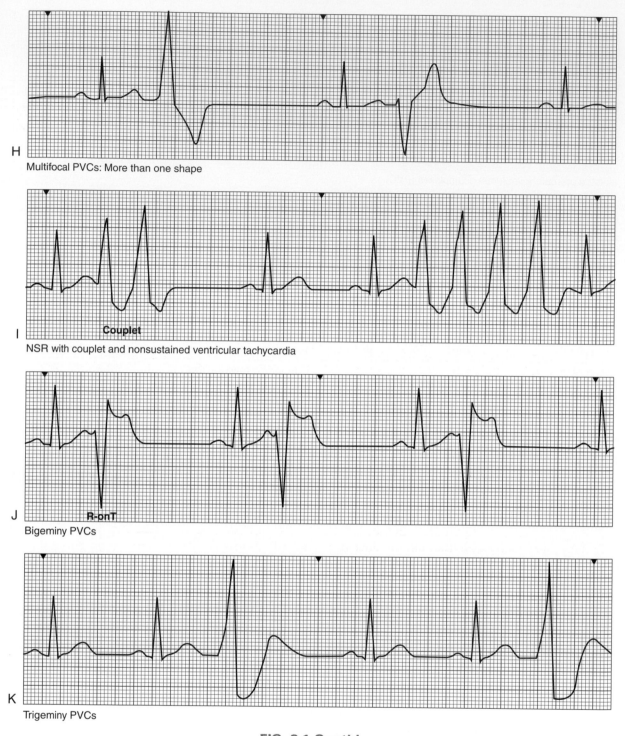

H Multifocal PVCs: More than one shape

I Couplet
NSR with couplet and nonsustained ventricular tachycardia

J R-onT
Bigeminy PVCs

K Trigeminy PVCs

FIG. 8.1 Cont'd

> **AUTHOR'S NOTE** Being able to differentiate a compensatory pause from a noncompensatory pause is vital in differentiating a premature atrial complex (PAC) from a premature junctional complex (PJC) or a PVC.

QRS Complex

The QRS complex of the PVC appears prematurely before the next expected QRS complex of the underlying rhythm. The QRS complex is always greater than 0.12 seconds because it takes longer for the electrical impulse to travel throughout the ventricles from the ectopic site. In addition, because of the abnormal direction and sequence of ventricular depolarization, the QRS complex is distorted and bizarre. It is often notched and appears quite different from the QRS complex of the underlying rhythm.

The QRS complex of the PVC is followed by an abnormally elevated or depressed ST segment and by a large, discordant

T wave. By *discordant* we mean that the wave is deflected in the direction opposite that of the major deflection of the QRS complex.

> **AUTHOR'S NOTE** We use the term *discordant* to describe a T wave that is deflected in the opposite direction from the QRS complex in any given lead and *concordant* to describe a T wave that is deflected in the same direction as the QRS complex. T waves associated with rhythms originating from the atrioventricular (AV) junction and above are *concordant*, whereas T waves of rhythms originating below the AV junction are *discordant*.

The shape of a PVC often resembles that of a right or left bundle-branch block. For example, the QRS complex of a PVC originating in the left ventricle resembles that of a right bundle-branch block because the impulse travels quickly through the left bundle branch but must travel backward through the conduction system to reach the right bundle branch. Likewise, a PVC originating in the right ventricle has a QRS complex resembling that of a left bundle-branch block. A PVC originating in the ventricles near the bifurcation of the bundle of His may appear relatively normal in shape, except that it will exceed 0.12 second in duration. See Chapter 13 for a detailed discussion of bundle-branch blocks.

PVCs that originate in the same ectopic pacemaker site are said to be *unifocal*. They have identical QRS complexes preceded by equal coupling intervals. When PVCs originate in two or more ectopic pacemaker sites, they are said to be *multifocal*. Multifocal PVCs have different QRS complexes with varying coupling intervals in the same lead.

When a PVC occurs while an electrical impulse of the underlying rhythm is attempting to depolarize the ventricles, depolarization occurs simultaneously in two different directions. In other words, impulses move from the PVC in one direction and from the underlying rhythm in the other. This produces not only a QRS complex with the characteristics of a PVC but also the QRS complex of the underlying rhythm. Such a QRS complex is called a *fusion beat*. The presence of fusion beats helps you determine that a premature ectopic complex originated in the ventricles rather than in the sinoatrial (SA) or AV node with aberrant ventricular conduction (for example, a PJC with aberrant conduction).

> ### fusion beat
> A QRS complex produced when a PVC occurs simultaneously with the QRS of the underlying rhythm. The resulting QRS complex, or fusion beat, possesses the characteristics of both the PVC and QRS of the underlying rhythm.

Frequency and Pattern

The following are the various forms in which PVCs may appear:
- **Infrequent**: Fewer than five per minute.
- **Frequent**: Five or more per minute.
- **Isolated**: Occurring singly.

- **Group beats**: Occurring in groups of two or more. The occurrence of two PVCs in a row is called a *couplet*. The occurrence of three or more consecutive PVCs is referred to as a *run of ventricular tachycardia*.
- **Repetitive beats**: If a PVC occurs after every QRS complex of the underlying rhythm, *bigeminy* is present. *Trigeminy* exists when one PVC occurs after every second QRS complex of the underlying rhythm. *Quadrigeminy* occurs when there is a PVC after every third QRS complex.
- **R-on-T phenomenon**: When a PVC occurs during the *relative refractory period* of ventricular repolarization, the PVC is superimposed on (appears on top of) the T wave. This is the most vulnerable period of ventricular repolarization. It coincides with the downslope of the T wave. During this period, a portion of the ventricular myocardium may have been completely repolarized, whereas other areas may have been only partially repolarized. Still others may be completely refractory—that is, the areas can't be depolarized. Stimulation of the ventricles at this point by the electrical impulse of the PVC may produce nonuniform conduction of the impulse through the muscle fibers. Some fibers will be able to conduct the impulse normally, whereas others will be able to conduct them only slowly or not at all. The result is a reentry mechanism that may trigger repetitive ventricular complexes, resulting in ventricular tachycardia (VT or V-tach) or ventricular fibrillation (VF or V-fib).
- **Interpolated PVCs**: A PVC that occurs between two normally conducted QRS complexes without greatly disturbing the underlying rhythm is called an *interpolated PVC*. Such a complex tends to occur when the underlying rhythm is relatively slow (less than 60 per minute). The R-R interval that includes the PVC is often slightly longer than that of the underlying rhythm. A compensatory pause does not occur.

Origin

The PVC originates in an ectopic site in the ventricles, bundle branches, Purkinje network, or ventricular myocardium. PVCs may originate in a single ectopic site or in multiple sites.

> **AUTHOR'S NOTE** Some refer to a PVC as a premature ventricular *contraction* instead of a *complex*. This is true only in the context of the physical examination of a patient. A premature ventricular contraction results in an unexpected heartbeat you can feel while taking a patient's pulse. However, because a premature complex can arise from sites other than the ventricles, as occurs with a PAC or PJC, we refer to a PVC as it relates to the ECG. Therefore it is technically a premature complex.

Causes

PVCs are caused either by enhanced automaticity of the cells within the ectopic site or by a reentry mechanism. They may occur in healthy people without apparent cause. However, when they occur frequently, the following are the most common causes:
- Increased activity of the sympathetic nervous system, such as occurs during physical or emotional stress

- Stimulants (caffeine, tobacco, amphetamine, or cocaine)
- Myocardial ischemia or infarction associated with acute coronary syndrome (ACS)
- Heart failure
- Excessive administration of digitalis or sympathomimetic drugs (for example, epinephrine, isoproterenol, or norepinephrine)
- Hypoxia
- Acidosis
- Hypokalemia
- Hypomagnesemia

Clinical Significance

Isolated PVCs in patients with no underlying heart disease are usually insignificant and require no treatment. They are more worrisome in the presence of heart disease associated with ACS and/or drug toxicity, such as digitalis toxicity. In that case, PVCs may warn of the onset of such life-threatening rhythms as V-tach or VF.

Remember that the presence of a QRS complex does not necessarily indicate that the ventricle has contracted with sufficient strength to eject blood into the circulatory system. The presence of a pulse must be verified and correlated with each QRS complex on the ECG. The lack of a pulse with a QRS could cause a substantial drop in blood pressure. For example, a patient with normal sinus rhythm at a rate of 60 beats/min may have normal blood pressure. If he or she were to develop ventricular bigeminy with no palpable pulse from the PVC, this person would effectively have a heart rate of 30 beats/min.

> **AUTHOR'S NOTE** At times, premature atrial and junctional complexes with aberrant ventricular conduction may mimic PVCs because their abnormally wide and bizarre-appearing QRS complexes resemble right or left bundle-branch block. The presence of P waves or a notch in the preceding T wave followed by a noncompensatory pause helps differentiate PACs from PVCs. PJCs with aberrant conduction may be indistinguishable from PVCs.

VENTRICULAR TACHYCARDIA

ventricular tachycardia (VT or V-tach)

Often referred to as *VT* or *V-tach,* this rhythm originates in an ectopic pacemaker in the bundle branches, Purkinje network, or ventricular myocardium; has a rate of 100 to 250 beats/min; and is characterized by an abnormally wide and bizarre QRS complex (Fig. 8.2).

Characteristics

Rate	100–250; usually 150–200
Regularity	Regular
P wave	Usually absent
PR interval	None, because the ectopic pacemaker originates below the AV node
R-R interval	Equal
Conduction ratio	AV dissociation
QRS complex	Greater than 0.12 sec
Origin	Ectopic pacemaker in the bundle branches, Purkinje network, or ventricular myocardium

Rate

More than 100 beats/min. Usually between 150 and 200 beats/min.

Regularity

Regular.

P Wave

A normal atrial P wave is absent.

PR Interval

Because the ectopic pacemaker originates below the AV node, there is no PR interval associated with this rhythm.

R-R Interval

Intervals are equal to one another but may vary slightly if the rate changes.

Conduction Ratio

Impulse originates below the AV node; the QRS complexes are unrelated to any atrial or junction impulse. Therefore there is AV dissociation.

QRS Complex

Exceeds 0.12 second and is usually distorted and bizarre—often notched. Followed by a large, discordant T wave. Usually, the QRS complexes are identical, but occasionally one or more will differ in size, shape, or direction, especially at the onset or termination of the rhythm. When this occurs, it is referred to as a *ventricular fusion* beat.

Occasionally, an electrical impulse of the underlying rhythm is conducted from the atria to the ventricles through the AV junction. This produces a normal-appearing QRS complex among the abnormal ones that characterize V-tach. Such a QRS complex is called a *capture beat* (Fig. 8.3). The R-R interval between the QRS complex of the V-tach before the capture beat and the QRS complex of the capture beat is usually shorter than the R-R interval of the V-tach. The presence of capture beats or ventricular fusion beats indicates that the tachycardia probably originated in the ventricles.

Origin

Begins in an ectopic pacemaker in the bundle branches, Purkinje network, or ventricular myocardium.

Forms of Ventricular Tachycardias

V-tach can take any of several forms, depending on the configuration of the QRS complex.

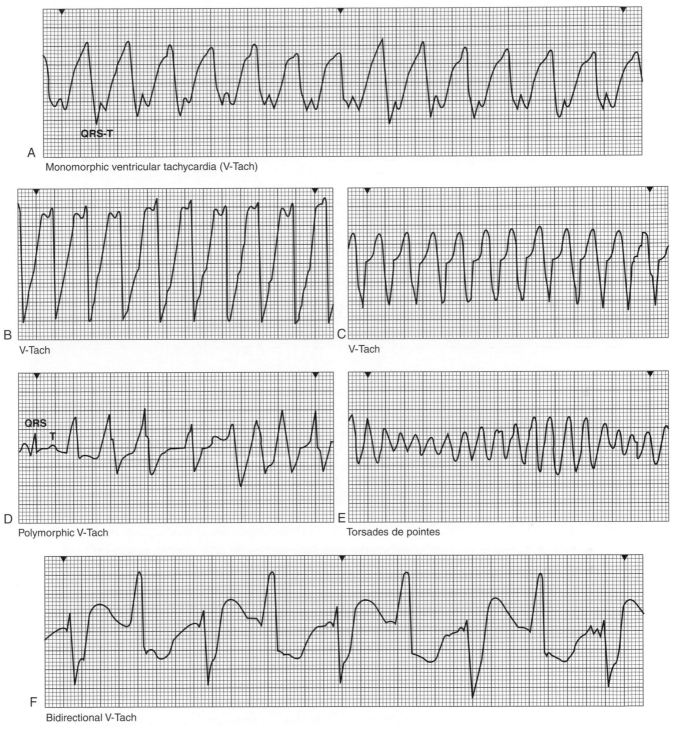

FIG. 8.2 Ventricular tachycardia.

A — Monomorphic ventricular tachycardia (V-Tach)
QRS-T

B — V-Tach

C — V-Tach

D — Polymorphic V-Tach
QRS
T

E — Torsades de pointes

F — Bidirectional V-Tach

MONOMORPHIC V-TACH

V-tach with QRS complexes that are of the same or almost the same shape, size, and direction.

BIDIRECTIONAL V-TACH

V-tach with two distinctly different, alternating QRS complexes. These complexes originate in two different ventricular ectopic sites.

POLYMORPHIC V-TACH

V-tach in which the QRS complexes differ markedly in shape, size, and direction from beat to beat. (Recall that *poly-* means "many," and *-morph* means "form.")

TORSADES DE POINTES

A form of polymorphic V-tach characterized by QRS complexes that gradually change back and forth from one shape, size, and

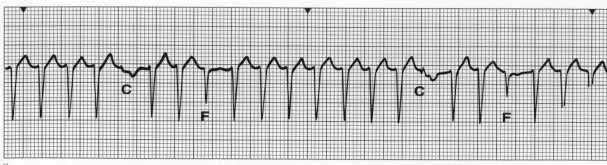

II

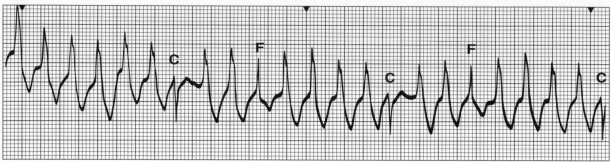

V1

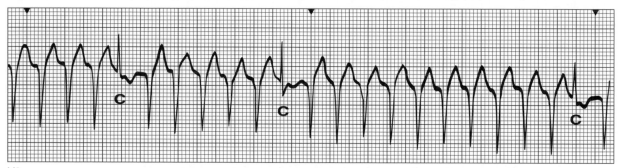

V6

FIG. 8.3 Fusion and capture beats during ventricular tachycardia (VT). The QRS complex is prolonged, and the R-R interval is regular except for occasional capture beats (C) that have a normal contour and are slightly premature. Complexes intermediate in contour represent fusion beats (F). Thus even though atrial activity is not clearly apparent, atrioventricular (AV) dissociation is present during VT and produces intermittent capture and fusion beats. (Modified from Mann, D. L., Zipes, D., Libby, P., & Bonow, R. [Eds.]. [2015]. *Braunwald's heart disease: A textbook of cardiovascular medicine* [10th ed.]. Saunders.)

direction to another over a series of beats. *Torsades de pointes (TdP)*, literally translated from the French, means "twisting around a point." It is commonly called *torsades*. This form of V-tach typically occurs when the QT interval of the underlying rhythm is abnormally prolonged (usually longer than 0.5 seconds) as a result of severely slowed myocardial repolarization.

> **AUTHOR'S NOTE** To make the clinical diagnosis of TdP, an ECG demonstrating a prolonged QT interval must be obtained either before TdP occurs or after it terminates in any given patient, because the QT interval cannot be determined during the episode of TdP. However, when an ECG demonstrates the typical cycle of QRS complexes changing shape, it is common to refer to the rhythm as *torsades*, but a more accurate interpretation would be polymorphic V-tach.

Differentiating Ventricular Tachycardia From Supraventricular Tachycardia With a Wide QRS Complex

At times, a supraventricular tachycardia (SVT)—for example, sinus, atrial, and junctional tachycardias; atrial flutter; and paroxysmal SVT—may mimic V-tach. If these rhythms have an intraventricular conduction disturbance, such as a bundle-branch block, aberrant ventricular conduction, or ventricular preexcitation, the resulting QRS will resemble that of V-tach. Atrial fibrillation with a wide QRS complex and a rapid ventricular rate may also mimic V-tach. Usually, though, the irregularly irregular rhythm of atrial fibrillation indicates its true identity.

The presence of certain features common to V-tach helps differentiate it from SVT with aberrant conduction. Chief among them are AV dissociation, a QRS complex lasting longer than 0.12 second, and capture or ventricular fusion beats (see Fig. 8.3). A 12-lead ECG or monitoring in lead V_1 or MCL_1 can also be useful in this situation by helping to determine whether a P wave is present and, if so, how it relates to the QRS complex. Once you learn to analyze the 12-lead ECG, as explained in Chapters 12, 13, and 14, you'll have more tools to assist in the differentiation of SVT from V-tach. See Chapter 14 for more information on distinguishing SVT from V-tach.

Causes

V-tach usually occurs in the presence of at least one of the following:

- Coronary artery disease, particularly in the setting of ACS, especially if hypoxia or acidosis is present (most common cause)
- Cardiomyopathy, mitral valve prolapse, or congenital heart disease
- Left ventricular hypertrophy, valvular heart disease, and congestive heart failure
- Digitalis toxicity
- QT interval prolonged by excessive administration of procainamide, disopyramide, sotalol, phenothiazine, or a tricyclic antidepressant. The TdP form of V-tach is particularly prone to occurring after the administration of such antiarrhythmic agents.
- Electrolyte disturbances (particularly hypokalemia and hypomagnesemia). The latter can enhance automaticity and is often seen in the TdP form of V-tach.
- Genetic conditions that cause prolonged QT syndrome

Another electrophysiologic mechanism sometimes responsible for V-tach is triggered activity. V-tach may be triggered during the vulnerable period of ventricular repolarization that coincides with the peak of the T wave. This is the R-on-T phenomenon described in the section on PVCs. However, V-tach may occur without preexisting or precipitating PVCs.

Clinical Significance

The onset and termination of V-tach may be abrupt or gradual. The rhythm may occur in bursts of three or more consecutive PVCs, or it may persist. V-tach lasting less than 30 seconds is called *nonsustained* or *paroxysmal V-tach*. When V-tach lasts longer than 30 seconds, it is called *sustained V-tach*.

---

sustained V-tach

V-tach lasting longer than 30 seconds.

---

nonsustained V-tach

V-tach lasting less than 30 seconds.

Symptoms of V-tach depend on ventricular rate, duration, and the presence and extent of underlying heart disease. V-tach can occur in several forms:

- Short, asymptomatic, nonsustained episodes
- Sustained, hemodynamically stable events, which generally occur at slower rates or in otherwise-normal hearts

- Unstable runs, often degenerating into VF. In some patients who have nonsustained V-tach initially, a sustained episode of V-tach or VF later develops.

The signs and symptoms of V-tach vary, depending on the nature and severity of the underlying cardiac disease, such as acute myocardial infarction (MI) or congestive heart failure. V-tach may cause or aggravate existing angina pectoris, acute MI, or congestive heart failure. Sometimes it produces hypotension or shock, or it terminates in VF or asystole. The patient with V-tach often experiences feelings of impending doom. The TdP form of V-tach tends to terminate and recur spontaneously.

In V-tach, there is little or no atrial contraction. This, coupled with the fast rate, markedly reduces cardiac output. Depending on the health of the heart, this may or may not result in a palpable pulse. Where there is no pulse, the rhythm is referred to as *pulseless V-tach.*

Because it often presents without a pulse, V-tach is one of the three most common cardiac-arrest rhythms. It is considered a life-threatening rhythm, often initiating or deteriorating into VF or asystole. V-tach and its underlying causes must therefore be treated immediately. Pulseless V-tach is treated the same as VF in cardiac arrest.

VENTRICULAR FIBRILLATION

---

ventricular fibrillation (VF or V-fib)

A rhythm that originates in numerous ectopic sites in the Purkinje network or ventricles and is characterized by very rapid, chaotic fibrillatory waves and an absent QRS complex (Figs. 8.4 and 8.5).

Characteristics

Rate	300–500
Regularity	Totally irregular
P wave	Absent
PR interval	Absent
R-R interval	Absent
Conduction ratio	AV dissociation
QRS complex	Chaotic fibrillatory waves
Origin	Multiple ectopic sites in Purkinje network and ventricular myocardium

---

Rate

No coordinated ventricular beats are present. The chaotic electrical impulses occur at a rate of 300 to 500 times a minute in an unsynchronized and uncoordinated manner.

Regularity

Totally irregular.

PR Interval

Absent.

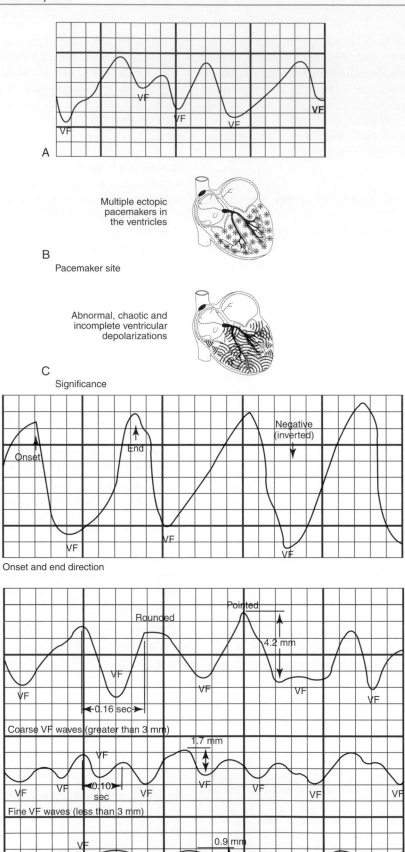

FIG. 8.4 Ventricular fibrillation waves.

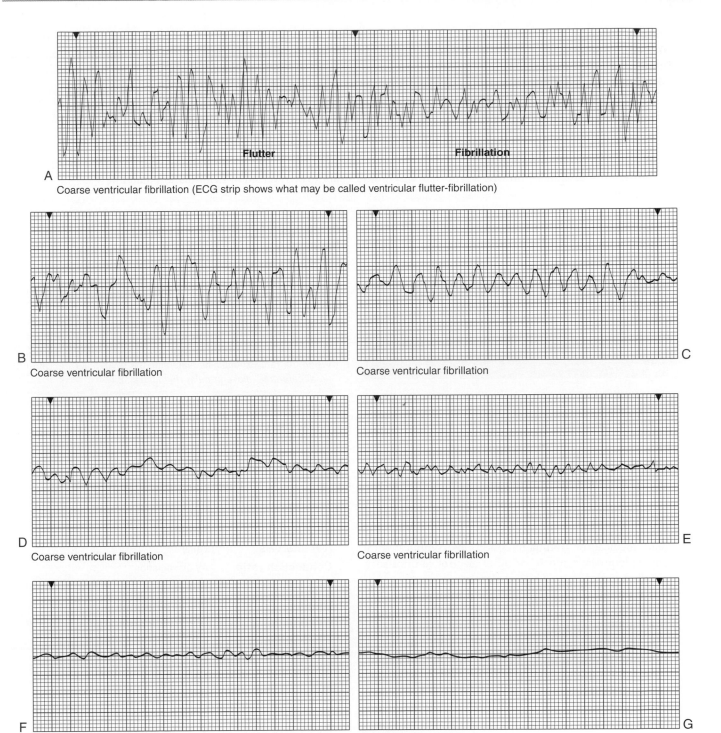

FIG. 8.5 Ventricular fibrillation.

R-R Interval

Absent.

Conduction Ratio

VF originates below the AV node and is not related to any atrial or AV-junction impulses. As a result, there is AV dissociation.

QRS Complex

Absent.

Characteristics of Ventricular Fibrillatory Waves

Relationship to Cardiac Anatomy and Physiology. Ventricular fibrillatory waves represent abnormal, chaotic, incomplete ventricular depolarization as a result of disorderly depolarization of small individual groups (or islets) of muscle fibers. Because organized depolarization of the atria and ventricles fails to occur, there is no evidence of any distinct P wave, QRS complex, ST segment, or T wave.

Onset and End. Cannot be determined with certainty.

Direction. Varies randomly from positive (upright) to negative (inverted).

Duration. Cannot be measured with certainty.

Amplitude. Varies from less than 1 mm to about 10 mm. Generally, if the fibrillatory waves are small (less than 3 mm), the rhythm is called *fine VF*. If the waves are large (greater than 3 mm), the pattern is called *coarse VF*. If the waves are so small or fine that they are not recorded, the ECG appears as a wavy or flat (isoelectric) line resembling asystole.

Shape. Markedly dissimilar, bizarre waves that vary from rounded to pointed.

Origin

Multiple ectopic sites in the Purkinje network and ventricular myocardium.

> **fine VF**
>
> A rhythm characterized by ventricular fibrillatory waves of less than 3 mm in height.

> **coarse VF**
>
> A rhythm characterized by ventricular fibrillatory waves of more than 3 mm in height.

Causes

VF usually occurs in the following:

- Coronary artery disease (myocardial ischemia and infarction associated with ACS is the most common cause of VF)
- Cardiomyopathy, mitral valve prolapse, or cardiac trauma (commonly blunt)
- Cardiac, medical, or traumatic conditions complicated by significant hypoxia, acidosis, or other electrolyte imbalance (especially hypokalemia or hyperkalemia)
- Excessive administration of digitalis or procainamide
- Accidental electrocution, or after an unsuccessful attempt by medical professionals to electrically convert another rhythm

The electrophysiologic mechanism responsible for VF is either enhanced automaticity or reentry. A PVC can initiate VF when the PVC occurs during the vulnerable period of ventricular repolarization coinciding with the peak of the T wave (R-on-T phenomenon). This is particularly likely when the heart's electrical stability has been compromised by ischemia or acute MI. Sustained V-tach may also precede the onset of VF. However, VF often begins without preexisting or precipitating PVCs or V-tach.

Clinical Significance

If one were able to visualize the heart in VF, it would resemble a bag of quivering worms. That's because chaotic depolarization of the myocardium produces ineffective ventricular contraction. Together, VF and V-tach are responsible for 30% of cardiac arrests because organized ventricular depolarization and contraction cease. Cardiac output plummets as a result, and pulse and blood pressure suddenly disappear. When VF occurs

in a patient who is awake, he or she will feel faint seconds before losing consciousness and becoming apneic (failing to breathe). If VF remains untreated, death is certain. *VF must be treated immediately!*

VF is treated by defibrillation. The goal is to stop all electrical activity, including that which is causing the VF, so that a normal pacemaker signal can awaken the heart and generate a rhythm that produces a pulse. Finding coarse VF is significant because it indicates a recent onset of the rhythm, which is therefore more apt to be reversed by defibrillation than fine VF.

VENTRICULAR ESCAPE RHYTHM (IDIOVENTRICULAR RHYTHM)

> **ventricular escape rhythm**
>
> Also called *idioventricular rhythm.* A rhythm originating in an ectopic pacemaker in the bundle branches, Purkinje network, or ventricular myocardium with a rate of less than 40 beats/min (Fig. 8.6). When the rate exceeds 40 beats/min, the rhythm is referred to as an *accelerated idioventricular rhythm* (Fig. 8.7).

Characteristics

Rate	Less than 40
Regularity	Regular
P wave	Usually absent (if present, unrelated to QRS [AV dissociation])
PR interval	Absent
R-R intervals	Equal
Conduction ratio	AV dissociation
QRS complex	Wide (greater than 0.12 sec) and bizarre
Origin	Ectopic pacemaker in bundle branches, Purkinje network, or ventricular myocardium

Rate

Less than 40 beats/min; usually between 20 and 40 beats/min, but it may be less.

Regularity

Regular.

P Wave

If present, it has no set relation to the QRS complex of the ventricular escape rhythm and appears independently at a rate different from that of the QRS complex. This represents AV dissociation.

PR Interval

Absent.

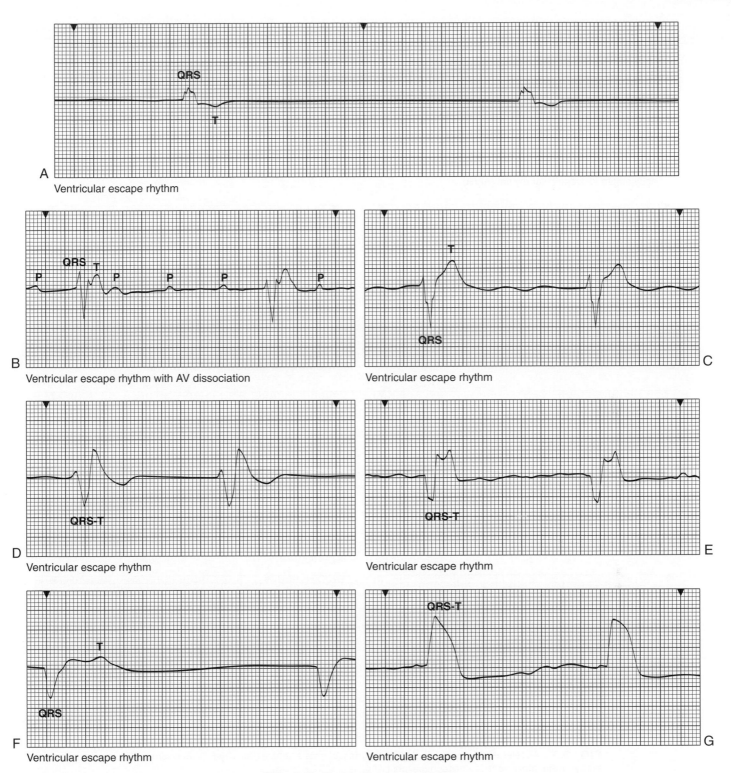

FIG. 8.6 Ventricular escape rhythm.

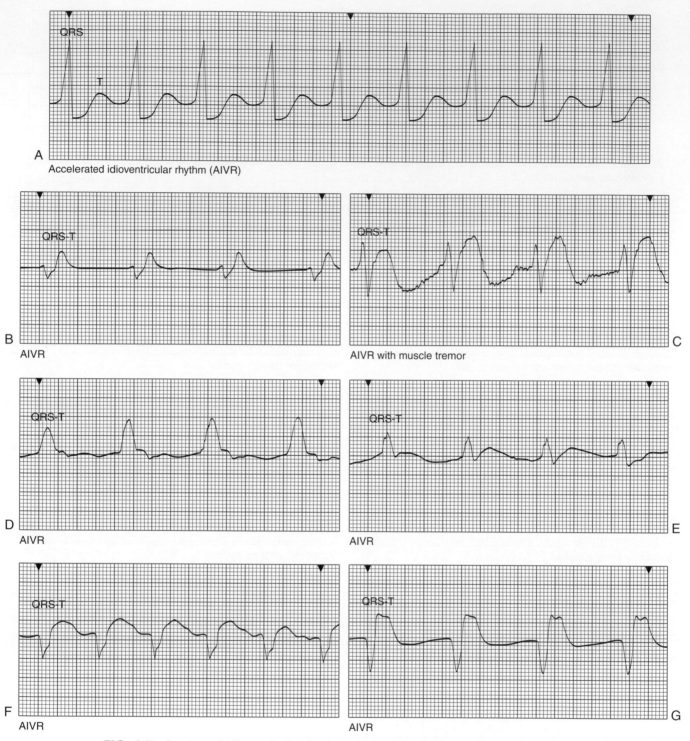

A
Accelerated idioventricular rhythm (AIVR)

B
AIVR

C
AIVR with muscle tremor

D
AIVR

E
AIVR

F
AIVR

G
AIVR

FIG. 8.7   Accelerated idioventricular rhythm (accelerated ventricular rhythm, idioventricular tachycardia, slow ventricular tachycardia [VT]).

R-R Interval

Intervals are equal to one another.

Conduction Ratio

The pacemaker is below the AV node and is unrelated to any atrial or AV junction impulses, if present. Therefore there is AV dissociation.

QRS Complex

The QRS complex exceeds 0.12 second and appears bizarre. Sometimes the shape of the QRS complex varies as the site of the ventricular impulse changes. The QRS complexes resemble those of PVCs.

Origin

Originates in an escape pacemaker in the bundle branches, Purkinje network, or ventricular myocardium.

> **AUTHOR'S NOTE** Accelerated idioventricular rhythm, also called *idioventricular tachycardia,* has the same characteristics as idioventricular rhythm except that the rate exceeds 40 beats/min. It is one of the most common rhythms that presents with the return of circulation after successful resuscitation from cardiac arrest.

Causes

The ventricular escape rhythm can occur under either of the following conditions:

- When the rate of impulse formation of the dominant pacemaker (usually the SA node) and of the escape pacemaker in the AV junction becomes less than that of the escape pacemaker in the ventricles
- When the electrical impulses from the SA node, atria, and AV junction fail to reach the ventricles because of a sinus arrest, SA exit block, or third-degree (complete) AV block

Generally, when an electrical impulse fails to arrive in the ventricles within 1.5 to 2.0 seconds, an escape pacemaker in the ventricles takes over at its inherent (natural) firing rate of 20 to 40 beats/min. The result is one or more ventricular escape beats or a ventricular escape rhythm.

When an untreated idioventricular rhythm is present (as may occur during unsuccessful cardiac arrest resuscitation), it progressively slows, and the QRS widens. This is referred to as *agonal rhythm.* It precedes the final, fatal rhythm—asystole.

Clinical Significance

In the hierarchy of cardiac pacemakers, the ventricular escape pacemaker is the lowest and slowest—the heart's last resort, you might say. If it fails to fire when needed, the result is asystole. Even when called upon, the ventricular escape rhythm is usually symptomatic because of its slow rate and the underlying poor condition of the heart. Hypotension with a marked reduction in cardiac output and decreased perfusion of the brain and other vital organs usually occurs, resulting in syncope (fainting), shock, or heart failure.

ASYSTOLE

asystole
The absence of all electrical activity within the ventricles.

Characteristics

Rate	Absent
Regularity	No electrical activity and therefore no pattern
P wave	Usually absent
PR intervals	Absent
R-R interval	Absent
Conduction ratio	None, because there is no electrical activity
QRS complex	None
Origin	Total lack of ventricular electrical activity; therefore no origin

Rate

Absent.

Regularity

There is no electrical activity and therefore no regular or irregular pattern.

P Wave

May be present or absent.

PR Interval

Absent.

R-R Interval

Absent.

Conduction Ratio

No ventricular activity. Therefore a conduction ratio is not clinically relevant.

QRS Complex

Absent.

Origin

There is no rhythm and therefore no origin. If a P wave is present, its pacemaker site is the SA node or an ectopic or escape pacemaker in the atria or AV junction.

> **AUTHOR'S NOTE** Asystole is often assumed to be present when no electrical activity is seen on the ECG. However, asystole also exists when there are P waves in the absence of ventricular activity for prolonged periods. This is referred to as *ventricular standstill.*

Causes

Asystole is present in one-third of cases of cardiac arrest (Fig. 8.8). It is the only true *arrhythmia* (absence of rhythm) because no electrical activity is present. It may occur in advanced cardiac disease as a primary event in the following situations:

- When the dominant pacemaker (usually the SA node) or the escape pacemaker in the AV junction or both fail to generate electrical impulses

- When the electrical impulses are blocked from entering the ventricles because of a third-degree (complete) AV block and an escape pacemaker in the ventricles fails to take over
- In the dying heart, asystole is usually the final event that occurs after V-tach and VF.

A short period of asystole may also follow the termination of various types of supraventricular or ventricular tachycardias after the administration of medications, defibrillation shocks, or synchronized cardioversion.

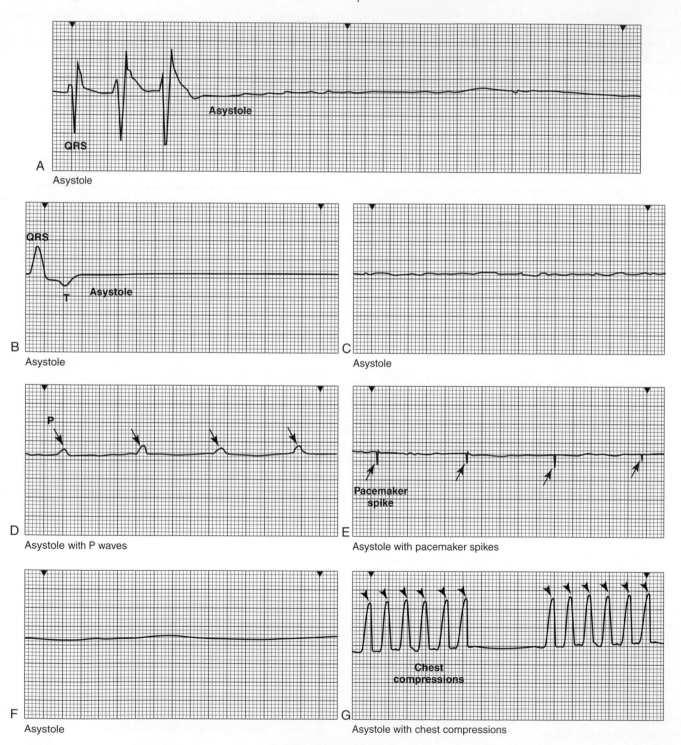

FIG. 8.8 Asystole.

Clinical Significance

Organized ventricular depolarization and contraction—and consequently, cardiac output and a palpable pulse—are absent in asystole. The occurrence of sudden asystole in a conscious person results in syncope, followed within seconds by loss of consciousness and, if untreated, death.

TAKE-HOME POINTS

- When an ectopic site below the AV node increases its automaticity or is stimulated by a reentry mechanism, a ventricular rhythm may develop. The presence of any ventricular rhythm is a cause for concern and should be treated promptly.
- A PVC is an extra, unexpected QRS complex that is usually wide and bizarre, occurs earlier than the next expected beat of the underlying rhythm, and is followed by a compensatory pause.
- A ventricular rhythm may present with solitary PVCs or multifocal PVCs.
- Frequent PVCs can significantly reduce cardiac output, leading to shock.
- The occurrence of a PVC during the T wave is called the *R-on-T phenomenon.* It can precipitate V-tach or VF.
- V-tach may be difficult to distinguish from SVT with a wide QRS complex. The occurrence of coupled and fusion beats may help differentiate the two rhythms, and a 12-lead ECG may provide further clues as to which rhythm is present.
- VF is a totally irregular rhythm that originates in numerous ectopic sites and is characterized by chaotic fibrillatory waves and rapid but unsynchronized and ineffective ventricular contraction.
- The ventricular fibrillatory waves in VF may be coarse or fine. Coarse waves indicate a more recent onset of the rhythm and thus a greater likelihood that it can be reversed.
- If the ectopic ventricular site generates an escape pacemaker, the rhythm is called an *idioventricular escape rhythm.* If greater than 40 beats/min, it is termed an *accelerated idioventricular rhythm* or *idioventricular tachycardia.*
- The idioventricular pacemaker is the last pacemaker in the heart's chain of escape pacemakers. An idioventricular rhythm should be treated promptly.
- Asystole, the absence of all electrical activity within the ventricles, is the only true arrhythmia.
- In asystole, there is an absence of organized ventricular depolarization and contraction and, consequently, an absence of cardiac output and a palpable pulse.
- Asystole occurs after V-tach, and VF is usually the final event before death.
- Table 8.1 summarizes the characteristics of the various ventricular rhythms discussed in this chapter.

TABLE **8.1**	Typical Diagnostic ECG Features of Ventricular Rhythms				
Rhythm	**Heart Rate (beats/min)**	**Rhythm**	**P Wave**	**PR Interval**	**QRS Complexes**
Ventricular tachycardia	110–250	Regular	Present or absent; unrelated to QRS complex	None	Abnormal, >0.12 sec
Ventricular fibrillation	None	None	Present or absent	None	Ventricular fibrillatory waves
Accelerated idioventricular rhythm	40–100	Regular	Present or absent; unrelated to QRS complex	None	Abnormal, >0.12 sec
Ventricular escape rhythm	>40	Regular	Present or absent; unrelated to QRS complex	None	Abnormal, >0.12 sec
Asystole	None	None	Present or absent	None	None

CHAPTER REVIEW QUESTIONS

1. Which term best describes an unexpected, abnormally wide, and bizarre QRS complex originating in an ectopic site in the ventricles?
   A. A PAC
   B. A PJC
   C. A nonconducted PJC
   D. A PVC

2. Which term best describes identical PVCs that originate from a single ectopic site?
   A. Isolated
   B. Multifocal
   C. Multiform
   D. Unifocal

3. A PVC may do what?
   A. Cause asystole
   B. Depolarize the SA node, momentarily suppressing it, so that the next P wave of the underlying rhythm appears earlier than expected
   C. Occur simultaneously with a normal QRS, forming an interpolated beat
   D. Trigger ventricular fibrillation if it occurs during ventricular repolarization

4. A PVC is followed by a compensatory pause. The R-R interval encompassing the PVC is how many times the duration of the preceding R-R interval?
   A. 1
   B. 2
   C. 3
   D. Variable

5. Which term best describes a QRS complex with characteristics of both the PVC and the QRS complex of the underlying rhythm?
   A. Fascicular PVC
   B. A capture beat
   C. Multifocal PVC
   D. A fusion beat

6. Which term best describes three PVCs in a row?
   A. A burst of PVCs
   B. A couplet of PVCs
   C. A run of V-tach
   D. A salvo of PVCs

7. Which term best describes a form of V-tach characterized by QRS complexes that gradually change back and forth from one shape and direction to another over a series of beats?
   A. Bigeminy
   B. Multiform VT
   C. Torsades de pointes
   D. Ventricular flutter

8. Successful defibrillation of VF is related to which of the following variables?
   A. The rate of the fibrillatory waves
   B. The presence of a P wave
   C. The size of the fibrillatory waves
   D. The underlying rhythm

9. Which of the following is true of an accelerated idioventricular rhythm?
   A. It is often associated with acute myocardial infarction.
   B. It should be treated immediately.
   C. It usually develops during second-degree (type II) AV block.
   D. The heart rate is usually more than 100 beats/min.

10. Which term best describes a ventricular rhythm with a rate of less than 40 beats/min?
    A. Accelerated idioventricular rhythm
    B. Pulseless electrical activity of the heart
    C. Ventricular asystole
    D. Ventricular escape rhythm

9

Atrioventricular Blocks

FIRST-DEGREE AV BLOCK

first-degree atrioventricular (AV) block

A rhythm in which there is a constant delay in the conduction of electrical impulses through the AV node. It is characterized by PR intervals that are consistent but prolonged to 0.20 second or more (Fig. 9.1).

Characteristics

Rate	Underlying rhythm
Regularity	Regular
P wave	Upright (lead II)
PR interval	>0.20 sec
P-P, R-R intervals	Equal
Conduction ratio	1:1
QRS complex	Normal unless conduction delay present
Origin	Sinus node

Rate

That of the underlying sinus or atrial rhythm. The atrial and ventricular rates are the same. The rate may be slow (40–60 beats/min), normal (60–100 beats/min), or fast (greater than 100 beats/min).

Regularity

Regular because it originates from the sinoatrial (SA) node.

P Wave

The P waves are identical to one another, and a P wave precedes each QRS complex. Waves are upright in lead II and have a normal shape and duration.

PR Interval

Prolonged (greater than 0.20 second) and of consistent duration.

R-R Interval

Regular and same as those of the underlying rhythm.

Conduction Ratio

There is a P wave for every QRS complex and a QRS complex for every P wave; therefore the conduction ratio is 1:1.

QRS Complex

Usually normal, but the QRS complex may be abnormal because of a preexisting intraventricular conduction disturbance (such as a bundle-branch block).

Origin

The SA node.

Causes

First-degree AV block represents a delay in the conduction of the electrical impulses through the AV node. Thus the QRS complexes are normal unless a preexisting intraventricular conduction disturbance, such as a bundle-branch block, is present. Infrequently, the AV block occurs below the AV node

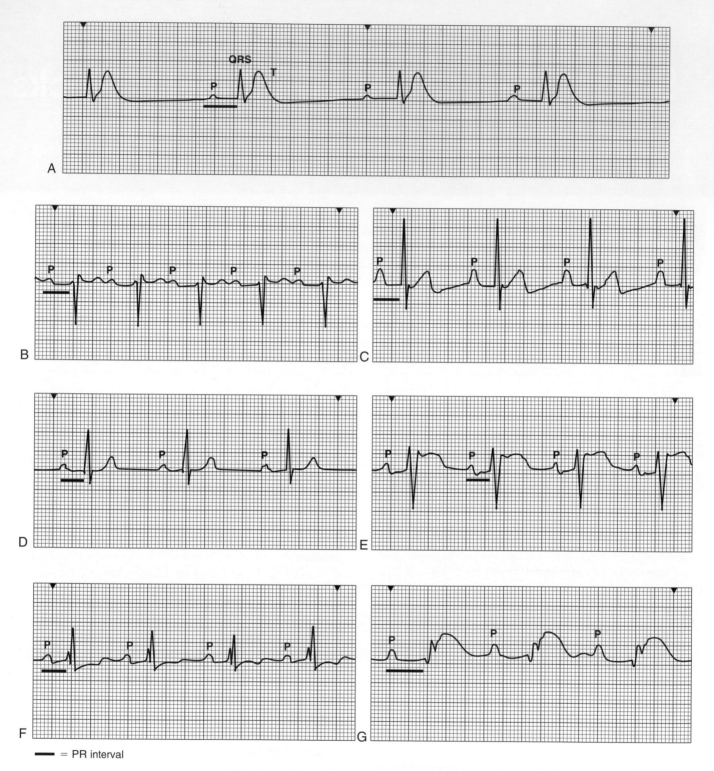

FIG. 9.1 First-degree atrioventricular (AV) block.

in the His–Purkinje system of the ventricles, such as in the bundle of His or bundle branches. This is called an *infranodal AV block*.

Although first-degree AV block may appear without any apparent cause, it can occur in the following circumstances:

- Acute inferior wall or right ventricular myocardial infarction (MI) as a result of an increased vagal (parasympathetic) tone and/or ischemia in the AV node

- Ischemic heart disease in general
- Excessive inhibitory vagal (parasympathetic) tone from whatever cause
- Digitalis toxicity
- Administration of certain drugs, such as amiodarone, beta blockers (for example, atenolol, metoprolol, propranolol), or calcium-channel blockers (for example, diltiazem, verapamil, nifedipine)

- Electrolyte imbalance, such as hyperkalemia
- Acute rheumatic fever or myocarditis

Clinical Significance

First-degree AV block produces no signs or symptoms and usually requires no specific treatment. However, any underlying cause should be corrected if possible. Rarely, first-degree AV block can progress to a higher-degree AV block under certain conditions, such as acute inferior wall MI, right ventricular MI, or excessive administration of beta blockers or calcium-channel blockers. In such cases, the patient may require observation and ECG monitoring.

SECOND-DEGREE TYPE I AV BLOCK (WENCKEBACH)

second-degree type I AV block (Wenckebach)

A rhythm in which a delay in conduction through the AV node progressively lengthens until conduction is completely blocked. The delay lengthens with each P-QRS-T cycle until a QRS complex fails to appear after the P wave.

Second-degree type I AV block is also referred to as *Mobitz I second-degree AV block, Wenckebach phenomenon,* or simply *Wenckebach.* It produces a repetitive sequence of incrementally increasing PR intervals until a QRS complex fails to occur (Fig. 9.2).

AUTHOR'S NOTE Working in the late 1800s, Karel Frederik Wenckebach was a Dutch anatomist for whom the term *Wenckebach* is named. Woldemar Mobitz, a Russian-German physician, was the first to publish his findings on the electrophysiology of second-degree heart block in the early 1900s—hence his name is often attached to this kind of block.

Characteristics

Rate	Underlying rhythm
Regularity	Patterned irregularity
P wave	Upright (lead II)
PR interval	Progressively longer until a QRS complex is dropped
P-P, R-R intervals	Equal P-P, unequal R-R (progressively shorter)
Conduction ratio	Variable (usually 4:3 or 3:2)
QRS complex	Normal unless conduction is delayed
Origin	SA node

Rate

That of the underlying sinus or atrial rhythm. The ventricular rate is less than the atrial rate because there are absent or dropped QRS complexes.

Regularity

Patterned irregularity, with a pattern of group beats. This occurs because the SA-node impulse is slowed progressively with each complex, lengthening each successive PR interval until the AV node is completely blocked, resulting in a dropped QRS complex.

P Wave

P waves are identical to one another and precede the QRS complex. The P wave associated with the dropped QRS complex is identical to all the other P waves.

PR Interval

Initially normal but may be longer. They gradually lengthen until a QRS complex fails to appear after a P wave (nonconducted P wave or dropped beat). After the pause produced by the nonconducted P wave, the sequence begins again. The PR interval after the nonconducted P is the same as the PR interval of the first P-QRS-T cycle in the pattern.

R-R Interval

Unequal. As the PR interval gradually lengthens, the R-R interval gradually decreases until the P wave is no longer conducted. The cycle then repeats itself. The reason for this progressive decrease is simple: the PR interval does not increase in large enough increments to maintain the R-R intervals at the same duration as that of the first one—the one that occurred immediately after the nonconducted P wave.

Rarely, the R-R interval remains constant until the P wave is no longer conducted. In this case the R-R interval that includes the nonconducted P wave is usually less than twice the duration of the R-R interval of the underlying rhythm.

Conduction Ratio

Usually 4:3 or 3:2, but it may be 5:4, 6:5, 7:6, and so forth. An AV conduction ratio of 5:4, for example, indicates that for every five P waves, four are followed by QRS complexes. The AV conduction ratio is usually fixed (remains the same) but may vary depending on the rate of the underlying rhythm. When the rate increases, the ratio decreases because the time needed to reach a sufficient delay in conduction to result in AV block decreases. For example, if the underlying rate is 60 beats/min, the conduction ratio might be 4:3, but when the rate increases to 100 beats/min, the ratio may decrease to 3:2.

QRS Complex

Usually normal in duration and shape, but it may be abnormal because of a preexisting intraventricular conduction disturbance (such as a bundle-branch block).

Origin

SA node.

AUTHOR'S NOTE The absent QRS complex at the point of the complete block of the P wave impulse is usually referred to as having been "dropped" because it's just simpler than referring to it as an "absent QRS complex resulting from a nonconducted P wave."

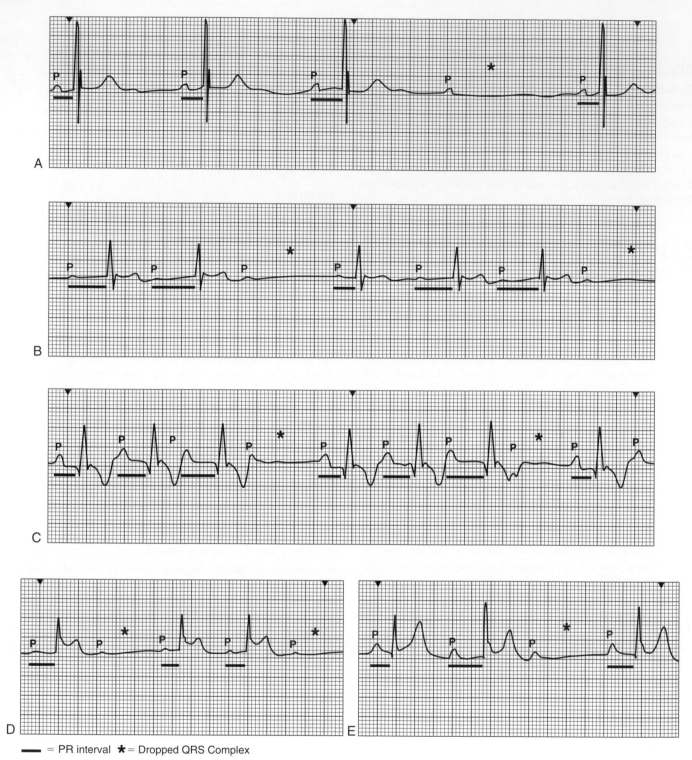

— = PR interval ✱ = Dropped QRS Complex

FIG. 9.2 Second-degree type I atrioventricular (AV) block (Wenckebach).

Causes

Second-degree type I AV block represents defective conduction of the electrical impulse through the AV node, a condition called *nodal AV block*. Thus the QRS complexes are typically normal unless a preexisting intraventricular conduction disturbance, such as a bundle-branch block, is present. The AV block occasionally occurs below the AV node in the His–Purkinje system of the ventricles, such as in the bundle of His or bundle branches. This is known as an *infranodal AV block*. When an infranodal AV block occurs, the QRS complex will last 0.10 to 0.12 second but will have a bizarre shape.

Type I second-degree AV block often occurs in the following conditions:

- Acute inferior wall or right ventricular MI caused by an increase in vagal (parasympathetic) tone and/or ischemia in the AV node
- Ischemic heart disease in general
- Excessive inhibitory vagal (parasympathetic) tone from whatever cause
- Digitalis toxicity
- Administration of certain drugs, such as amiodarone, beta blockers (for instance, atenolol, metoprolol, propranolol), or calcium-channel blockers (for example, diltiazem, verapamil, nifedipine)
- Electrolyte imbalance, such as hyperkalemia
- Acute rheumatic fever or myocarditis

Clinical Significance

Second-degree type I AV block is usually transient and reversible. Although it produces few or no symptoms, it can progress to a higher-degree AV block. As a result, the patient requires observation and ECG monitoring. If it's necessary to increase the heart rate, type I AV block does respond to the administration of atropine.

SECOND-DEGREE TYPE II AV BLOCK

second-degree type II AV block

A rhythm characterized by an intermittent, yet complete, block of electrical conduction below the AV node (infranodal conduction). This pattern produces an AV block characterized by absent (dropped) QRS complexes, usually producing an AV conduction ratio of 4:3 or 3:2. Second-degree type II AV block is also referred to as *Mobitz type II second-degree AV block* (Fig. 9.3).

Characteristics

Rate	Underlying rhythm
Regularity	Patterned irregularity
P wave	Upright (lead II)
PR interval	Normal and constant until a QRS complex is dropped
P-P, R-R intervals	Equal P-P, unequal R-R
Conduction ratio	Variable (usually 3:2, 4:3)
QRS complex	Usually greater than 0.12 sec
Origin	SA node or atrial pacemaker

Rate

That of the underlying sinus or atrial rhythm. The ventricular rate is less than the atrial rate because there are nonconducted P waves.

Regularity

Patterned (regular) irregularity of conducted and nonconducted P waves.

P wave

P waves are identical to one another. When present, the P wave precedes the QRS complex. The P wave associated with the dropped QRS complex is identical to all the other P waves.

PR Interval

Usually normal and of consistent duration.

R-R Interval

Equal to one another except for those that include the nonconducted P wave where the QRS complex is absent. These intervals are equal to or slightly less than twice the R-R interval of the underlying rhythm.

Conduction Ratio

Usually 4:3 or 3:2, but it may be 5:4, 6:5, 7:6, and so forth. More specifically, there is always one more P wave than QRS complex across the pattern. An AV conduction ratio of 4:3, for example, indicates that for every four P waves, three are followed by QRS complexes. The AV conduction ratio may be fixed or variable.

> **AUTHOR'S NOTE** Second-degree type II AV block, in contrast to advanced AV block, always has only one more P wave than QRS complex.

A nonconducted premature atrial complex (PAC; see Chapter 6) can be confused with second-degree type II block. However, the P′ of the PAC will occur prematurely and often has a shape significantly different from that of the underlying rhythm P wave. Additionally, the PAC is usually an infrequent event on the ECG and lacks the typical pattern of dropped beats characteristic of second-degree type II AV block.

QRS Complex

The block may occur in the bundle of His, resulting in a normal QRS, but more commonly occurs when a complete block of one bundle branch is accompanied by an intermittent block in the other bundle branch, resulting in a QRS duration of greater than 0.12 seconds and a shape characteristic of either a right or left bundle-branch block. See Chapter 13.

Origin

SA node or atrial pacemaker.

Causes

Second-degree type II AV block usually occurs below the bundle of His in the bundle branches. This is called an *infranodal AV block*. It represents an intermittent block of electrical conduction through one bundle branch and a complete block of electrical impulses in the other. This produces an intermittent AV block with an abnormally wide and bizarre QRS complex.

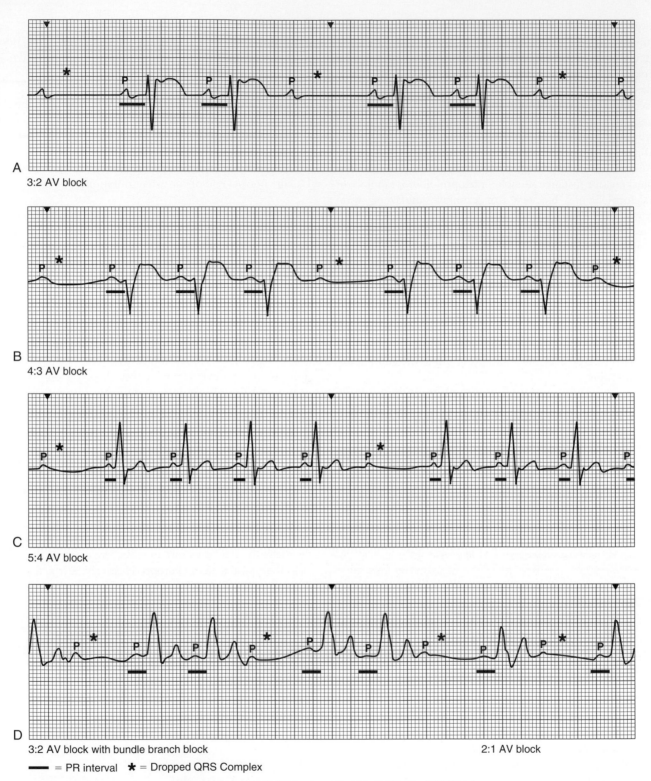

A

3:2 AV block

B

4:3 AV block

C

5:4 AV block

D

3:2 AV block with bundle branch block   2:1 AV block

▬ = PR interval   ✱ = Dropped QRS Complex

FIG. 9.3 Second-degree type II atrioventricular (AV) block.

Second-degree type II AV block is often the result of extensive damage to the bundle branches after an acute anterior wall MI.

Clinical Significance

The signs and symptoms of second-degree type II AV block with excessively slow heart rate are the same as those in symptomatic sinus bradycardia. Because second-degree type II AV block is more serious than type I AV block, often progressing to third-degree block, a standby cardiac pacemaker is indicated even for asymptomatic patients. Temporary cardiac pacing is required immediately for symptomatic patients, especially in the setting of an acute anterior wall

MI. Atropine is usually not effective in reversing type II AV block.

SECOND-DEGREE 2:1 AND ADVANCED AV BLOCK

second-degree 2:1 and advanced AV block

Rhythm caused by the defective conduction of electrical impulses through the AV node or the bundle branches (or both), producing a high-grade AV block characterized by regularly absent QRS complexes, resulting in an AV conduction ratio of 2:1, 3:1, or greater. This sequence of conduction ratios distinguishes both of these blocks from the classic second-degree type I and type II AV blocks (Fig. 9.4).

Characteristics

Rate	Underlying rhythm
Regularity	Patterned irregularity
P wave	Upright (lead II)
PR interval	Normal but consistent until a QRS complex is dropped
P-P, R-R intervals	Equal P-P, unequal R-R
Conduction ratio	Variable (usually 2:1, 3:1, 4:1) Two or more consecutive nonconducted P waves
QRS complex	Usually greater than 0.12 sec
Origin	SA node

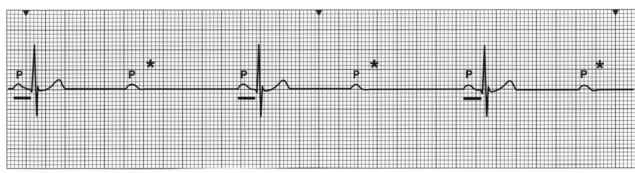

A   2:1 AV block

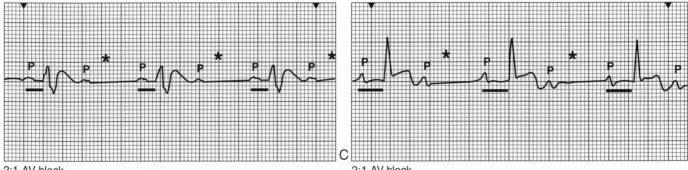

B   2:1 AV block   C   2:1 AV block

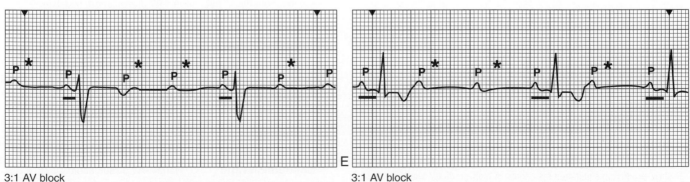

D   3:1 AV block   E   3:1 AV block

━━ = PR interval   ✱ = Dropped QRS Complex

FIG. 9.4 Second-degree 2:1 and advanced atrioventricular (AV) block.

Rate

That of the underlying sinus rhythm. The ventricular rate is less than the atrial rate because of nonconducted P waves and dropped QRS complexes.

Regularity Patterned (regular) irregularity of conducted and nonconducted P waves.

P Wave

The P waves are identical to one another and precede the QRS complex. The P waves associated with the dropped QRS complexes are identical to all the other P waves.

PR Interval

Normal and of consistent length.

> **AUTHOR'S NOTE** Second-degree 2:1 AV block can mimic second-degree type I AV block. In the typical type I AV block, the PR will become progressively longer, such that the dropped QRS complex occurs after three to six cardiac cycles. If the PR is initially very long, the subsequent cycle may be long enough to result in AV block, causing a dropped QRS complex after the second P wave. If the PR interval is normal and the conduction ratio is 2:1, then the rhythm is most likely second-degree 2:1 AV block.

R-R Interval

Unequal over the period of dropped QRS complexes and usually a multiple of the R-R interval of the underlying rhythm.

Conduction Ratio

The ratio is 2:1—hence the name. With advanced AV block, the conduction ratio is 3:1, 4:1, or greater. An AV conduction ratio of 4:1, for example, indicates that for every four P waves, one is followed by a QRS complex. In other words, three consecutive P waves are not followed by QRS complexes, and then a P wave is followed by a QRS complex. The AV conduction ratio may be either fixed or variable.

QRS Complex

In second-degree block, the conduction delay causing the block usually occurs in the bundle branches, which results in a wider-than-normal QRS. It will have an abnormal shape consistent with the bundle-branch block that is causing the AV block. See Chapter 13. If the block occurs in the bundle of His, the QRS complex duration will be 0.10 to 0.12 second.

Origin

The SA node.

> **AUTHOR'S NOTE** We say that this is a "high-grade" AV block because the conduction ratio is so great that the resulting heart rate is often very slow, producing significant symptoms. A high-grade AV block can easily become a third-degree AV block if the remaining functioning bundle branch stops conducting the atrial impulse.

Causes

Narrow QRS 2:1 and advanced AV blocks with a narrow QRS complex usually represent defective conduction of the electrical impulse through the bundle of His. These blocks are often seen in the following circumstances:

- Acute inferior-wall or right ventricular MI as a result of the effect of an increase in vagal (parasympathetic) tone and/or ischemia on the AV node
- Ischemic heart disease in general
- Excessive inhibitory vagal (parasympathetic) tone from whatever cause
- Digitalis toxicity
- Administration of certain drugs, such as amiodarone, beta blockers (such as atenolol, metoprolol, or propranolol), or calcium-channel blockers (such as diltiazem, verapamil, or nifedipine)
- Electrolyte imbalance, such as hyperkalemia
- Acute rheumatic fever or myocarditis

Clinical Significance

When the heart rate is excessively slow in 2:1 and advanced second-degree AV blocks, the signs and symptoms are the same as those in symptomatic sinus bradycardia. A 2:1 or advanced AV block with a normal QRS complex is often transient, whereas one with a wide QRS is usually permanent. Atropine may be effective in treating 2:1 AV block, but it is ineffective in advanced AV block.

Because a 2:1 or advanced AV block with a wide QRS complex often progresses to a third-degree AV block or even asystole, a standby cardiac pacemaker is indicated for asymptomatic patients. Temporary cardiac pacing is required immediately for symptomatic patients, especially in the setting of an acute anterior MI.

THIRD-DEGREE AV BLOCK

> **third-degree (complete) AV block**
>
> A rhythm caused by the complete absence of conduction of the electrical impulse through the AV node, bundle of His, and bundle branches and characterized by P wave and QRS complexes that are independent of each other (AV dissociation) (Fig. 9.5).

Characteristics

Rate	Underlying rhythm
Regularity	Regular
P wave	Upright (lead II), f or F waves
PR interval	Variable
P-P, R-R intervals	Equal P-P, equal R-R
Conduction ratio	None—AV dissociation
QRS complex	Usually greater than 0.12 sec
Origin	AV node or idioventricular

Rate

The atrial rate is that of the underlying sinus or atrial rhythm. The ventricular rate is typically 40 to 60 beats/min. However, it may be as slow as 30 or less. The ventricular rate is less than that of the atrial rate.

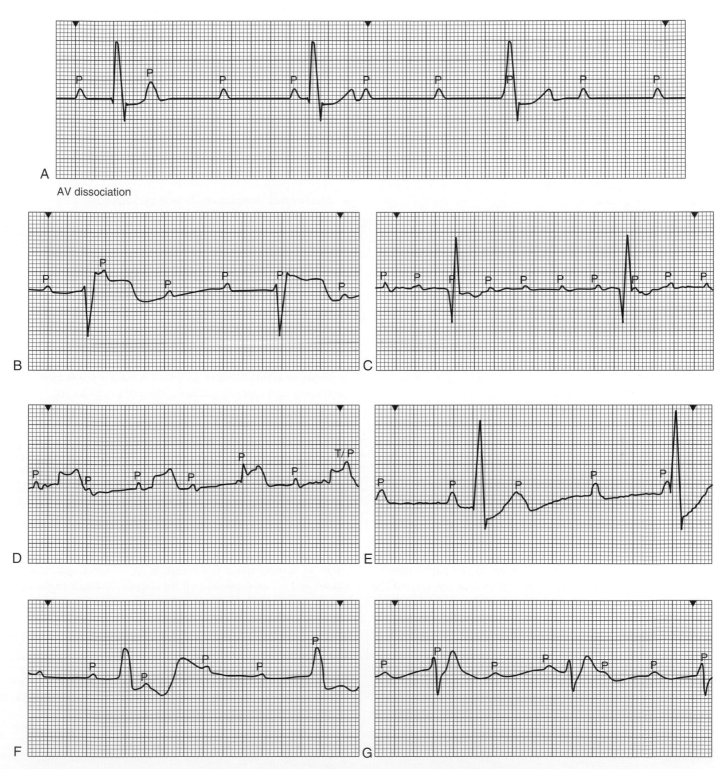

FIG. 9.5 Third-degree (complete) atrioventricular (AV) block.

Regularity

The atrial rhythm may be regular or irregular, depending on the underlying sinus or atrial rhythm. The ventricular rhythm is regular. The atrial and ventricular rhythms are independent of each other (AV dissociation). Atrial fibrillation with complete AV block will be regular instead of irregularly irregular.

P Wave

P waves, atrial flutter, or atrial fibrillation waves may be present. When present, the P wave is not related to the QRS complex, appearing independently at a rate different from that of the QRS complex (AV dissociation). Atrial flutter or fibrillation in the context of complete AV block will have the characteristic f or F waves but with a wide QRS complex. Atrial flutter in the context of complete AV block will have F waves that occur at the same time as the QRS complex.

PR Interval

The PR interval varies widely because the P wave and QRS complex occur independently.

R-R and P-P Interval

Both intervals will be constant but independent of each other. Occasionally the intervals will be similar, making it difficult to detect the dissociation. When this occurs, the key to interpretation in the clinical setting is to examine multiple rhythm strips.

Conduction Ratio

The atrial rate and the ventricular rate are independent of each other. Consequently, there is no conduction ratio (AV dissociation).

QRS Complex

Typically exceeds 0.12 second. The shape is bizarre depending on where in the bundle branches or ventricular myocardium the ventricular escape rhythm arises. May be of normal duration if the pacemaker site is in the bundle of His or AV junction.

Origin

If P waves are present, they may have originated in the SA node or in an ectopic or escape pacemaker in the atria. The pacemaker site of the QRS complex is an escape pacemaker in the AV junction, bundle branches, Purkinje network, or ventricular myocardium.

Generally, if the third-degree AV block is at the level of the AV node, the escape pacemaker is infranodal, in the bundle of His. If the AV block is at the level of the bundle branches, the escape pacemaker is in the Purkinje network or ventricles distal to the site of the AV block. If the escape pacemaker is in the AV junction, a junctional escape rhythm results, and the heart rate is 40 to 60 beats/min. If the escape pacemaker is in the ventricles, such as the bundle branches, Purkinje network, or ventricular myocardium, a ventricular escape rhythm is seen, and the heart rate is 20 to 40 beats/min or less.

Causes

Third-degree AV block represents a complete block of electrical conduction from the atria to the ventricles at the level of the AV node (nodal AV block), bundle of His, or bundle branches (infranodal AV block). It may be transient and reversible or permanent.

Transient and reversible third-degree AV block is usually associated with a narrow QRS complex and a heart rate of 40 to 60 beats/min. It is typically characterized by a junctional escape rhythm caused by a complete block of conduction of electrical impulses through the AV node. This block can be seen in the following conditions:

- Acute inferior-wall or right ventricular MI as a result of the effect of an increase in vagal (parasympathetic) tone and/or ischemia in the AV node
- Ischemic heart disease in general
- Excessive inhibitory vagal (parasympathetic) tone from whatever cause
- Digitalis toxicity
- Administration of certain drugs, such as amiodarone, beta blockers (such as atenolol, metoprolol, or propranolol), or calcium-channel blockers (such as diltiazem, verapamil, or nifedipine)
- Electrolyte imbalance, such as hyperkalemia
- Acute rheumatic fever or myocarditis

Permanent or chronic third-degree AV block is usually associated with a wide QRS complex and a heart rate of 20 to 40 beats/min or less. It is normally characterized by a ventricular escape rhythm caused by a complete block of conduction of electrical impulses through both bundle branches. This rhythm is usually preceded by one or more of the following:

- Acute anterior wall MI
- Chronic degenerative changes in the bundle branches that occur in the elderly

Permanent third-degree AV block is usually not the result of increased vagal (parasympathetic) tone or drug toxicity.

Clinical Significance

The signs and symptoms of third-degree AV block are the same as those in symptomatic sinus bradycardia. Third-degree AV block can be more ominous, however, especially when it produces wide and bizarre QRS complexes. If an AV junctional or ventricular escape rhythm does not take over after a sudden onset of third-degree AV block, asystole will occur. This causes light-headedness, followed within seconds by loss of consciousness and death.

Temporary cardiac pacing is required immediately for treatment of symptomatic third-degree AV block (regardless of cause) and for asymptomatic third-degree AV block in the setting of an acute anterior wall MI.

TAKE-HOME POINTS

- *Heart block* is the general term for AV conduction disturbances that occur when transmission of the P wave impulse through the AV junction is delayed or blocked.
- The key to recognizing an AV block is to evaluate the PR interval carefully.
- If the PR interval is greater than 0.20 second yet consistent and always followed by a QRS complex, then first-degree AV block is present.

- If a QRS complex does not follow a given P wave, the PR interval is absent for that beat. Such a pattern indicates a blockage of electrical conduction through the AV node, bundle of His, or bundle branches into the ventricles. If QRS complexes follow some P waves and not others, a second-degree AV block is present. There are two kinds of second-degree AV blocks.
- If the PR intervals are unequal, check for a progressive lengthening of their duration until you see a P wave that is not followed by a QRS complex. This is called a *nonconducted P wave* or *dropped QRS complex*. It indicates a progressive delay in conduction through the AV node or, less commonly, the bundle of His or bundle branches into the ventricles, until the signal becomes completely blocked. This is a second-degree type I AV block (Wenckebach phenomenon).

- If the PR intervals are equal and there is one more P wave than QRS complex across the pattern of the rhythm, a second-degree type II AV block is present. The AV conduction ratio will be 2:1, 3:2, 4:3, or greater.
- If the PR intervals are equal and there are two or more P waves than QRS complexes across the pattern of the rhythm, a second-degree 2:1 or advanced AV block exists. The AV conduction ratio will be 2:1, 3:1, 4:1, or greater.
- If QRS complexes are present but are not associated with any of the P waves, a third-degree (complete) AV block is present. These QRS complexes tend to be abnormally wide.
- Fig. 9.6 provides an algorithm that can assist in the determination of the degree and type of AV block.
- Table 9.1 summarizes the ECG characteristics of AV blocks.

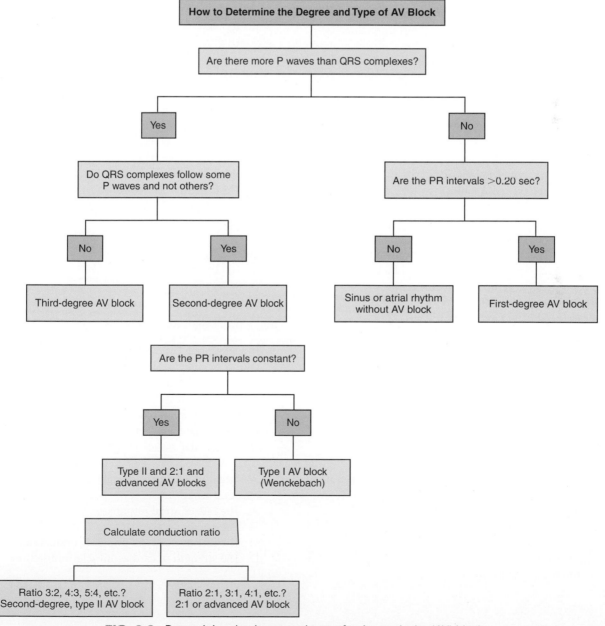

FIG. 9.6 Determining the degree and type of atrioventricular (AV) block

TABLE 9.1	Typical Diagnostic ECG Features of First-, Second-, and Third-Degree AV Blocks		
AV Block	**PR Intervals**	**AV Conduction Ratio**	**QRS Complex**
First-degree	Prolonged, constant	1:1	Usually normal
Second-degree type I (Wenckebach)	Gradually lengthening	5:4, 4:3, 3:2 or 6:5, 7:6, etc.	Usually normal
Type II	Consistent	3:2, 4:3, 5:4, etc.	Typically abnormal
2:1	Consistent	2:1	Normal or abnormal
Advanced	Consistent	3:1, 4:1, 5:1, etc.	Normal or abnormal
Third-degree	No relationship of P wave to QRS complex	None	Normal or abnormal

CHAPTER REVIEW QUESTIONS

1. Which rhythm often occurs in acute inferior wall MI because of the effect of increased vagal (parasympathetic) tone or ischemia or both in the AV node?
   A. First-degree AV block
   B. Second-degree type II AV block
   C. Chronic third-degree AV block
   D. Ventricular tachycardia

2. Which rhythm is characterized by a progressively lengthening delay in electrical conduction through the AV node after each P wave until conduction is completely blocked?
   A. First-degree AV block
   B. Second-degree type I AV block
   C. Second-degree type II AV block
   D. Third-degree AV block

3. If second-degree type I AV block is usually transient and reversible, why must the patient be monitored and observed?
   A. It can progress to a higher-degree AV block.
   B. It can progress to ventricular tachycardia.
   C. It is usually symptomatic.
   D. It is often associated with anterior wall MI.

4. Which rhythm is characterized by a complete block of electrical conduction in one bundle branch and an intermittent block in the other?
   A. First-degree AV block
   B. Second-degree type I AV block
   C. Second-degree type II AV block
   D. Third-degree AV block

5. If a second-degree type II AV block occurs in the setting of acute anterior wall MI, which immediate treatment is given in a symptomatic patient?
   A. Dopamine infusion
   B. Isoproterenol drip
   C. Epinephrine
   D. Temporary cardiac pacing

6. Which of the following ratios is consistent with the conduction ratio of advanced AV block?
   A. 4:3
   B. 3:2
   C. 3:1
   D. 1:1

7. Which AV block is characterized by the absence of electrical conduction through the AV node, bundle of His, or bundle branches, producing independent contraction of the atria and ventricles?
   A. Second-degree type I AV block
   B. Second-degree type II AV block
   C. Third-degree AV block
   D. First-degree AV block

8. An escape pacemaker in the AV junction has a firing rate of how many beats/min?
   A. 100 to 120
   B. 80 to 100
   C. 60 to 80
   D. 40 to 60

9. If a junctional or ventricular escape pacemaker does not take over after a sudden onset of third-degree AV block, asystole will occur, causing what?
   A. Cardiac arrest
   B. Bundle-branch block
   C. Junctional escape rhythm
   D. Ventricular escape rhythm

10. AV heart blocks are clinically significant because of their effect on what?
    A. The rate of atrial response
    B. The rate of ventricular response
    C. The rate of electrical impulse conduction
    D. The strength of cardiac muscle contraction

10 Implanted Pacemaker Rhythms

PACEMAKERS

A pacemaker is a battery-powered device whose primary purpose is to stimulate the heart with electricity. Such a device is helpful for patients with chronically slow heart rhythms or rhythms that can at times become slow. The most common indications for pacemaker placement are listed in ECG Keys Box 10.1.

A pacemaker has two major components:
1. A controller pack that contains the battery and programmable hardware
2. Wire electrode(s) that are attached to the heart chamber(s) being stimulated

Pacemakers are either temporary or permanent (implanted). With temporary pacemakers, the pacing wire is connected to a controller outside the body, and the electrode is run through a transvenous catheter into the heart. With long-term, implanted pacemakers, the controller is inserted subcutaneously, usually under the chest wall. With both types, the pacemaker wire is threaded through a vein into the right ventricular cavity. This allows the pacemaker electrode to stimulate the endocardium of the right ventricle (Fig. 10.1). During an emergency and before central vascular access can be obtained, transcutaneous pacing of the heart may be performed using the same self-adhesive pads used for defibrillation. Whether temporary or permanent, you will need to be able to interpret the ECG rhythm of a patient with a pacemaker.

Along the pacemaker wire are two sensors, one in the atria and one in the ventricle, which we refer to as the *pacemaker leads*, that permit the pacemaker to detect the electrical impulses in the heart. The pacemaker wire also has two electrodes, again, one for the atria and one at the wire's end in the right ventricle. This allows the pacemaker to stimulate the atria, the ventricle, or both depending on the pacemaker's programming.

Regardless of type, all current pacemaker leads are capable of performing two functions:
1. Sensing atrial and/or ventricular electrical activity
2. Pacing, during which the electrode generates an electrical discharge to depolarize the myocardium of the right atria and/or ventricle

TYPES OF PACEMAKERS

Fixed Rate or Demand

There are two basic kinds of pacemakers: *fixed rate* and *demand*. Fixed-rate pacemakers are designed to fire constantly at a preset rate without regard to the heart's own electrical activity. The first pacemakers on the market could provide only a fixed rate of pacing and are rare today. Demand pacemakers, on the other hand, have a sensing device that detects the heart's electrical activity and fires at a preset rate only when the heart's activity drops below a predetermined rate. Current pacemakers are demand pacemakers.

A demand pacemaker, then, incorporates two distinct features:
1. A sensing mechanism designed to inhibit the pacemaker when the heart rate is adequate
2. A pacing mechanism designed to trigger the pacemaker when no intrinsic P and/or QRS complex occurs within a predetermined period

Present-day demand-type pacemakers can also be programmed by placing a special telemetry device on the chest wall to communicate with the pacemaker. Besides programming,

| **Most Common Indications for Pacemaker Placement**

- Symptomatic sinus bradycardia
- Atrioventricular (AV) block associated with one of the following:
  - Third-degree AV block that produces symptoms
  - Third-degree AV block with pauses of longer than 3 seconds or with an escape rate of less than 40 beats/min in an awake patient
  - Postoperative AV block that is not expected to resolve
  - Second-degree AV block that produces symptoms
  - Chronic bifascicular or trifascicular block with an intermittent third-degree AV block or type II second-degree AV block or alternating bundle-branch block
- AV block associated with myocardial infarction and one or more of the following:
  - Second- or third-degree AV block in the His–Purkinje system
  - Transient second- or third-degree infranodal AV block and associated bundle-branch block
  - Persistent, symptomatic second- or third-degree AV block
- Sinus node dysfunction
  - Symptomatic sinus bradycardia or sinus pauses
  - Symptomatic sinus arrest
- Carotid sinus syndrome: recurrent syncope or near-syncope as a result of carotid sinus syndrome

the device can check the pacemaker to determine how well it is picking up the heart's electrical activity and can download a log of the pacemaker's activity.

fixed-rate pacemaker

A pacemaker that does not sense the intrinsic firing of the heart's electrical system and instead generates electrical impulses at a preset rate. This type is rare today.

Each time a demand pacemaker senses a spontaneous QRS complex, it inhibits the generation of a pacemaker pulse. Demand pacemakers fire only when the spontaneous heart rate is slower than the preset rate of the pacemaker. This rate is usually 60 to 70 beats/min. When the pacemaker does fire, it generates a sharp spike on the ECG. The spike appears before each QRS complex (Fig. 10.2).

demand pacemaker

A pacemaker that senses the intrinsic firing of the heart's electrical system and generates an impulse only when the rate of the heart's rhythm drops below a preset rate.

The timing cycle of a demand pacemaker consists of a defined lower rate (LR) limit and a ventricular refractory period (VRP). The LR is the period of time the pacemaker will wait for an intrinsic electrical discharge from the heart before initiating a pulse. The VRP begins when the pacemaker senses a QRS complex or the pacemaker generates an impulse (Fig. 10.3). During the refractory period, a demand pacemaker does not sense electrical activity. In the absence of a sensed intrinsic ventricular impulse, a pacing spike is delivered when the LR limit is reached. If an intrinsic QRS occurs, the LR time begins at that point. A VRP begins with any sensed or paced ventricular activity.

Single or Dual Chamber

Pacemakers can be either *single-chamber* units, which pace either the ventricles or the atria, or *dual-chamber* devices that pace both the atria and ventricles. The Intersociety Commission for Heart Disease (ICHD) code is a systematic method of denoting how a given pacemaker senses, what it senses, and in which chamber(s) it generates an impulse. Although there are

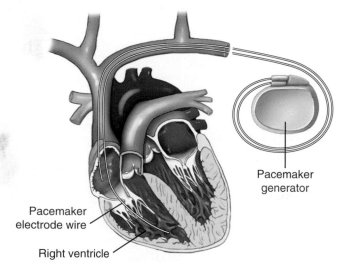

Pacemaker generator

Pacemaker electrode wire

Right ventricle

FIG. 10.1 Implanted pacemaker.

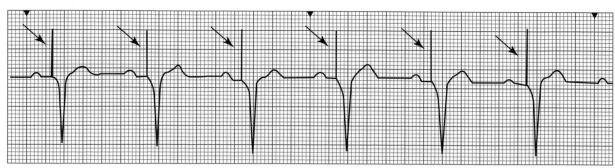

FIG. 10.2 Pacer spikes on ECG. *Arrows,* pacer spikes.

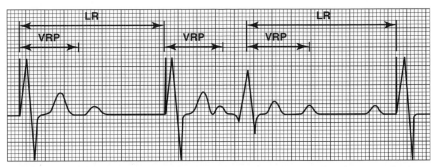

FIG. 10.3 Lower rate and ventricular refractory period of demand pacemaker. *LR,* Lower rate; *VRP,* ventricular refractory period. (Modified from Mann, D. L., Zipes, D., Libby, P., & Bonow, R. [Eds.]. [2015]. *Braunwald's heart disease: A textbook of cardiovascular medicine* [10th ed.]. Saunders.)

TABLE 10.1	Five-Letter Pacemaker Code			
Letter 1	**Letter 2**	**Letter 3**	**Letter 4**	**Letter 5**
Chamber paced	Chamber sensed	Sensing response	Programmability	Antitachycardia functions
A = atrium	A = atrium	T = triggered	P = simple	P = pacing
V = ventricle	V = ventricle	I = inhibited	M = multiprogrammable	S = shock
D = dual	D = dual	D = dual (A and V inhibited)	R = rate adaptive	D = dual (shock + pace)
0 = none	0 = none	0 = none	C = communicating	
			0 = none	

The letter in the first position indicates the chamber(s) being paced—the atrium (A), ventricle (V), or both (D). The letter in the second position indicates the chamber(s) in which sensing occurs—again, the atrium (A), ventricle (V), or both (D). Finally, the letter in the third position refers to the mode of response of the pacemaker—triggered (T), inhibited (I), or dual (D).

BOX 10.1	Deciphering ICHD Pacemaker Codes

- The first letter of the code indicates which chamber is paced (A, atria; V, ventricles; D, both atria and ventricles).
- The second letter indicates which chamber is sensed (A, atria; V, ventricles; D, both atria and ventricles).
- The third letter indicates the mode of sensing or the response of the pacemaker to a P wave or QRS complex (I, pacemaker impulse is inhibited by the P wave or QRS complex; D, pacemaker impulse is inhibited by a QRS complex and triggered by a P wave).
- The fourth letter indicates the programmability of the pacemaker even after it is surgically implanted in the patient.
- The fifth letter indicates whether it has the ability to defibrillate the heart if a potentially lethal rhythm develops.

ICHD, Intersociety Commission for Heart Disease.

five letters in the code, not all are used for every pacemaker. In general, the first three letters provide sufficient information about the pacemaker's function to allow a clinician to interpret its associated ECG rhythm. Table 10.1 provides a full list of the codes. Box 10.1 shows how the codes can be deciphered.

SINGLE CHAMBER

Atrial Demand Pacemaker (AAI)

An AAI pacemaker senses spontaneously occurring P waves and paces the atria when they do not appear (Fig. 10.4). The AAI timing cycle consists of a defined LR limit and an atrial refractory period (ARP). During the ARP, the pacemaker will not sense any additional atrial electrical activity. When the LR limit is reached, a pacing impulse is delivered to the right atrium. This impulse acts like an ectopic atrial impulse and is conducted to the AV node and then to the ventricles. If an intrinsic P wave occurs, the LR timer is reset. The ARP begins with any sensed or paced atrial activity. The purpose of the ARP is to prevent the firing of a pacemaker impulse before a sufficient time has elapsed to permit an intrinsic or pacemaker-delivered impulse to be conducted to the ventricles.

The AAI timing cycle is not affected by impulses generated in the ventricles. Therefore if a premature ventricular complex (PVC) occurs, it is not sensed by the AAI pacemaker, and the atrial pacing spike may occur during the T wave of the PVC. This can cause ventricular tachycardia (V-tach) or ventricular fibrillation (V-fib). The AAI should not be used in patients with atrioventricular (AV) blocks because the atrial impulse generated by the pacemaker will not be conducted to the ventricles.

Ventricular Demand Pacemaker (VVI)

A VVI pacemaker senses spontaneously occurring QRS complexes and paces the ventricles when they do not appear. The VVI pacemaker protects the patient from potentially lethal slow bradycardias. However, the VVI pacemaker, like the AAI pacemaker, does not promote a coordinated depolarization of the atria and ventricles. Thus it is rarely used for long-term pacing.

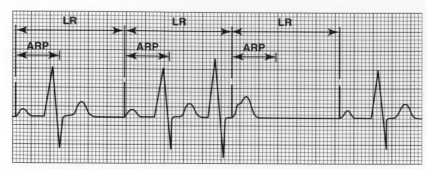

FIG. 10.4 Single-chamber atrial demand pacemaker (AAI). *ARP,* Atrial refractory period; *LR,* lower rate. (Modified from Mann, D. L., Zipes, D., Libby, P., & Bonow, R. [Eds.]. [2015]. *Braunwald's heart disease: A textbook of cardiovascular medicine* [10th ed.]. Elsevier.)

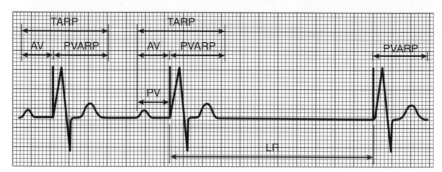

FIG. 10.5 Dual-chamber pacemaker (VDD). *AV,* Atrioventricular interval; *PVARP,* postventricular atrial refractory period; *TARP,* total atrial refractory period. (Modified from Libby, P. [2008]. *Braunwald's heart disease: A textbook of cardiovascular medicine* [8th ed.]. Saunders.)

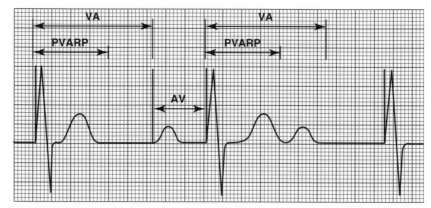

FIG. 10.6 Dual-chamber atrioventricular sequential pacemaker (DDI). *AV,* Atrioventricular interval; *PVARP,* postventricular atrial refractory period; *VA,* ventricular activation. (Modified from Mann, D. L., Zipes, D., Libby, P., & Bonow, R. [Eds.]. [2015]. *Braunwald's heart disease: A textbook of cardiovascular medicine* [10th ed.]. Elsevier.)

See Fig. 10.3, which shows the ECG of a patient with a VVI pacemaker.

DUAL CHAMBER

Atrial Synchronous Pacemaker (VDD). A VDD pacemaker paces only in the ventricle but does so in a synchronized manner with the heart's atrial electrical impulse (P wave). It senses spontaneously occurring P waves and QRS complexes and paces the ventricles, but not the atria, when a QRS complex fails to appear after a spontaneously occurring P wave. Patients with second-degree type II and complete AV block would benefit

from a VDD pacemaker because the pacing of the ventricles is synchronized with the P waves. This coordination ensures that ventricular depolarization follows atrial depolarization in the normal physiologic sequence (Fig. 10.5).

Atrioventricular Sequential Pacemaker (DDI)

A DDI pacemaker senses spontaneously occurring QRS complexes and paces both the atria and the ventricles. It sequentially paces the atria first; then, after a short delay, it paces the ventricles when QRS complexes fail to appear (Fig. 10.6). The timing cycle in DDI pacing consists of an LR limit, an AV interval, a VRP, and an ARP. The VRP is initiated by any sensed or paced ventricular activity, and the ARP is initiated by any sensed or paced atrial activity. The DDI pacemaker is infrequently used. However, patients with fast heart rhythms, such as atrial fibrillation with rapid ventricular response and occasional episodes of significant slow ventricular response, may benefit from a DDI pacemaker. In this case the LR limit is not reached even if the spontaneous sinoatrial (SA) node rate occurs at a faster rate than the LR limit, and the DDI pacemaker assures that there is ventricular pacing when the ventricular rate is slow.

Optimal Sequential Pacemaker (DDD)

A DDD pacemaker senses spontaneously occurring P waves and QRS complexes and responds as follows:
1. Paces the atria when P waves fail to appear, as in sinus node dysfunction
2. Paces the ventricles when QRS complexes fail to appear after spontaneously occurring or paced P waves (Fig. 10.7)

The timing cycle in DDD consists of an LR limit, an AV interval, a post-VPR/ARP (PVARP), and an upper rate limit. The AV interval and PVARP together make up the total atrial refractory period (TARP). If intrinsic atrial and ventricular activity occur before the LR times out, both channels are inhibited, and no pacing occurs. If no intrinsic atrial or ventricular activity occurs, an atrial spike is generated. This spike is followed, after an appropriate delay, by a ventricular spike. If no atrial activity is sensed before the ventriculoatrial (VA) interval is completed, an atrial pacing spike is delivered. This spike initiates the AV interval. If intrinsic ventricular activity occurs before the AV interval terminates, the ventricular output of the pacemaker is inhibited. If a P wave is sensed before the VA interval ends, output from the atrial channel is inhibited. If no ventricular activity is sensed before the AV interval ends, a ventricular pacing spike is generated.

The DDD pacemaker is most appropriate for patients with sinus rhythm disturbances and AV blocks.

AUTHOR'S NOTE There are biventricular pacemakers, which pace both ventricles. They are used in certain conditions to optimize cardiac output.

PACEMAKER RHYTHM

pacemaker rhythm

The pattern of waves and complexes produced on an ECG as a pacemaker discharges spikes of electromechanical energy, stimulating the ventricles to contract. This pattern is regular in a continuous pacemaker but may be irregular in a demand pacemaker.

Characteristics

Rate

Usually 60 to 70 beats/min, depending on its preset rate of firing. If the pacemaker rate is greater than 90 beats/min, it is probably malfunctioning.

Rhythm

Regular if the pacemaker is pacing continuously. The ventricular rate may be irregular when the pacemaker is pacing on demand—for example, pacing only when a P wave or QRS complex fails to appear.

AUTHOR'S NOTE The pacemaker spikes may be difficult to detect on the ECG monitor and/or the printed ECG. Turning up the gain on the monitor will usually make these spikes more discernible. Current ECG monitors/defibrillators often include automatic sensing of pacer spikes and note their presence on the ECG rhythm strip and monitor with arrows.

P Wave

If present, they may occur spontaneously or be induced by a pacemaker lead positioned in one of the atria. When not followed by an intrinsic QRS complex, a spontaneously occurring

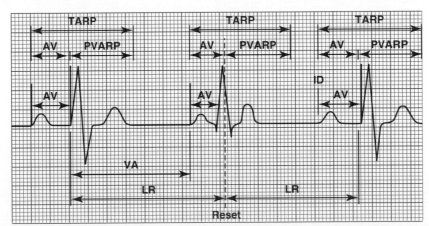

FIG. 10.7 Dual-chamber optimal sequential pacemaker (DDD). *AV,* Atrioventricular interval; *LR,* lower rate; *PVARP,* postventricular atrial refractory period. *TARP,* total atrial refractory period. (Modified from Mann, D. L., Zipes, D., Libby, P., & Bonow, R. [Eds.]. [2015]. *Braunwald's heart disease: A textbook of cardiovascular medicine* [10th ed.]. Elsevier.)

P wave is usually followed by a pacemaker-induced QRS complex. This indicates that a dual-chamber VDD or DDD pacemaker is present. A narrow, often biphasic pacemaker spike precedes the pacemaker-induced P wave (Fig. 10.8). With the pacemaker electrode placed in the right atrium, a pacemaker spike (A) is seen before each P wave. The QRS complex is normal because the ventricle is not being paced. Such a P wave may be followed by the inherent QRS complex or by a pacemaker-induced QRS complex, as seen in dual-chamber DDI or DDD pacemakers. A ventricular pacemaker usually does not produce a retrograde, inverted P wave.

PR Interval

The PR interval in atrial synchronous and dual-paced AV sequential pacemakers is within normal limits.

R-R Interval

Intervals are equal if the pacemaker is pacing constantly. When the pacemaker-induced QRS complexes are interspersed among the patient's normally occurring QRS complexes, the R-R intervals are unequal.

QRS Complex

The pacemaker-induced QRS complex is typically longer than 0.12 second (Fig. 10.9).

On the 12-lead ECG, the QRS will have a left bundle-branch block pattern. This is because the electrode is in the right ventricle. Therefore the conduction moves through the right bundle branch first before moving toward the left bundle branch. This delay produces the characteristic left bundle-branch block pattern. See Chapter 13, Bundle-Branch and Fascicular Blocks.

If only the atria are paced, the resulting QRS complex is that of the underlying rhythm and is normal unless a preexisting intraventricular conduction disturbance, such as a bundle-branch block or ventricular preexcitation, is present.

Pacemaker Site

The pacemaker site of a cardiac pacemaker is an electrode. It is usually located in the tip of the pacemaker lead. The lead is usually positioned in the apex of the right ventricular cavity (ventricular pacemaker), in the right atrium (atrial pacemaker), or in both (dual-chamber pacemaker). These rhythms are referred to as *pacemaker-induced rhythms,* denoting both the site of the pacemaker that generated the rhythm and the origin of the rhythm.

Clinical Significance

A pacemaker rhythm indicates that the patient's heart is being artificially paced. Cardiac pacemakers are permanently implanted in patients in order to treat underlying second- or third-degree AV block or symptomatic sinus bradycardia, such as marked sinus bradycardia and sinus arrest, slow junctional rhythms, or atrial fibrillation or flutter with an excessively slow ventricular response.

Temporary pacemakers are often employed during cardiac emergencies when an extremely slow rhythm occurs. For example, such a device might be used to treat AV block associated with myocardial infarction. They are also used immediately after open-heart surgery or during cardiac arrest when the ECG shows a slow escape rhythm that is unresponsive to drug therapy. Occasionally, a temporary pacemaker is needed for a patient in whom digitalis or other drug toxicity has caused profound bradycardia.

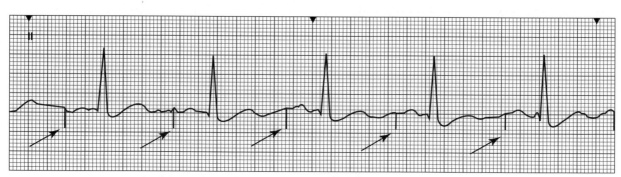

FIG. 10.8 Atrial pacemaker spikes. *Arrows,* Pacemaker spikes.

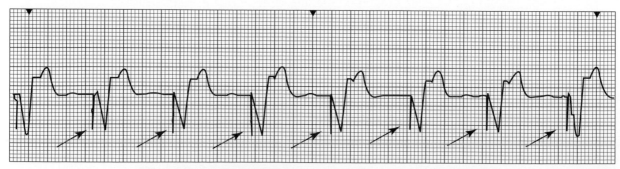

FIG. 10.9 Ventricular pacemaker spikes. *Arrows,* Pacemaker spikes.

PACEMAKER MALFUNCTION

Pacemaker spikes followed by QRS complexes indicate that the patient's heart rate is being regulated by a cardiac pacemaker. When a QRS complex follows every pacemaker spike or every paced P wave (as seen in single-chamber pacing) or every pair of pacemaker spikes (as seen in dual-chamber pacing), the pacemaker is functioning normally even if the patient's own P waves and QRS complexes are interspersed among the pacemaker spikes and associated QRS complexes.

Most problems with pacemakers can be categorized as failure to sense, failure to capture, or both.

Failure to Sense

To function properly, the pacemaker must be able to sense the presence of the underlying P waves and QRS complexes. For example, in Fig. 10.10, you will see a series of sinus beats with a prolonged PR interval after the first two paced complexes. If the pacemaker unit fails to sense these intrinsic QRS complexes, it will generate inappropriate pacemaker spikes (•), which sometimes fall on T waves. Three of these spikes do not capture the ventricle because they occur during the refractory period of the cardiac cycle.

There are two common causes of failure to sense (without actual battery failure):

1. **Dislodgment of the pacemaker pacing wire.** If the pacemaker wire is dislodged, the sensing electrode is no longer in direct contact with the heart.
2. **Excessive scarring (fibrosis) around the tip of the pacing wire.** Scarring occurs because the electrode is embedded in the heart's muscle tissue. As the heart beats, the contact points of the pacemaker electrode scar the muscle. This scarring insulates the tissue around the electrode so that it can no longer receive electrical signals. The result is the pacemaker's failure to sense.

Failure to Capture

The presence of pacemaker spikes that are not followed by P waves or QRS complexes indicates that the electrical impulses are unable to stimulate the heart to depolarize. This is referred to as *failure to capture*. It is most often caused by either a low output of electrical current from the pacemaker or as a result of scarring that insulates the heart muscle from being stimulated. In Fig. 10.11, you'll notice that beats 1, 3, and 4 show pacemaker spike (s on the strip) and normally paced, wide QRS complexes and T waves. The remaining beats show only pacemaker spikes without capture. (R represents the patient's slow spontaneous QRS complexes, which the pacemaker also fails to sense.)

Pacemaker malfunction in patients with temporary pacemakers should always prompt an immediate search for loose connections between the battery and the pacing wire or for a faulty battery or dislodged wire.

> **AUTHOR'S NOTE** To determine whether the pacemaker is functioning and generating pacer spikes, an insulated circular magnet is placed over the pacemaker generator. This causes the pacemaker to go into the default (fixed-rate) mode, resulting in pacer spikes at the preset rate. These can then be seen on the ECG strip.

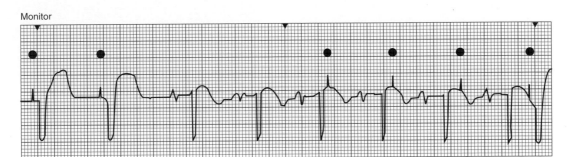

FIG. 10.10 Failure to sense. •, Pacer spike. (Modified from Goldberger, A. L., Goldberger, Z. D., & Shvilkin, A. [Eds.]. (2012). *Goldberger's clinical electrocardiography: A simplified approach* [8th ed.]. Saunders. Adapted from Conover, M. B. [1996]. *Understanding electrocardiography* [4th ed.]. Mosby.)

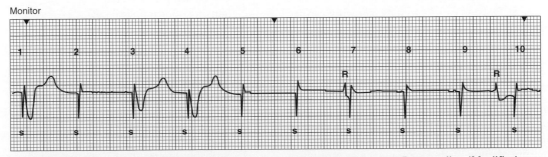

FIG. 10.11 Failure to capture. Note that 1, 3, and 4 have capture. *, Pacer spike. (Modified from Goldberger, A. L., Goldberger, Z. D., & Shvilkin, A. [Eds.]. [2012]. *Goldberger's clinical electrocardiography: A simplified approach* [8th ed.]. Saunders.)

IMPLANTABLE CARDIOVERTER-DEFIBRILLATOR THERAPY

Sudden cardiac arrest is often caused by the abrupt onset of V-fib, often preceded by a run of V-tach. The goal in modern cardiology is to prevent or interrupt episodes of ventricular rhythms that can lead to sudden cardiac arrest in high-risk patients.

The three major approaches to this problem are as follows:
1. Antidysrhythmic drug therapy that consists of medication like amiodarone to suppress the occurrence of lethal V-tach and fibrillation
2. Radiofrequency catheter ablation that is designed to physically destroy areas of the ventricles that generate ectopy
3. Implantable cardioverter-defibrillators (ICDs)

ICD therapy, as the name implies, involves the internal placement of a device, resembling a pacemaker, capable of delivering electrical shocks to the heart to terminate (cardiovert or defibrillate) a life-threatening run of V-tach or V-fib. This approach is modeled on conventional external cardioversion/defibrillation devices used in advanced cardiopulmonary resuscitation (CPR), which deliver an electrical shock via paddles placed on the chest wall.

The clinical indications for ICD therapy are shown in ECG Keys Box 10.2.

ICD Devices

ICD devices resemble pacemakers and have two major components: a lead system and a pulse generator (Fig. 10.12). The device is very similar to a pacemaker. However, instead of a simple electrode in the right ventricle, an ICD has a special electrode that touches more surface area of the endocardium. This electrode delivers a life-saving shock to the heart if a lethal ventricular rhythm develops.

Contemporary ICD devices have many programmable features, including the capacity to automatically deliver *tiered* therapy. In a tiered device, the shock energy level escalates when a dangerous tachycardia is detected (Fig. 10.13). These devices also have a function to terminate fast heart rhythms through a process called *antitachycardia pacing* (ATP). When the tachycardia reaches a preprogrammed upper rate, the ICD delivers a pacing spike with slightly higher energy levels than the standard pacing spike but significantly lower energy levels than those used for defibrillation.

Most ICD models also function as pacemakers in the case of bradycardia. The ICD units can store data, allowing cardiac electrophysiologists to check the device periodically to obtain a detailed record of any abnormal rhythm sensed and any pacing spikes or shocks delivered.

ICD Malfunction

ICD devices malfunction for many of the same reasons that pacemakers do. In addition, because of their ability to defibrillate the heart, they suffer from the following malfunctions:
- Increase or abrupt change in shock frequency as a result of poor sensing

---

BOX 10.2 ECG KEYS | **Indications for Implantable Cardioverter-Defibrillator Therapy**

- Cardiac arrest resulting from ventricular fibrillation (V-fib) or ventricular tachycardia (V-tach) not produced by a transient or reversible cause
- Spontaneous sustained V-tach in association with structural heart disease
- Syncope of undetermined origin with clinically relevant, hemodynamically significant sustained V-tach or V-fib induced during electrophysiologic study
- Nonsustained V-tach in patients with coronary artery disease, prior myocardial infarction, left ventricular dysfunction, and inducible V-fib or sustained V-tach during electrophysiologic study
- Spontaneous sustained V-tach in patients without structural heart disease and that is not amenable to other treatments
- Patients with impaired left ventricular ejection fraction, 30% or less, after myocardial infarction

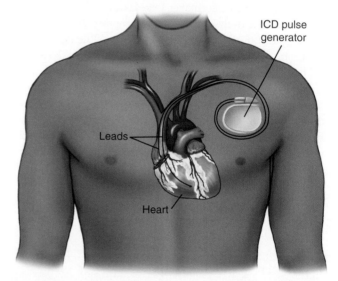

FIG. 10.12 An implantable cardioverter-defibrillator (ICD). (Modified from Goldberger, A. L., Goldberger, Z. D., & Shvilkin, A. [Eds.]. [2012]. *Goldberger's clinical electrocardiography: A simplified approach* [8th ed.]. Saunders.)

- Sensing and shock of suspected supraventricular tachydysrhythmia, resulting in the following:
  1. Oversensing of T waves
  2. Sensing noncardiac signals
  3. Syncope, near-syncope, and dizziness
- Low shock strength (lead problem, change in defibrillation threshold), leading to the following:
  1. Hemodynamically significant supraventricular tachydysrhythmia
  2. Inadequate backup pacing for bradydysrhythmia (spontaneous or drug induced)
- Cardiac arrest
  1. Probably as a result of V-fib that failed to respond to programmed shock parameters

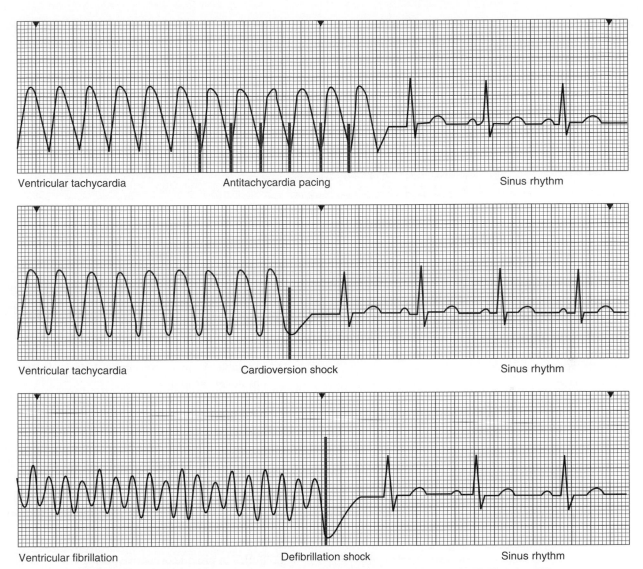

FIG. 10.13 Tiered dysrhythmia therapy and implanted cardioverter-defibrillators (ICDs). (Modified from Goldberger, A. L., Goldberger, Z. D., & Shvilkin, A. [Eds.]. [2012]. *Goldberger's clinical electrocardiography: A simplified approach* [8th ed.]. Saunders.)

A patient may report that he or she can feel the ICD firing. Patients may sense the shock, which sometimes is painful. They will also notice the heavy beating of the heart when the ICD fires. An ICD rarely fires unnecessarily, because malfunctions are rare. Therefore, if it's firing, the most conservative reason is because it is working properly, and the patient is experiencing a potentially lethal cardiac rhythm. The first step in determining whether or not the ICD is functioning appropriately is to attach the patient to a cardiac monitor so that the rhythm being defibrillated can be interpreted.

▌TAKE-HOME POINTS

- Pacemakers are battery-powered devices used to stimulate the heart electrically, particularly when the patient's heart rate is excessively slow.

- Pacemakers consist of a control box and electrodes that are inserted into an atrial or ventricular chamber. They can be used either for the temporary treatment of an AV block associated with myocardial infarction accompanying cardiac arrest or for the permanent treatment of persistent rhythm disturbances.

- Cardiac pacing can be done in a fixed-rate or demand mode. Demand pacemakers are inhibited when the heart rate is faster than the LR of the pacemaker, whereas fixed-rate pacemakers discharge constantly at a preset rate.

- Pacemakers are either single chamber or dual chamber. Single-chamber pacemakers sense and pace the activity of only one chamber and are rarely used. Dual-chamber pacemakers can sense and pace the atria and ventricles. Dual-chamber pacemakers promote a more normal physiologic contraction of the heart.

- When the pacemaker fires, it produces a narrow spike on the ECG. This pacer spike may be seen either before a P wave, before the QRS complex, or both, depending on the type of pacemaker. A ventricular pacemaker spike generates a QRS complex that resembles a left bundle-branch block because the pacing electrode is within the endocardium of the right ventricle.

- The most common pacemaker malfunctions are failure to sense, failure to capture, or a combination of the two.

The ECG can be used to detect both types of malfunctions.

- ICD therapy involves the internal placement of a device capable of delivering electrical shocks to the heart to interrupt a life-threatening run of V-tach or V-fib, thereby preventing syncope or sudden death. The ICD usually has the additional ability to pace the heart.

CHAPTER REVIEW QUESTIONS

1. Which of the following is the primary indication for the placement of a permanent pacemaker?
   A. Digitalis toxicity
   B. History of multiple prior myocardial infarctions
   C. Symptomatic bradydysrhythmias
   D. Ventricular bigeminy

2. Fibrosis around the pacemaker electrode primarily results in which of the following?
   A. Failure to sense
   B. Failure to pace
   C. Failure to sense and pace
   D. Normal pacemaker function with a ventricular premature beat

3. Which kind of pacemaker fires only when the heart rate falls below a set limit?
   A. Demand pacemaker
   B. Dual-chamber pacemaker
   C. Fixed-rate pacemaker
   D. Overdrive pacemaker

4. The QRS complex generated by an implanted pacemaker has which of the following characteristics?
   A. Duration less than 0.12 second
   B. Appearance of left bundle-branch block
   C. Normal P wave preceding the QRS complex
   D. Appearance of right bundle-branch block

5. Which code denotes a pacemaker that senses and paces both the atria and the ventricles?
   A. AVI
   B. DDD
   C. DVI
   D. VVI

6. The period after the pacer spike in a VVI pacemaker, during which time a pacer spike will not discharge, is called what?
   A. Absolute refractory period
   B. Lower set limit
   C. Relative refractory period
   D. VRP

7. The application of a circular magnet over the controller of an implanted pacemaker will cause it to do what?
   A. Go into demand mode
   B. Go into fixed-rate mode
   C. Increase the power of the discharges to overcome poor capture
   D. Stop functioning completely

8. ICD therapy is contraindicated in which condition?
   A. Inducible V-fib or sustained V-tach during electrophysiological study
   B. Spontaneous sustained V-tach in association with structural heart disease
   C. Sustained V-tach secondary to digitalis toxicity
   D. Syncope of undetermined origin with clinically relevant, hemodynamically significant sustained V-tach

9. Modern pacemakers and ICDs have what in common?
   A. Both can be checked by an external controller to determine how well they are functioning.
   B. Both can cardiovert ventricular tachycardia.
   C. Both can provide overdrive pacing when needed.
   D. They have the same type of electrode attached to the endocardium.

10. A patient complains that he can feel his ICD firing in his chest. What is your conclusion?
    A. He is obviously mistaken because he is awake and not in cardiac arrest.
    B. He most likely has a severe bradycardia.
    C. He should be immediately placed on a cardiac monitor.
    D. His pacemaker probably has a dead battery.

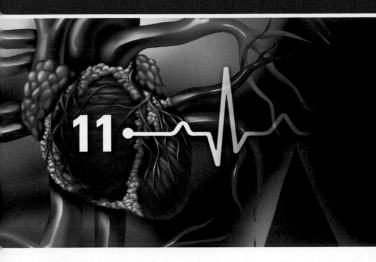

11   Treatment of Rhythm Disturbances

OUTLINE

ASSESSING THE PATIENT

The first question to ask when assessing the patient with an ECG rhythm disturbance is whether the patient is symptomatic. If so, the next question is whether or not the symptoms are caused by the dysrhythmia, or is the rhythm disturbance itself a symptom of an underlying condition such as myocardial infarction (MI). It is beyond the scope of this text to explore all possible combinations of signs and symptoms, so we'll assume that any symptoms discussed are caused by the dysrhythmia. We've outlined the various symptoms associated with each rhythm in earlier chapters.

Some symptoms are mild, whereas others are profound. The question for the clinician, then, is when to treat the rhythm. Aggressive treatment of minimally symptomatic rhythms may lead to complications because the medications used to treat these conditions are not without their hazards. Therefore for patients with milder symptoms, it is smart to take a less aggressive approach while performing diagnostic testing and trying to correct underlying causes. As symptoms worsen, treating them

becomes more urgent. At that point, the decision comes down to which of the two modalities, pharmacologic or electrical, is more likely to stabilize the heart.

Stable Versus Unstable

It's accepted practice to use electrical therapy such as transcutaneous pacing (TCP), cardioversion, and defibrillation in the unstable patient and reserve pharmacologic therapy for the stable patient. The unstable patient typically has the following:

- Signs and symptoms of decreased cardiac output (for example, decreased level of consciousness)
- Chest pain or dyspnea
- Hypotension (systolic blood pressure less than 90 mm Hg)
- Congestive heart failure or pulmonary edema

Although it's true that each of these signs and symptoms indicates that the patient's condition may significantly deteriorate, we must also take into account the clinical context of the patient's care. Is the patient being cared for in the prehospital setting, far from a fully staffed emergency department, or is he or she in an intensive care unit surrounded by a resuscitation team? As described later, the patient often must be sedated when electrical therapy is administered, requiring potentially complex airway management. Additionally, there is a risk that after cardioversion, the patient's condition may deteriorate. In the worst-case scenario, she or he may be in cardiac arrest and require more resources than are immediately available. Thus the degree of patient stability a clinician is willing to accept depends on many factors and is not simply a matter of whether the patient exhibits a given set of symptoms.

In the end, each clinician—prehospital providers, nurses, and physicians alike—must decide what constitutes instability based on available resources.

TREATING THE PATIENT

Once the rhythm has been interpreted and the stability of the patient determined, you must decide what treatment to use. For some rhythms, such as ventricular fibrillation (VF or V-fib), electrical therapy is the only option. For most rhythms, however, electrical and pharmacologic therapy both have their own merits.

Electrical Therapy

CARDIOVERSION AND DEFIBRILLATION

It is beyond the scope of this text to describe the procedure for performing cardioversion and defibrillation because the procedure differs with the make and model of each device. However, we can outline some general similarities and differences (Table 11.1).

The primary difference between cardioversion and defibrillation is the energy level and timing of the energy delivery. Cardioversion is synchronized to the relative refractory period of the QRS-T complex by sensing the R or S waves. The operator pushes the discharge button, and the machine delivers the energy at the proper time during the absolute refractory period, which occurs during the QRS complex. This is to prevent the energy from being delivered during the relative refractory period, which could result in the rhythm deteriorating to ventricular tachycardia (VT or V-tach) or V-fib. Defibrillation is not synchronized, resulting in the immediate delivery of the shock at the moment the discharge button is pressed.

> **synchronized cardioversion**
>
> The delivery of energy to the heart during the absolute refractory period of the QRS-T complex.

Although there is ongoing debate regarding the optimal energy to terminate a particular rhythm, the following guidelines are consistent with current literature.

> **AUTHOR'S NOTE** When performing cardioversion or TCP, it is important to remember that this procedure will cause the patient pain and anxiety. Therefore you should establish vascular access in order to administer analgesics and sedatives.

Transcutaneous Pacing

TCP is performed using the same pads used for cardioversion and defibrillation. The differences are as follows:

1. Significantly smaller energy levels are used.
2. The energy is delivered to the heart in a rhythmic manner. The goal of TCP is to deliver energy to the heart in order to stimulate the ventricular walls to contract.

TCP tends to be less effective in the clinical settings of severe hypothermia, hyperkalemia, metabolic acidosis, and cardiac arrest.

INDICATIONS

The indications for TCP are as follows:

- Used or the treatment of all symptomatic bradycardias resistant to pharmacologic therapy
- Considered in the initial treatment of symptomatic bradycardia associated with acute coronary syndrome (ACS) and in situations in which vascular access is difficult or delayed
- Treatment of choice in symptomatic bradycardia in patients with heart transplants because atropine is usually ineffective in such patients. It is reasonable, however, to try a pharmacologic agent such as epinephrine or dopamine while preparing the transcutaneous pacemaker.
- Control of polymorphic VT with prolonged QT interval, such as torsades de pointes. Once capture is obtained, the pacing is lowered to a sustainable rate. This process is referred to as *overdrive pacing*.

TABLE 11.1	Comparison of Cardioversion and Defibrillation	
	Cardioversion	**Defibrillation**
Goal	Goal is to stop all electrical activity in the heart momentarily in order to allow a pacemaker site to awaken and resume control of the heart's rhythm	
Administration	Requires that special adhesive pads be applied to the body to conduct the energy in the defibrillator to the chest and toward the heart when the discharge (shock) button is pushed	
Timing of energy delivery	Synchronized mode	Unsynchronized mode, with immediate delivery of energy when the shock button is pushed
Indications	Used when there is an underlying organized rhythm	Reserved for life-threatening rhythms
Energy level	Less energy delivered	More energy delivered

- Initial treatment of the following symptomatic bradycardias (those with wide QRS complexes) when vascular access is delayed or the rhythm is resistant to pharmacologic therapy:
  1. Second-degree type II atrioventricular (AV) block
  2. Second-degree 2:1 and advanced AV block with wide QRS complexes
  3. Third-degree AV block with wide QRS complexes

Pharmacologic Therapy

ATROPINE

Atropine blocks the influence of the parasympathetic nervous system on the heart. The vagus nerve provides this influence by inhibiting the sinoatrial (SA) node, causing it to fire at a slower rate. Therefore atropine increases the heart rate by blocking the vagus nerve, which allows the SA node to fire more rapidly.

> **chronotropic**
>
> Refers to any drug or condition that influences the heart rate.

Atropine is administered by intravenous (IV) bolus. Never administer atropine slowly because it may cause paradoxical slowing of the heart that can last several minutes.

Atropine may or may not be effective or indicated in treating symptomatic bradycardias, depending on the cause and the site of the AV block.

Indications

Atropine is usually effective in treating the following symptomatic bradycardias and is indicated in their initial treatment:

- Sinus bradycardia and sinus arrest/SA exit block resulting from an increase in vagal (parasympathetic) tone on the SA node secondary to an inferior or right ventricular wall MI and/or SA node dysfunction. This is usually caused by an acute right ventricular wall MI.
- AV blocks caused by an increase in vagal (parasympathetic) tone on the AV node and/or an AV node dysfunction secondary to an acute inferior or right ventricular wall MI:
  1. Second-degree type I AV block (Wenckebach)
  2. Second-degree 2:1 and advanced AV block *with narrow QRS complexes*
  3. Third-degree AV block with narrow QRS complexes

Contraindications, End Points, and Adverse Effects

Observe the following contraindications and cautions when administering atropine:

- Atropine is usually not indicated in treating bradycardias that result from disruption of the electrical conduction system below the AV node secondary to an acute anterior wall MI. In this setting, with AV blocks (which tend to progress rapidly to complete third-degree AV block without warning) and third-degree AV blocks, the attachment of a transcutaneous pacemaker is indicated immediately, whether or not the bradycardia is symptomatic.

- Second-degree 2:1 and advanced AV block with wide QRS complexes.
- Third-degree AV block with wide QRS complexes.
- Use atropine with caution in patients with acute MI. The heart rate may increase excessively, which may increase ischemia and lead to V-tach or V-fib. TCP is preferred in such patients and in those in whom IV access is difficult or delayed.
- Atropine is usually ineffective in treating bradycardia in patients with heart transplants. That's because parasympathetic activity has no influence on the transplanted heart's rate because the vagus nerve is severed during the transplantation procedure. Without an intact vagus nerve, there is no direct influence on the SA node. Therefore TCP is the treatment of choice in symptomatic bradycardias in such patients. Drugs such as dopamine and epinephrine are also effective in treating symptomatic bradycardias in patients with transplanted hearts.

> **AUTHOR'S NOTE** In the guidelines and algorithms that follow, the IV route of administration is listed for all medications. Depending on the clinical scenario, vascular access may be obtained via a peripheral or central vein or through the insertion of an intraosseous (IO) needle (IO route). All the agents listed may be administered by IO without changing the concentration or dosage. The administration of medication via endotracheal tube is not recommended.

Vasopressors

Vasopressors are drugs that cause constriction in the arterioles and venous circulatory system. This constriction increases peripheral vascular resistance, which can improve blood pressure and coronary and cerebral blood flow. These drugs also increase cardiac output by increasing the heart rate and strengthening cardiac muscle contraction, referred to as an *inotropic effect*.

EPINEPHRINE

Epinephrine (adrenaline) is a naturally occurring drug produced as norepinephrine and then metabolized by the body into epinephrine. The release of norepinephrine from the adrenal gland mediates the sympathetic nervous system. In addition, sympathetic nerves release norepinephrine to exert their adrenergic (adrenaline-like) effect. There are two different adrenergic receptors: alpha and beta. Stimulation of alpha-receptors in the peripheral vessels constricts the arterioles. There are two types of beta-receptors. Beta$_1$-receptors in heart muscle are stimulated by epinephrine to increase the force of muscular contraction and the spontaneous rate of discharge of pacemaker and cardiac cells. Beta$_2$-receptors in the pulmonary, cerebral, and coronary arteries are stimulated to constrict to a lesser degree by epinephrine.

Epinephrine may be considered to treat symptomatic bradycardia when atropine is ineffective. TCP should be prepared in the event epinephrine is also ineffective. However, epinephrine must be used cautiously because it stimulates the heart muscle directly and may increase the heart rate too much, thus increasing myocardial oxygen demand, which can cause irritability, premature ventricular complexes (PVCs), or potentially lethal rhythms, such as V-tach or V-fib.

In patients with stable yet symptomatic bradycardia, epinephrine should be administered via a diluted infusion. Concentrated bolus administration is more likely to cause complications and should be reserved for the unstable patient.

VASOPRESSIN

Vasopressin is a nonadrenergic peripheral vasoconstrictor that also causes coronary and renal vasoconstriction. Vasopressin has been found to be equivalent to epinephrine in treating the following conditions:

- Shock-refractory V-fib/V-tach
- Asystole
- Pulseless electrical activity (PEA)

Vasopressin is administered as a single dose of 40 units IV or IO and may replace the first or second dose of epinephrine in the cardiac arrest treatment algorithms.

> **inotropic**
>
> Refers to the strength of ventricular contraction.

DOPAMINE

Dopamine is a naturally occurring precursor of norepinephrine in the body. At medium (5–10 mcg/kg/min) dosages, it stimulates the $beta_1$-receptors, resulting in increased SA-node discharge (positive chronotropic), improved myocardial contractility (positive inotropic), and faster impulse conduction through the myocardium. At high dosages (10–20 mcg/kg/min), dopamine stimulates both $alpha_1$- (arteriole) and $alpha_2$- (venule) receptors, resulting in vasoconstriction and increased heart rate.

Dopamine may be considered in treating symptomatic bradycardia. Caution must be taken to avoid causing tachycardia, which will increase myocardial oxygen demand. Administration of dopamine is by IV infusion only.

NOREPINEPHRINE

Norepinephrine is a naturally occurring, potent vasoconstrictor and inotropic agent. It may be effective for the management of patients with severe hypotension (systolic blood pressure <70 mm Hg) and in those who fail to respond to less potent adrenergic drugs, such as dopamine or epinephrine.

Norepinephrine is ordinarily not indicated in patients with low blood volume. In addition, because it may increase myocardial oxygen requirements, it should be used with caution in patients with ischemic heart disease.

DOBUTAMINE

Dobutamine is a synthetic drug that is often used for the treatment of severe systolic heart failure. Dobutamine is a potent inotropic agent. Dobutamine is administered at a rate of 10 to 20 mcg/min titrated to hemodynamic response, such as heart rate and/or blood pressure.

ISOPROTERENOL

Isoproterenol is a beta-adrenergic agent with $beta_1$ and $beta_2$ effects that increases the heart rate and, to a lesser extent, causes vasodilation in the pulmonary and coronary arteries. An infusion of 2 to 10 mcg/min is titrated to heart rate.

Antidysrhythmics

> **antidysrhythmics**
>
> Drugs that can terminate abnormal rhythms by influencing the route and rate of electrical conduction within the heart.

ADENOSINE

Adenosine is a naturally occurring agent that briefly depresses the activity of the SA and AV nodes.

Indications

Adenosine is indicated for the following conditions:

- Narrow-complex AV-node or sinus-node reentry tachycardias (supraventricular tachycardia [SVT])
- Unstable SVT while preparing for cardioversion
- Undefined, stable, narrow-complex SVT, as a combination therapeutic and diagnostic maneuver
- Stable, wide-complex tachycardia in patients with a recurrence of a known reentry pathway
- Stable, regular, monomorphic, wide-complex tachycardia, as a therapeutic and diagnostic maneuver

Contraindications, End Points, and Adverse Effects

Adenosine should not be used for the treatment of an SVT with Wolf–Parkinson–White (WPW) syndrome because it may result in a paradoxical increase in accessory pathway conduction, leading to V-tach or V-fib. Administration usually results in the patient feeling a warm and sometimes distressing sensation in the chest, which resolves quickly.

> **AUTHOR'S NOTE** Adenosine usually does not terminate rhythms such as atrial flutter, atrial fibrillation, atrial tachycardia, or V-tach because these rhythms are not caused by reentry mechanisms involving the SA or AV node. However, it may produce a transient AV block, resulting in a slowing of the rate and thus revealing the underlying rhythm.

AMIODARONE

IV amiodarone affects sodium, potassium, and calcium channels. It also has alpha- and beta-adrenergic blocking properties.

Indications

Amiodarone is indicated in the following conditions:

- Tachycardia
  1. For narrow-complex tachycardias caused by a reentry mechanism (SVT) if the rhythm is not terminated by adenosine and vagal maneuvers
  2. Stable monomorphic and polymorphic V-tach
  3. Wide-complex tachycardia of uncertain origin

- Cardiac arrest
- V-fib or pulseless V-tach unresponsive to defibrillation, cardiopulmonary resuscitation (CPR), and a vasopressor

Contraindications, End Points, and Adverse Effects

The major adverse effects of amiodarone are hypotension and bradycardia, which can be prevented by slowing the rate of drug infusion.

LIDOCAINE

Lidocaine is an antidysrhythmic of long-standing use and widespread familiarity. It has fewer immediate side effects than many other antidysrhythmic agents, such as amiodarone and procainamide.

Indications

The indications for the use of lidocaine include the following:
- Stable monomorphic V-tach (alternative agents are preferred)
- Polymorphic V-tach with normal baseline QT interval when ischemia is treated and electrolyte imbalance corrected

Contraindications, End Points, and Adverse Effects

Toxic reactions and side effects include slurred speech, altered consciousness, muscle twitching, seizures, and bradycardia.

PROCAINAMIDE

Procainamide suppresses both atrial and ventricular rhythm disturbances by slowing electrical conduction through myocardial tissue.

Indications

Procainamide may be considered in the following conditions:
- Stable monomorphic V-tach
- Control of heart rate in atrial fibrillation or atrial flutter with rapid ventricular response
- Conversion of rhythm in atrial fibrillation or atrial flutter in patients with known preexcitation (WPW) syndrome
- Paroxysmal supraventricular tachycardia (PSVT) if rhythm is uncontrolled by adenosine and vagal maneuvers and the patient's ventricular function is normal

Contraindications, End Points, and Adverse Effects

The administration of procainamide must be stopped when specific end points have been reached. These are listed in ECG Keys Box 11.1.

BOX 11.1 ECG KEYS	Clinical End Points for the Administration of Procainamide

- Tachycardia is suppressed.
- A total dose of 17 mg/kg of procainamide has been administered (1.2 g of procainamide for a 70-kg [154-lb] patient).
- Side effects of the procainamide appear (such as hypotension).
- The QRS complex widens by 50% of its original width.

MAGNESIUM

Magnesium is an electrolyte required for normal physiologic function. It is involved in neurochemical transmission and muscular excitability. Administration of magnesium is indicated in treating torsades de pointes.

IBUTILIDE

Ibutilide is a short-acting drug that prolongs the action potential and increases the refractory period of the myocardium. Ibutilide has minimal effects on blood pressure and heart rate. Its major limitation is a relatively high incidence of ventricular rhythms such as polymorphic V-tach, including torsades de pointes. Before administering ibutilide, hyperkalemia or hypomagnesemia must be corrected. Monitor patients receiving ibutilide *continuously* for rhythm changes at the time of its administration and for *at least 4 to 6 hours* thereafter. Ibutilide is not indicated if the baseline QT interval is greater than 440 msec.

Indications

Ibutilide may be used in the following conditions:
- Pharmacologic conversion of atrial fibrillation or atrial flutter in stable patients when the duration of the rhythm's onset is <48 hours
- Control of atrial fibrillation or atrial flutter rate when calcium-channel blockers or beta blockers are ineffective
- Pharmacologic conversion of atrial fibrillation or atrial flutter in stable patients with WPW syndrome when the duration of the rhythm's onset is <48 hours

Calcium Channel Blockers

Verapamil and diltiazem are calcium-channel blockers that slow conduction time through the AV node. These actions may terminate reentrant rhythms and control the ventricular response rate in patients with a variety of atrial tachycardias.

Indications

These medications are indicated in the following circumstances:
- Stable, narrow-complex reentry mechanism tachycardias (SVT) if rhythm remains uncontrolled or unconverted by adenosine or vagal maneuvers
- Atrial fibrillation or atrial flutter with rapid ventricular response

Contraindications, End Points, and Adverse Effects

Calcium-channel blockers should not be given to patients with atrial fibrillation or atrial flutter associated with known preexcitation (WPW) syndrome because this may result in a complete heart block. ECG Keys Box 11.2 lists other contraindications for the administration of calcium-channel blockers. Calcium-channel blockers should not be used for the treatment of a PSVT with WPW because it may result in a paradoxical increase in accessory pathway conduction, leading to V-tach or V-fib.

Verapamil and, to a lesser extent, diltiazem may decrease myocardial contractility and critically reduce cardiac output in

BOX 11.2 ECG KEYS	Administration of Calcium-Channel Blockers

Calcium-channel blockers are not indicated in the following situations:
- If hypotension or cardiogenic shock is present
- If second- or third-degree AV block, sinus-node dysfunction, or atrial flutter or fibrillation associated with ventricular or atrio–His preexcitation or a wide-QRS-complex tachycardia is present
- If beta blockers are being administered intravenously
- If there is a history of bradycardia

Calcium-channel blockers should be used cautiously, if at all, in patients with congestive heart failure and those receiving oral beta blockers.

The patient's blood pressure and pulse must be monitored frequently during and after the administration of a calcium-channel blocker.
- If hypotension occurs with a calcium-channel blocker, place the patient in a Trendelenburg position and administer 1 gram of calcium chloride IV slowly, IV fluids, and a vasopressor.
- If bradycardia, AV block, or asystole occurs, refer to the appropriate treatment protocol.

BOX 11.3 ECG KEYS	Contraindications for Administration of Beta Blockers

- If bradycardia (heart rate <60 beats/min) is present
- If hypotension (systolic blood pressure <100 mm Hg is present)
- If PR interval >0.24 second or second- or third-degree AV block is present
- Presence of ventricular preexcitation such as Wolff–Parkinson–White (WPW) syndrome
- If severe congestive heart failure (left and/or right heart failure) is present
- If bronchospasm or a history of asthma is present (relative contraindication)
- If severe chronic obstructive pulmonary disease (COPD) is present
- If intravenous (IV) calcium-channel blockers have been administered within a few hours (caution advised):
  - The patient's blood pressure and pulse must be monitored frequently during and after the administration of a beta blocker.
  - If hypotension occurs with a beta blocker, place the patient in a Trendelenburg position and administer a vasopressor.
- If bradycardia, AV block, or asystole occurs, refer to the appropriate treatment protocol.

patients with severe left ventricular dysfunction and result in hypotension.

> **AUTHOR'S NOTE** Diltiazem is cited as the calcium-channel blocker of choice throughout this text. However, some clinicians prefer verapamil.

Beta Blockers

The beta-blocking agents atenolol, metoprolol, and esmolol reduce the effects of circulating adrenaline, decreasing the heart rate and blood pressure.

Indications

For acute tachycardia, these agents are indicated for rate control under the following conditions:
- Stable, narrow-complex tachycardia originating from either a *reentry mechanism* (SVT) or an *ectopic focus* (junctional, ectopic, or multifocal tachycardia) uncontrolled by vagal maneuvers and adenosine
- Rate control in atrial fibrillation and atrial flutter if the patient is stable
- Conversion of V-tach when used in conjunction with amiodarone or procainamide

Contraindications, End Points, and Adverse Effects

Contraindications to the use of beta blockers are listed in ECG Keys Box 11.3.

Side effects of beta-blocker administration include bradycardia, AV conduction delay, and hypotension.

Oxygen

All cells require oxygen and glucose to perform their metabolic activities. The application of high-flow oxygen has been the traditional therapy for all ill patients, regardless of cause. However, recent research has revealed that high concentrations of oxygen in the human body can cause harm. It has been proposed that hyperoxemia (elevated levels of oxygen saturation) worsens the neurologic outcome from cardiac arrest and may extend the size of myocardial ischemia. The mechanism of harm is not fully known but is thought to relate to the creation of "free radicals," which are solitary oxygen atoms that are highly disruptive to cellular metabolism.

Indications

The current guidelines for oxygen administration are as follows:
- Supplemental oxygen via nasal cannula at 2 to 4 L/min only if the patient is in respiratory distress, is in heart failure, is cyanotic, or has documented hypoxemia with an oxygen saturation of less than 94%
- Titration of oxygen concentration after return of spontaneous circulation in cardiac arrest to a saturation of 94% to 98%

BRADYCARDIA (FIG. 11.1)

A bradycardia with a heart rate between 50 and 59 beats/min (*mild bradycardia*) usually does not produce symptoms by itself. If the heart rate slows to 30 to 45 beats/min or less (*marked bradycardia*), the cardiac output may drop significantly, causing the systolic blood pressure to fall to 80 to 90 mm Hg or less and signs and symptoms of decreased perfusion of the body, especially of the vital organs, to appear. The skin may become pale, cold, and clammy; the pulse may be weak or absent; and the patient may be agitated, light-headed, confused, or unconscious. The patient may experience chest pain and develop trouble breathing (dyspnea).

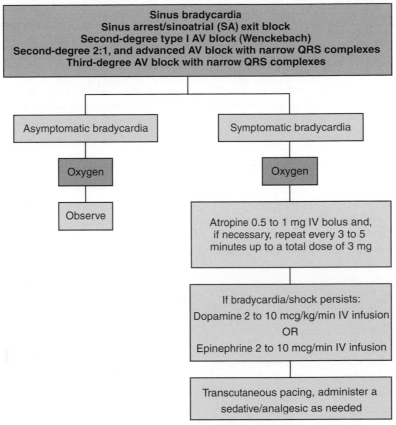

FIG. 11.1 Sinus bradycardia, sinoatrial (SA) exit block, and heart block with narrow QRS complex.

In the setting of ACS, mild bradycardia may actually be beneficial to some patients because a slower heart rate reduces the workload of the heart, which reduces the oxygen requirements of the myocardium, minimizes the extension of the infarction, and lessens the predisposition to develop a life-threatening rhythm. This is referred to as a *cardioprotective* characteristic. Marked bradycardia, however, may result in hypotension, with a marked reduction of cardiac output leading to congestive heart failure, loss of consciousness, and shock, and predispose the patient to more serious rhythms, such as PVCs, V-tach, or V-fib.

If sinus arrest or an SA exit block is prolonged, or if a second-degree AV block suddenly progresses to a third-degree AV block, and if an escape pacemaker in the AV junction (junctional escape rhythm) or ventricles (ventricular escape rhythm) does not take over, asystole will follow.

INDICATIONS FOR TREATMENT

Treatment of bradycardia, regardless of cause, is indicated immediately if the heart rate is less than 60 beats/min and the patient is unstable.

Occasionally, treatment to increase the heart rate may also be indicated if the heart rate is somewhat above 60 beats/min and the patient is symptomatic. This may result if the heart rate is too slow relative to the existing metabolic needs.

CONTRAINDICATIONS FOR TREATMENT, END POINTS, AND ADVERSE EFFECTS

Treatment may not be indicated even if the heart rate falls below 60 beats/min under the following conditions:

- The systolic blood pressure remains greater than 100 mm Hg and the patient is stable
- Absence of congestive heart failure, chest pain, and dyspnea
- Absence of agitation, light-headedness, confusion, or loss of consciousness
- Frequent PVCs do not occur

Symptomatic Bradycardia

TREATMENT

For the treatment of sinus bradycardia, sinus arrest/SA exit block, and all AV heart blocks with narrow QRS complex:

- Oxygen if indicated
- Administer atropine 0.5 to 1 mg IV. Repeat every 3 to 5 minutes until the heart rate increases to 60 to 100 beats/min. If the patient remains symptomatic after 3 mg of atropine, begin TCP.

AND/OR

Initiate TCP if immediately available. If the patient is unable to tolerate TCP, consider sedation and analgesia.
- If the bradycardia, hypotension, or both persist:
1. Start an IV infusion of epinephrine at an initial rate of 2 to 10 mcg/min and adjust the rate of infusion to increase

the heart rate to 60 to 100 beats/min and the systolic blood pressure to within normal limits.

OR

2. Start an IV infusion of dopamine at an initial rate of 2 to 10 mcg/kg/min and adjust the rate of infusion up to 20 mcg/kg/min to increase the heart rate to 60 to 100 beats/min and the systolic blood pressure to within normal limits.

- Insert a temporary transvenous pacemaker as soon as possible.

Second- or Third-Degree Heart Block With Wide QRS Complex (Fig. 11.2)

Asymptomatic second- or third-degree AV block associated with acute anterior wall MI, including the following conditions:
- Second-degree type II AV block
- Second-degree 2:1 and advanced AV block with narrow QRS complexes
- Third-degree AV block with narrow QRS complexes

TREATMENT

Treatment may include the following:
- Oxygen if indicated
- Attach a transcutaneous pacemaker, test for ventricular capture and patient tolerance, and put on standby.
- If the bradycardia is or becomes symptomatic, initiate TCP and consider sedation and analgesia.

> **AUTHOR'S NOTE** If TCP is not available, consider administering atropine; however, it is usually not effective in second- and third-degree AV blocks.

- If the bradycardia, hypotension, or both persist:
  1. Start an IV infusion of dopamine at an initial rate of 2 to 10 mcg/kg/min and adjust the rate of infusion up to

20 mcg/kg/min to increase the heart rate to 60 to 100 beats/min and the systolic blood pressure to within normal limits.

OR

2. Start an IV infusion of epinephrine at an initial rate of 2 to 10/min and adjust the rate of infusion to increase the heart rate to 60 to 100 beats/min and the systolic blood pressure to within normal limits.

OR

3. Insert a temporary transvenous pacemaker as soon as possible.

Junctional Escape Rhythm and Ventricular Escape Rhythm (Fig. 11.3)

TREATMENT

Treat junctional and ventricular escape rhythms as follows:
- Oxygen if indicated
- Initiate TCP and consider sedation and analgesia. Insert a temporary transvenous pacemaker as soon as possible.
- If the bradycardia, hypotension, or both persist:
  1. Start an IV infusion of dopamine at an initial rate of 2 to 10 mcg/kg/min. Adjust the rate of infusion up to 20 mcg/kg/min to increase the heart rate to 60 to 100 beats/min and the systolic blood pressure to within normal limits.

OR

2. Start an IV infusion of epinephrine at an initial rate of 2 to 10 mcg/min and adjust the rate of infusion to increase the heart rate to 60 to 100 beats/min and the systolic blood pressure to within normal limits.

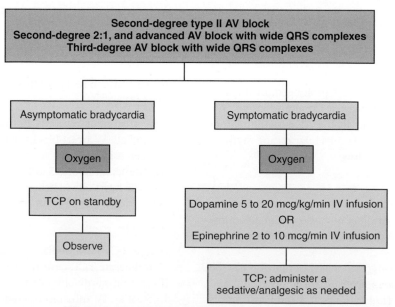

FIG. 11.2 Heart block with wide QRS complex.

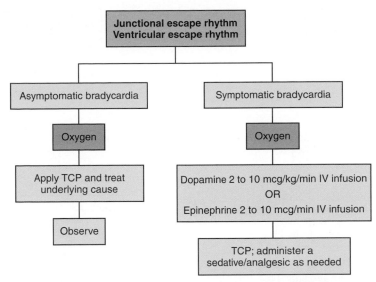

FIG. 11.3 Junctional and ventricular escape rhythms.

TACHYCARDIA

The signs and symptoms of tachycardia depend on the presence or absence of heart disease, the nature of the heart disease, the ventricular rate, and the duration of the tachycardia. Tachycardia is often accompanied by palpitations, nervousness, or anxiety.

Tachycardia with a heart rate over 150 beats/min may cause cardiac output to drop significantly because the ventricles are unable to fill completely during the extremely short diastole that results from the very rapid beating of the heart. Consequently, the systolic blood pressure may fall to 90 mm Hg or less, and signs and symptoms of decreased perfusion of the body, especially of the brain and other vital organs, may occur:

- The skin may become pale, cold, and clammy.
- The pulse may become weak or disappear.
- The patient may become agitated, confused, light-headed, or unconscious.
- He or she or may experience chest pain and have trouble breathing.

Perfusion of the coronary arteries occurs during diastole, and if the heart rate is too high, coronary perfusion can be compromised.

In addition, because a rapid heart rate increases the workload of the heart, tachycardia usually increases the oxygen requirements of the myocardium. Thus in addition to the consequences of decreased cardiac output, tachycardia in the setting of ACS may be characterized by the following:

- Increase in myocardial ischemia and the frequency and severity of chest pain
- Extension of the infarct
- Congestive heart failure
- Hypotension
- Cardiogenic shock
- Greater likelihood of serious ventricular rhythms

Contributing to the low cardiac output in certain tachycardias, such as atrial flutter, atrial fibrillation, and PSVT, is the loss of the normal atrial contraction preceding each ventricular contraction (the so-called *atrial kick*). The ventricles do not fill completely during diastole, reducing cardiac output by as much as 25%.

INDICATIONS FOR TREATMENT

Specific treatment of atrial tachycardia without block, atrial flutter, atrial fibrillation, PSVT, and junctional tachycardia is indicated if the heart rate is greater than 150 beats/min or even as low as 120 beats/min, particularly if signs and symptoms of decreased cardiac output or increased workload of the heart are associated with the tachycardia.

Treatment of V-tach, however, is indicated immediately, regardless of whether signs and symptoms of decreased cardiac output are present, because of its potential for initiating or degenerating into V-fib.

No specific treatment of sinus tachycardia and atrial tachycardia with block is indicated.

Sinus Tachycardia (Fig. 11.4)
TREATMENT

No specific treatment of sinus tachycardia is indicated:

- Treat the underlying cause of the tachycardia (anxiety, exercise, pain, fever, congestive heart failure, hypoxemia, hypovolemia, hypotension, or shock).
- Discontinue administration of drugs such as atropine, epinephrine, or other vasopressors.

Atrial Tachycardia With Block (Fig. 11.5)
TREATMENT

No specific treatment of atrial tachycardia with block is indicated:
- Treat the underlying cause of the tachycardia.
- Discontinue digitalis if digitalis toxicity is suspected or confirmed.
- Administer Digibind if digitalis toxicity is confirmed.

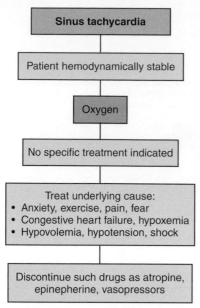

FIG. 11.4 Sinus tachycardia.

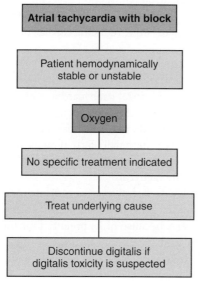

FIG. 11.5 Atrial tachycardia with block.

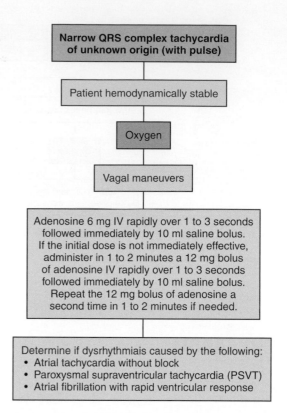

FIG. 11.6 Narrow-QRS-complex tachycardia of unknown origin.

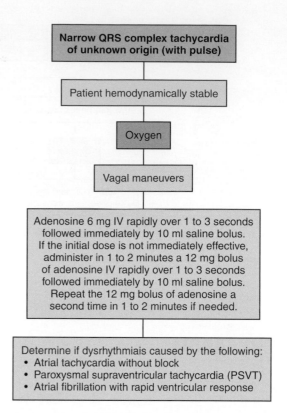

> **vagal maneuvers**
>
> Physical maneuvers performed to stimulate baroreceptors in the internal carotid artery and the aortic arch. This stimulation produces a reflexive slowing of the heart rate.

AUTHOR'S NOTE Use *extreme caution* when applying carotid sinus pressure to older patients because it may result in stroke. *Never* apply bilateral carotid pressure or exceed 10 seconds in duration. Be prepared with vascular access and continuous ECG monitoring, and have a defibrillator ready.

Narrow-QRS-Complex Tachycardia of Unknown Origin (With Pulse) (Fig. 11.6)

TREATMENT

Treat narrow QRS tachycardia as follows:

- Oxygen if indicated
- Attempt vagal maneuvers such as the following:
  1. Having the patient bear down as if having a bowel movement (Valsalva maneuver)
  2. Cold stimulation to the face with an ice water–soaked washcloth or ice pack
  3. Coughing, squatting, or breath-holding
  4. Carotid sinus pressure applied at the angle of the jaw, preferably on the right, for 5 seconds

If the vagal maneuvers are unsuccessful and the patient remains stable, administer a 6-mg bolus of adenosine IV rapidly over 1 to 3 seconds, followed immediately by a 10- to 20-mL saline bolus. If the initial dose is not immediately effective, administer a 12-mg bolus of adenosine IV rapidly over 1 to 3 seconds, followed immediately by a 10- to 20-mL saline bolus. Repeat the 12-mg bolus of adenosine a second time 1 to 2 minutes later if needed.

Conversion to normal sinus rhythm confirms that PSVT was present. Continue treatment after the next appropriate state in the Paroxysmal Supraventricular Tachycardia With Narrow QRS Complexes section later in this chapter.

If the heart rate slows sufficiently to allow the detection of atrial or junctional tachycardia, continue with the treatment plans outlined in either the Atrial Tachycardia Without Block section (following section) or the Junctional Tachycardia section (later in this chapter), as appropriate.

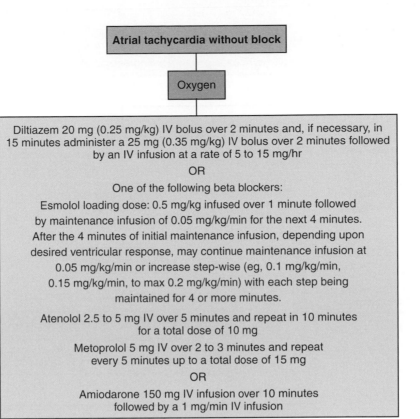

FIG. 11.7 Atrial tachycardia without block.

If the heart rate slows sufficiently to allow for the detection of atrial fibrillation or atrial flutter, continue with the treatment plans outlined in the Atrial Flutter/Fibrillation section (later in this chapter) as appropriate.

Atrial Tachycardia Without Block (Fig. 11.7)

TREATMENT

If no block is present, treat as follows:
- Oxygen if indicated
- Administer a calcium-channel blocker such as diltiazem; a beta blocker such as esmolol, atenolol, or metoprolol; or an antidysrhythmic such as amiodarone.
- For the calcium-channel blocker:
  1. Administer a 20-mg (0.25-mg/kg) dose of diltiazem IV slowly over 2 minutes. If the initial dose is not effective in 15 minutes and no adverse effects have occurred, give a second 25-mg (0.35-mg/kg) dose of diltiazem IV slowly over 2 minutes. (Exception: In patients over age 60, administer the dose of diltiazem slowly over 3–4 minutes.)

  AND

  2. Start a maintenance IV infusion of diltiazem at a rate of 5 to 15 mg/hr to maintain the heart rate within normal limits.
- For the beta blocker:
  1. Administer a 0.5-mg/kg dose of esmolol IV over 1 minute, followed by an IV infusion of esmolol at 0.05 mg/kg/min. Repeat the 0.5-mg/kg dose of esmolol IV twice at 5-minute

intervals while increasing the IV infusion of esmolol 0.05 mg/kg/min after each dose of esmolol if the response is inadequate, up to a maximum infusion of 0.2 mg/kg/min, if necessary. Then titrate the esmolol infusion to maintain the heart rate within normal limits. Do not exceed the maximum infusion of 0.2 mg/kg/min.

OR

  2. Administer 2.5 to 5 mg atenolol IV over 5 minutes. Repeat every 10 minutes as needed, up to a total dose of 10 mg, if needed.

OR

  3. Administer 5 mg metoprolol IV over 2 to 5 minutes. Repeat twice at 5-minute intervals, up to a total dose of 15 mg, if needed.

AND

  4. Monitor pulse, blood pressure, and ECG while administering the drug. Stop administering the beta blocker if the systolic blood pressure falls below 100 mm Hg.
- For the antidysrhythmic:
  1. Administer amiodarone with a loading dose of 150 mg IV over 10 minutes.

AND

  2. Start an IV infusion of amiodarone at a rate of 1 mg/min for 6 hours. Then decrease to 0.5 mg/min for 18 hours.

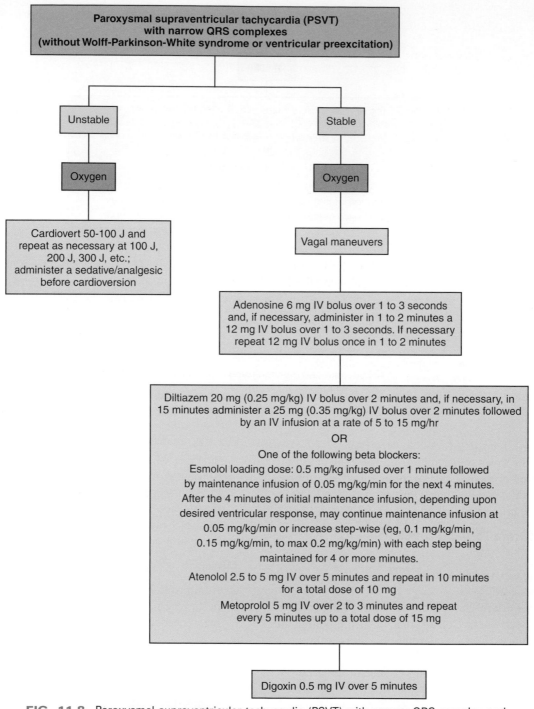

FIG. 11.8 Paroxysmal supraventricular tachycardia (PSVT) with narrow QRS complex and without Wolff–Parkinson–White (WPW) syndrome.

Paroxysmal Supraventricular Tachycardia With Narrow QRS Complexes Without WPW (Fig. 11.8)

TREATMENT

Treat as follows:

If unstable:

- Oxygen
- Cardiovert 50 to 100 J and repeat at 100 J, 200 J, and 300 J as needed

If stable:

- Oxygen if indicated
- Attempt vagal maneuvers.
- If the vagal maneuvers are unsuccessful and the patient remains stable, administer an AV-node depressant such as adenosine; a calcium-channel blocker such as diltiazem; or a beta blocker such as esmolol, atenolol, or metoprolol.

- For adenosine:
  1. Administer a 6-mg bolus IV rapidly over 1 to 3 seconds, followed immediately by a 10- to 20-mL saline bolus. If the initial dose is not immediately effective, administer a 12-mg bolus of adenosine IV rapidly over 1 to 3 seconds, followed immediately by a 10- to 20-mL saline bolus. Repeat the 12-mg bolus of adenosine in 1 to 2 minutes if needed.
- For the calcium-channel blocker:
  1. Administer a 20-mg (0.25-mg/kg) dose of diltiazem IV slowly over 2 minutes. If the initial dose is not effective in 15 minutes and no adverse effects have occurred, give a second dose of 25 mg (0.35 mg/kg) IV slowly over 2 minutes. (Exception: In patients >60 years of age, administer the dose slowly over 3–4 minutes.)

AND

  2. Start a maintenance IV infusion of diltiazem at a rate of 5 to 15 mg/hr to maintain the heart rate within normal limits.
- For the beta blocker:
  1. Administer a 0.5-mg/kg dose of esmolol IV over 1 minute, followed by an IV infusion of esmolol at 0.05 mg/kg/min. If the response is inadequate, repeat the 0.5-mg/kg dose of esmolol IV twice, at 5-minute intervals while increasing the IV infusion of esmolol 0.05 mg/kg/min after each dose, up to a maximum infusion of 0.2 mg/kg/min, if

necessary. Then titrate the esmolol infusion to maintain the heart rate within normal limits. Do not exceed the maximum infusion rate of 0.2 mg/kg/min.

OR

  2. Administer 2.5 to 5 mg atenolol IV over 5 minutes, and repeat every 10 minutes as needed, up to a total dose of 10 mg, if needed.

OR

  3. Administer 5 mg metoprolol IV over 2 to 5 minutes. Repeat twice, at 5-minute intervals, up to a total dose of 15 mg, if needed.

AND

  4. Monitor the pulse, blood pressure, and ECG while administering the drug. Stop administering the beta blocker if the systolic blood pressure falls below 100 mm Hg.

Paroxysmal Supraventricular Tachycardia With Narrow QRS Complexes With WPW (Fig. 11.9)

TREATMENT

Treat as follows:

If unstable:
- Oxygen
- Cardiovert 50 to 100 J and repeat at 100 J, 200 J, and 300 J as needed

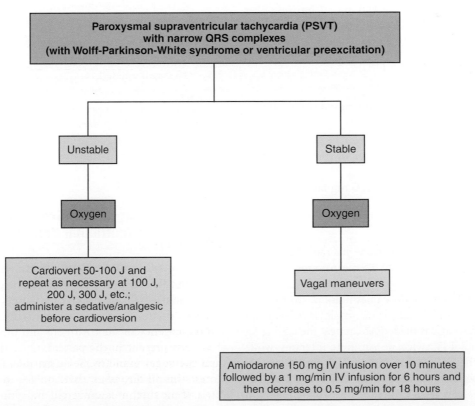

FIG. 11.9 Paroxysmal supraventricular tachycardia (PSVT) with narrow QRS complex and Wolff–Parkinson–White (WPW) syndrome.

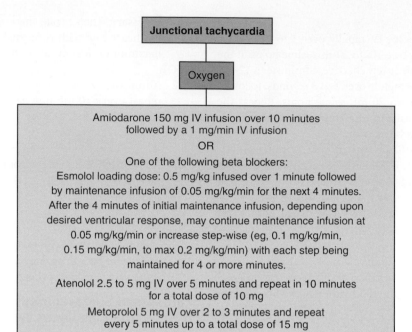

FIG. 11.10 Junctional tachycardia.

If stable:
- Oxygen if indicated.
- Attempt vagal maneuvers.

If the vagal maneuvers are unsuccessful and the patient remains stable, administer amiodarone 150 mg IV infusion over 10 minutes followed by a 1-mg/min IV infusion for 6 hours and then decrease to 0.5 mg/min for 18 hours.

Junctional Tachycardia (Fig. 11.10)

TREATMENT

Follow this algorithm in patients with junctional tachycardia:
- Oxygen if indicated
- Administer an antidysrhythmic drug such as amiodarone or a beta blocker such as esmolol, atenolol, or metoprolol.
  1. For the antidysrhythmic:
     - Administer a loading dose of 150 mg amiodarone IV over 10 minutes.

AND

  - Start an IV infusion of amiodarone at a rate of 1 mg/min for 6 hours. Then decrease to 0.5 mg/min for 18 hours.
  2. For the beta blocker:
     - Administer a 0.5-mg/kg dose of esmolol IV over 1 minute, followed by an IV infusion of esmolol at 0.05 mg/kg/min. If the response is inadequate, repeat the 0.5-mg/kg dose of esmolol IV twice, at 5-minute intervals, while increasing the IV infusion rate to 0.05 mg/kg/min after each dose, up to a maximum infusion of 0.2 mg/kg/min, if necessary. Then titrate the infusion to maintain the heart rate within normal limits. Do not exceed the maximum infusion rate of 0.2 mg/kg/min.

OR

  - Administer 2.5 to 5 mg atenolol IV over 5 minutes. Repeat every 10 minutes as needed, up to a total dose of 10 mg, if needed.

OR

- Administer 5 mg metoprolol IV over 2 to 5 minutes. Repeat twice, at 5-minute intervals, up to a total dose of 15 mg, if needed.

AND

- Monitor the pulse, blood pressure, and ECG while administering the drug. Stop administering the beta blocker if the systolic blood pressure falls below 100 mm Hg.

Atrial Flutter/Atrial Fibrillation (Without WPW Syndrome or Ventricular Preexcitation) (Fig. 11.11)

There are two options for the treatment of atrial flutter and atrial fibrillation: either the rate can be controlled to improve the patient's cardiac output, or attempts can be made to convert the rhythm to normal sinus rhythm. The choice depends on the urgency of the treatment and the duration the rhythm has been present in the patient. Over time, atrial fibrillation and flutter can result in the formation of a blood clot, referred to as a *mural thrombus,* that adheres to the inner wall of the atria. If the rhythm is converted and a mural thrombus is present, there is a risk that the thrombus could break free, causing a stroke. To avoid this, it is recommended that atrial fibrillation

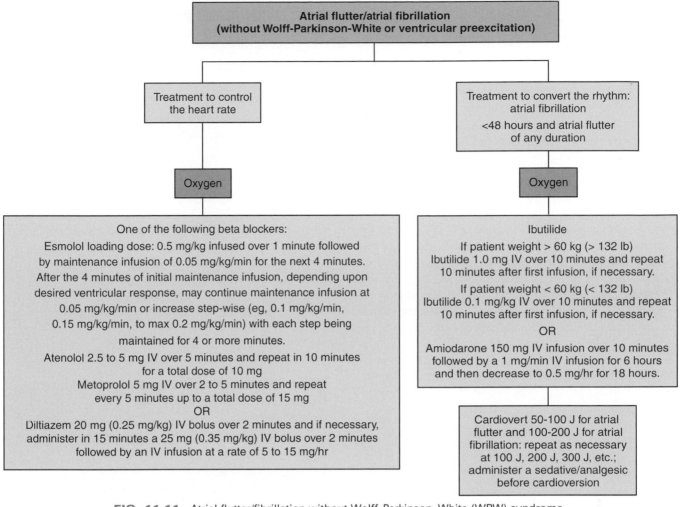

FIG. 11.11 Atrial flutter/fibrillation without Wolff–Parkinson–White (WPW) syndrome.

and flutter not be converted until the presence of a mural thrombus is excluded by performing an echocardiogram (ECHO), which is an ultrasound of the heart. If a mural thrombus is present, the patient must be placed on anticoagulants (blood thinners) until the threat posed by the mural thrombus has been minimized.

TREATMENT TO CONTROL RATE IF HEMODYNAMICALLY STABLE

- Oxygen if indicated
- Administer a beta blocker or a calcium-channel blocker:
  1. For the beta blocker:
     - Administer a 0.5-mg/kg dose of esmolol IV over 1 minute, followed by an IV infusion of esmolol at 0.05 mg/kg/min. If the response is inadequate, repeat the 0.5-mg/kg dose of esmolol IV twice at 5-minute intervals while increasing the IV infusion of esmolol 0.05 mg/kg/min after each dose, to a maximum infusion of 0.2 mg/kg/min (if necessary). Then titrate the esmolol infusion to maintain the heart rate within normal limits. Do not exceed the maximum infusion rate of 0.2 mg/kg/min.

OR

- Administer 2.5 to 5 mg atenolol IV over 5 minutes and repeat every 10 minutes as needed, up to a total dose of 10 mg, if needed.

OR

- Administer 5 mg metoprolol IV over 2 to 5 minutes. Repeat twice, at 5-minute intervals, up to a total dose of 15 mg, if needed.

AND

- Monitor the pulse, blood pressure, and ECG while administering the drug. Stop administering the beta blocker if the systolic blood pressure falls below 100 mm Hg.
  2. For the calcium-channel blocker:
     - Administer a 20-mg (0.25-mg/kg) dose of diltiazem IV slowly over 2 minutes. If the initial dose is not effective in 15 minutes and no adverse effects have occurred, give a second 25-mg (0.35-mg/kg) dose of diltiazem IV slowly over 2 minutes. (Exception: In patients over age 60, administer the doses of diltiazem slowly over 3–4 minutes.)

AND

　□ Start a maintenance IV infusion of diltiazem at a rate of 5 to 15 mg/hr to maintain the heart rate within normal limits.

> **AUTHOR'S NOTE** Calcium channel blockers are not indicated for atrial fibrillation and atrial flutter in the presence of WPW syndrome.

TO CONVERT THE RHYTHM (ONSET <48 HOURS AGO AND HEMODYNAMICALLY STABLE)

- Oxygen if indicated
- Administer a short-acting antidysrhythmic such as ibutilide:
  1. *If the patient weighs more than 60 kg (132 lb),* administer 1 mg of ibutilide IV over 10 minutes. Repeat in 10 minutes if necessary, after completion of the first infusion.
  2. *If the patient weighs less than 60 kg (132 lb),* administer 0.1 mg/kg of ibutilide IV over 10 minutes. Repeat in 10 minutes if necessary, after completion of the first infusion. Do not exceed the maximum of 2 mg of ibutilide.

OR

- Administer an antidysrhythmic drug such as amiodarone:
  1. Administer a loading dose of 150 mg of amiodarone IV over 10 minutes.

AND

  2. Start an IV infusion of amiodarone at a rate of 1 mg/min for 6 hours. Then decrease to 0.5 mg/min for 18 hours.

OR

- Administer an antidysrhythmic drug such as procainamide:
  1. Start an IV infusion of procainamide at a rate of 20 to 30 mg/min (up to 50 mg/min, if necessary). Continue the infusion of procainamide until reaching the end point listed in ECG Keys Box 11.1.

OR

  2. Perform immediate synchronized cardioversion. Cardiovert at 100 to 200 joules.

TO CONVERT THE RHYTHM IF HEMODYNAMICALLY UNSTABLE

- Oxygen if indicated
- Rhythm conversion is not indicated until the patient has been anticoagulated with heparin. There is an increased risk of a thromboembolic stroke because of thrombus formation that may have occurred during the period of atrial fibrillation. If the patient becomes unstable, perform immediate synchronized cardioversion.
  1. For atrial fibrillation:
     □ Cardiovert at 100 to 120 joules.
     □ Escalate subsequent shock doses as required.
  2. For atrial flutter:
     □ Cardiovert at 50 to 100 joules.

Atrial Flutter/Atrial Fibrillation (With WPW Syndrome or Ventricular Preexcitation) (Fig. 11.12)

TREATMENT

- Oxygen if indicated
- To control the heart rate and/or convert the rhythm of any duration
- Administer an antidysrhythmic drug such as amiodarone.
  1. Administer a loading dose of 150 mg amiodarone IV over 10 minutes.

AND

  2. Start an IV infusion of amiodarone at a rate of 1 mg/min for 6 hours. Then decrease to 0.5 mg/min for 18 hours.
- To convert the rhythm of less than 48 hours' duration or if hemodynamically unstable:
  1. Perform immediate synchronized cardioversion.
     □ For atrial fibrillation:
       ▸ Cardiovert at 100 to 120 joules.
       ▸ Escalate subsequent shock doses as required.
     □ For atrial flutter:
       ▸ Cardiovert at 50 to 100 joules.
- Escalate subsequent shock doses as required.

Wide-QRS-Complex Tachycardia of Unknown Origin (With Pulse) (Fig. 11.13)

TREATMENT

Treat wide QRS complex tachycardia of unknown origin (with pulse) as follows:
- Oxygen if indicated
- If unstable, consider immediate cardioversion or administration of an antidysrhythmic drug.
  1. Deliver a cardioversion (100 J).
     □ Repeat the cardioversion as often as necessary at progressively increasing energy levels (200, 300, and 360 J).

OR

  2. Administer an antidysrhythmic drug such as amiodarone:
     □ Administer a loading dose of 150 mg of amiodarone IV over 10 minutes.

AND

     □ Start an IV infusion of amiodarone at a rate of 1 mg/min for 6 hours. Then decrease to 0.5 mg/min for 18 hours.

OR

  3. If the wide-QRS-complex tachycardia persists and the patient is or becomes hemodynamically unstable and has a pulse, continue with an antidysrhythmic drug such as amiodarone while continuing the delivery of cardioversions.

Ventricular Tachycardia, Monomorphic (With Pulse) (Fig. 11.14)

TREATMENT

Treat monomorphic V-tach with pulse as follows:
- Oxygen if indicated

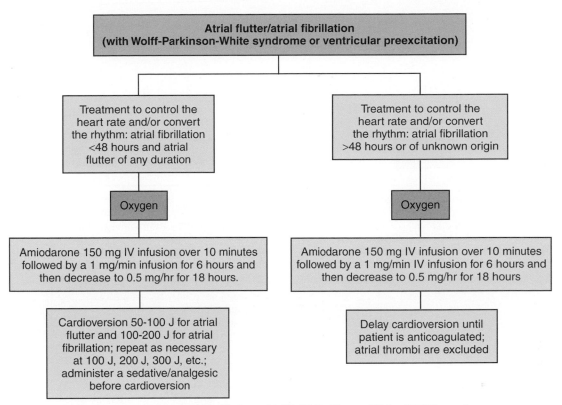

FIG. 11.12 Atrial flutter/fibrillation with Wolff–Parkinson–White (WPW) syndrome.

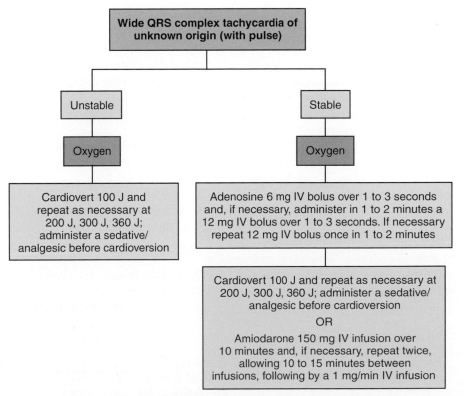

FIG. 11.13 Wide-QRS-complex tachycardia of unknown origin.

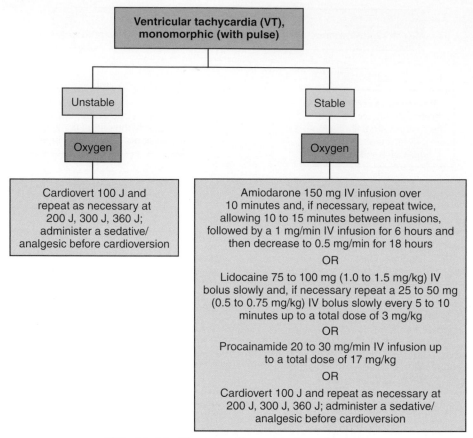

FIG. 11.14 Monomorphic ventricular tachycardia.

- If unstable, consider immediate cardioversion or administration of an antidysrhythmic drug. Deliver a cardioversion (100 J). Repeat the cardioversion as often as necessary at progressively increasing energy levels (200, 300, and 360 J).
  1. If V-tach persists and the patient is or becomes hemodynamically unstable and has a pulse, administer an antidysrhythmic drug such as amiodarone, lidocaine, or procainamide, as described later, while continuing the delivery of cardioversions.
- If stable, administer an antidysrhythmic drug such as amiodarone, lidocaine, or procainamide:
  1. Administer a loading dose of 150 mg of amiodarone IV over 10 minutes, and repeat two to three times, if necessary, allowing 10 to 15 minutes between infusions.

AND

  2. Start an IV infusion of amiodarone at a rate of 1 mg/min for 6 hours, and then decrease to 0.5 mg/min for 18 hours.

OR

  3. Administer a 1.0- to 1.5-mg/kg bolus (75–100 mg) of lidocaine IV slowly, and repeat a 0.5- to 0.75-mg/kg bolus (25–50 mg) of lidocaine IV slowly every 5 to 10 minutes

until the V-tach is suppressed or a total dose of 3 mg/kg of lidocaine has been administered.

AND

  4. Start a maintenance infusion of lidocaine at a rate of 1 to 4 mg/min to prevent the recurrence of the V-tach.

OR

  5. Start an IV infusion of procainamide at a rate of 20 to 30 mg/min (up to 50 mg/min, if necessary) and continue until reaching the end point listed in Box 11.1.

AND

- Start a maintenance IV infusion of procainamide at a rate of 1 to 4 mg/min.
  1. If amiodarone, lidocaine, or procainamide is unsuccessful in suppressing V-tach, or if at any time the patient's condition becomes hemodynamically unstable and cardioversions were not delivered initially:
     □ Immediately deliver a cardioversion (100 J).

AND

     □ Repeat the cardioversion as often as necessary at progressively increasing energy levels (200, 300, and 360 J).

Ventricular Tachycardia, Polymorphic (With Pulse), Normal Baseline QT Interval

TREATMENT

In polymorphic V-tach with pulse and a normal baseline QT interval, treat as monomorphic V-tach, as noted earlier.

Ventricular Tachycardia, Polymorphic (With Pulse), Prolonged Baseline QT Interval (See Fig. 11.14)

TORSADES DE POINTES (WITH PULSE) (FIG. 11.15)

Treatment

- Oxygen if indicated
  1. Administer a dose of 1 to 2 grams (8–16 mEq) of magnesium sulfate, diluted with 50 to 100 mL of D$_5$W, IV over 5 to 60 minutes.

AND

2. Follow with a maintenance IV infusion of 0.5 to 1 gram (4–8 mEq) of magnesium sulfate, diluted with 100 mL of D$_5$W, IV to run for 1 hour.

AND/OR

3. Initiate transcutaneous overdrive pacing, if appropriate.
4. Withhold administration of such antidysrhythmic agents as amiodarone, disopyramide, procainamide, quinidine, and sotalol or other agents that prolong the QT interval, such as phenothiazines and tricyclic antidepressants.

AND

5. Correct any electrolyte imbalance.

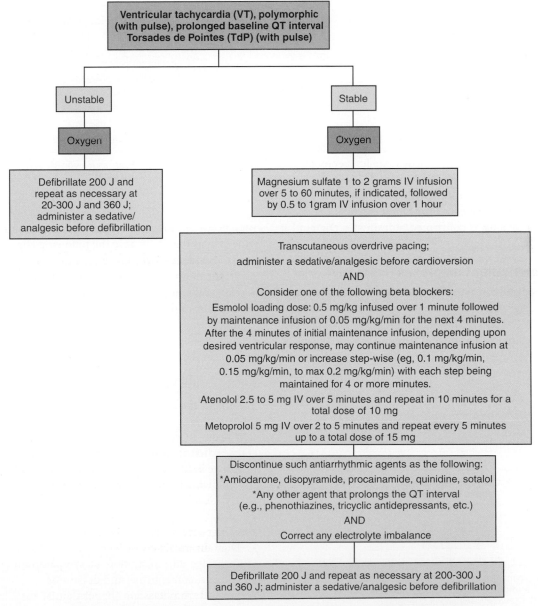

FIG. 11.15 Polymorphic ventricular tachycardia with prolonged QT interval.

6. If polymorphic V-tach or torsades de pointes persists and the patient is or becomes unstable:
   □ Deliver a defibrillation (360 J).

   AND

   □ Repeat the defibrillation as often as necessary at 360 joules.

PREMATURE ECTOPIC BEATS

Premature Atrial and Junctional Complexes (Fig. 11.16)

Single, isolated premature atrial complexes (PACs) or premature junctional complexes (PJCs) are not significant. Frequent PACs and PJCs may indicate the presence of enhanced atrial or junctional automaticity, respectively; an atrial or junctional reentry mechanism; or both and herald impending atrial rhythm, such as atrial tachycardia, atrial flutter, and atrial fibrillation, and PSVT. The most common cause is elevated sympathetic tone from stress, pain, anxiety, or stimulant drugs or agents. Hypoxia must also be considered.

INDICATIONS FOR TREATMENT

Treatment may be indicated if the premature atrial and junctional complexes are frequent (8–10 per minute), occur in groups of two or more, or alternate with the QRS complexes of the underlying rhythm (bigeminy).

If stimulants (such as caffeine, tobacco, or alcohol) or excessive amounts of sympathomimetic drugs (such as epinephrine or dopamine) have been administered:

- Discontinue the stimulants and sympathomimetic drugs.
- If digitalis toxicity is suspected, withhold digitalis.
- Once digitalis toxicity is confirmed, administer Digibind if indicated.

Premature Ventricular Complexes (Fig. 11.17)

Single PVCs, especially in patients who have no heart disease, are generally not significant. In patients with an ACS or an ischemic episode, PVCs may indicate the presence of enhanced ventricular automaticity, a ventricular reentry mechanism, or both and herald the appearance of a life-threatening dysrhythmia, such as V-tach or V-fib. Although these lethal rhythms

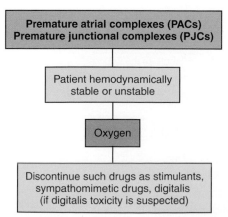

FIG. 11.16   Premature atrial and junctional complexes.

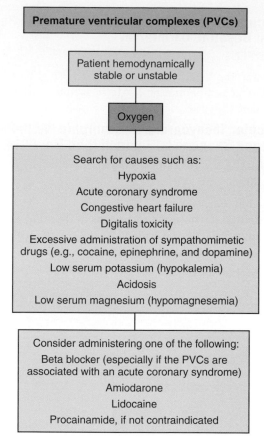

FIG. 11.17   Premature ventricular complexes.

may occur without warning, they are often initiated by PVCs, especially if the PVCs have the following characteristics:

- Are frequent (six or more per minute)
- Occur in groups of two or more (group beats)
- Have different QRS configurations (multiform)
- Arise from different ventricular ectopic pacemakers (multifocal)
- Are closely coupled
- Fall on the T wave (R-on-T phenomenon)

INDICATIONS FOR TREATMENT

Treatment should be considered for PVCs in patients in whom an acute MI or ischemic episode is suspected, except for those that occur in conjunction with bradycardias. In such circumstances, first treat the underlying bradycardia. Refer to the appropriate bradycardia treatment. If feasible, identify and correct the following underlying causes of PVCs:

- Hypoxia
- ACS
- Congestive heart failure
- Digitalis toxicity
- Excessive administration of sympathomimetic drugs (e.g., cocaine, epinephrine, and dopamine)
- Low serum potassium (hypokalemia)
- Acidosis
- Low serum magnesium (hypomagnesemia)

TREATMENT

- If the PVCs are associated with an ACS:
  1. Treat the ACS (see Chapter 17).

  AND

  2. Consider the administration of a beta blocker such as esmolol, atenolol, or metoprolol.
- If the PVCs are not associated with an ACS:
  1. Identify and correct any underlying causes of the PVCs.

  AND

- Consider administering an antidysrhythmic drug such as amiodarone, procainamide, or lidocaine.

TAKE-HOME POINTS

The following is a summary of the rhythm treatment algorithms presented in this chapter:
- Bradycardias
  1. Sinus bradycardia
  2. Sinus arrest/SA exit block
  3. Second-degree type I AV block (Wenckebach)
  4. Second-degree 2:1 and advanced AV block with narrow QRS complexes
  5. Third-degree AV block with narrow QRS complexes
     □ Oxygen
     □ Atropine sulfate

     OR

     □ Dopamine or epinephrine infusion

     AND/OR

  6. TCP
  7. Second-degree type II AV block
  8. Second-degree 2:1 and advanced AV block with wide QRS complexes
  9. Third-degree AV block with wide QRS complexes
     ▪ Oxygen
     ▪ TCP
     ▪ Dopamine or epinephrine infusion
     ▪ Transvenous pacemaker
  10. Junctional escape rhythm
  11. Ventricular escape rhythm
     ▪ Oxygen
     ▪ TCP
     ▪ Dopamine or epinephrine infusion
- Tachycardias
  1. Sinus tachycardia
  2. Atrial tachycardia with block
     □ No specific treatment
     □ Treat underlying cause.
     □ Discontinue any drugs responsible for the block.
     □ Narrow QRS complex tachycardia of unknown origin (with pulse)
     □ Oxygen
     □ Vagal maneuvers

     □ Adenosine
     □ Determine whether rhythm is:
       ‣ PSVT
       ‣ Atrial tachycardia without block
       ‣ Junctional tachycardia
       ‣ Atrial flutter/fibrillation
  3. Atrial tachycardia without block
     □ Oxygen
     □ Diltiazem or beta blocker (esmolol, atenolol, or metoprolol) or amiodarone
  4. PSVT with narrow QRS complexes
     □ Oxygen
     □ Vagal maneuvers
     □ Adenosine, diltiazem, or beta blocker (esmolol, atenolol, or metoprolol)
     □ Digoxin
     □ Cardioversion
  5. Junctional tachycardia
     □ Oxygen
     □ Amiodarone or beta blocker (esmolol, atenolol, or metoprolol)
  6. Atrial flutter/atrial fibrillation
     □ Treatment to control the heart rate
       ‣ Oxygen
       ‣ Beta blocker (esmolol, atenolol, or metoprolol) or diltiazem
       ‣ Digoxin
     □ Treatment to convert the rhythm
       ‣ Atrial fibrillation <48 hours
         ▹ Oxygen
         ▹ Ibutilide, amiodarone, or procainamide
         ▹ Cardioversion
       ‣ Atrial fibrillation >48 hours or of unknown duration
     □ Oxygen
     □ Delay cardioversion until the patient is anticoagulated and atrial thrombi are excluded.
     □ Cardioversion and amiodarone if patient unstable
  7. Wide-QRS-complex tachycardia of unknown origin (with pulse)
     □ Oxygen
     □ Cardioversion
     □ Adenosine or amiodarone
  8. Ventricular tachycardia, monomorphic (with pulse)
     □ Oxygen
     □ Cardioversion
     □ Amiodarone, lidocaine, or procainamide
  9. VT, polymorphic (with pulse) normal baseline QT interval
     □ Same as monomorphic V-tach
  10. VT, polymorphic (with pulse) prolonged baseline QT interval torsades de pointes (with pulse)
     □ Oxygen
     □ Magnesium sulfate
     □ TCP and beta blocker (esmolol, atenolol, or metoprolol)
     □ Defibrillation
     □ Discontinue amiodarone, procainamide, beta blockers, or agents that prolong QT interval.

11. Premature atrial and junctional complexes
    - Discontinue any stimulants and sympathomimetic drugs.
    - Withhold digitalis (if digitalis toxicity is suspected).
    - Digibind if digitalis toxicity confirmed
12. PVCs
    - Oxygen
    - Identify and   correct any underlying causes of the PVCs.

□ Consider one of the following:
  ‣ Beta blocker (esmolol, atenolol, or metoprolol) if PVCs are associated with an ACS
  ‣ Amiodarone
  ‣ Lidocaine
  ‣ Procainamide

CHAPTER REVIEW QUESTIONS

1. In an unstable patient with symptomatic bradycardia and an ECG showing a second-degree type II AV block, you should administer oxygen, start an IV line, and administer or begin which of the following?
   A. A dopamine infusion
   B. Atropine
   C. Lidocaine
   D. TCP

2. Patients with symptomatic sinus tachycardia should be treated with
   A. appropriate treatment for the underlying cause of the tachycardia.
   B. diltiazem.
   C. dopamine.
   D. epinephrine.

3. If a patient is stable and has an ECG showing PSVT after administering oxygen and starting an IV line, you should do which of the following?
   A. Administer adenosine.
   B. Administer diazepam.
   C. Administer diltiazem.
   D. Attempt vagal maneuvers.

4. Your patient presents with chest pain and signs and symptoms of an acute MI. His ECG shows multifocal PVCs. After administering oxygen and starting an IV line, you should immediately consider
   A. a cardioversion of 50 joules.
   B. a loading dose of amiodarone.
   C. an adenosine bolus.
   D. transcutaneous pacing.

5. The administration of adenosine for a narrow-complex tachycardia
   A. may reveal the underlying rhythm to be atrial fibrillation or atrial flutter.
   B. must be administered slowly to avoid hypotension.
   C. should only be performed if the diagnosis of SVT is known.
   D. will always convert SVT to normal sinus rhythm.

6. A patient with atrial fibrillation of less than 48 hours in duration who is hemodynamically unstable and hypotensive should receive which treatment?
   A. Amiodarone alone
   B. Ibutilide followed by cardioversion
   C. Immediate cardioversion and amiodarone
   D. Immediate cardioversion alone

7. Your patient is conscious and hemodynamically stable with a pulse and an ECG showing monomorphic V-tach. After administering oxygen and starting an IV, you should do which of the following?
   A. Administer 1 mg of epinephrine.
   B. Administer a 150-mg loading dose of amiodarone IV.
   C. Deliver a cardioversion of 100 joules.
   D. Start an infusion of epinephrine.

8. If your patient in question No. 7 begins to complain of chest pain and then becomes pulseless, you should immediately
   A. administer a lidocaine bolus.
   B. begin TCP.
   C. deliver a cardioversion of 100 joules.
   D. deliver defibrillation of 360 joules.

9. Which of the following is *not* contraindicated in the treatment of PSVT with WPW?
   A. Adenosine
   B. Calcium-channel blocker
   C. Beta blocker
   D. Amiodarone

10. When may attempts to convert atrial fibrillation to normal sinus rhythm be undertaken?
    A. At any time, regardless of its duration
    B. After anticoagulation if its duration is longer than 48 hours
    C. As long as the patient is stable
    D. After the administration of a calcium-channel blocker

The 12-Lead ECG: Leads and Axis

12

The 12-lead ECG permits the clinician to more closely examine the electrical activity of the heart and the various conditions that can alter it. The primary role of the 12-lead ECG is to detect the presence of myocardial ischemia and infarction. The specific 12-lead ECG findings associated with these conditions will be discussed in Chapter 16.

Another role of the 12-lead ECG is to assist in the differentiation of various cardiac rhythms, particularly those that have similar appearances in lead II (the most common lead used to interpret ECG rhythms and monitor the heart).

LEADS

The 12-lead ECG, as its name implies, consists of 12 leads, 6 limb leads and 6 precordial leads, that examine the heart simultaneously from multiple angles (Fig. 12.1):
- Six limb leads
  1. Three standard (bipolar) limb leads: leads I, II, and III
  2. Three augmented (unipolar) leads: leads aVR, aVL, and aVF
- Six precordial (unipolar) leads: leads V1, V2, V3, V4, V5, and V6

> **12-lead ECG**
>
> An ECG that produces 12 views of the heart's electrical activity to assist in heart rhythm interpretation.

Standard (Bipolar) Limb Leads

The monitoring of leads I, II, and III was discussed in Chapter 2. The same three leads are used in a 12-lead ECG and are obtained using a *positive electrode* and a *negative electrode* to detect the electrical current generated by the depolarization and repolarization of the heart. An additional electrode, the *ground*

electrode, is often attached to the right leg (or any other location on the body) to provide a path of least resistance for electrical interference in the body (Fig. 12.2 and Table 12.1).

Lead Axis

> **axis**
>
> In the context of an ECG, the axis of a lead (lead axis) is a hypothetical line joining the poles of a lead.

A hypothetical line joining the poles of a bipolar lead is known as the *axis of the lead* (or *lead axis*) (Fig. 12.3). The axis runs from the negative to the positive pole of the lead. The location of the positive and negative poles in a lead determines the orientation (or direction) of the axis of the lead.

In addition, each lead axis has a perpendicular axis or, simply, the *perpendicular*. It is usually depicted as a line intersecting or connecting with the lead axis at 90 degrees (or a right angle), midway along the axis between the two poles. This is considered the "zero" point of the lead axis. The perpendicular divides the lead axis into two halves. The positive half is on the side of the perpendicular closest to the positive pole. The negative half is on the side closest to the negative pole.

The relationships of the standard limb leads are such that the sum of the electrical impulses recorded in leads I and III equals the sum of the electrical impulses recorded in lead II. This is called *Einthoven's law*, named after the developer of three-lead electrocardiography.

Einthoven's law is expressed mathematically as follows:

$$\text{Lead I} + \text{Lead III} = \text{Lead II}$$

Because the positive electrodes of the three bipolar limb leads are electrically the same distance from the heart, an

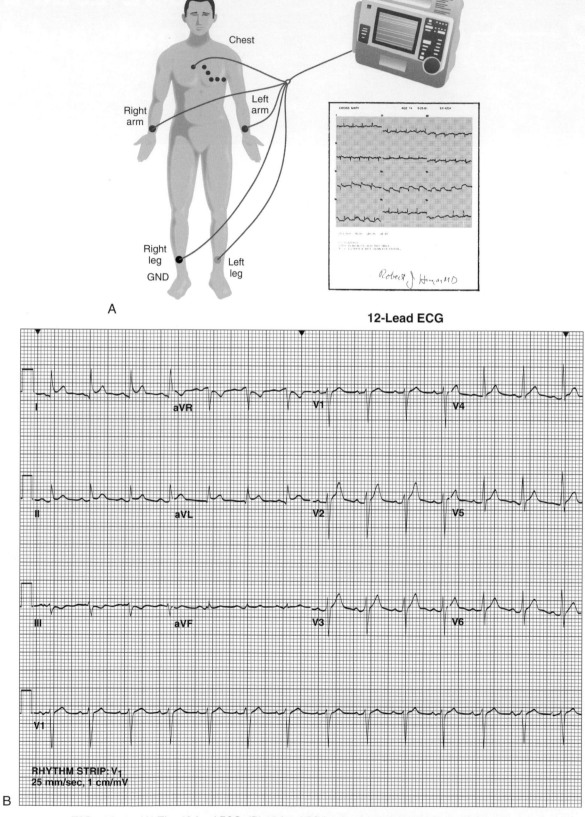

FIG. 12.1 (A) The 12-lead ECG. (B) 12-lead ECG printout with a lead V₁ rhythm strip.

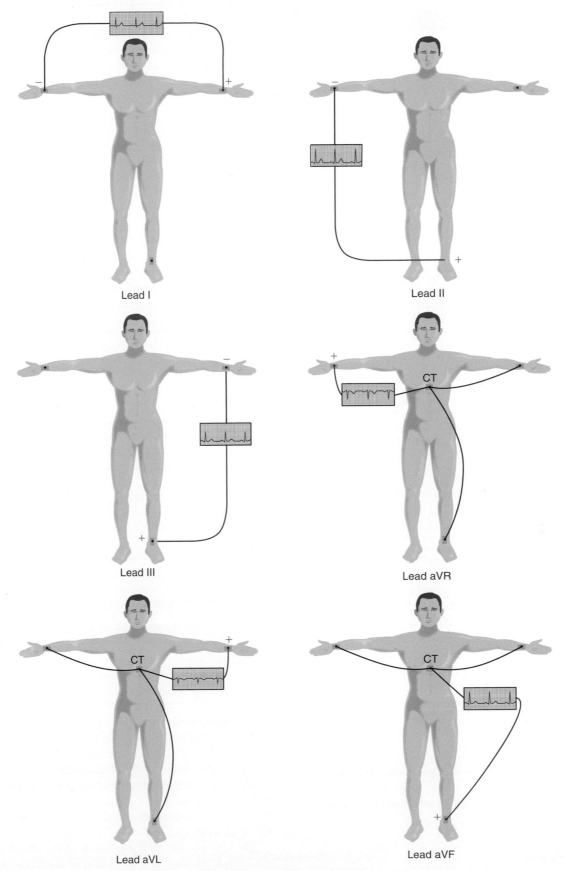

Lead I

Lead II

Lead III

Lead aVR

Lead aVL

Lead aVF

FIG. 12.2   Standard limb leads.

TABLE 12.1	Electrodes of the Standard Limb Leads	
Lead	**Positive Electrode**	**Negative Electrode**
I	Left arm	Right arm
II	Left leg	Right arm
III	Left leg	Left arm

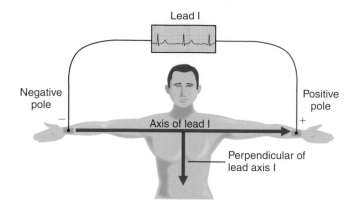

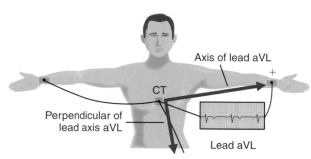

FIG. 12.3 Axis of a lead and its perpendicular.

equilateral triangle (Einthoven's equilateral triangle; Fig. 12.4) can be depicted in the body's frontal plane using their axes as each side of the triangle. The positive terminal of lead I is 0°, lead II is 60°, and lead III is 120°. This creates the triaxial reference figure for leads I, II, and III. The negative halves of the lead axis are usually depicted as dotted or dashed lines, as shown in Fig. 12.5.

The ECG machine uses the mathematics of Einthoven's triangle to calculate a theoretical point in the center of the heart that is electrically neutral. This is called the *central terminal*. It can be mathematically visualized in the heart as a point just left of the interventricular septum and below the atrioventricular (AV) junction.

> **AUTHOR'S NOTE** The central terminal is not an actual lead or electrode but is instead an imaginary point of "electrical neutrality" calculated by the ECG machine. Although it may appear labeled on figures, it is not an actual physical location.

Electrical Planes

Planes are imaginary surfaces that divide the body from front to back, top to bottom, and side to side. Envisioning these abstract surfaces helps us picture the body's organs, including the heart, in three dimensions. The 12 leads represent the heart's electrical activity in two different electrical planes: frontal and horizontal. These planes intersect to give us a three-dimensional view of the heart.

FRONTAL PLANE

The three standard limb leads (I, II, and III) and the three augmented leads (aVR, aVL, and aVF) measure the electrical activity of the heart in the two-dimensional *frontal plane*. This imaginary surface runs from head to toe, dividing the body into front and back halves (Fig. 12.6).

HORIZONTAL PLANE

The six precordial leads (V_1, V_2, V_3, V_4, V_5, and V_6) measure the electrical activity of the heart at a right angle to the frontal plane, the *horizontal plane*. The center of each of the radiating points on both the frontal and horizontal planes is the previously described central terminal.

> **AUTHOR'S NOTE** To remember which way the horizontal plane divides the heart, picture the horizon, which marks the line between land and sky.

Unipolar Leads

> **unipolar lead**
>
> A lead that has only one (positive) electrode.

A lead that has only one electrode (which is positive) is called a *unipolar lead*. It does not have a corresponding negative lead; instead, the "view" of the electrode is in relation to the central terminal. Consequentially the limb leads *must* be attached to the patient to record the precordial leads. Without the bipolar limb lead, the central terminal cannot be calculated by the machine.

AUGMENTED (UNIPOLAR) LEADS

> **augmented limb leads**
>
> The three unipolar augmented limb leads—aVR, aVL, and aVF—detect the electrical potential between a positive electrode attached to one of three extremities and the central terminal.

The augmented unipolar leads exist at 90-degree angles (perpendicular) to the axis of the limb leads. aVR is perpendicular to limb lead III, aVL is perpendicular to limb lead II, and aVF is perpendicular to limb lead I. Because the electrical current (and size) of the waves and complexes in the ECG obtained in this manner is so small, these signals are increased, or "augmented," by the ECG machine. Hence the name "augmented," which is the "a" in *aVR*, *aVL*, and *aVF*.

The lead axis for an augmented lead is a line drawn between the central terminal and its extremity electrode, with the central terminal designated as the negative pole and the extremity electrode as the positive pole (Fig. 12.7, *A*, and Table 12.2). The

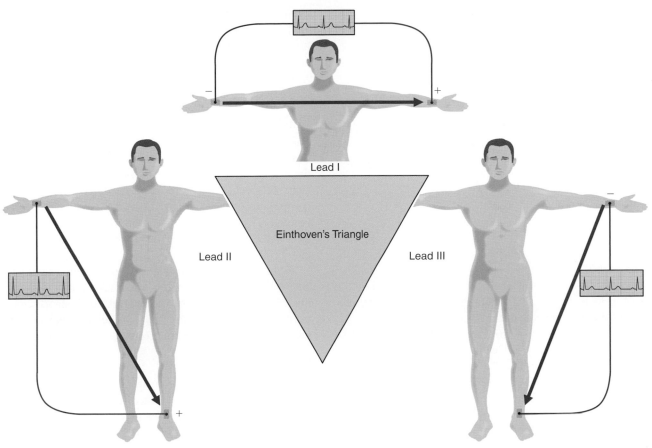

FIG. 12.4 Standard (bipolar) limb leads I, II, and III; their axes; and Einthoven's triangle.

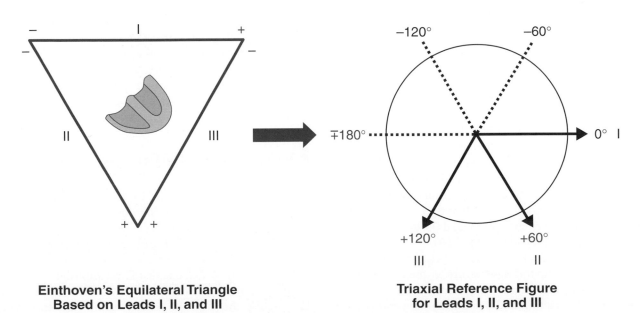

Einthoven's Equilateral Triangle Based on Leads I, II, and III

Triaxial Reference Figure for Leads I, II, and III

FIG. 12.5 Einthoven's triangle and triaxial reference figure.

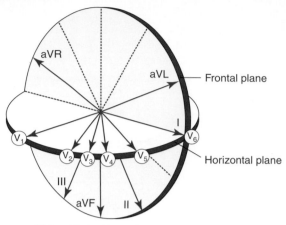

FIG. 12.6 Frontal and horizontal planes.

augmented leads use the same physical electrodes used by the limb leads. However, the ECG machine treats each extremity electrode as the positive pole of the augmented lead.

The positive electrodes of the three augmented leads, like those of the three standard limb leads, are also electrically equidistant from the central terminal of the heart. The augmented lead *triaxial reference figure* (Fig. 12.7, *B*) formed in the body's frontal plane by the axes of the three augmented leads is similar to that of the standard limb leads, with its lead axes 60 degrees apart but rotated 30 degrees around the zero reference point. The augmented lead axis is usually depicted with its negative half extended as a dotted, dashed, or shaded line.

When the triaxial reference figures of the standard limb leads and the augmented leads are superimposed, they form a *hexaxial reference figure* (Fig. 12.8). Each augmented lead axis is perpendicular to a standard limb lead axis so that the limb leads and augmented leads are spaced 30 degrees apart around the hexaxial reference figure. The hexaxial reference figure is used to plot the electrical axis of the heart in the body's frontal plane and will be described in greater detail later in the chapter.

PRECORDIAL (UNIPOLAR) LEADS

The precordial leads V_1, V_2, V_3, V_4, V_5, and V_6 are unipolar leads obtained by attaching the positive electrode to prescribed areas over the anterior chest wall (Fig. 12.9, *A*). A precordial lead thus measures the difference in electrical potential between a positive chest electrode and the central terminal.

The individual chest electrodes are positioned across the anterior chest wall from right to left so that they overlie the right ventricle, the interventricular septum, and the anterior and lateral surfaces of the left ventricle (Table 12.3).

The chest electrodes for leads V_1 and V_2 (the right precordial [or septal] leads) overlie the right ventricle, the electrodes for leads V_3 and V_4 (the mid-precordial [or anterior] leads) overlie the interventricular septum and part of the left ventricle, and those for leads V_5 and V_6 (the left precordial [or lateral] leads) overlie the rest of the left ventricle.

The lead axis for each precordial lead is drawn from the central terminal to the specific chest electrode, with the central

terminal designated as the negative pole and the electrode as the positive pole (Fig. 12.9, *B*). A transverse (cross-sectional) outline of the chest wall showing the central terminal, the six chest electrodes, and the six precordial lead axes is called a *precordial reference figure*. It is used in plotting the heart's electrical activity in the body's horizontal plane.

Right-Sided Chest Leads

The precordial leads of the standard 12-lead ECG record the heart's electrical activity primarily over the left ventricle. To determine the electrical activity over the right ventricle, right-sided chest leads must be used. These leads are not a component of the standard 12-lead ECG. Instead, leads designated V_{2R} through V_{6R} are obtained by attaching positive electrodes to specific locations on the right chest (Fig. 12.10 and Table 12.4).

Right-sided chest leads are used to rule out a right ventricular myocardial infarction after the initial finding of an inferior myocardial infarction. In the majority of instances, only one right-sided chest lead, lead V_{4R}, is needed to make the diagnosis. This will be discussed in greater detail in Chapter 16.

Facing Leads

Facing leads view specific surfaces of the heart (Fig. 12.11). Except for lead aVR, which faces the interior or endocardial surface of the ventricles, the remaining 11 leads view the epicardial or other surface of the heart. Because the left ventricle comprises the largest muscle mass of the heart and represents the predominant electrical component of the QRS complex, the views are referred to from the perspective of the left ventricle.

Leads I and aVL and the precordial leads V_5 and V_6 view the lateral wall of the left ventricle, leads II, III, and aVF view the inferior (diaphragmatic) wall, and leads V_1 through V_4 view the anterior wall of the left ventricle. The right-sided precordial lead—lead V_{4R}—views the right ventricle. No leads face the posterior surface of the heart (Table 12.5).

> **AUTHOR'S NOTE** No leads face the posterior surface of the heart. It is important to know the facing leads in determining the location of an acute myocardial infarction!

ELECTRICAL IMPULSE

An electrical impulse flowing parallel to or along the axis of a lead, the hypothetical line joining the negative and positive poles of a lead, produces either a positive or negative deflection on an ECG, depending on the direction of its flow. An electrical impulse flowing toward the positive pole produces a positive deflection on the ECG; one that flows toward the negative pole produces a negative deflection. The greater the magnitude of the impulse, the larger the deflection, and vice versa. When the flow of the impulse is perpendicular to the axis of a lead, no deflection is produced because it is neither positive nor negative. Subsequently, it is referred to as *isoelectric*. Fig. 12.12, *A*, shows the relationship between the direction of flow of an

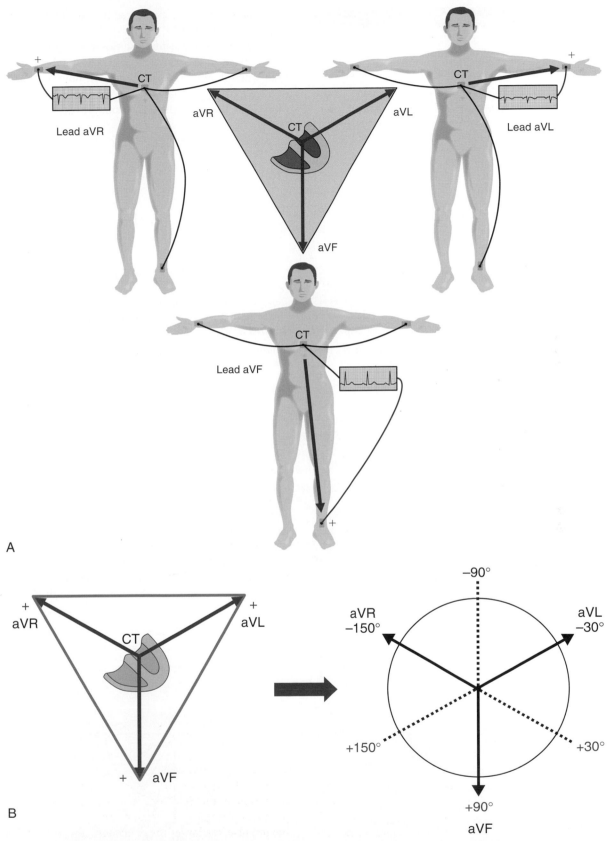

FIG. 12.7 (A) Augmented leads aVR, aVL, and aVF and their axes. (B) Triaxial reference figure for the augmented leads.

TABLE 12.2	Electrodes of Augmented Limb Leads	
Lead	**Positive Electrode**	**Negative Electrode**
aVR	Right arm	Central terminal (left arm and left leg)
aVL	Left arm	Central terminal (right arm and left leg)
aVF	Left leg	Central terminal (right arm and left arm)

electrical impulse, as represented by a vector, and the deflection it produces on an ECG.

When an electrical impulse flows in a direction other than exactly parallel, at an angle to the axis, the deflection is smaller than when the same electrical current flows parallel to the axis of a lead. The more parallel the electrical impulse is to the axis of the lead, the larger the deflection; the more perpendicular, the

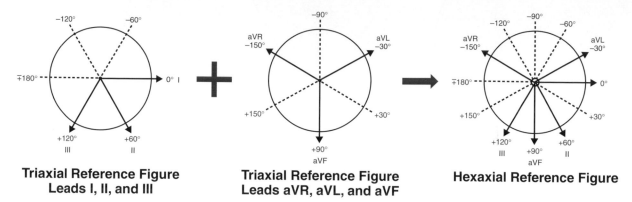

Triaxial Reference Figure Leads I, II, and III + **Triaxial Reference Figure Leads aVR, aVL, and aVF** → **Hexaxial Reference Figure**

FIG. 12.8 Hexaxial reference figure.

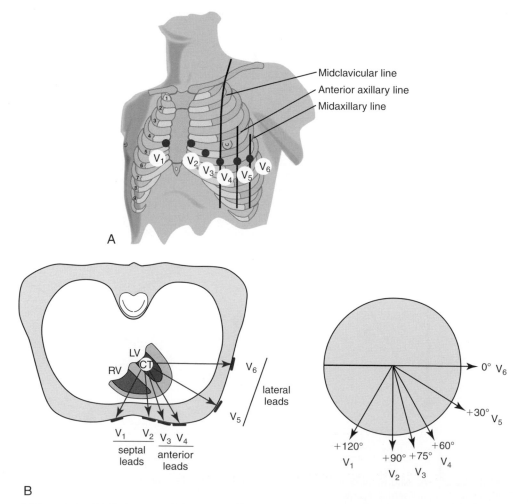

A

B

FIG. 12.9 (A) Placement of the precordial electrodes. (B) Precordial lead axes and reference figure.

TABLE 12.3	Placement of Chest Electrodes		
Lead	**Name**	**Placement**	**Anatomic Landmarks**
V_1	Right precordial (septal) leads	Over the right ventricle	Right side of the sternum in the fourth intercostal space
V_2			Left side of the sternum in the fourth intercostal space
V_3	Mid-precordial (anterior) leads	Over the interventricular septum and part of the left ventricle	Midway between V_2 and V_4
V_4			Left midclavicular line in the fifth intercostal space
V_5	Left precordial (or lateral) leads	Over the rest of the left ventricle	Left anterior axillary line at the same level as V_4
V_6			Left midaxillary line at the same level as V_4

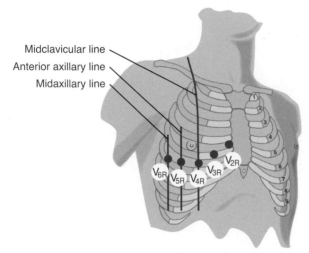

Midclavicular line
Anterior axillary line
Midaxillary line

FIG. 12.10 Right-sided chest leads.

TABLE 12.4	Placement of Right-Sided Chest Leads
V_{2R}	Right side of the sternum in the fourth intercostal space
V_{3R}	Midway between V_{2R} and V_{4R}
V_{4R}	Right midclavicular line in the fifth intercostal space
V_{5R}	Right anterior axillary line at the same level as V_{4R}
V_{6R}	Right midaxillary line at the same level as V_{4R}

smaller the deflection. This is true whether the electrical impulse is flowing toward or away from the positive pole (Fig. 12.12, *B*).

Another way to think of this is to imagine yourself standing on the edge of a train track. As the approaching train sounds its horn, the sound grows loudest if you are directly in the path of the train. The farther you move perpendicular to the track and away from the train, the sound of the approaching train and the receding train cancel out, and the net change in the level of the train noise is zero.

In the heart, numerous electrical impulses are firing in many directions (vectors) throughout the cardiac cycle. The placement of the lead is analogous to the person standing directly on or at some angle to the track. The difference is that in the heart, because there are multiple trains traveling in many directions (vectors) simultaneously, the ECG lead measures the average of all the vectors it detects.

When an electrical impulse flows partly toward and then partly away from the positive pole over time, a bidirectional electrical current is present. It is represented by a single mean vector. The mean vector is an average of all the positive and negative electrical impulses (or vectors) present. Such an electrical impulse produces a biphasic deflection on the ECG—one that is partly positive and partly negative. The size of the components of the deflection depends on the magnitude of the individual electrical impulse. If the sum of the directions (that is, the amount positive and amount negative) is positive, no matter by how little, the deflection is said to be positive; if the sum of the directions is negative, the deflection is said to be negative.

Using the train example, if at first a train comes toward me, I note the loud rising sound of the approaching train. As it passes, a second train on a nearby track moves away from me, and I note the sound of the receding horn. If three trains were to come toward me and one away, then over the course of the period of observation, I have recorded more approaching trains than departing ones.

The QRS normally extends over a period of 0.12 second. During that period, the vectors of impulses move through many directions; however, the sum of the vectors is recorded and results in the deflection of the QRS complex. At certain points in the recording, the sum will be negative, resulting in a negative deflection. At other times, it will be positive, resulting in a positive deflection. When the QRS complex consists of both positive and negative deflections, it is referred to as *biphasic*. The overall vector of the QRS complex is the sum of its positive and negative deflections (Fig. 12.12, *C*).

The more parallel the overall vector of a biphasic deflection is to the axis of the lead, the more positive the biphasic deflection; the closer the orientation of the overall vector is to the perpendicular, the less positive the biphasic deflection. When the positive and negative deflections are equal in magnitude, an equiphasic deflection is present, and the sum of the deflections is zero. In this case, the mean vector is perpendicular to the lead axis (Fig. 12.12, *D*).

A mostly positive QRS complex in a given lead indicates that the positive pole of the vector of the QRS axis lies somewhere on the positive side of the lead axis. Conversely, a mostly negative QRS complex in a lead indicates that the positive pole of the vector of the QRS axis lies somewhere on the negative side of the lead axis (Fig. 12.12, *E*).

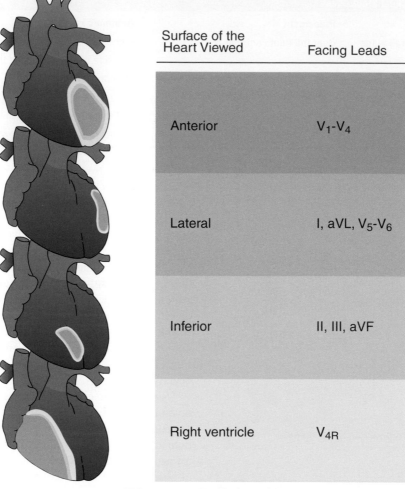

Surface of the Heart Viewed	Facing Leads
Anterior	V_1-V_4
Lateral	I, aVL, V_5-V_6
Inferior	II, III, aVF
Right ventricle	V_{4R}

FIG. 12.11 The facing leads.

TABLE 12.5	Facing Leads	
General View of the Heart	**Surface of the Heart Viewed**	**Lead**
Lateral	Outside wall of the left ventricle	I
		aVL
		V_5
		V_6
Inferior	Diaphragmatic wall	II
		III
		aVF
Anterior	Front wall of the left ventricle	V_1
		V_2
		V_3
		V_4
Rightward	Right ventricle	V_{4R}

ELECTRICAL AXIS AND VECTORS

The electrical impulse generated by the depolarization or repolarization of the atria or ventricles at any given moment produces an *instantaneous cardiac vector*. It is usually depicted as an arrow that has magnitude, direction, and polarity (Fig. 12.13). The vector is described by its magnitude, direction, and polarity:

- **Magnitude.** The longer the shaft of the arrow, the greater the magnitude, or force, of the electrical impulse.
- **Direction.** The direction in which the current is flowing is indicated by the position or orientation of the arrow compared with a reference axis.
- **Polarity (positivity or negativity).** The tip of the arrow represents the positive pole of the electrical current, and the tail is the negative pole.

The sequence of electrical impulses produced by the depolarization of the ventricles during one cardiac cycle, for example, can be depicted as a series of cardiac vectors, each representing the real-time electrical impulses generated by depolarization of a small segment of the ventricular wall (Fig. 12.14).

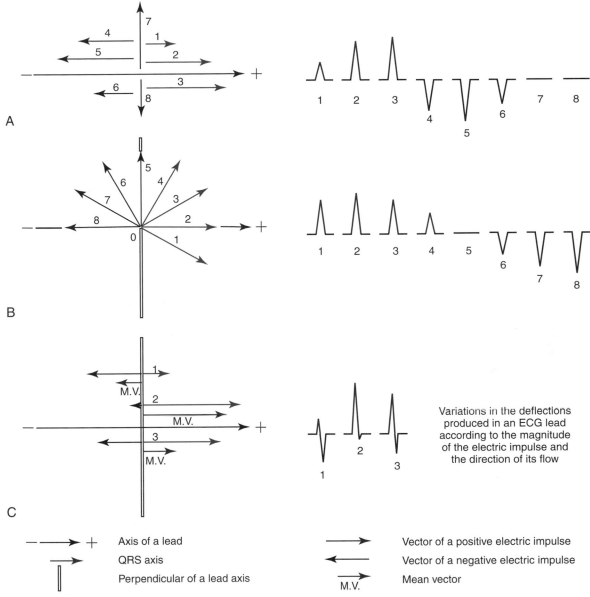

FIG. 12.12 The axis of a lead, its perpendicular, and the direction of flow of electrical impulses.

1. The first cardiac vector represents the depolarization of the interventricular septum. It moves from left to right. It is followed immediately by a sequence of vectors flowing from the inner to the outer ventricular wall as it depolarizes.
2. The electrical impulses flow from the right and left ventricles near the apex of the heart, close to the septum.
3. The impulses continue to move through the thin wall of the right ventricle and the thick lateral wall of the left ventricle.
4. The impulses end in the lateral and posterior portion of the left ventricle near its base.

The vectors arising in the right ventricle are directed mostly to the right when viewed in the frontal plane; those in the left ventricle are directed mostly to the left. The thick, muscular left ventricular wall generates larger, more persistent vectors than those produced by the smaller right ventricle.

mean QRS axis

The mean (or average) of all vectors that result from ventricular depolarization, generating a composite view of the direction in which the heart's electrical impulses are moving.

Taken together, the vectors give us a composite view that tells us the general direction in which the heart's electrical impulses are flowing. The mean (or average) of all vectors that result from ventricular depolarization is a single large vector called the *mean QRS axis*, or simply the *QRS axis*. We call it an *axis* rather than a *vector* because it is static. It has direction but no magnitude or polarity. Normally, the QRS axis points to the left and downward, reflecting the dominance of the left ventricle over the right. The QRS axis is the most important and the most

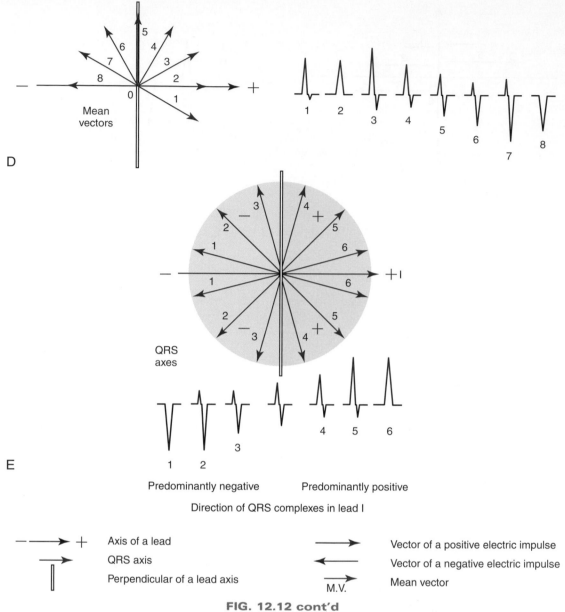

D Mean vectors

E QRS axes

Predominantly negative   Predominantly positive

Direction of QRS complexes in lead I

--—→ + Axis of a lead

--→ QRS axis

▯ Perpendicular of a lead axis

——→ Vector of a positive electric impulse

←—— Vector of a negative electric impulse

——→ Mean vector
M.V.

FIG. 12.12 cont'd

A cardiac vector, depicted as an arrow, has:

1. |←— Magnitude —→|

2. Direction
——————→

3. Polarity   Negative pole   Positive pole
   − ——————→ +

FIG. 12.13 The cardiac vector.

frequently determined axis. Commonly, when the term *axis* is used alone, it refers to the QRS axis.

The QRS complex normally extends over a period of 0.12 second. During that period, the vectors of impulses move through many directions of the compass; however, the average of the vectors is recorded and results in the deflection of the

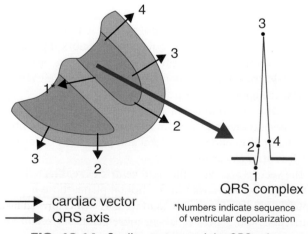

——▶ cardiac vector
——▶ QRS axis

QRS complex

*Numbers indicate sequence of ventricular depolarization

FIG. 12.14 Cardiac vectors and the QRS axis.

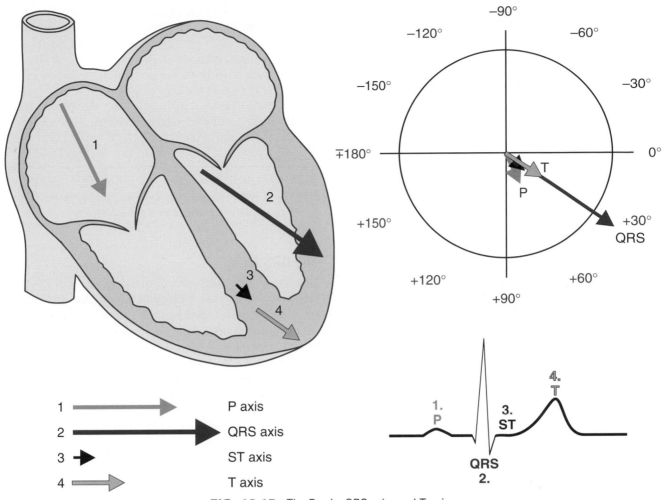

FIG. 12.15 The P axis, QRS axis, and T axis.

QRS complex. This average will be positive, negative, or biphasic (both positive and negative).

The mean of all vectors generated during the depolarization of the atria is the *P axis*; those generated during repolarization of the ventricles are the *T axis* (Fig. 12.15).

The P axis is rarely determined. The T axis is determined in certain conditions, such as myocardial ischemia and acute myocardial infarction, in which there is a significant shift in the direction of the T axis. Determination of the shift in the T axis helps localize the affected area of the myocardium. The QRS axis is the most important and most frequently determined axis.

> **AUTHOR'S NOTE** When the term *axis* is used alone, it usually refers to the QRS axis.

HEXAXIAL REFERENCE FIGURE

The word *hexaxial* simply means "six axes"—it is formed by laying one triangle on top of another, rotated 30 degrees from the bottom triangle. As previously stated, one of the triangles is

formed from the three standard limb leads (I, II, III). The other is formed from the three augmented leads (aVR, aVL, aVF; Fig. 12.16, *A*). The six lead axes are arranged like spokes on a wheel, with the central terminal as the hub or zero point. The positions of the lead axes are consistent with their actual direction and polarity in the frontal plane, so their positive and negative poles are spaced 30 degrees apart around the rim of the wheel.

The hexaxial reference figure is divided into four quadrants by the bisection of lead axis I and aVF (Fig. 12.16, *B*). Although there are several different ways to designate the quadrants, the following designation is used in this book:

DEGREES	QUADRANT
0° to −90°	I
0° to +90°	II
+90° to +180°	III
−90° to +180°	IV

Each lead axis is perpendicular, 90 degrees, from another lead. Any vector between the poles of the perpendicular axis

The purpose of the hexaxial reference figure is to aid in the determination of the direction of the QRS axis in the frontal plane.

Each positive and negative pole is assigned a degree number ranging from 0° to 180°. The poles around the rim of the upper half of the wheel are labeled with negative numbers: −30°, −60°, −90°, −120°, −150°, and ±180°; those around the lower half of the rim have positive numbers: +30°, +60°, +90°, +120°, +150°, and ±180° (Table 12.7).

> **AUTHOR'S NOTE** The negative and positive degrees should not be confused with the negative and positive poles of the lead axis. They merely indicate the position of each spoke in the figure.

The QRS Axis

Determining the QRS axis is a vital component of 12-lead ECG interpretation because it provides information on the health of the ventricles as reflected by their ability to depolarize.

The normal QRS axis, as determined using the hexaxial reference figure, lies between −30° and +90° in the frontal plane (see Fig. 12.17). A change or shift in the direction of the QRS axis from normal to one between −30° and −90° is considered *left axis deviation (LAD)*; a shift of the QRS axis to one between +90° and +180° is *right axis deviation (RAD)*. A QRS axis rarely falls between −90° and −180°. If it does, it is referred to as *indeterminate (IND)* because there are no known physiologic conditions that can result in such an extreme RAD (Fig. 12.18).

> **AUTHOR'S NOTE** Some texts refer to the indeterminate axis as *extreme RAD*. However, because it is not associated with any known physiological condition, it is essentially a hypothetical area. Therefore *indeterminate axis* is a more proper classification.

A QRS complex with LAD is always abnormal. A QRS complex with RAD may or may not be abnormal, depending on the age and body build of the patient. RAD of up to +120° or more may be present in newborns and infants, and RAD of up to about +110° may be present in young adults with long, narrow chests.

In the majority of adults, however, RAD is seldom present without some cardiac abnormality. For this reason, such a disorder should be suspected whenever RAD is present in adults.

In general, the most common causes of an abnormal shift of the QRS axis to the left or right are (1) ventricular enlargement and hypertrophy and (2) bundle-branch and fascicular blocks. These conditions will be presented in Chapter 13.

DETERMINING THE QRS AXIS

Although there are many methods to determine the QRS axis, the steps in this chapter will outline a rapid method that results in a general approximation of the axis.

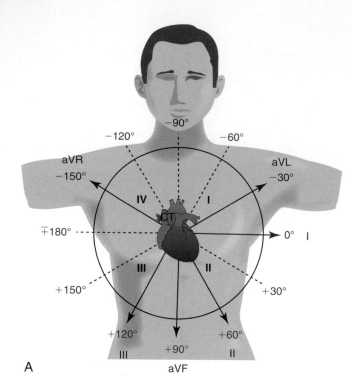

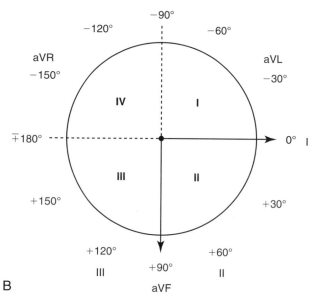

FIG. 12.16 (A) The hexaxial reference figure. (B) The four quadrants of the hexaxial reference figure.

that is closer to the positive electrode of the lead defines the positive side of the lead axis. For example, the lead axis perpendicular to the axis of lead II is the axis of lead aVL. The axis of aVL has one pole at −30° and the other at +150°. Any vector between −30° and +150° that is closer to the positive side of lead II falls within the positive half of the lead II axis. Fig. 12.17 defines the negative and positive side of each lead axis and its perpendicular.

Table 12.6 summarizes the location of the negative and positive poles of the lead axis and their perpendiculars.

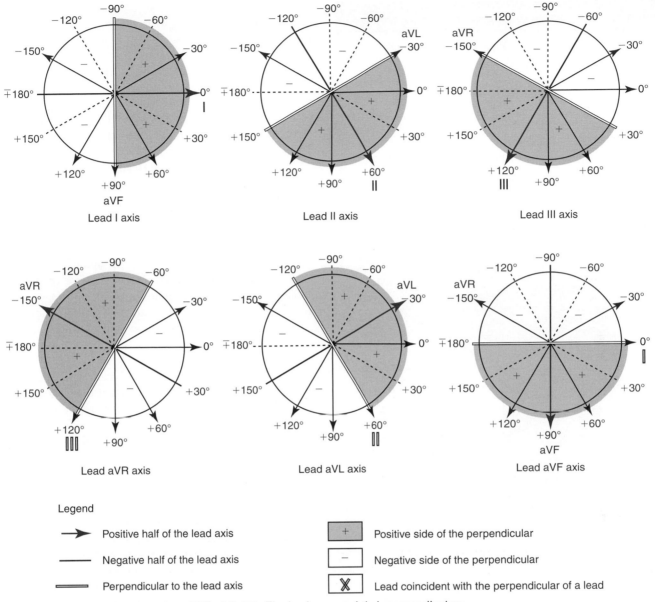

FIG. 12.17 The lead axes and their perpendiculars.

TABLE 12.6	Negative and Positive Poles of the Lead Axis and Their Perpendiculars				
	LOCATION OF LEAD AXIS POLES		**LOCATION OF THE POLES OF THE PERPENDICULAR (AND ITS COINCIDENT LEAD AXIS)**		
Lead	**−Pole**	**+Pole**	**−Pole**	**+Pole**	**Perpendicular Lead**
I	±180°	0°	−90°	+90°	aVF
II	−120°	+60°	+150°	−30°	aVL
III	−60°	+120°	+30°	−150°	aVR
aVR	+30°	−150°	−60°	+120°	III
aVL	+150°	−30°	−120°	+60°	II
aVF	−90°	+90°	±180°	0°	I

TABLE 12.7	Positive and Negative Poles of Lead Axes in the Hexaxial Reference Figure	
	−Pole	+Pole
Standard leads		
Lead I	±180°	0°
Lead II	−120°	+60°
Lead III	−60°	+120°
Augmented leads		
aVR	+30°	−150°
aVL	+150°	−30°
aVF	−90°	+90°

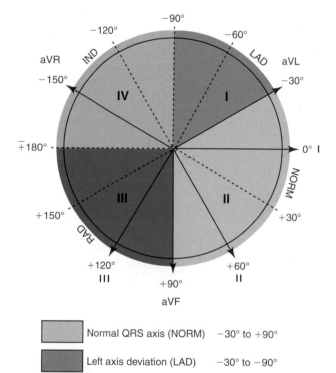

	Normal QRS axis (NORM)	−30° to +90°
	Left axis deviation (LAD)	−30° to −90°
	Right axis deviation (RAD)	+90° to +180°
	Indeterminate axis (IND)	−90° to −180°

FIG. 12.18 Normal and abnormal QRS axes.

Rapid Method

The fastest method is simply to determine in which quadrant the QRS axis lies:

- First, determine the net positivity or negativity of the QRS complexes in certain limb leads (that is, whether the QRS complexes are predominantly positive or negative).
- Then, by using this information and knowing the perpendiculars to these leads, determine the approximate QRS axis on the hexaxial reference figure and determine in which quadrant the QRS axis resides.

Lead I is evaluated first, then lead II. Between the two, it can be determined whether the QRS axis is normal or LAD or RAD is present. Depending on the findings at this point, one or more of the other leads (that is, leads III, aVF, aVR, and, rarely, aVL) are evaluated to determine the location of the QRS axis with greater accuracy.

Important points to remember in rapidly determining the QRS axis using the hexaxial reference figure are outlined in Table 12.8 and include the following:

1. Positive QRS complexes in lead I and lead II indicate that the QRS axis is in the lower portion of quadrant I or in quadrant II and therefore is normal (−30° to +90° = normal axis) (Fig. 12.19, *A*).
2. A positive QRS complex in lead I associated with a negative QRS complex in lead II indicates that the QRS axis is in the upper portion of quadrant I, and therefore LAD (−30° to −90° LAD) is present (Fig. 12.19, *B*).
3. Positive QRS complexes in lead aVF and lead I indicate that the QRS axis lies in quadrant II and therefore is normal (0° to +90° normal; Fig. 12.20).
4. A positive QRS complex in lead aVF associated with a negative QRS complex in lead I indicates that the QRS axis is in quadrant III and that RAD (+90° to +180° RAD) is present (Fig. 12.21, *A*).
5. A negative QRS complex in lead aVF and lead I indicates that the QRS axis is in quadrant IV (−90° to −180° IND) and that an indeterminant axis is present (Fig. 12.21, *B*).

Although there are many points to consider, in reality, the process is simple. Approach the QRS axis determination systematically. First, determine whether lead I is positive or negative. Second, determine whether lead II is positive or negative, and finally, do the same with aVF. The information in Table 12.9

TABLE 12.8	Basic Points to Remember in Determining the QRS Axis				
LEADS			**AXES**		
I	II	aVF	QRS Axis Range	Quadrant	Axis
Positive	Positive		−30° to +90°		Normal
Positive	Negative		−30° to −90°		LAD
Positive		Positive	0° to +90°	II	Normal
Positive		Negative	0° to −90°	I	LAD, Normal
Negative		Positive	+90° to ±180°	III	RAD
Negative		Negative	−90° to ±180°	IV	IND

LAD, Left axis deviation, *IND,* indeterminate; *RAD,* right axis deviation.

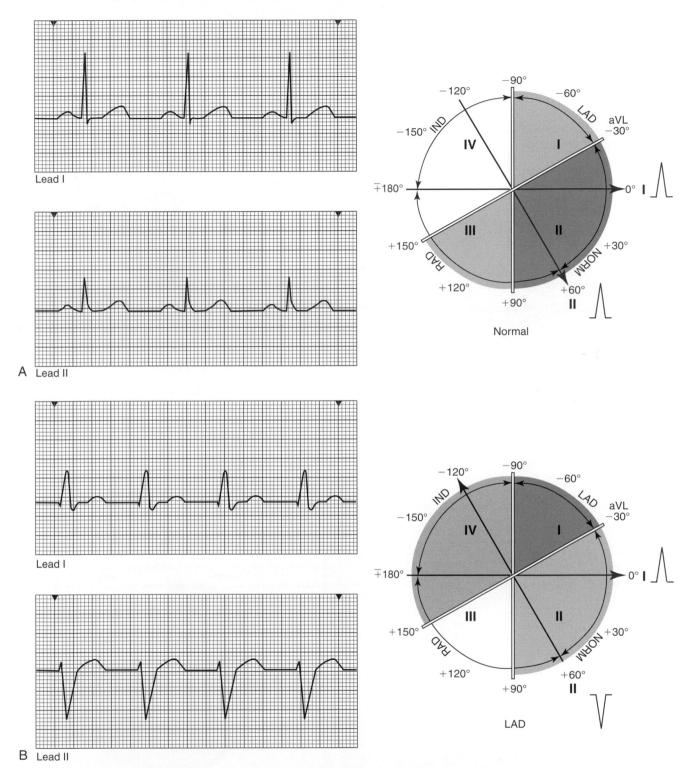

FIG. 12.19 (A) Normal QRS axis based on leads I and II. (B) Left axis deviation.

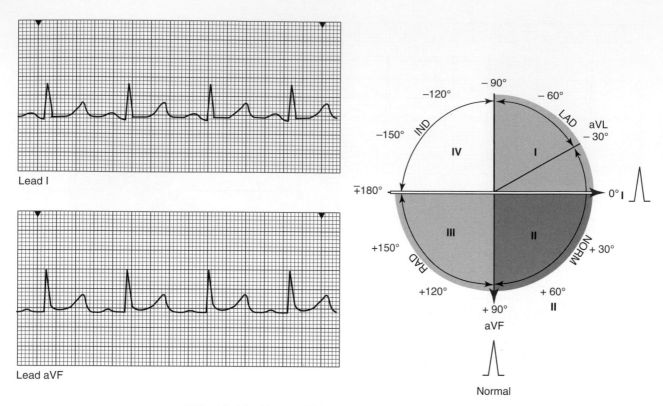

FIG. 12.20 Normal QRS axis, based on leads I and aVF.

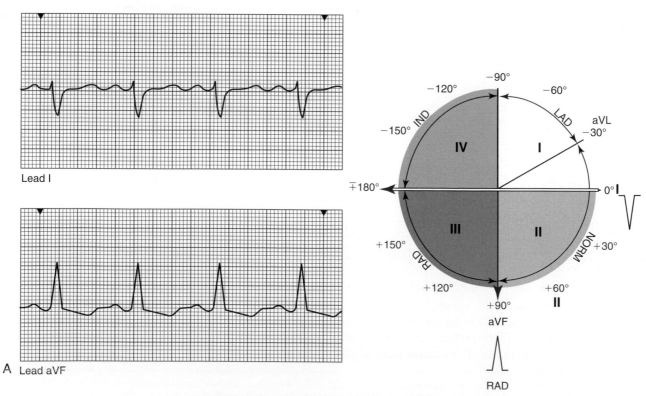

FIG. 12.21 (A) Right axis deviation (RAD).

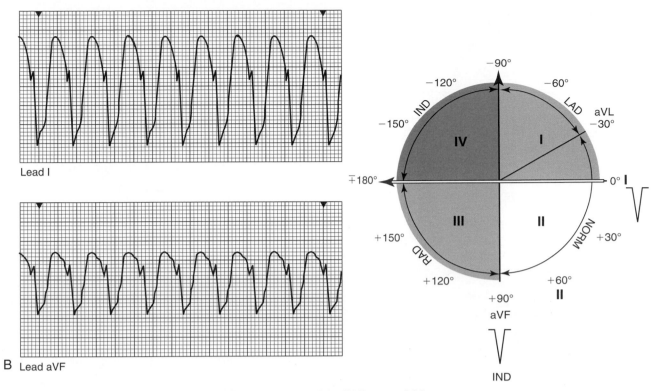

Lead I

B Lead aVF

FIG. 12.21 cont'd   (B) Extreme RAD.

TABLE 12.9	QRS Characteristics in Various Leads and Associated QRS Axis

LEADS						EQUIPHASIC LEADS						
I	II	aVF	III	aVR	Location of QRS Axis	I	II	aVF	III	aVR	aVL	Location of QRS Axis
+	+	+	+		+30° to +90°	±	−	−	−	+		−90
+	+	+	+		0° to +30°	+	−	−	−	±		−60
+	+	−	−		0° to −30°	+	±	−	−	−		−30
+	−	−	−		−30° to −90°	+	+	±	−	−		0
−	+	+	+		±90° to +120°	+	+	+	±	−	±	+30
−	+	+	+	+	+120° to +150°	+	+	+	+	−	±	+60
−	−	−	−		−90° to −150°	±	+	+	+	−		+90
						−	+	+	+	±		+120
						−	±	+	+	+		+150
						−	−	±	+	+		±180
						−	−	−	±	+		−150
						−	−	−	−	±	±	−120

+, Predominantly positive; −, predominantly negative; ±, equiphasic.

shows that the combination of these results places the QRS axis in one of the four quadrants. The only value of examining lead II is to determine whether the QRS axis is normal or there is LAD.

Accurate Measurement

There are three steps in determining an accurate QRS axis, as described next.

Step 1

Determine the net positivity or negativity of the QRS complexes in lead I.

A. If the QRS complexes are predominantly *positive* in lead I, the QRS axis lies between −90° and +90° (that is, in quadrant I or II). The QRS axis may be between −30° and +90° (normal QRS axis) or between −30° and −90° (LAD).

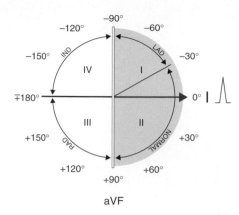

B. If the QRS complexes are predominantly *negative* in lead I, the QRS axis is greater than +90° (lying between +90° and −90°), indicating RAD. Most likely, the QRS axis lies in quadrant III and, rarely, in quadrant IV.

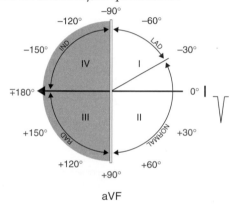

Note: If the QRS complexes are predominantly positive in lead I, proceed to Step 2. If the QRS complexes are predominantly negative in lead I, proceed to *Step 3*.

Step 2

If the QRS complexes are predominantly *positive* in lead I:

Determine the net positivity or negativity of the QRS complexes in one or more of the following three leads (II, aVF, and III):

1. Lead II

    A. If the QRS complexes are predominantly *positive* in lead II, the QRS axis is between +30° and +90° (normal QRS axis).

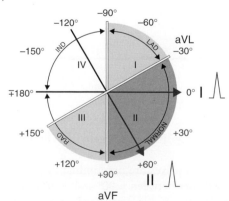

B. If the QRS complexes are predominantly *negative* in lead II, the QRS axis is between −30° and −90° (LAD).

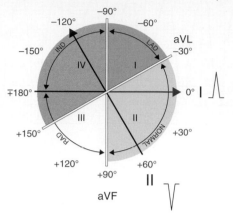

2. Lead aVF

    I. If the QRS complexes are predominantly *positive* in lead aVF, the QRS axis is between 0° and +90° (quadrant II).

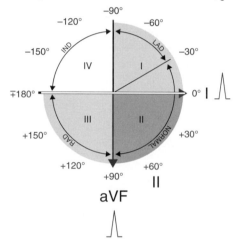

II. If the QRS complexes are predominantly *negative* in lead aVF, the QRS axis is between 0° and −90° (quadrant I).

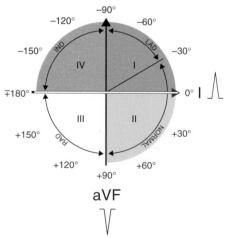

3. Lead III
   A. If the QRS complexes are predominantly *positive* in lead III, the QRS axis is between +30° and +90°.

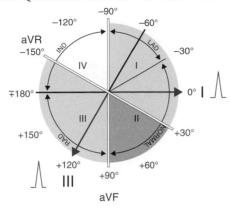

   B. If the QRS complexes are predominantly *negative* in lead III, the QRS axis is between +30° and −90°.

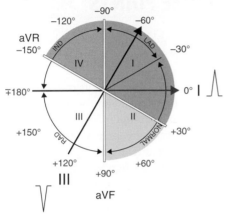

Step 3

If the QRS complexes are predominantly *negative* in lead I:

- Determine the net positivity or negativity of the QRS complexes in one or more of the following four leads (II, aVF, III, and aVR):

1. Lead II
A. If the QRS complexes are predominantly *positive* in lead II, the QRS axis is between +90° and +150°.

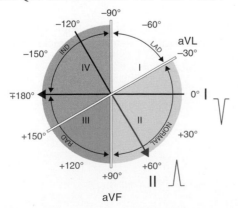

B. If the QRS complexes are predominantly *negative* in lead II, the QRS axis is greater than +150°.

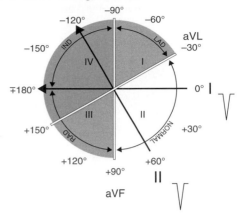

2. Lead aVF
I. If the QRS complexes are predominantly *positive* in lead aVF, the QRS axis is between +90° and +180° (quadrant III).

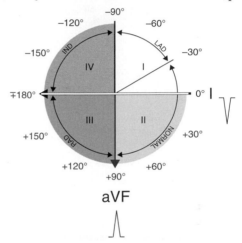

II. If the QRS complexes are predominantly negative in lead aVF, the QRS axis is between −90° and −180° (quadrant IV).

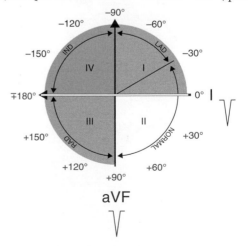

3. Lead III

A. If the QRS complexes are predominantly *positive* in lead III, the QRS axis is between +90° and −150°.

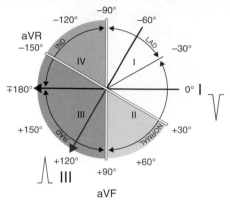

B. If the QRS complexes are predominantly *negative* in lead III, the QRS axis is between −90° and −150°.

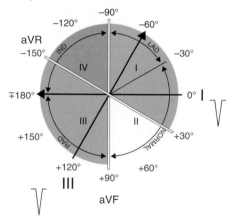

4. Lead aVR

A. If the QRS complexes are predominantly *positive* in lead aVR, the QRS axis is greater than +120° (severe RAD).

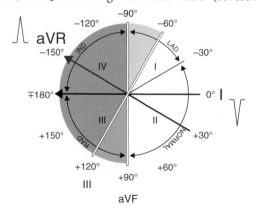

B. If the QRS complexes are predominantly *negative* in lead aVR, the QRS axis is between +90° and +120° (mild to moderate RAD).

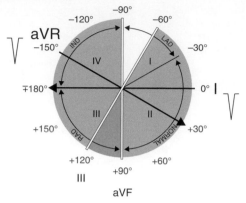

TAKE-HOME POINTS

- The three limb leads are bipolar leads, whereas the augmented leads are unipolar leads. Combined, they view the heart in the frontal plane.
- Each lead has a unique axis and its own perpendicular.
- The axes of the limb leads and the augmented leads, when joined, form a triaxial reference figure, with each lead separated from the next by an angle of 60 degrees.
- When the two triaxial reference figures are combined, they form a hexaxial reference figure, with each lead in the frontal plane separated by an angle of 30 degrees.
- The precordial unipolar leads view the heart in the horizontal plane.
- The 12-lead ECG is used to provide specific views of the heart.
- The electrical impulses of the heart can be described as having both a magnitude and an axis, which we call a *vector*.
- The ECG records numerous simultaneous vectors and generates results on the screen that represent the averaged cardiac vectors for the P wave, QRS complex, and T wave.
- The axis, or direction of the QRS complex, can be calculated by using the hexaxial reference figure generated by the limb leads.
- The QRS axis can be affected by multiple conditions. Therefore it is important to determine quickly whether it is normal.

CHAPTER REVIEW QUESTIONS

1. Which lead represents the difference in electrical potential between a positive and a negative electrode?
   A. Bipolar
   B. Central
   C. Terminal
   D. Unipolar

2. In leads aVR, aVL, and aVF, what does the "a" stand for?
   A. Alternative
   B. Arterial
   C. Atrial
   D. Augmented

3. The relationships of the standard limb leads are such that the electrical impulses of lead _____ + lead _____ = lead _____.
   A. I, II, III
   B. I, III, II
   C. II, III, I
   D. II, III, IV

4. To obtain lead aVL, the positive electrode is attached to the _____ arm and the other two electrodes to the _____, which, when combined, form the central terminal.
   A. left; right and left arms
   B. left; right arm and left leg
   C. right; left arm and left leg
   D. right; right and left legs

5. Which lead measures the difference in electrical potential between a chest electrode and the central terminal?
   A. Bipolar
   B. Precordial
   C. Terminal
   D. Nonpolar

6. The V_4 positive chest electrode is placed where?
   A. In the anterior axillary line at the fifth intercostal space
   B. In the midaxillary line at the sixth intercostal space
   C. Left side of the sternum in the fourth intercostal space
   D. Midclavicular line in the fifth intercostal space

7. An electrical impulse flowing toward the positive pole of a lead produces what on the ECG?
   A. Elongated deflection
   B. Negative deflection
   C. Parallel deflection
   D. Positive deflection

8. The more parallel the electrical impulse is to the axis of the lead, the _____ the deflection.
   A. larger
   B. more oblique
   C. more regular
   D. smaller

9. A predominantly negative QRS complex in a given lead indicates that the _____ pole of the vector of the QRS axis lies somewhere on the _____ side of the perpendicular axis.
   A. positive; positive
   B. positive; negative
   C. negative; negative
   D. negative; positive

10. If the QRS complexes are predominantly positive in leads I and aVF, the QRS axis is between
    A. $-30°$ and $+90°$.
    B. $0°$ and $+90°$.
    C. $0°$ and $-90°$.
    D. $-30°$ and $-90°$.

Bundle-Branch and Fascicular Blocks

ANATOMY AND PHYSIOLOGY OF THE BUNDLE-BRANCH CONDUCTION SYSTEM

Anatomy

As described in Chapter 1, the impulse-conduction system located below the atrioventricular (AV) node is called the His–Purkinje system. It consists of the bundle of His, the right and left bundle branches, and the Purkinje network. It terminates in the ventricular myocardium through a network of extremely fine Purkinje fibers. Take a moment to locate these structures in Fig. 13.1 as we review the path of electrical conduction through the heart:

- After leaving the AV node, an impulse travels through the bundle of His. This bundle then divides into the right and left bundle branches.
  1. The long, thin, round right bundle branch runs down the right side of the interventricular septum (the wall between the ventricles), conducting the electrical impulses to the right ventricle.
  2. The left bundle branch consists of a short, thick, flat bundle of nervous tissue. It divides into two smaller branches called *fascicles:*
     □ The relatively long, thin left anterior fascicle occupies the anterior portion of the interventricular septum. It conducts the electrical impulse from the left bundle branch to the anterior (front) and lateral (side) walls of the left ventricle.

     □ The short, broad left posterior fascicle runs down the posterior wall of the interventricular septum. It conducts the electrical impulse to the posterior wall of the left ventricle.

> **AUTHOR'S NOTE** The word *fascicle* comes from the Latin word *fascia,* meaning "band," especially a band wrapped around a bundle.

BLOOD SUPPLY

The AV node artery is the primary blood supply of the AV node and proximal part of the bundle of His (Fig. 13.2). Like the posterior descending artery (PDA), it arises from the right coronary artery (RCA) in 85% to 90% of hearts. In the other 10% to 15%, it arises from the left circumflex coronary artery (LCx). In most hearts, the left anterior descending (LAD) artery is the primary blood supply to the distal part of the bundle of His.

The LAD branch of the left coronary artery (LCA) supplies the anterior two-thirds of the interventricular septum. The PDA supplies the posterior third of the interventricular septum. The PDA arises from the RCA in 85% to 90% of hearts and from the LCx of the LCA in the other 10% to 15%. Therefore the entire right bundle branch, the main portion of the left bundle branch, and the left anterior fascicle are supplied with blood from the LAD. The left posterior fascicle is supplied by both the LAD and the PDA.

Myocardial infarction (MI) from an occlusion of these arteries injures not only the heart muscle but also the electrical conduction system the arteries supply.

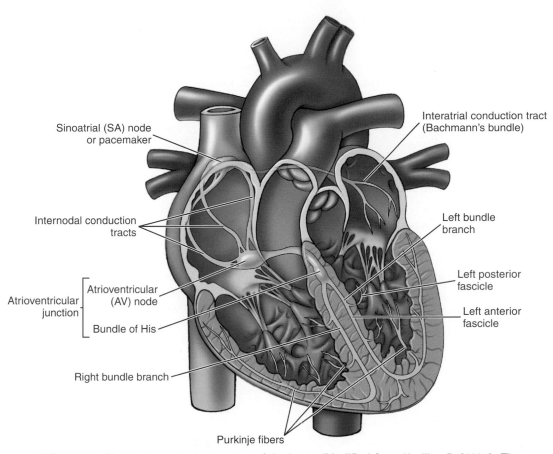

FIG. 13.1 Electrical conduction system of the heart. (Modified from Herlihy, B. [2001]. *The human body in health and illness* [4th ed.]. Saunders.)

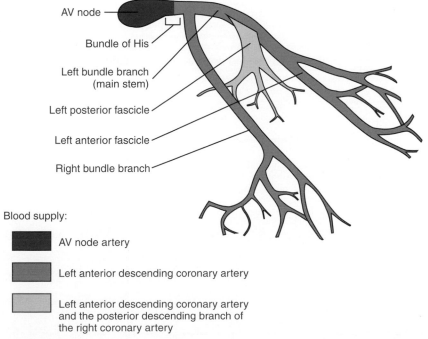

FIG. 13.2 The electrical conduction system and its blood supply in most hearts.

Table 13.1 summarizes the blood supply to the various parts of the bundle-branch conduction system.

Physiology

Normally, the electrical impulses progress through the right bundle branch and left bundle branch and its fascicles simultaneously

TABLE 13.1	Blood Supply of the His–Purkinje Conduction System	
Portion	**Primary Blood Supply**	**Alternative Blood Supply**
AV node	AV node artery	None
Proximal bundle of His	AV node artery	None
Distal bundle of His	LAD	PDA
Proximal right bundle branch	LAD	PDA
Distal right bundle branch	LAD	None
Main stem of left bundle branch	LAD	PDA
Left anterior fascicle	LAD	None
Left posterior fascicle	LAD and PDA	None

AV, Atrioventricular; *LAD,* left anterior descending artery by way of the septal perforator arteries; *PDA,* posterior descending coronary artery.

(Fig. 13.3). This first depolarizes the interventricular septum from left to right (1) and then simultaneously depolarizes the right and left ventricles (2). However, the left ventricle is much larger than the right. Therefore the electrical activity generated by the left ventricle during depolarization exceeds that of the right ventricle. For this reason, the QRS complex primarily reflects the depolarization of the left ventricle. The QRS typical of normal bundle-branch conduction is shown in Fig. 13.3.

The normal conduction of the bundle branch can be impaired by the chronic effects of atherosclerotic heart disease and diabetes. It can also be impaired when an MI occurs that involves the portion of the heart through which it travels. Table 13.2 lists the types of bundle-branch blocks associated with particular MIs.

When normal bundle-branch conduction is blocked, two components of the QRS are affected: the *ventricular activation time* (VAT) and the *intrinsicoid deflection*. The VAT is the time it takes for depolarization of the interventricular septum and the portion of the ventricles progressing toward any given lead (Fig. 13.4). The VAT is measured from the onset of the QRS complex to the peak of the last R wave in the QRS complex.

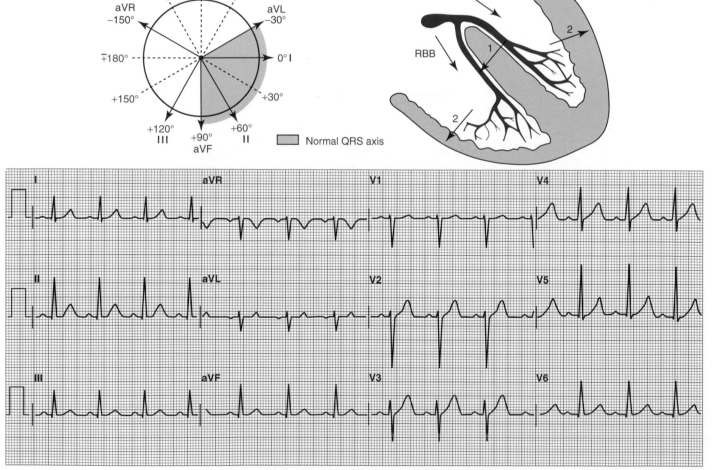

FIG. 13.3 Normal sinus rhythm with normal bundle-branch conduction.

The time taken to depolarize the interventricular septum and ventricles. Normal is less than 0.035 second in leads V_1 and V_2 and 0.055 second in leads V_5 and V_6.

Normally, it is less than 0.035 second in leads V_1 and V_2 and less than 0.055 second in leads V_5 and V_6. When there is a bundle-branch block of any kind, the VAT will be prolonged.

The intrinsicoid deflection, sometimes referred to as the "terminal forces" of the QRS, is the upward or downward component of the R or S wave as it returns to the baseline (ST segment).

TABLE 13.2	Bundle-Branch and Fascicular Blocks and the Acute Myocardial Infarctions That Usually Cause Them
Bundle-Branch and Fascicular Block	**Acute Myocardial Infarction (Coronary Artery Involved)**
Right bundle-branch block	Anteroseptal (LAD) OR Right ventricular (RCA) (rare)
Left bundle-branch block	Anteroseptal (LAD) OR Inferior (LCx) (rare)
Left anterior fascicular block	Anteroseptal (LAD)
Left posterior fascicular block	Anteroseptal (LAD) AND Right ventricular (RCA) OR Inferior (distal RCA or LCx)

LAD, Left anterior descending coronary artery; *LCx,* left circumflex coronary artery; *RCA,* right coronary artery.

It represents the final stages of ventricular depolarization. When a bundle-branch block occurs, the right and left ventricles do not depolarize simultaneously, and the ventricle affected by the blocked bundle depolarizes slightly slower than the other.

The abrupt upward or downward component of the R or S wave as the QRS complex returns to the ST segment.

RIGHT BUNDLE-BRANCH BLOCK

In a right bundle-branch block (RBBB), electrical impulses are prevented from traveling through the right bundle branch to the ventricles (Fig. 13.5). Instead, the impulses travel rapidly down the left bundle branch into the left side of the interventricular septum and Purkinje network of the left ventricle. At some point beyond the block, the impulses in the septum slowly cross from left to right and enter the right ventricle. This slow progression across the septum delays right ventricular depolarization.

Consequently, the interventricular septum and left ventricle depolarize normally because their impulse is not blocked. The septum depolarizes from left to right (1), and then the left ventricle depolarizes from right to left (2). After the left ventricle depolarizes and the impulse has slowly crossed the interventricular septum beyond the block, the right ventricle depolarizes in a normal direction, from left to right (3).

Because of the delay, the QRS complex is longer than 0.12 second in duration and has a bizarre shape and appearance compared with the normal QRS complex. The delay is identified by a prolonged VAT in the precordial leads overlying the anterior portion of the septum and right ventricle.

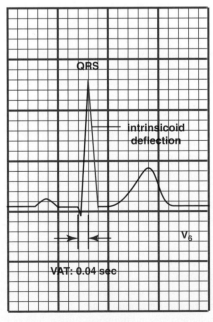

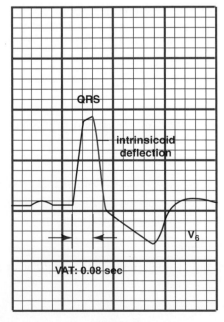

Normal

Abnormal

FIG. 13.4 The ventricular activation time and intrinsicoid deflection.

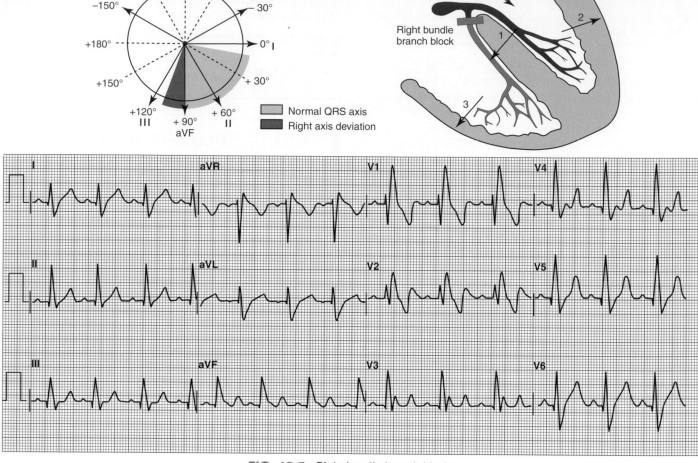

FIG. 13.5 Right bundle-branch block.

The characteristics of RBBB are outlined next and summarized in ECG Keys Box 13.1.

Characteristics

QRS COMPLEX

Duration

Greater than 0.12 second; 0.10 to 0.12 second in incomplete RBBB. VAT exceeds 0.035 second in leads V_1 and V_2.

Axis

May be normal or have a slight right axis deviation (between +90° and 110°). This shift to the right occurs because left ventricular depolarization precedes right ventricular depolarization.

Ventricular Activation Time

Greater than 0.035 second (1 small box) in the precordial leads V_1 and V_2.

PATTERN

Characteristically has a "rabbit-ears" appearance with small q waves, rSR′ in V_1 to V_2, and slurring of the last 0.04 second

---

BOX 13.1 ECG KEYS | **ECG Characteristics of Right Bundle-Branch Block**

Leads V_1 to V_2
Wide QRS complex with a classic rSR′ rabbit-ears pattern
- Initial small r wave
- Deep, slurred S wave
- Tall R′ wave
ST-segment depression
T-wave inversion
Leads I, aVL, V_5 to V_6
Wide QRS complex with a qRS pattern
- Initial small q wave
- Tall R wave
- Slurred S wave
QRS Axis
Normal or right axis deviation (+90° to +110°)
Ventricular Activation Time
Prolonged beyond the upper normal limit of 0.035 second in the right precordial leads V_1 and V_2

of the QRS complex, resulting in a large S wave in leads I, V_5, and V_6. The intrinsicoid deflection is downward as the R′ wave returns to the ST segment.

Q Wave

Normal small septal q waves may be present in leads I, aVL, and V_5 to V_6, reflecting the normal depolarization of the interventricular septum.

R Wave

Small r waves are present in the right precordial leads V_1 to V_2, reflecting the normal depolarization of the interventricular septum. Wide, slurred, and tall R waves are present in lead aVR and the right precordial leads V_1 to V_2. This produces the classic rabbit-ears pattern of the rSR′ pattern in leads V_1 to V_2.

S wave

Deep and slurred S waves are present in leads I and aVL and the left precordial leads V_5 to V_6. This produces the typical qRS pattern of RBBB in leads V_5 to V_6.

ST SEGMENT

ST segment depression may be present in leads V_1 to V_2.

T WAVE

T-wave inversion may be present in leads V_1 to V_2.

The ST segments and T waves are *discordant*. That means they deflect in the opposite direction of the overall deflection of the QRS. Therefore they are inverted (negative) in leads V_1 and V_2 and upright (positive) in leads V_5 and V_6 and in leads I and aVL. If they both deflect in the same direction, the T wave is termed *concordant*, which indicates underlying ischemia.

discordant and concordant

The deflection of the T wave or ST segment opposite the overall deflection of the QRS. Concordant deflection exists when the T wave and/or ST segment deflect in the same direction of the QRS complex.

Causes

RBBB may be present without any apparent cause in otherwise-healthy people with normal hearts. Common pathologic causes of RBBB include the following:

- Coronary and hypertensive heart disease
- Anteroseptal MI
- Pulmonary embolism or infarction
- Heart failure
- Pericarditis or myocarditis

Clinical Significance

The presence of a new RBBB in the context of an acute coronary syndrome is highly suggestive of an anterior MI. This will be discussed in greater detail in Chapter 16. The progression of RBBB to complete AV block occurs twice as often as that of left bundle-branch block (LBBB), especially when RBBB is

associated with a fascicular block. However, complete AV block as a result of MI is usually temporary, lasting 1 to 2 weeks.

Treatment

Only rarely does RBBB require treatment. In the event of a complete AV block, a temporary pacemaker may be used until the block resolves.

LEFT BUNDLE-BRANCH BLOCK

In LBBB, the electrical impulses are prevented from traveling through the left bundle branch (Fig. 13.6). The electrical impulses travel rapidly down the right bundle branch into the right ventricle normally. Meanwhile, they progress slowly across the interventricular septum from right to left into the left ventricle. Consequently, the septum depolarizes first in an abnormal way, from right to left (1), and either anteriorly or posteriorly. This is followed by the depolarization of the right ventricle in a normal way, left to right (2), and then depolarization of the left ventricle in a normal direction from right to left (3).

The electrical impulses enter the left ventricle from the right, through the interventricular septum instead of the left bundle branch. As a result, depolarization of the left ventricle occurs slightly behind schedule.

Because of this delay, the VAT is greater than 0.055 second in the facing precordial leads (V_5 and V_6). The QRS complex is greater than 0.12 second and has an abnormal shape and appearance.

The characteristics of LBBB are outlined next and summarized in ECG Keys Box 13.2.

Characteristics

QRS COMPLEX

Duration

Greater than 0.12 second; 0.10 to 0.12 second in incomplete LBBB. VAT exceeds 0.035 second in leads V_1 and V_2.

Pattern

In LBBB, depolarization of the left ventricle occurs much later than that of the right ventricle. The impulses of depolarization of the left ventricle are directed leftward and last more than 40 msec (0.04 second), producing the typical broad R and S waves in the various leads. The combined impulses of the right ventricular depolarization and delayed left ventricular depolarization produce the typical wide, monophasic QRS complexes of LBBB. They are said to be monophasic because they are solely negative or positive. The intrinsicoid deflection is upward as the S wave returns to the ST segment.

Q Wave

Septal q waves are absent in leads I and aVL and in the left precordial leads (V_5 to V_6), where they normally occur. They are absent because of depolarization of the interventricular septum in an abnormal direction, from right to left.

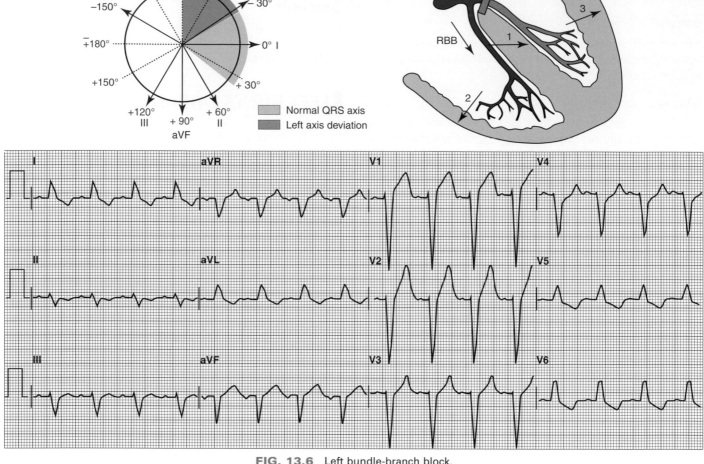

FIG. 13.6   Left bundle-branch block.

Box 13.2 ECG KEYS	**ECG Characteristics of Left Bundle-Branch Block**

Leads V₁ to V₃
Wide QRS complex with an rS or QS pattern
- Initial small r or absent R wave
- Deep wide S wave

ST-segment elevation
T-wave concordant with QRS complex

Leads I, aVL, V₅ to V₆
Wide QRS complex with an R pattern
- Absent initial small q wave
- Tall, wide, slurred R wave, with or without notching, and a prolonged VAT

ST-segment depression
T-wave inversion concordance

QRS Axis
Normal QRS axis or left axis deviation (−30° to −90°)

Ventricular Activation Time
Prolonged beyond the upper normal limit of 0.055 second in the left precordial leads V₅ and V₆

R Wave

Small, narrow r (small r) waves are present in leads V_1 to V_3 when the interventricular septum depolarizes from right to left and anteriorly. This occurs in about two-thirds of LBBBs. The R waves in leads V_1 to V_3 show very minimal increases from one lead to the other. This is referred to as *poor R-wave progression*, a hallmark of LBBB and old anteroseptal infarctions. In the other third of LBBBs, in which the interventricular septum depolarizes from right to left and posteriorly, R waves are absent in leads V_1 to V_3. Tall, wide, slurred R waves are present in leads I and aVL and in the left precordial leads (V_5–V_6). These R waves may be notched, particularly near their peaks. The VAT is prolonged up to 0.07 second or more, particularly in lead aVL and the left precordial leads V_5 to V_6.

S Wave

Deep, wide S waves are present in leads V_1 to V_3, producing the typical rS or QS complexes. Because of these wide S waves, an anteroseptal MI may be mistakenly diagnosed. S waves are absent in leads I and aVL and the left precordial leads V_5 to V_6.

ST SEGMENT

ST-segment depression is present in leads I and aVL and in the left precordial leads (V_5 to V_6). ST-segment elevation is present in leads V_1 to V_3.

T WAVE

T-wave inversion is present in leads I and aVL and in the left precordial leads (V_5 to V_6). The T wave is upright in leads V_1 to V_3. The T waves are *disconcordant,* which means that the QRS complex and the T wave deflect in opposite directions. This is normal for LBBB. If they both deflect in the same direction, the T wave is termed *concordant,* which indicates underlying ischemia.

Causes

In general, LBBB is more common than is RBBB. Common causes of LBBB include the following:

- Hypertensive heart disease (the most common cause) and coronary artery disease
- Cardiomyopathy and myocarditis
- Anteroseptal MI
- Heart failure
- Pericarditis or myocarditis
- Acute cardiac trauma
- Administration of such drugs as beta blockers and calcium-channel blockers

Clinical Significance

The presence of a new LBBB in the context of an acute coronary syndrome is highly suggestive of an anteroseptal MI. This will be discussed in greater detail in Chapter 16. The progression of LBBB to complete AV block is uncommon.

Treatment

Only rarely does LBBB require treatment. In the event of a complete AV block, a temporary pacemaker may be needed until the block resolves.

HEMIBLOCK

The left bundle branch splits into the anterior and posterior fascicles. Electrical impulse conduction can become blocked in either fascicle. When only one fascicle is blocked, the condition is called a *hemiblock*—recall that the prefix *hemi-* means "half." Because the conduction block affects only a portion of the left bundle branch, the QRS complex is not prolonged.

LEFT ANTERIOR FASCICULAR BLOCK (LEFT ANTERIOR HEMIBLOCK)

In a left anterior fascicular block (LAFB; Fig. 13.7), electrical impulses are prevented from directly entering the anterior and lateral walls of the left ventricle. Instead, the impulses travel rapidly down the left posterior fascicle into the interventricular septum and posterior wall of the left ventricle. Then, after a very slight delay, they progress into the anterior and lateral walls of

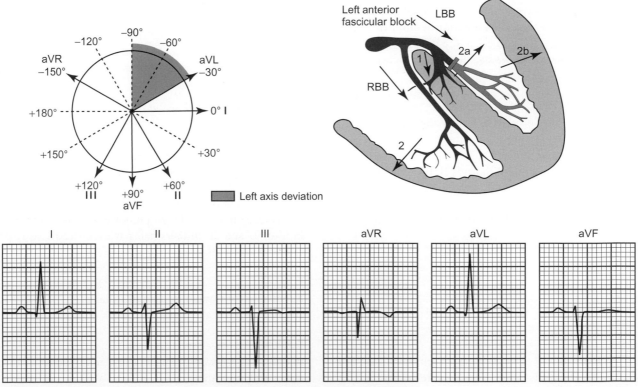

FIG. 13.7 Left anterior fascicular block.

the left ventricle. At the same time, electrical impulses travel down the right bundle branch into the right ventricle in a normal way.

The interventricular septum depolarizes first in a normal direction, from left to right (1). This is followed by the depolarization of the right ventricle (2) and the posterior wall of the left ventricle (2a), followed almost instantaneously by depolarization of the anterior and lateral walls of the left ventricle (2b).

Because there is little delay between the depolarization of the posterior and anterolateral walls of the left ventricle, the QRS complex is of normal duration. The electrical impulses generated by the slightly delayed depolarization of the anterior and lateral walls of the left ventricle travel in an upward and leftward direction, producing a marked left axis deviation. LAFB can occur alone or with RBBB.

Characteristics

QRS COMPLEX

Duration

Normal; less than 0.12 second in duration.

Axis

Left axis deviation (−30° to −90°) caused by the delayed depolarization of the anterior and lateral walls of the left ventricle upward and leftward, obscuring the rest of the QRS complex.

Pattern

Appears normal, without unusual notching or any delay in the VAT. The presence of an initial small q wave in lead I coupled with an initial small r wave in lead III (q_1r_3 pattern) indicates LAFB. The QRS complex of a left anterior hemiblock typically has an rS pattern in II, III, and aV, and a qR pattern in lead I. Even in the presence of Q waves, the overall deflection will point toward left axis deviation.

Q wave

Initial small q waves are present in leads I and aVL.

R wave

Initial small r waves are present in leads II, III, and aVF.

S wave

Usually deep; larger than the R waves in leads II, III, and aVF.

ST SEGMENT

Normal.

T WAVE

Normal.

Causes

Because the LAD supplies blood to the left anterior fascicle, the most common cause of LAFB is an acute anteroseptal MI.

LEFT POSTERIOR FASCICULAR BLOCK (LEFT POSTERIOR HEMIBLOCK)

In a left posterior fascicular block (LPFB; Fig. 13.8), electrical impulses are prevented from directly entering the interventricular septum and posterior wall of the left ventricle. Instead, electrical impulses travel rapidly down the left anterior fascicle into the anterior and lateral walls of the left ventricle. Then, after a very slight delay, they advance to the posterior wall of the left ventricle. At the same time, electrical impulses travel down the right bundle branch into the right ventricle in a normal way.

Subsequently, the interventricular septum depolarizes. This occurs first in an abnormal direction, from right to left, anteriorly and superiorly (1). This is followed by the depolarization of the right ventricle (2) and the anterior and lateral walls of the left ventricle (2a), followed almost instantaneously by depolarization of the posterior wall of the left ventricle (2b).

> **AUTHOR'S NOTE** These findings relative to the QRS complex are significant only in the absence of other causes of right axis deviation, such as right ventricular hypertrophy, which will be discussed in Chapter 14.

Because there is little delay between the depolarization of the anterolateral and posterior walls of the left ventricle, the QRS complex is of normal duration. The impulses generated by the slightly delayed depolarization of the posterior wall of the left ventricle travel in a downward and rightward direction, producing a marked right axis deviation.

Characteristics

QRS COMPLEX

Duration

Normal (less than 0.12 second).

Axis

Right axis deviation (+90° to +180°).

Pattern

The QRS complexes appear normal, without unusual notching or any delay in the VAT. The presence of an initial small q wave in lead III and an initial small r wave in lead I (q_3r_1 pattern) indicates an LPFB.

Q Wave

Initial small q waves are present in leads II, III, and aVF and absent in leads I, aVL, and V_5 to V_6.

R Wave

Initial small r waves are present in leads I and aVL, and tall R waves are present in leads II, III, and aVF.

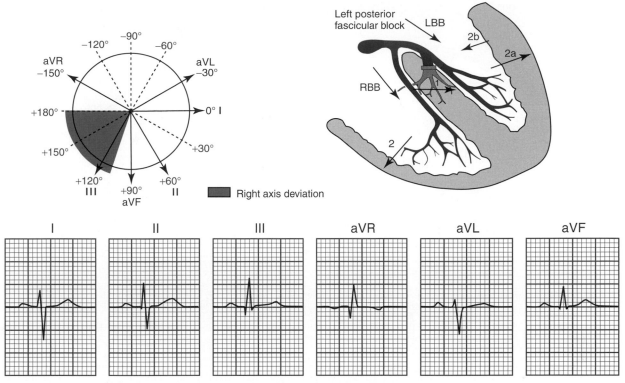

FIG. 13.8   Left posterior fascicular block.

S Wave

Deep S waves are present in leads I and aVL.

ST SEGMENT

Normal

T WAVE

Normal

Causes

LPFB is rare because the nerve fibers of the posterior fascicle are not as organized and discrete as those of anterior fascicle, and it therefore requires a more significant area of the heart to be injured to result in its being blocked. It can occur in an acute anteroseptal MI. LPFB can occur alone or with RBBB.

BIFASCICULAR BLOCK

As we have discussed, either of the hemiblocks can occur alone or with an RBBB. When they occur with an RBBB, this is termed a *bifascicular block.*

Because LAFB is more common, the combination of RBBB and LAFB is the usual presentation of bifascicular block. It can deteriorate into complete heart block, particularly in the setting of MI, if the posterior fascicle is involved. As demonstrated in Fig. 13.9, the characteristics of RBBB and LAFB include the following:

- RSR' pattern in V1 and slurred S in V6
- QRS-complex duration of longer than 0.12 second

- Left axis deviation and rS pattern in lead III (typical of LAFB) compared with right axis deviation (RBBB alone)

The ischemia required to injure the posterior fascicle also injures the RBBB. Fig. 13.10 depicts findings characteristic of RBBB and LPFB:

- Typical configuration of RBBB with RSR' pattern in V1 and slurred S in V6
- QRS-complex duration of longer than 0.12 second
- Significant right axis deviation (between +110° and +180°)
- Small q wave in lead III, compared with slight right axis deviation in RBBB alone

> **AUTHOR'S NOTE** LAFB alone is not uncommon, and in combination with RBBB, it is the most common bifascicular block. On the other hand, LPFB rarely occurs alone and will be accompanied by a RBBB block.

NONSPECIFIC INTRAVENTRICULAR CONDUCTION DELAY

Not all intraventricular conduction delays (IVCDs) will meet the strict criteria presented in this chapter. Some ECGs exhibit QRS complexes that have the characteristic pattern of a bundle-branch block yet appear in only one or two leads or last less than 0.12 second. This is called a *nonspecific intraventricular conduction delay.*

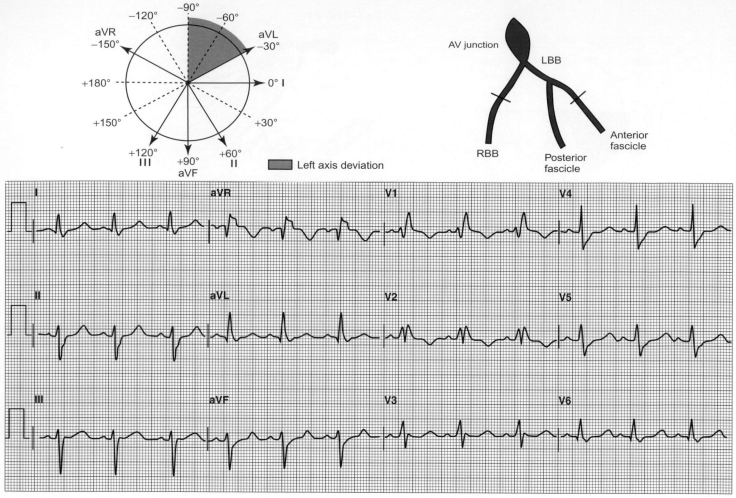

FIG. 13.9 Bifascicular block, right bundle-branch block, and left anterior hemiblock. (Modified from Goldberger, A. L., Goldberger, Z. D., & Shvilkin, A. [Eds.]. (2012). *Goldberger's clinical electrocardiography: A simplified approach* [8th ed.]. Saunders.)

The delay may be localized, seen in only one or two leads, or it may appear throughout the 12-lead ECG. Localized IVCD is often seen in lead III. It is of no clinical significance. However, a generalized IVCD of longer than 0.12 second that does not meet the criteria of any of the bundle-branch or fascicular blocks indicates a possible electrolyte abnormality, such as hyperkalemia (high blood potassium).

DIFFERENTIATING BETWEEN SUPRAVENTRICULAR TACHYCARDIA AND VENTRICULAR TACHYCARDIA

At times, a supraventricular tachycardia (such as sinus, atrial, or junctional tachycardia; atrial flutter; or paroxysmal supraventricular tachycardia) with a wide QRS complex caused by a preexisting intraventricular conduction disturbance (such as a bundle-branch block), aberrant ventricular conduction, or ventricular preexcitation may mimic ventricular tachycardia

(V-tach). Atrial fibrillation with a wide QRS complex and a rapid ventricular rate may also mimic V-tach. Usually, however, the grossly irregular rhythm of atrial fibrillation provides a clue to its true identity.

Certain features common to V-tach help differentiate it from supraventricular tachycardia with a wide QRS complex:
- AV dissociation
- A QRS complex with a duration longer than 0.12 second (especially if it is longer than 0.14 second)
- Capture or ventricular fusion beats

A 12-lead ECG or evaluation of lead MCL₁ is also useful in this situation by helping to determine whether a P wave is present and, if so, what its relationship is to the QRS complex. Analysis of specific QRS shapes can also be helpful in diagnosing V-tach and localizing its site of origin. For example, QRS shapes suggesting V-tach include left axis deviation in the frontal plane and a QRS duration exceeding 0.14 second. In precordial leads with an RS pattern, if the duration of the onset of the R to the bottom of the S exceeds 0.10 second, V-tach is a likely diagnosis. During V-tach with an RBBB appearance, (1) the QRS

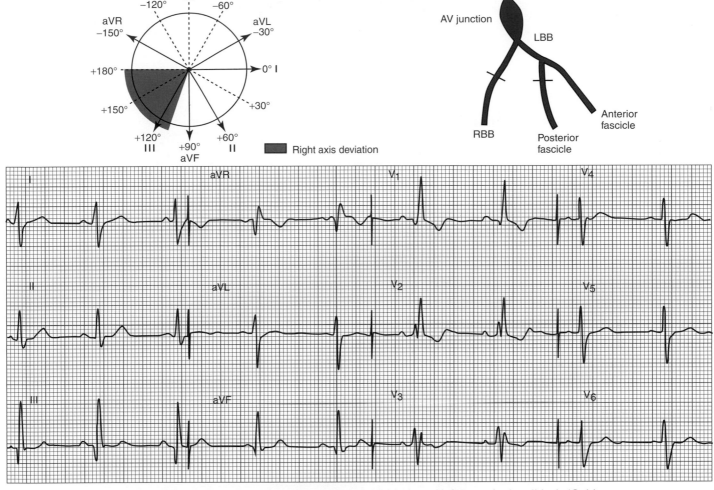

FIG. 13.10 Bifascicular block, right bundle-branch block, and left posterior hemiblock. (Goldberger, A. L., Goldberger, Z. D., & Shvilkin, A. [Eds.]. (2012). *Goldberger's clinical electrocardiography: A simplified approach* [8th ed.]. Saunders.)

complex is monophasic or biphasic in V_1, with an initial deflection different from that of the sinus-initiated QRS complex; (2) the amplitude of the R wave in V_1 exceeds the R′; and (3) a small R and large S wave or a QS pattern in V_6 may be present. With a V-tach that has an LBBB contour, (1) the axis can be rightward, with negative deflections deeper in V_1 than in V_6; (2) a broad, prolonged (longer than 0.04 second) R wave can be noted in V_1; and (3) a small Q or QS pattern in V_6 can exist. A QRS complex that is similar in V_1 through V_6—either all negative or all positive—favors a ventricular origin.

Supraventricular QRS complexes with aberrant conduction often have a triphasic pattern in V_1. A grossly irregular, wide QRS tachycardia with a ventricular rate exceeding 200 beats/min is more consistent with atrial fibrillation with conduction through an accessory pathway. In the presence of a preexisting bundle-branch block, a wide QRS tachycardia with a QRS shape different from the shape exhibited during sinus rhythm is most likely ventricular tachycardia.

Based on these criteria, several algorithms have been proposed for distinguishing ventricular tachycardia from supraventricular tachycardia with aberrancy (see Fig. 14.18). Exceptions exist to all the aforementioned criteria, especially in patients who have preexisting conduction disturbances or preexcitation syndrome. When in doubt, rely on your clinical judgment, and consider the ECG as only one of several helpful ancillary tests.

Fig. 13.11 provides an algorithm that may be used to differentiate supraventricular tachycardia and ventricular tachycardia.

TAKE-HOME POINTS

- Once the electrical impulse reaches the AV node or the AV node fires independently, the impulse is conducted to the ventricles through the right and the left bundle branches.
- The left bundle branch is divided into a small left anterior fascicle and a larger posterior fascicle.
- Both the right and left bundle branches, as well as the fascicles of the left bundle branch, receive their blood supply from specific coronary arteries. Disruption of this blood

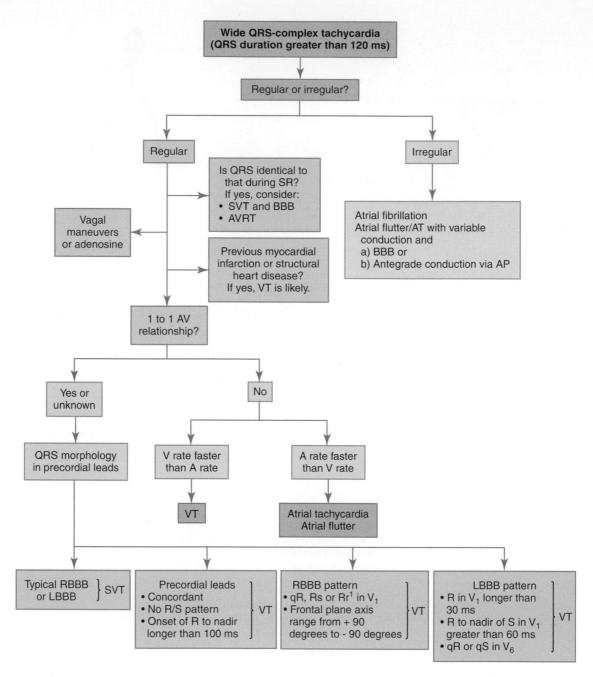

SR = Sinus rhythm, SVT = Supraventricular tachycardia, BBB = Bundle branch block, V = Ventricular, A = Atrial, AVRT = Atrioventricular reentrant tachycardia, AP = Accessory pathway

FIG. 13.11 Algorithm for distinguishing supraventricular tachycardia from ventricular tachycardia. (Redrawn from Mann, D. L., Zipes, D., Libby, P., & Bonow, R. [Eds.]. [2015]. *Braunwald's heart disease: A textbook of cardiovascular medicine* [10th ed.]. Saunders.)

supply during MI can result in a block of the conduction through the affected pathway.

- The VAT is the time it takes for depolarization of the interventricular septum and the portion of the ventricles progressing toward any given lead and is measured from the onset of the QRS complex to the peak of the last R wave in the QRS complex.
- LBBB is more common than RBBB, and either can be caused by an anteroseptal MI.

- The RBBB typically presents with a "rabbit-ears" shape in leads V_1 to V_3.
- LBBB typically presents with an RS pattern in leads V_1 to V_3.
- Bundle-branch blocks and fascicular blocks (hemiblocks) can also occur as a result of other conditions, such as cardiovascular disease and ventricular hypertrophy.
- The clinical significance of bundle-branch blocks and hemiblocks is variable, and their presence can make the detection of an ST-elevation MI more difficult.

- LAFB is the most common hemiblock because its fibers are much larger and more well organized than those of the posterior fascicle.
- Left axis deviation with an initial small q wave in lead I coupled with an initial small r wave in lead III (q_1r_3 pattern) indicates an LAFB.

- Right axis deviation with an initial small q wave in lead III and an initial small r wave in lead I (q_3r_1 pattern) is an indication of an LPFB.
- RBBB with LAFB is the most common bifascicular block. It is evidenced by the typical RBBB QRS shape in the precordial leads, combined with right axis deviation.

Chapter Review Questions

1. Which term best describes the time from the onset of the QRS complex to the peak of the R wave in the QRS complex?
   A. Depolarization threshold
   B. Interventricular conduction delay
   C. Preintrinsicoid deflection
   D. Ventricular activation time

2. Which artery supplies the anterior portion of the interventricular septum?
   A. AV node artery
   B. Left anterior descending coronary artery
   C. Posterior descending coronary artery
   D. Right coronary artery

3. In most hearts, the main blood supply to the AV node and proximal part of the bundle of His is the AV node artery, which arises from where?
   A. Circumflex coronary artery
   B. Left anterior descending artery
   C. Posterior descending coronary artery
   D. Right coronary artery

4. Common causes of bundle-branch and fascicular blocks include which of the following?
   A. Electrolyte abnormality, specifically hyperkalemia
   B. Ischemic heart disease
   C. Severe right ventricular hypertrophy
   D. Stroke and seizures

5. RBBBoccurs primarily in which kind of acute MI?
   A. Anteroseptal MI
   B. Inferior MI
   C. Lateral MI
   D. Posterior MI

6. Which of the following can be said of patients with acute MI with bundle-branch block, compared with patients who have no such block?
   A. A temporary transcutaneous pacemaker is less frequently indicated.
   B. The incidence of pump failure and ventricular dysrhythmias is higher.
   C. The incidence of supraventricular tachycardia is higher.
   D. The incidence of ventricular fibrillation is lower.

7. Which of the following are common causes of chronic RBBB?
   A. Congestive heart failure, stroke, and seizures
   B. Hyperventilation, acute coronary syndrome, and diabetes
   C. Myocarditis, cardiomyopathy, and cardiac surgery
   D. Ventricular hypertrophy

8. Which of the following best describes the QRS complex in lead V_1 in an RBBB?
   A. Narrow with a QRS pattern
   B. Wide with a classic triphasic rSR′ pattern
   C. With a tall R wave
   D. Wide with deep QS pattern

9. When electrical impulses are prevented from directly entering the anterior and lateral walls of the left ventricle, which condition is present?
   A. Bifascicular block
   B. Left anterior fascicular block
   C. Left lateral hemiblock
   D. Left posterior fascicular block

10. Which bifascicular block is the most common?
    A. RBBB and left anterior fascicular block
    B. LBBB and left anterior fascicular block
    C. RBBB and left posterior fascicular block
    D. LBBB and right posterior hemiblock

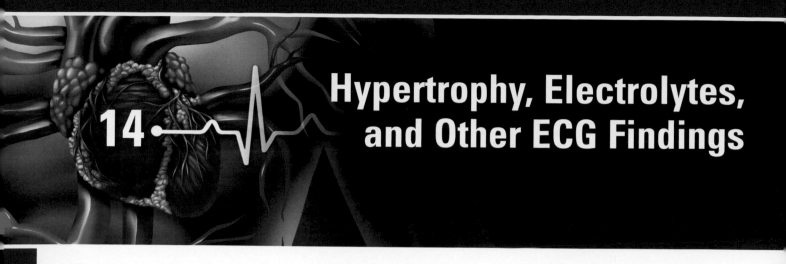

HEART CHAMBER ENLARGEMENT

Enlargement of the atria and ventricles often occurs when heart disease forces them to accommodate greater-than-normal pressure and/or volume. Enlargement of the heart chamber occurs by distention and hypertrophy.

DISTENTION

Distention refers to the dilatation of an individual heart chamber. Distention is also referred to as *enlargement*. It may be acute or chronic. Acute distention is usually not associated with hypertrophy of the chamber wall, whereas chronic distention often is. Common causes of acute distention include heart failure and pulmonary embolism. Common causes of chronic distention, on the other hand, include aortic and mitral valve disease.

When heart failure develops, the ventricles cannot accept the blood ejected from the atria. The pressure in the atria increases, causing distention. When a pulmonary embolus occurs, the pressure increases in the right ventricle, causing distention.

When the mitral or aortic valve becomes stenotic (stiff from scarring), greater pressure is required to open it. Over time, this elevated pressure distends the left atria, in the case of the mitral valve, and the left ventricle, in the case of the aortic valve. In some cases, the valves can fail to close completely. This allows blood to continue to be pumped into the already-full chamber. This condition is referred to as *valvular insufficiency*. The result is atrial and ventricular distention.

HYPERTROPHY

Hypertrophy in the context of cardiac disease refers to an increase in the size of the heart muscle. It occurs in chronic conditions of the heart and is characterized by an increase in the thickness of a chamber's myocardial wall secondary to the increase in the size of the muscle fibers. Unfortunately, myocardial hypertrophy does not strengthen muscle but instead only thickens it. This thicker muscle intrudes into the chamber, limiting the volume of blood it can hold. Examples of chamber hypertrophy include the following:

- Left ventricular hypertrophy (LVH) in aortic valve stenosis or insufficiency and systemic hypertension

- Right ventricular hypertrophy in pulmonary valve stenosis and chronic obstructive pulmonary disease (COPD)
- Left atrial enlargement in mitral valve stenosis and insufficiency and LVH from any cause
- Right atrial enlargement in tricuspid valve stenosis and insufficiency and right ventricular hypertrophy from any cause

Distention and hypertrophy affect the ECG differently. Distention stretches the walls of the myocardium, changing the normal conduction pathway. The impulse must travel a longer distance. This requires more time. Therefore distention exerts its effect on the ECG by prolonging the duration of the affected wave. Myocardial hypertrophy involves the depolarization of a greater number of muscle fibers. This increased number of depolarizations increases the amplitude of the waveform on the ECG.

> **AUTHOR'S NOTE** *Hypertrophy* is an increase in mass of the chamber walls, whereas *distention* is an increase in chamber size. Both describe an enlargement of the heart.

RIGHT ATRIAL ENLARGEMENT

Right atrial enlargement (generally more distention than hypertrophy) is usually caused by increased pressure in the right atrium. This is referred to as *right atrial overload*. It occurs in the following conditions:

- Pulmonary valve stenosis
- Tricuspid valve stenosis and insufficiency (relatively rare)
- Pulmonary hypertension from various causes, such as the following:
  1. COPD
  2. Status asthmaticus
  3. Pulmonary embolism
  4. Pulmonary edema
  5. Mitral valve stenosis or insufficiency
  6. Congenital heart disease

Characteristics (Fig. 14.1)

The typical result of right atrial enlargement is a tall, symmetrically peaked P wave. This waveform is referred to as *P pulmonale*.

P WAVE

Duration

Usually normal (0.10 second or less).

Shape

Typically tall and symmetrically peaked P wave (P pulmonale) in leads II, III, and aVF.

- Sharply peaked biphasic P wave in leads V_1 and V_2

Direction

Positive (upright) in leads II, III, and aVF and biphasic (having both upright and inverted components) in V_1 and V_2, with the initial deflection greater than the terminal deflection.

Amplitude

2.5 mm or greater in leads II, III, and aVF.

P pulmonale

Tall, symmetrically peaked P waves characteristic of right atrial distention.

LEFT ATRIAL ENLARGEMENT

Left atrial enlargement (generally more distention than hypertrophy) is usually caused by increased pressure in the left atrium—a condition referred to as *left atrial overload*. It occurs in the following conditions:

- Mitral valve stenosis and insufficiency
- Acute myocardial infarction (AMI)
- Left heart failure
- LVH from various causes, such as the following:
  1. Aortic valve stenosis or insufficiency
  2. Systemic hypertension
  3. Hypertrophic cardiomyopathy

Characteristics (Fig. 14.2)

The result of left atrial enlargement is usually a wide, notched P wave referred to as *P mitrale*. Such a P wave may also arise from a delay or block of the progression of the electrical impulses through the interatrial conduction tract (Bachmann's bundle) between the right and left atria.

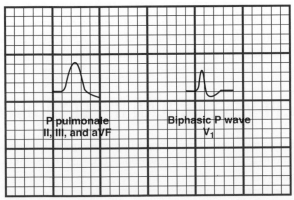

Right atrial enlargement

FIG. 14.1 Right atrial enlargement.

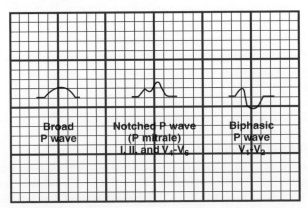

Left atrial enlargement

FIG. 14.2 Left atrial enlargement.

P WAVE

Duration

Usually longer than 0.10 second.

Shape

A broad, positive (upright) P wave, 0.10 second or longer in duration, in any lead.

- A wide, notched P wave with two humps that appear 0.04 second or more apart—the P mitrale. The first hump represents the depolarization of the right atrium. The second hump represents the depolarization of the distended left atrium. The P mitrale is best detected in leads I, II, and V_4 to V_6.

- A biphasic P wave, longer than 0.10 second in total duration, with the terminal, negative component 1 mm (0.1 mV) or more deep and 1 mm (0.04 second) or more in duration (that is, 1 small square or greater). The initial, positive (upright) component of the P wave represents the depolarization of the right atrium. The terminal, negative component represents the depolarization of the distended left atrium. Such biphasic P waves are best detected in leads V_1 to V_2.

Direction

Positive (upright) in leads I, II, and V_4 to V_6 and biphasic in leads V_1 to V_2. The P wave may be negative in leads III and aVF.

Amplitude

Usually normal (0.5–2.5 mm).

mitrale

Wide, notched P waves characteristic of left atrial distention.

> **AUTHOR'S NOTE** It is not uncommon for both the left and right atria to be enlarged at the same time. This will appear as a P wave with the characteristics of both P mitrale and P pulmonale. The resulting P wave consists of two notches, with the first one tall and peaked.

RIGHT VENTRICULAR HYPERTROPHY

Right ventricular hypertrophy (RVH) is caused by increased pressure in the right ventricle. This condition is called *right ventricular overload*. It occurs in the following conditions:
- Pulmonary valve stenosis and other congenital heart defects (for example, atrial and ventricular septal defects)
- Tricuspid valve insufficiency (relatively rare)
- Pulmonary hypertension from various causes, such as the following:
  1. COPD
  2. Pulmonary embolism
  3. Mitral valve stenosis or insufficiency

Characteristics (Fig. 14.3)

Right ventricular hypertrophy produces abnormally large rightward electrical forces that travel toward lead V_1 and away from the left precordial leads V_5 to V_6. The sequence of depolarization of the ventricles remains normal. However, because the left ventricle is normally much larger than the right and contributes the majority of the QRS amplitude, right ventricular hypertrophy must be severe to produce ECG changes.

P WAVE

Changes indicative of right atrial enlargement may be present (that is, tall, symmetrically peaked P waves [P pulmonale] in leads II, III, and aVF and sharply peaked biphasic P waves in leads V_1 and V_2). However, the P wave may be normal.

QRS COMPLEX

Duration

Normal, 0.12 second or less.

QRS axis

A right axis deviation of $+90°$ or more is usually present.

Ventricular Activation Time

The ventricular activation time (VAT) is prolonged beyond the upper normal limit of 0.035 second in the right precordial leads V_1 and V_2.

QRS PATTERN

R Wave

A tall R wave is present in leads II, III, and V_1. This R wave is usually 7 mm or more (0.7 mV) in height in lead V_1. It is equal to or greater than the S wave in depth in this lead. A relatively tall R wave is also present in the adjacent precordial leads V_2 to V_3.

S Wave

A relatively deeper-than-normal S wave is present in lead I and the left precordial leads V_4 to V_5. In lead V_6, the depth of the S wave may be greater than the height of the R wave.

ST SEGMENT

Downsloping ST-segment depression of 1 mm or more may be present in leads II, III, aVF, and V_1 and sometimes in leads V_2 and V_3.

T WAVE

T-wave inversion is often present in leads II, III, aVF, and V_1 and sometimes in leads V_2 and V_3.

> **AUTHOR'S NOTE** The downsloping ST-segment depression and the T-wave inversion together form the so-called *strain pattern* characteristic of long-standing right or left ventricular hypertrophy. This pattern gives the noted "hockey stick" appearance to the QRS-T complex.

LEFT VENTRICULAR HYPERTROPHY

LVH is usually caused by increased pressure in the left ventricle, referred to as *left ventricular overload*. It occurs in the following conditions:
- Mitral valve insufficiency
- Aortic valve stenosis or insufficiency

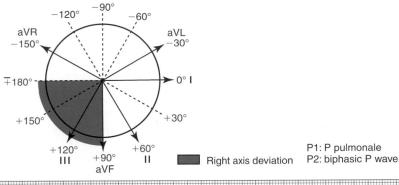

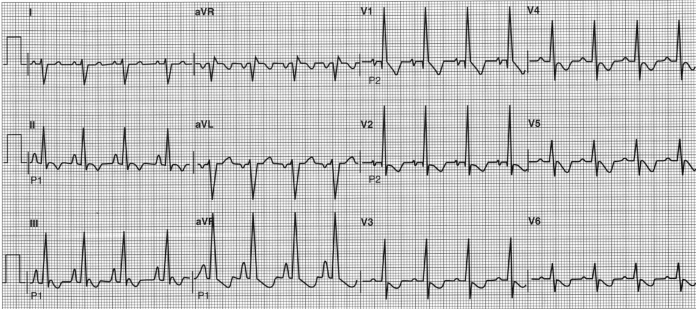

FIG. 14.3 Right ventricular hypertrophy with right atrial enlargement.

- Systemic hypertension
- AMI
- Hypertrophic cardiomyopathy

Characteristics (Fig. 14.4)

LVH produces abnormally large leftward electrical forces that travel toward the left precordial leads V_5 to V_6 and away from lead V_1. The sequence of depolarization of the ventricles, however, remains normal.

> **AUTHOR'S NOTE** There are several criteria for right and left ventricular hypertrophy because much research has been undertaken to find criteria that will definitively indicate that hypertrophy is present. The criteria presented in this text are highly specific. That is, when the criteria are present in the ECG, the heart does, in fact, have ventricular hypertrophy. Unfortunately, almost half of all hearts found to have hypertrophy on exam do not have ECG evidence of hypertrophy.

P WAVE

Changes indicative of left atrial enlargement are often present with a wide, notched P wave (P mitrale) in leads I, II, and V_4

and V_6 and biphasic P waves in leads V_1 and V_2. However, the P wave may be normal.

QRS COMPLEX

Duration

Normal (0.12 second or less).

QRS Axis

Usually normal, but it may have a slight left axis deviation of greater than $-30°$.

Ventricular Activation Time

Prolonged beyond the upper normal limit of 0.04 to 0.05 second or more in the left precordial leads V_5 and V_6.

QRS PATTERN

R Wave

A tall R wave is present in leads I and aVL and in the left precordial leads V_5 to V_6. The following criteria concerning the amplitude of the R wave in various leads are often used to diagnose left ventricular hypertrophy:

- An R wave of 20 mm (2.0 mV) or more in lead I

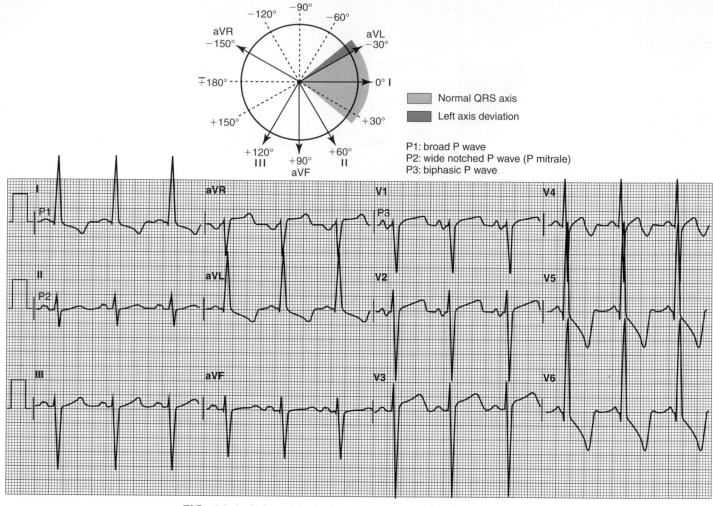

FIG. 14.4 Left ventricular hypertrophy with left atrial enlargement.

- An R wave of 11 mm (1.1 mV) or more in lead aVL
- An R wave of 30 mm (3.0 mV) or more in lead V_5 or V_6

S Wave

A deep S wave is present in lead III and in the right precordial leads V_1 and V_2. The following criteria concerning the depth of the S wave in various leads are often used to diagnose LVH:

- An S wave of 20 mm (2.0 mV) or more in lead III
- An S wave of 30 mm (3.0 mV) or more in lead V_1 or V_2

Sum of R and S Waves

The sum of the height of the R waves and the depth of the S waves (in mm) in the leads in which these two waves are most prominent is often used to determine the presence of LVH. LVH is considered present if any one of the following summations is exceeded:

- The sum of any R wave and any S wave in any of the limb leads I, II, or III is 20 mm (2.0 mV) or more:

  R (I, II, or III) + S (I, II, or III) ≥ 20 mm (= 2.0 mV)

- The sum of the R wave in lead I and the S wave in lead III is 25 mm (2.5 mV) or more:

  R I + S III ≥ 25 mm (= 2.5 mV)

- The sum of the S wave in lead V1 or V2 and the R wave in lead V5 or V6 is 35 mm (3.5 mV) or more:

  S V_1 (or S V_2) + R V_5 (or R V_6) ≥ 35 mm (= 3.5 mV)

ST SEGMENT

Downsloping ST-segment depression of 1 mm or more is often present in leads I, aVL, and V_5 to V_6, and upsloping ST segment elevation of 1 mm or more is often present in V_1 to V_3.

T WAVE

T-wave inversion is often present in leads I, aVL, and V_5 to V_6.

AUTHOR'S NOTE ST elevation because of LVH is one of the most common "mimics" of ST-segment elevation myocardial infarction (STEMI). This will be discussed in Chapter 16.

Table 14.1 summarizes the criteria for the height or depth of R and S waves used to diagnose LVH on the 12-lead ECG.

PERICARDITIS

Pericarditis is an inflammatory disease of the pericardium, directly involving the epicardium, with deposition of inflammatory cells and a variable amount of serous, fibrous, purulent, or hemorrhagic fluid within the pericardial sac.

Unlike acute coronary syndromes, which pericarditis may mimic, pericarditis often occurs in younger patients without cardiac risk factors who are not suspected of having coronary artery disease. Other signs and symptoms of acute pericarditis include the following:

- Chest pain
- Dyspnea
- Tachycardia
- Fever
- Malaise

TABLE 14.1	Diagnosis of Left Ventricular Hypertrophy Using Height or Depth of R and S Waves				
	LEAD				
Wave	**I**	**III**	**aVL**	**V$_1$ or V$_2$**	**V$_5$ or V$_6$**
R wave	≥20 mm		≥11 mm		≥30 mm
S wave		≥20 mm		≥30 mm	
Summation R (I, II, or III) + S (I, II, or III) ≥20 mm (≥20 mV)					
	R I + S III ≥25 (≥2.5 mV)				
	S V$_1$ or V$_2$ + R V$_5$ or V$_6$ ≥35 mm (≥35 mV)				

R wave	I	aVL	V$_5$-V$_6$

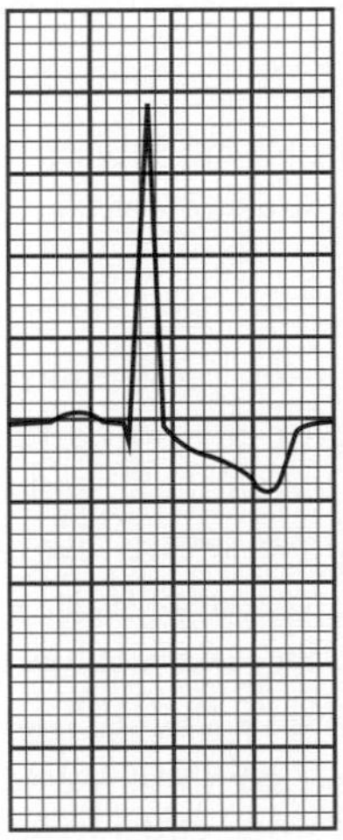

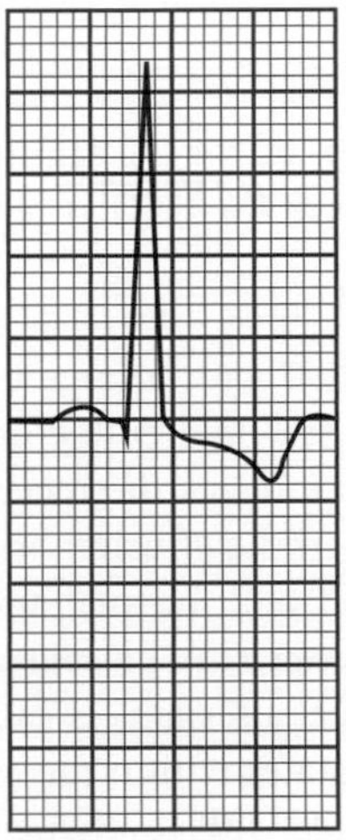

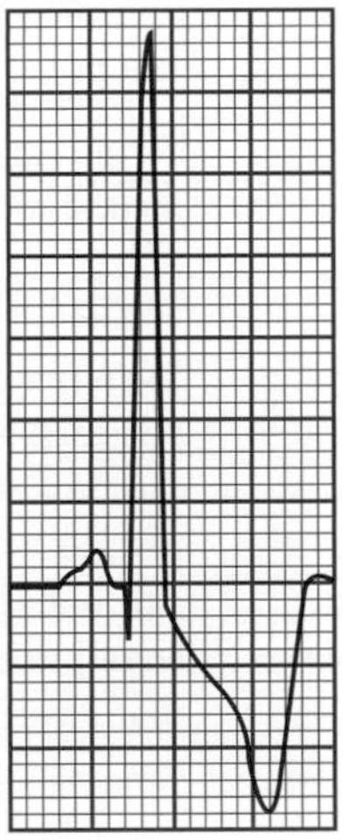

S wave	III	V1–V2

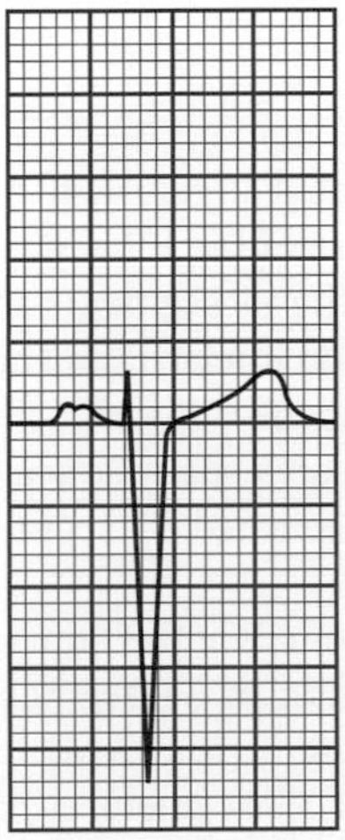

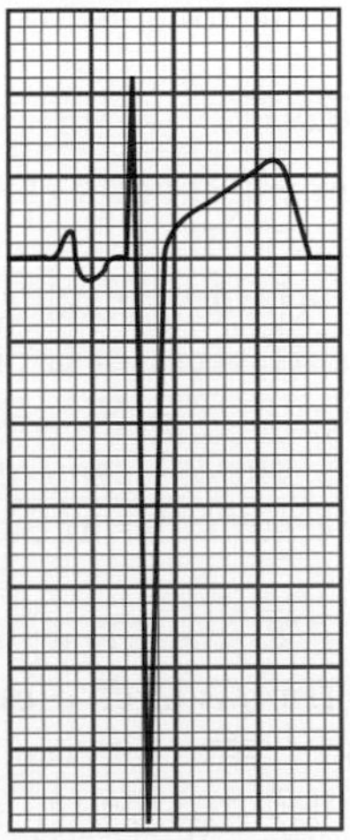

TABLE 14.1	Diagnosis of Left Ventricular Hypertrophy Using Height or Depth of R and S Waves—Con't					
	LEAD					
Wave	**I**	**III**	**aVL**	**V₁ or V₂**	**V₅ or V₆**	
Summation	R PLUS	S OR	RI PLUS	S III OR	SV₁/V₂ PLUS	R V₅/V₆
	(I, II, III)	(I, II, III)				

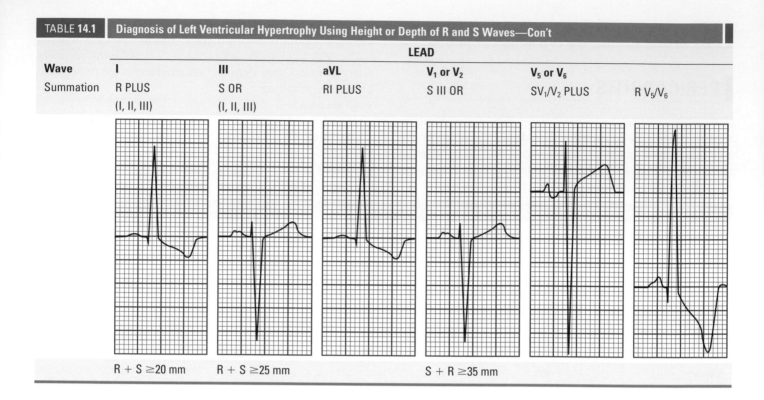

R + S ≥20 mm	R + S ≥25 mm	S + R ≥35 mm

- Weakness
- Chills

The chest pain, which can mimic that of AMI, is sharp and severe, with radiation to the neck, back, left shoulder, and, occasionally, the arm. Characteristically, the pain is present along the sternum, made worse by lying flat, and relieved by sitting up or leaning forward. Often, the pain is pleuritic (made worse by breathing), especially during inspiration. Unlike the pain of AMI, the pain may last for days and not be relieved with rest.

A pericardial friction rub is the sound of the inflamed pericardial sac rubbing against the inflamed outer surface of the heart during the cardiac cycle. It can be heard and even felt along the lower left sternal border. Characteristic ECG findings are present in 90% of patients with pericarditis.

Characteristics (Fig. 14.5)

The ECG changes characteristic of pericarditis occur because the inflamed pericardium is in direct contact with the outer surface of the heart.

PR SEGMENT

The PR segment is elevated in lead aVR and depressed in leads I, II, III, V₅, and V₆. These changes are attributable to the proximity of the atria to the inflamed pericardium and how that inflammation affects the repolarization of the atria. The PR and ST segments typically elevate or depress in opposite directions from each other. For example, in lead aVR, the PR segment is elevated; therefore the ST segment is depressed.

Additionally, the PR segment slopes downward toward the QRS complex. The depressed and downsloping PR segment accentuates the appearance of the ST-segment elevation. This accentuation of the ST-segment elevation can result in misinterpretation of the ECG as representing myocardial infarction.

QRS COMPLEX

In pericarditis with a large effusion (collection of fluid in the pericardial sac), the QRS complex is of low amplitude because the fluid suppresses the reception of the impulses by the electrodes. When the effusion becomes severe, the QRS complexes alternate between normal and low amplitude, a condition referred to as *electrical alternans* (Fig. 14.6). It has been proposed that electrical alternans is caused by the QRS axis changing as the heart rotates within the enlarged pericardial sac. Although it is associated with severe pericardial effusion and cardiac tamponade, it is present in only 10% to 15% of patients with a clinically significant effusion.

ST SEGMENT

The ST segment appears elevated in most, if not all, leads—except lead aVR. This is because of the PR-segment depression in those same leads is making the ST segments appear elevated. Because the ST segment is often longer than the PR segment, the elevation in the ST segment appears to dominate the 12-lead ECG. The ST segments are usually concave in shape but may be convex, similar to the elevated ST segments present in AMI.

In lead aVR, the ST segment is either normal or slightly depressed. This wide distribution of ST-segment elevation in pericarditis helps to differentiate it from AMI, in which there is more limited distribution of ST-segment elevation over the specific portion of the heart affected by the infarction. As the pericarditis resolves, the ST segments return to normal.

PR1: Down Sloping PR segment depression   PR2: Up Sloping PR segment elevation   ST: ST segment elevation

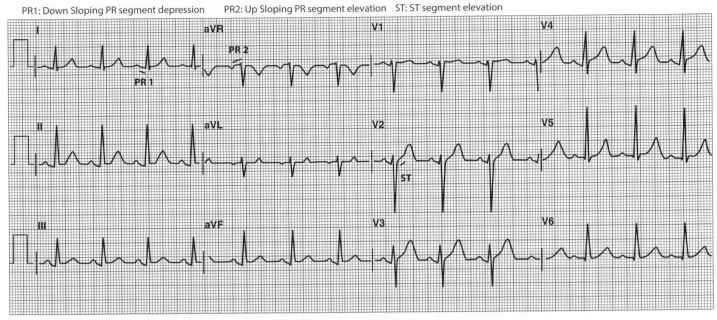

FIG. 14.5 Pericarditis.

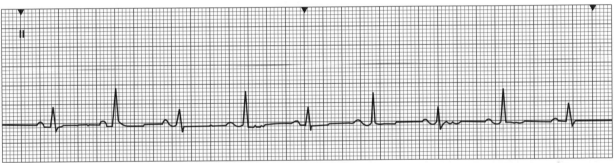

FIG. 14.6 Electrical alternans. (Modified from Goldberger, A. L., Goldberger, Z. D., & Shvilkin, A. [Eds.]. (2012). *Goldberger's clinical electrocardiography: A simplified approach* [8th ed.]. Saunders.)

T WAVE

The T wave is elevated during the early phase of pericarditis. As it resolves, the T wave first becomes inverted in the leads that had ST-segment elevation and then returns to normal.

electrical alternans

Alternating large- and small-amplitude QRS complexes on the ECG associated with pericardial effusion.

AUTHOR'S NOTE Misinterpretation of the ST elevation in pericarditis as evidence of myocardial infarction is one of the most common 12-lead interpretation errors. To distinguish pericarditis from infarction, place a ruler across the TP segments of the ECG strip and examine the PR and ST segments. Downsloping PR-segment depression will be seen in almost every lead in pericarditis, whereas ST segments will be elevated only in a few specific leads in myocardial infarction.

ELECTROLYTE IMBALANCE

HYPERKALEMIA

Potassium is an element that is required to promote the movement of sodium back and forth across the myocardial cell membrane during depolarization and repolarization. Alterations in the level of potassium in the body therefore have significant consequences on impulse transmission through the heart and contraction and relaxation of the myocardium.

When the potassium level in the blood exceeds the normal range of 3.5 to 5.0 milliequivalents per liter (mEq/L), *hyperkalemia* exists. The most common causes of hyperkalemia are kidney failure and certain diuretics, such as triamterene, that cause the body to retain potassium. Characteristic ECG changes occur as levels of potassium increase. The first changes occur to repolarization and are therefore seen in the T wave and ST

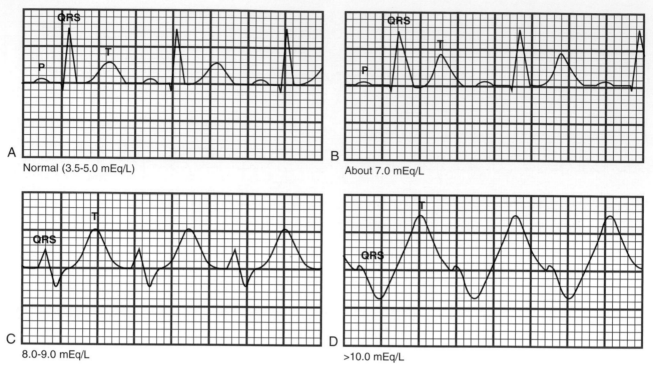

FIG. 14.7 Hyperkalemia.

segments. As the levels continue to rise, depolarization abnormalities occur, distorting the QRS complex. Sinus arrest may occur when the serum potassium level reaches about 7.5 mEq/L, and ventricular fibrillation or asystole may occur at about 10 to 12 mEq/L. Early recognition of the peaking of the T wave in hyperkalemia, as described next, may be lifesaving.

Characteristics (Fig. 14.7)

> **AUTHOR'S NOTE** The ECG changes seen with hyperkalemia may occur at different levels in any given patient. The levels presented in this text should be considered average for hyperkalemic ECG changes.

P WAVE

Begins to flatten out and become wider when the serum potassium level reaches about 6.5 mEq/L. As the potassium level exceeds 7 to 9 mEq/L, the P wave disappears as a result of the loss of sinus-node and atrial pacemaker activity.

PR INTERVAL

May be normal or prolonged (longer than 0.20 second). The PR interval is absent when the P wave is absent.

QRS COMPLEX

Begins to widen when the serum potassium level reaches about 6 to 6.5 mEq/L. As it widens, the QRS complex resembles a left bundle-branch block (LBBB), with the typical rS pattern in leads V_1 and V_2, whereas in leads I and V_6, it looks like a right bundle-branch block (RBBB), with a deep, slurred S wave. As the potassium level approaches 10 mEq/L, the QRS complex

becomes markedly slurred and abnormally widened. The QRS complex may widen to the point that it merges with the following T wave. The result is an oscillating sine-wave QRS-T pattern.

> **AUTHOR'S NOTE** The presence of an interventricular conduction delay with LBBB and RBBB characteristics is highly suggestive of hyperkalemia.

ST SEGMENT

Disappears as the serum potassium level reaches about 10 mEq/L.

T WAVE

Becomes characteristically narrow, tall, and peaked when the serum potassium level reaches about 5.5 to 6.5 mEq/L. This tentlike T wave reaches a height of at least 50% of the total height of the QRS complex. The peaking of the T wave is symmetrical, with the highest point at the midpoint of the duration of the T wave. The earliest T-wave changes are best seen in leads II, III, and V_2 to V_4.

QT INTERVAL

Not affected by hyperkalemia. However, because renal failure is one of the most common causes of hyperkalemia, the ECG may demonstrate QT-interval prolongation secondary to associated hypocalcemia.

HYPOKALEMIA

Hypokalemia is present when the serum potassium level is below the normal range of 3.5 to 5 mEq/L. The most common

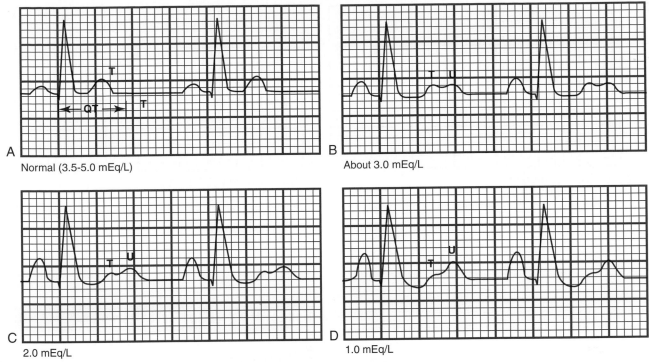

A Normal (3.5-5.0 mEq/L)

B About 3.0 mEq/L

C 2.0 mEq/L

D 1.0 mEq/L

FIG. 14.8 Hypokalemia.

cause of hypokalemia is renal failure, or the loss of potassium in the urine because of diuretic antihypertensive medications. Other causes include loss of body fluids through vomiting, gastric suctioning, and sweating.

Symptoms of hypokalemia, such as polyuria and frequent urination, occur in mild cases and progress to muscle weakness in more severely affected patients. Digitalis, a drug often given for cardiac rhythm disturbances, such as atrial fibrillation and flutter, in the presence of hypokalemia may precipitate serious ventricular rhythm disturbances, including the torsades de pointes form of ventricular tachycardia (V-tach).

Characteristics (Fig. 14.8)

P WAVE

In severe hypokalemia (about 2 mEq/L or less), the P wave becomes typically tall and symmetrically peaked, with an amplitude of 2.5 mm or greater in leads II, III, and aVF. Because these P waves resemble those of P pulmonale, they are called *pseudo–P pulmonale*.

QRS COMPLEX

Begins to widen when the serum potassium level drops to about 3 mEq/L.

ST SEGMENT

May become depressed by 1 mm or more.

T WAVE

Begins to flatten when the serum potassium level drops to about 3 mEq/L. Continues to become smaller as the U wave increases in size. The T wave may either merge with the U wave or become inverted.

U WAVE

Begins to increase in size, becoming as tall as the T wave when the serum potassium level drops to about 3 mEq/L. It becomes taller than the T wave at about 2 mEq/L. The U wave is considered to be prominent when it is equal to or taller than the T wave in the same lead. The U wave reaches a giant size and fuses with the T wave at a potassium level of 1 mEq/L or less.

QT INTERVAL

The QT interval may appear to be prolonged when the U wave becomes prominent and fuses with the T wave.

▌HYPERCALCEMIA

Hypercalcemia is the elevation of serum calcium levels above the normal range of 8.5 to 10.2 mg/dL. Common causes of serious hypercalcemia include the following:

- Adrenal insufficiency
- Hyperparathyroidism
- Kidney failure
- Cancers involving the bone, such as multiple myeloma, breast, and lung cancer
- Sarcoidosis
- Hyperthyroidism
- Vitamin A and D intoxication

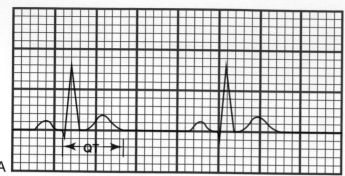

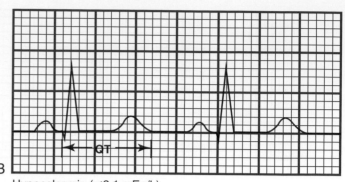

A
Hypercalcemia (>2.6 mEq/L)
Abnormal QT interval: 0.30 sec
(below QT$_C$ range of 0.32-0.39 sec for a heart rate of 80)

B
Hypocalcemia (<2.1 mEq/L)
Abnormal QT interval: 0.44 sec
(above QT$_C$ range of 0.32-0.39 sec for a heart rate of 80)

FIG. 14.9 (A) Hypercalcemia. (B) Hypocalcemia.

Although it is rare, severe hypercalcemia is life threatening. It can cause torsades de pointes, V-tach, and third-degree heart block.

Characteristics (Fig. 14.9, *A*)

QT INTERVAL

Shorter than normal for the heart rate. The shortening of the QT interval is primarily a result of shortening of the ST segment. This may result in the fusing of the T wave to the end of the QRS complex, giving the impression of ST-segment elevation.

HYPOCALCEMIA

Hypocalcemia is present when the level of serum calcium falls below the normal range of 8.5 to 10.2 mg/dL. Common causes of significant hypocalcemia include the following:

- Low albumin (protein) levels from chronic malnutrition, cirrhosis, and chronic illness
- Diuretics (such as furosemide)
- Hypomagnesemia (possibly because of lack of parathyroid hormone)
- Vitamin D deficiency
- Hypoparathyroidism

Characteristics (Fig. 14.9, *B*)

ST SEGMENT

Prolonged.

QT INTERVAL

Prolonged beyond the normal limits for the heart rate because of the prolongation of the ST segment. As the QT progressively lengthens, there is an increasing likelihood of a premature ectopic ventricular beat occurring during the relative refractory period of the T wave. This can cause ventricular tachycardia or fibrillation.

OTHER ECG FINDINGS

DRUG EFFECTS

Many pharmaceutical agents have electrophysiologic effects on the heart, including many agents whose primary purpose is not for the treatment of heart conditions. Table 14.2 contains a list of some of the more common cardiac drugs. Drugs are classified by their mechanism of action on the heart muscle (Table 14.3).

The reader should consult a toxicology text for a full description of their effects on the heart. However, two of the most common drug-induced cardiac rhythm disturbances will be presented here.

DIGITALIS

Digitalis administered within the therapeutic range produces characteristic changes in the ECG. This is often referred to as the *digitalis effect*. In addition, when given in excess, digitalis toxicity occurs, causing excitatory or inhibitory effects on the heart and its electrical conduction system.

Excitatory effects include the following:
- Premature atrial complexes
- Atrial tachycardia, with or without block
- Nonparoxysmal junctional tachycardia
- Premature ventricular complexes
- Ventricular tachycardia
- Ventricular fibrillation

Inhibitory effects include the following:
- Sinus bradycardia
- Sinoatrial (SA) exit block
- Atrioventricular (AV) block

Characteristics (Fig. 14.10)

The ECG changes characteristic of digitalis are as follows.

TABLE **14.2**	Common Cardiac Drugs
Class	**Specific Agents**
Class I antiarrhythmic: sodium-channel blockers	1. Cardiovascular drugs: procainamide, quinidine, disopyramide, flecainide, tocainide 2. Psychiatric drugs: antidepressants: carbamazepine, amitriptyline, doxepin, nortriptyline 3. Other drugs: amantadine (antiviral), diphenhydramine (antihistamine), propoxyphene (narcotic)
Class II antiarrhythmics: beta blockers	Propranolol, metoprolol, and atenolol

Class III antiarrhythmics: potassium-channel blockers	1. Cardiovascular drugs: disopyramide, quinidine, procainamide, flecainide, amiodarone, sotalol
	2. Psychiatric drugs:
	  A. Antipsychotics: chlorpromazine, droperidol, haloperidol, risperidone
	  B. Antidepressants: amitriptyline, imipramine
	3. Antibiotics: ciprofloxacin, levofloxacin, clarithromycin, erythromycin, azithromycin

Class IV antiarrhythmics: calcium-channel blockers	Nicardipine, nifedipine, nimodipine, diltiazem, verapamil
Cardiac glycosides: sodium–potassium pump blockers	Digoxin

PR INTERVAL

The PR intervals are prolonged over 0.2 second.

ST SEGMENT

The ST segments are depressed 1 mm or more in many of the leads, with a characteristic scooped-out appearance.

T WAVE

The T waves may be flattened, inverted, or biphasic.

QT INTERVAL

The QT intervals are shorter than normal for the heart rate.

> **AUTHOR'S NOTE** Digitalis toxicity can cause almost every rhythm disturbance presented in this textbook. Therefore it has no classic ECG rhythm presentation.

PROCAINAMIDE

Procainamide administered within the therapeutic range produces characteristic changes in the ECG. In addition,

when given in excess, procainamide toxicity occurs, causing excitatory or inhibitory effects on the heart and its electrical conduction system.

Excitatory effects include the following:
- Premature ventricular complex
- V-tach in the form of torsades de pointes (occurrence less common than in quinidine administration)
- Ventricular fibrillation
Inhibitory effects include the following:
- Depression of myocardial contractility, which may cause hypotension and congestive heart failure
- AV block
- Asystole

Characteristics (Fig. 14.11)

PR INTERVAL

May be prolonged.

QRS COMPLEX

Duration may be increased beyond 0.12 second. Widening is a sign of toxicity. The R wave may be decreased in amplitude.

T WAVE

May be decreased in amplitude. Occasionally the T wave may be widened and notched because of the appearance of a U wave.

ST SEGMENT

May be depressed 1 mm or more.

QT INTERVAL

May occasionally be prolonged beyond the normal limits for the heart rate. Prolongation of the QT interval is a common sign of procainamide toxicity.

PULMONARY EMBOLISM

Pulmonary embolism occurs when a blood clot (thromboembolus) or other foreign matter (solid, liquid, or gaseous) lodges in a pulmonary artery and causes obstruction of blood flow to the lung segment supplied by the occluded artery. The thromboemboli originate most often in the deep leg veins or the pelvic veins and occasionally in the veins of the upper extremities or in the right atria or ventricle.

If the area of the pulmonary circulation affected by pulmonary embolization is small, the symptoms, if any, are minimal, such as sinus tachycardia and dyspnea. If pulmonary embolization shuts off a large portion of the pulmonary circulation, it is considered a massive pulmonary embolism.

Because of the increased pressure in the pulmonary artery (pulmonary hypertension) caused by the severe obstruction of blood flow through the pulmonary circulation, the right ventricle and atrium become distended and unable to function properly, leading to right heart failure. This condition is called *acute cor pulmonale*.

TABLE 14.3	Cardiac Agents and Their Mechanisms of Action	
Agent	**Mechanism of Action**	**Effect at Toxic Levels**
Class I antiarrhythmics: sodium channel blockers	These agents inhibit the rapid influx of sodium during phase 0 of the action potential. This decreases the speed and amplitude of the action potential. At therapeutic levels, these drugs suppress ventricular ectopy.	Slowed or complete SA-node block Right bundle-branch block Prolonged QT interval Widens QRS complex, sometimes causing ventricular tachycardia or fibrillation
Class II antiarrhythmics: beta blockers	These agents inhibit sympathetic nervous system stimulation on the SA and AV nodes. At proper levels, this controls heart rate.	• Effects of the parasympathetic nervous system become more dominant, causing sinus bradycardia • Slowed automaticity of SA node and Purkinje system • AV node block
Class II antiarrhythmics: potassium-channel blockers	These drugs inhibit the outward flow of potassium in the cell. This slows the rate of repolarization and, at therapeutic levels, suppresses ventricular ectopy.	• Can slow overall rate of impulse movement: SA node, atrium, AV node, Purkinje system, and ventricles • AV block • Widened QRS • Prolonged QT interval • PVCs followed by torsades de pointes • Ventricular tachycardia or fibrillation
Class III antiarrhythmics: calcium-channel blockers	These agents inhibit the very sensitive slow calcium channels within the cell membrane. These channels control the depolarization of the SA and AV nodes. They are most often used to control heart rate.	• Severe bradycardia • AV node block • Sinus arrest with AV junctional rhythm • Widened QRS
Cardiac glycosides: sodium–potassium pump blockers	Affect the heart by inhibiting the active transport of sodium and potassium across the cell membrane. This increases the level of calcium ions inside the cell. The result is stronger cell contraction and increased automaticity.	• AV block and ventricular automaticity (most common manifestations) • Sinus bradycardia • Sinus arrest with AV junctional rhythm • Widened QRS

AV, Atrioventricular; *PVC,* premature ventricular complex; *SA,* sinoatrial.

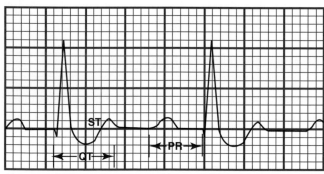

Abnormal QT interval: 0.30 sec   Abnromal PR interval: > 0.20 sec
(below QT$_c$ range of 0.32-0.39 sec for a heart rate of 80)

FIG. 14.10 Digitalis effect.

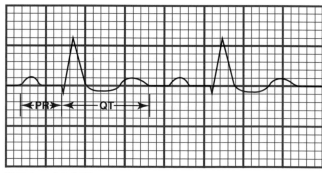

PR interval: >0.20 sec
QT interval: Prolonged, 0.45 sec
(above QT$_C$ range of 0.32-0.39 sec for a heart rate of 80)
QRS complex: Widened, >0.12 sec

FIG. 14.11 Procainamide toxicity.

In minimally to moderately significant pulmonary emboli, the ECG may be normal. However, in massive pulmonary embolism (acute cor pulmonale), the ECG shows a P pulmonale and a characteristic $S_1Q_3T_3$ pattern.

acute cor pulmonale

The combination of ECG findings of P pulmonale and S wave in lead 1, Q wave in lead III, and inverted T wave in lead III ($S_1Q_3T_3$ pattern).

Characteristics (Fig. 14.12)

P WAVE

Evidence of right atrial enlargement is present (tall, symmetrically peaked P waves [P pulmonale] in leads II, III, and aVF and sharply peaked biphasic P waves in leads V_1 and V_2).

QRS COMPLEX

An S wave in lead I, a Q wave in lead III, and an inverted T wave in lead III (the $S_1Q_3T_3$ pattern) may occur acutely. In addition, an RBBB may occur.

Pulmonary Embolism (Acute)

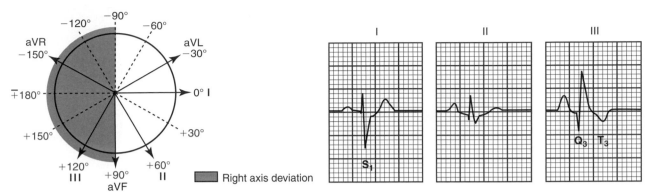

FIG. 14.12 Pulmonary embolism.

QRS AXIS

Right axis deviation is present with a QRS axis greater than +90°.

ST SEGMENT/T WAVE

A right ventricular strain pattern may be present (inverted T wave in leads V_1 to V_3 and ST-segment elevation in aVR).

> **AUTHOR'S NOTE** The $S_1Q_3T_3$ pattern is not always seen in patients with clinically significant pulmonary emboli, but its presence should raise your suspicion that a pulmonary embolus exists.

CHRONIC COR PULMONALE

Chronic cor pulmonale is the enlargement of the right ventricle (dilatation and/or hypertrophy). It is usually accompanied by right heart failure. It is usually the end-stage result of prolonged pulmonary hypertension that occurs with many diseases of the lung, including COPD and recurrent pulmonary embolization.

Chronic cor pulmonale is often associated with atrial rhythm disturbance, including the following:

- Premature atrial complexes
- Wandering atrial pacemaker
- Multifocal atrial tachycardia
- Atrial flutter
- Atrial fibrillation

Characteristics (Fig. 14.13)

P WAVE

Changes indicative of right atrial enlargement are present (tall, symmetrically peaked P waves [P pulmonale] in leads II, III, and aVF and sharply peaked biphasic P waves in leads V_1 and V_2).

QRS COMPLEX

Changes indicative of right ventricular hypertrophy are present.

QRS AXIS

Right axis deviation is present with a QRS axis greater than +90°.

ST SEGMENT/T WAVE

A right ventricular strain pattern is present (inverted T wave in leads V_1–V_3).

> **AUTHOR'S NOTE** In a small percentage of patients with chronic cor pulmonale, especially those with severe lung hyperinflation, the ECG shows S waves in leads I, II, and III (the $S_1S_2S_3$ pattern), along with a P pulmonale and a QRS axis in the 90° to 150° range. Patients with this type of ECG pattern have been shown to have a poor survival rate.

EARLY REPOLARIZATION

Early repolarization is a term used to describe an ST segment that is elevated or depressed 1 to 2 mm above or below the baseline but not associated with any underlying cardiovascular disease. The ST elevation is most often seen in leads I, II, and aVF and the precordial leads V_2 to V_6. ST depression may be present in lead aVR. Early repolarization occurs most often in normal healthy young people. The ST elevation can mimic the ECG pattern seen in AMI and pericarditis.

The ST-segment elevation present in early repolarization is similar to that seen during the early phase of acute anterior, lateral, and inferior MIs. However, there are no typical ST depressions in the leads facing the opposite side of the heart (reciprocal ST depression). Unlike the elevated ST segment in early acute coronary syndromes that later returns to the baseline, this ST elevation persists. Another difference is that the ST segment of early repolarization tends to be concave in shape, whereas that of ischemia is convex. One final hallmark of early repolarization is called *J-point elevation*. The J point is the point at which the QRS complex meets the ST segment. In early repolarization, the last segment (terminal forces) of the QRS complex will be slightly positive. This causes a small J-point elevation before the ST-segment elevation.

Differentiating between the ST elevation of early repolarization and that seen in acute pericarditis is often difficult. The only clues are that early repolarization ST segments do not return to baseline and that the T waves do not invert as they do over time in resolving pericarditis.

Cor pulmonale

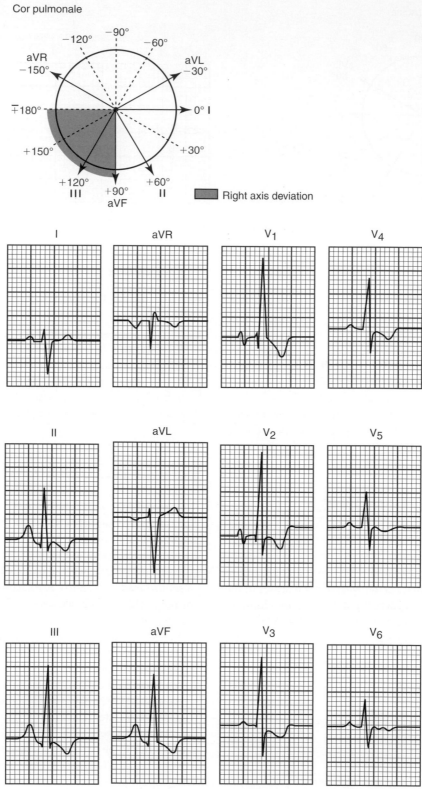

FIG. 14.13 Cor pulmonale.

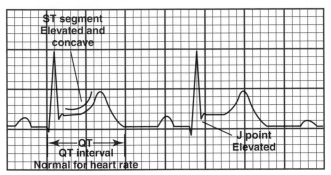

FIG. 14.14 Early repolarization.

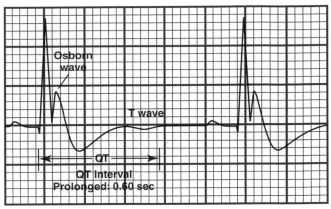

FIG. 14.15 Hypothermia.

Characteristics (Fig. 14.14)

QRS COMPLEX

Abnormal Q wave is usually absent.

ST SEGMENT

Elevated by about 0.5 to 1 mm in leads I, II, and aVF and less than 2 mm in the mid-precordial leads V_2 to V_5. May be depressed in lead aVR. The ST segment is concave. The J point is elevated before the ST segment.

T WAVE

Usually normal.

HYPOTHERMIA

In the majority of hypothermic patients with a core body temperature of 89° F or less, a distinctive narrow, positive wave—the Osborn wave (also referred to as the *J wave*, the *J deflection*, or the *camel's hump*)—occurs at the junction of the QRS complex and the ST-segment J point. Other ECG changes associated with severe hypothermia include prolonged PR and QT intervals and widening of the QRS complex.

Sinus bradycardia and junctional and ventricular rhythms also occur in hypothermia. The abnormal ECG changes and rhythms noted here are reversed after normalization of the body's temperature.

Characteristics (Fig. 14.15)

PR INTERVAL

May occasionally be longer than 0.20 second.

QRS COMPLEX

May occasionally be abnormally wide (longer than 0.12 second).

QT INTERVAL

The corrected QT interval (QTc interval) is usually prolonged.

OSBORN WAVE

An Osborn wave is present, typically in the leads facing the left ventricle (leads II, III, aVF, V_5, and V_6). It is a narrow positive deflection closely attached to the end of the R or S wave of the QRS complex, at the point where the QRS complex joins the ST segment—the J point.

ACCESSORY CONDUCTION PATHWAYS AND PREEXCITATION SYNDROMES

Several distinct pathways in the heart conduct electrical impulses from the atria to the ventricles, bypassing the AV node, the bundle of His, or both. These accessory conduction pathways (Fig. 14.16) activate the ventricles earlier than if they had progressed down the His–Purkinje system normally. These pathways exist in all hearts but under certain conditions can lead to premature contraction of the ventricles. We call this *ventricular preexcitation* or *preexcitation syndrome*. Not only can these pathways conduct electrical impulses forward (antegrade), but most of them can also conduct impulses backward (retrograde). This flexibility may facilitate the development of reentry mechanisms such as paroxysmal supraventricular tachycardia.

preexcitation syndrome

Depolarization syndrome that occurs when electrical impulses travel from the atria or AV junction into the ventricles through accessory conduction pathways, causing the ventricles to depolarize earlier than normal.

ACCESSORY ATRIOVENTRICULAR PATHWAYS (WOLFF–PARKINSON–WHITE)

The accessory AV pathways (also known as the *bundles of Kent*) consist of bundles of conductive myocardial fibers that bridge

the fibrous layer, insulating the atria from the ventricles. Such accessory pathways have been found in the following locations:
- Between the posterior free wall of the left atrium and that of the left ventricle (type A Wolff–Parkinson–White [WPW] conduction pathway)

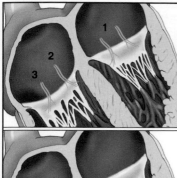
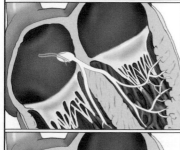
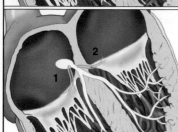

A. Accessory AV pathways (Bundles of Kent)
1. Type A
2. Posteroseptal
3. Type B

B. Atrio-His fibers (James fibers)

C. Mahaim fibers
1. Nodoventricular fibers
2. Fasciculoventricular fibers

FIG. 14.16 Accessory conduction pathways.

- Between the posterior atrial and ventricular walls in the septal region (posteroseptal WPW conduction pathway)
- Between the anterior free wall of the right atrium and that of the right ventricle (type B WPW conduction pathway)

These accessory AV pathways are responsible for accessory AV pathway conduction, also known as *WPW conduction.* They cause an abnormally wide QRS complex, the classic form of ventricular preexcitation. When this type of AV conduction is associated with a paroxysmal supraventricular tachycardia, it is known as the *WPW syndrome.*

Characteristics (Fig. 14.17, A)

PR INTERVAL

The PR intervals are usually shortened to less than 0.12 second, between 0.09 and 0.12 second.

QRS COMPLEX

The duration of the QRS complex is greater than 0.12 second. It is abnormally shaped, with a delta wave (the slurring of the onset of the QRS complex). The QRS complex may also develop larger-than-normal voltages because of the altered process of depolarization.

ST SEGMENT/T WAVE

The ST segment and T wave may deflect in the opposite direction as the QRS complex—that is, they are *discordant.*

ATRIO–HIS PATHWAY (LOWN–GANONG–LEVINE PREEXCITATION)

The atrio–His accessory conduction pathway (also known as the *James fibers*) connects the atria with the lowermost part of the AV node near the origin of the bundle of His, bypassing the

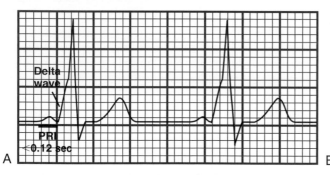
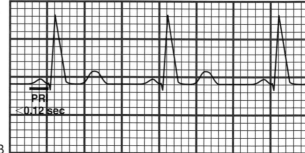

A. Ventricular preexcitation
B. Atrio-His preexcitation
C. Nodoventricular/fasciculoventricular preexcitation

FIG. 14.17 Preexcitation syndromes.

AV node. This form of anomalous AV conduction is classified as *atrio–His preexcitation* or *Lown–Ganong–Levine preexcitation*.

Characteristics (Fig. 14.17, B)

PR INTERVAL

The PR intervals are usually shortened to less than 0.12 second.

QRS COMPLEX

Duration is normal: 0.12 second or less in adults and 0.08 second or less in children. A delta wave is not present.

NODOVENTRICULAR/FASCICULOVENTRICULAR PATHWAY

The nodoventricular and fasciculoventricular fibers (also known as the *Mahaim fibers*) are accessory conduction pathways that provide bypass channels between the AV junction and the ventricles in the following locations:

- Between the lower part of the AV node and the right ventricle (the nodoventricular fibers)
- Between the bundle of His and the ventricles (the fasciculoventricular fibers)

Such anomalous AV conduction is called *nodoventricular/ fasciculoventricular preexcitation*.

Characteristics (Fig. 14.17, C)

PR INTERVAL

Usually normal (0.12 second or longer).

QRS COMPLEX

Duration longer than 0.12 second and abnormally shaped, with a delta wave (the slurring of the onset of the QRS complex) in both of these preexcitation syndromes.

> **AUTHOR'S NOTE** The preexcitation syndromes can best be differentiated by remembering that WPW has a delta wave and short PR interval, Lown–Ganong–Levine has a short PR interval and no delta wave, and the rare nodofascicular type has a delta wave and a normal PR interval.

SUPRAVENTRICULAR VERSUS VENTRICULAR TACHYCARDIA

Differentiating ventricular tachycardia from supraventricular tachycardia (SVT) can be difficult because both rhythms can present with a wide QRS complex. Recognizing that no criteria can rule out one or the other 100% of the time, there are some features that can help in making the diagnosis. They include the following:

- **AV dissociation:** As with third-degree heart block, V-tach has complete dissociation between the P waves pacing the atria and the QRS complexes being paced by an ectopic pacemaker in the ventricles. Close examination of the ECG can sometimes reveal P waves at a slower rate than the ventricles. They are usually buried in the QRS complex. Only a small minority of ECGs contain clear evidence of AV dissociation. When it is present, the rhythm is almost always

ventricular tachycardia. However, the absence of AV dissociation does not rule it out.

- **Shape of the QRS in V₁ to V₂ and V₆:** A QRS complex resembling a typical RBBB with a typical rSRR′ pattern in lead V₁ is often SVT, whereas a broad R wave or qR, QR, or RS pattern strongly suggests V-tach. When the QRS complex has the appearance of that seen in an LBBB, with a long (0.04 second or longer) and notched R wave and/or a QR pattern in lead V₆, the rhythm is more likely to be V-tach.
- *QRS duration:* Longer than 0.14 second with an RBBB pattern or longer than 0.16 second and an LBBB pattern suggests V-tach. Cardiac drugs such as procainamide and conditions such as hyperkalemia that widen the QRS complex lessen the value of this criterion.

In the clinical setting, it may be impossible to reliably differentiate V-tach from SVT. In this case, you must rely on clinical judgment. Hypotension and shock are more common with V-tach, but not all patients with V-tach will be hypotensive. Use the algorithm in Fig. 14.18 to differentiate V-tach from SVT.

> **AUTHOR'S NOTE** V-tach is the most worrisome cause of a tachycardia with a wide QRS complex. Although there are other causes, such as SVT with aberrant conduction and sinus tachycardia with bundle-branch block, it is reasonable to approach the care of the rhythm as if it were V-tach.

BRUGADA SYNDROME

In 1992, physicians and brothers Drs. Pedro and Josep Brugada described a new genetic syndrome with the following diagnostic features:

- ST-segment elevation in the right precordial leads (V1–V3) in the absence of acute coronary syndrome
- RBBB
- Susceptibility to V-tach
- A structurally normal heart
- A significantly higher rate of sudden cardiac arrest

The prevalence of this condition is unclear, but in parts of Asia (the Philippines, Thailand, and Japan), Brugada syndrome is the most common natural cause of death in men under age 50. It has been proposed that the genetic abnormality in Brugada syndrome alters normal repolarization of the ventricle.

The rhythm disturbance typical of Brugada syndrome is a rapid polymorphic V-tach. This rhythm often degenerates into ventricular fibrillation. An increased tendency to develop atrial fibrillation has also been documented in patients with Brugada syndrome. Despite the fact that this syndrome is genetically determined, its clinical manifestations (syncope or cardiac arrest) are rare during childhood. The manifestations become more severe in the third to fourth decades of life. Remarkably, the syndrome is eight times more common among men compared with women. The reasons for such age- and gender-dependent risk are not yet understood. Cardiac events in people with Brugada syndrome may occur during sleep or at rest. Fever, the use of

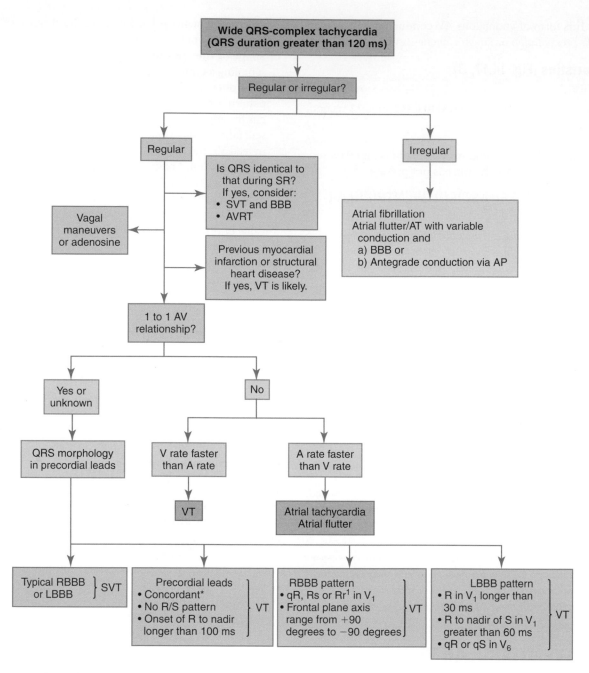

SR = Sinus rhythm, SVT = Supraventrencular tachycardia, BBB = Bundle branch block, V = Ventricular
A = Atrial, AVRT = Atrioventrencular reentrant tachycardia, AP = Accessory pathway

FIG. 14.18 Differentiating ventricular tachycardia from supraventricular tachycardia.

tricyclic antidepressants, and the use of cocaine have been identified as specific triggers for events in some patients.

The incidence of premature sudden cardiac arrest is estimated to be as high as 30% for those with Brugada syndrome. They are often diagnosed only after suffering a syncopal (fainting) episode. The only treatment proven to reduce the risk of death in patients with Brugada syndrome is the placement of an internal automatic defibrillator.

Characteristics (Fig. 14.19)

QRS COMPLEX

Significant J point elevation in the QRS complex in V_1 to V_2.

ST SEGMENT

The ST segment associated with the abnormal QRS complex in the precordial leads has a nonischemic concave elevation pattern, with no similar findings in the reciprocal leads.

Brugada Pattern

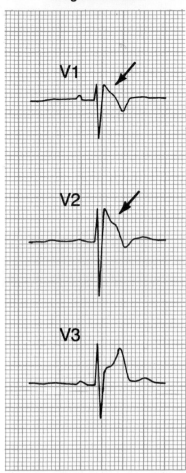

FIG. 14.19 Brugada syndrome. Arrows denote nonischemic downsloping ST-segment elevation. (Modified from Goldberger, A. L., Goldberger, Z. D., & Shvilkin, A. [Eds.]. (2012). *Goldberger's clinical electrocardiography: A simplified approach* [8th ed.]. Saunders.)

T WAVE

Inverted in V_1 to V_2.

TAKE-HOME POINTS

- The two physiologic changes to the myocardium that affect conduction are distention and hypertrophy. Distention increases the size of the chamber, and hypertrophy is an increase in the mass of the muscle.
- Evidence of left atrial enlargement appears as P mitrale, whereas evidence of right atrial enlargement appears as P pulmonale.
- Pericarditis can mimic STEMI because its characteristic PR depression may cause the ST segments to appear elevated.
- Electrical alternans is seen in cases of pericardial effusion.
- Significant elevation or depression of levels of electrolytes such as potassium and calcium causes characteristic ECG changes. Potassium is associated with T-wave changes, whereas calcium is associated with changes in the QT interval.
- Pulmonary embolism may result in the presence of $S_1Q_3T_3$ and ST-segment elevation and T-wave inversion.
- Certain drugs, particularly those used to treat cardiac rhythm disturbances, can cause significant cardiac conduction changes at toxic levels.
- The Osborn wave is the ECG characteristic of hypothermia.
- Accessory conduction pathways predispose the heart to tachycardias such as paroxysmal supraventricular tachycardia. The type depends on the particular pathway involved.
- V-tach and SVT may be difficult to differentiate. V-tach is characterized as having AV dissociation, an RBBB pattern, and wider QRS than SVT.
- The delta wave is characteristic of an accessory atrioventricular conduction known as *WPW syndrome*.
- Brugada syndrome is a genetic cause of sudden cardiac death and possesses a unique set of ECG findings.

CHAPTER REVIEW QUESTIONS

1. Which chronic condition is characterized by thickened chamber walls as a result of enlarged muscle fibers?
   A. Atrophy
   B. Dilatation
   C. Hypertrophy
   D. Stenosis

2. Which diagnosis is most likely to apply to a patient with mitral valve insufficiency or left heart failure?
   A. Left atrial and ventricular enlargement
   B. Left ventricular enlargement alone
   C. Right atrial and ventricular enlargement
   D. Right ventricular enlargement alone

3. Left ventricular hypertrophy, a condition usually caused by increased pressure or volume in the left ventricle, is often associated with which condition?
   A. COPD
   B. Pulmonary hypertension
   C. Systemic hypertension
   D. Ventricular septal defect

4. Which condition is an inflammatory disease involving the epicardium, with deposition of inflammatory cells and serous, fibrous, purulent, or hemorrhagic exudate within the sac surrounding the heart?
   A. Cardiac tamponade
   B. Electrical alternans
   C. Myocarditis
   D. Pericarditis

5. In pericarditis, the ST segment is elevated in which leads?
   A. All leads except aVR and V_1
   B. Leads aVR, aVL, and aVF
   C. The bipolar leads only
   D. The precordial leads V_1 through V_4

6. Which term describes a serum potassium level above the normal range of 3.5 to 5.0 mEq/L?
   A. Hypercalcemia
   B. Hypercarbia
   C. Hyperkalemia
   D. Hypernatremia

7. Which ECG change is characteristic of an elevated potassium level?
   A. Distorted appearance of U wave
   B. Prolonged QT interval
   C. Shortened PR interval
   D. Tall, peaked T wave and widened QRS complex

8. Which medication often prescribed for atrial fibrillation or flutter can cause a broad range of rhythm disturbances?
   A. Digitalis
   B. Furosemide
   C. Procainamide
   D. Verapamil

9. Which ECG change occurs in acute pulmonary embolism?
   A. A QRS axis of greater than +90°
   B. A right ventricular strain pattern in leads V_5 and V_6
   C. An $S_3Q_1T_3$ pattern in leads I and III
   D. Left axis deviation

10. The Osborn wave is a sign of which condition?
    A. Hyperthermia
    B. Hypothermia
    C. Pericarditis
    D. Ventricular preexcitation

Coronary Heart Disease and the 12-Lead ECG

CORONARY CIRCULATION

The coronary circulation (Fig. 15.1) consists of the *left* and *right coronary arteries.* The left coronary artery arises from the base of the aorta just above the left coronary cusp of the aortic valve. The right coronary artery (RCA) arises from the aorta just above the right aortic coronary cusp. During systole, blood is ejected out of the left ventricle, through the open aortic valve, and into the aorta. During diastole, the ventricles relax and the aortic valve closes, allowing blood to enter the coronary arteries.

> **AUTHOR'S NOTE** It is important to recognize that coronary blood flow occurs during the relaxation phase (diastole) of the cardiac cycle. Fast cardiac rhythms limit the period of diastole, which can reduce coronary blood flow to harmful levels.

Left Coronary Artery

The left coronary artery consists of the *left main coronary artery,* a short main stem of about 2 to 10 mm in length that usually divides into two equal major branches; the *left anterior descending coronary artery* (LAD); and the *left circumflex coronary artery* (LCx). Sometimes, a third major branch, the *intermediate diagonal coronary artery,* arises from the left main coronary artery.

> **AUTHOR'S NOTE** The term *artery* is used interchangeably with the term *branch* in this chapter as they relate to the coronary circulation.

The LAD travels anteriorly and downward within the interventricular groove over the interventricular septum. It circles the apex of the heart and ends in the inferior portion of the heart. The LAD gives rise to at least one and often up to six diagonal branches: three to five septal perforator branches and sometimes one or more right ventricular branches.

The diagonal branches course over the anterior and lateral surface of the left ventricle. The septal perforator arteries arise at a right angle from the LAD and run directly into the interventricular septum. The right ventricular arteries branch off of the LAD and course over the anterior surface of the right ventricle.

The LAD supplies blood to the anterior two-thirds of the interventricular septum, most of the right and left bundle branches, the anterior and lateral walls of the left ventricle, and sometimes portions of the right ventricle.

The LCx arises from the left main coronary artery at an obtuse angle (between 90 and 180 degrees). It runs posteriorly along the left atrioventricular (AV) groove, ending as the distal circumflex coronary artery supplying the posterior wall of the left ventricle in nearly all hearts. In the remaining hearts, the LCx continues along the AV groove to become the posterior left ventricular arteries, where it supplies the inferior wall of the left ventricle.

The LCx gives rise to the sinoatrial (SA) nodal artery in about half of hearts. The SA nodal artery supplies blood to the SA node. The LCx then gives rise to one or two left atrial circumflex branches, the left obtuse marginal, and the distal left circumflex artery.

The LCx supplies blood to the left atrial wall and to the lateral and posterior walls of the left ventricle. In 10% to 15% of hearts,

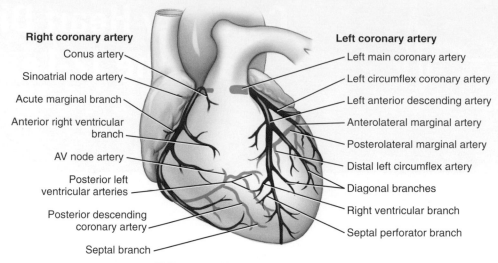

Right coronary artery
- Conus artery
- Sinoatrial node artery
- Acute marginal branch
- Anterior right ventricular branch
- AV node artery
- Posterior left ventricular arteries
- Posterior descending coronary artery
- Septal branch

Left coronary artery
- Left main coronary artery
- Left circumflex coronary artery
- Left anterior descending artery
- Anterolateral marginal artery
- Posterolateral marginal artery
- Distal left circumflex artery
- Diagonal branches
- Right ventricular branch
- Septal perforator branch

FIG. 15.1 The coronary circulation.

when the posterior left ventricular arteries, AV nodal artery, and *posterior descending artery* (PDA) arise from the LCx, the LCx also supplies the inferior wall of the left ventricle, the AV node, the proximal bundle of His, and the posterior one-third of the interventricular septum. When this occurs, the entire interventricular septum is supplied by the left coronary artery.

The anterolateral marginal artery runs over the anterolateral surface of the left ventricular wall toward the apex, lateral to the diagonal branches of the LAD. The posterolateral marginal arteries run down the posterolateral wall of the left ventricle, and the distal left circumflex artery runs down the left AV groove.

Right Coronary Artery

The RCA travels downward and then posteriorly in the right AV groove, giving rise to the *conus artery,* the *SA nodal artery* in about half of hearts, several anterior right ventricular branches, the right atrial branch, and the acute marginal branch.

In most hearts, the RCA gives rise to the AV nodal artery and the posterior descending artery (PDA), which runs down the posterior interventricular groove. From there, the RCA continues along the left AV groove, terminating at the posterior left ventricular arteries.

The RCA supplies blood to the walls of the right atrium and right ventricle, the AV node, the proximal bundle of His, the posterior one-third of the interventricular septum, and the inferior wall of the left ventricle in most hearts and the SA node in about half of hearts.

The RCA gives rise to both the PDA and the posterior left ventricular arteries in most hearts.

> **AUTHOR'S NOTE** To better appreciate the coronary circulation, it is helpful to follow the course of each artery on an illustration of the heart, such as Fig. 15.1. Doing so makes it easier to picture the portions of the heart each artery is traveling over and therefore which part of the heart it supplies with blood.

Table 15.1 summarizes the coronary circulation.

CORONARY HEART DISEASE

Cardiovascular disease is the leading cause of death in the United States. It comprises coronary heart disease (CHD), stroke, heart failure, hypertension, and atherosclerosis. CHD was previously referred to as *coronary artery disease.* It represents more than half of all annual deaths from cardiovascular disease in the United States. The name change reflects a better understanding of the pathophysiology of the disease and recognizes that although the primary site of pathology rests in the arteries, the entire cardiovascular system is affected.

As of 2012, the prevalence of CHD in adults over 20 in the United States was estimated to be 26.6 million, representing 11% of the U.S. population. The distribution between men and women is close to equal. CHD is the most common cause of death for both men and women, killing 610,000 per year—that is, 1 in 4 deaths. In 2014, 735,000 Americans suffered a heart attack. Of those, 525,000 were first-time heart attacks. The average age of a person having his or her first heart attack is 64.5 for men and 70.4 for women. In 2010, there were more than 1 million hospitalizations in the United States for heart failure, and it causes 1 in 5 deaths in this country. A sudden cardiac arrest occurs every 26 seconds, causing one death per minute.

Although the death rate from CHD remains high, it has continued to decline over the past two decades. The falling rate can be attributed primarily to increased awareness of the signs and symptoms of CHD and aggressive treatment of modifiable risk factors. The major modifiable risk factors for CHD are the following:

- Cigarette smoking
- Diabetes mellitus
- Hypertension
- Elevated lipid blood levels
- Obesity
- Lack of exercise
- Stress
- Illicit drug (stimulant) use

TABLE 15.1	Coronary Circulation		
Coronary Artery		**Branches**	**Region Supplied**
Left coronary artery	Left anterior descending coronary artery	Diagonal	Anterolateral wall of the left ventricle
		Septal perforator	Anterior two-thirds of the interventricular septum
		Right ventricular	Anterior portion of the right ventricle
	Left circumflex artery	SA nodal artery (40%–60% of hearts)	SA node
		Atrial LCx artery	Left atrium
		Anterolateral marginal artery	Anterolateral wall of the left ventricle
		Posterolateral marginal artery	Posterolateral wall of the left ventricle
		Distal LCx artery	Posterior wall of the left ventricle
		Posterior descending artery (10%–15% of hearts)	Posterior one-third of the interventricular septum
		AV nodal artery (10%–15% of hearts)	AV node
			Proximal bundle of His
		Posterior left ventricular artery (10%–15% of hearts)	Inferior wall of the left ventricle
Right coronary artery		Conus artery	Portions of the right ventricle
		SA nodal artery (50%–60% of hearts)	SA node
		Anterior right ventricular artery	Anterolateral wall of the right ventricle
		Right atrial artery	Right atrium
		Acute marginal artery	Lateral wall of the right ventricle
		PDA (85%–90% of hearts)	Posterior one-third of the interventricular septum
		AV nodal artery (85%–90% of hearts)	AV node
			Proximal bundle of His
		Posterior left ventricular artery (85%–90% of hearts)	Inferior wall of the left ventricle

AV, Atrioventricular; *LCx,* left circumflex artery; *PDA,* posterior descending coronary artery; *SA,* sinoatrial.

Coronary atherosclerosis, a form of arteriosclerosis (hardening of the arteries), is the primary disease process involved in CHD. It is responsible for the formation of atheromatous plaques in large and medium-size coronary arteries. Plaque formation is often followed by plaque disruption, thrombosis, and coronary artery occlusion. The consequence of coronary atherosclerosis is a group of clinical syndromes called *acute coronary syndrome* (ACS):

- Unstable angina
- Non–ST-segment-elevation myocardial infarction (NSTEMI)
- ST-segment-elevation myocardial infarction (STEMI)

acute coronary syndrome

As the name implies, a syndrome is a collection of signs and symptoms associated with a particular condition. Unstable angina, NSTEMI, and STEMI are all ACSs. A patient experiencing chest pain/discomfort may be suffering from any of the three and may progress from one to the other, depending on the underlying cause.

Coronary Atherosclerosis and Thrombosis

The first phase in the evolution of coronary atherosclerosis is the appearance of *atherosclerotic plaques* within the inner layer of the coronary arteries (Fig. 15.2, stage 1) that develop after damage to the *endothelium.* An inflammatory response by the myocardial cells (Fig. 15.2, stage 2) results in the deposition of low-density lipoproteins (LDLs) from the plasma into the intima of the vessel. There they evolve into small clumps of lipid-filled foam cells. These cells appear as yellow dots or streaks on the internal surface of the artery. Over time, the lesion progresses to form large plaques (Fig. 15.2, stage 3). These plaques consist of a soft, gruel-like lipid and cholesterol-rich atheromatous core and an external fibrous cap (Fig. 15.2, stage 4) composed primarily of smooth muscle cells and collagen. The volume and composition of the atheromatous core and the thickness of the fibrous cap vary from plaque to plaque, even within the same coronary artery. Atherosclerotic plaques may remain stable for years without causing any symptoms.

endothelium

Refers to the lining of epithelial cells that covers the inner surface of every component of the circulatory system, including arteries, veins, atria, and ventricles. This endothelium comprises the intima, or inner surface, of the artery.

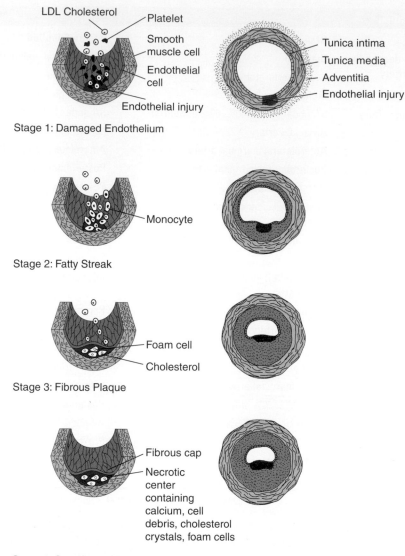

FIG. 15.2 Plaque formation. (From Libby, P. [2015]. The vascular biology of atherosclerosis. In D. L. Mann, D. Zipes, P. Libby, & R. Bonow [Eds.], *Braunwald's heart disease: A textbook of cardiovascular medicine* [10th ed.]. Saunders.)

Stable, Vulnerable, and Unstable Plaques

Any atherosclerotic plaque can rupture, totally occluding the coronary artery. Atherosclerotic plaques are categorized as *stable* if they are less prone to rupture. A stable coronary artery plaque (Fig. 15.3) has a lipid core separated from the arterial lumen by a thick fibrous cap. The lipid core does not stretch the arterial wall but instead intrudes into the lumen of the artery. Over time, it may narrow the lumen to the point that symptoms of *angina* (chest pain) occur. This pain occurs because the plaque limits blood flow to the myocardium. Acute myocardial infarction (MI) can sometimes occur with stable plaques that significantly narrow the arterial lumen.

Vulnerable plaques (see Fig. 15.3) are coronary lesions that have a thin fibrous cap. Over time, these vulnerable plaques become inflamed, resulting in a process called *remodeling*. Positive remodeling enlarges the artery as it compensates for the plaque. These plaques are referred to as *nonstenotic lesions* because they do not narrow the lumen of the artery. Negative remodeling causes calcification and further fat accumulation that narrows the arterial lumen. The lumen must be narrowed by greater than 50% to cause a clinically significant reduction in blood flow. These lesions occasionally result in ACS.

Vulnerable plaques are often located at branch points, or bends, in the coronary arteries. Because of the thinness of the fibrous cap, these plaques are susceptible to erosion and rupture, which can lead to thrombus formation and ACS. The leading edge of the vulnerable plaque can become inflamed as blood flows over it. This inflammation further weakens the plaque, making it more prone to rupture. At this point, the plaque is referred to as *unstable*.

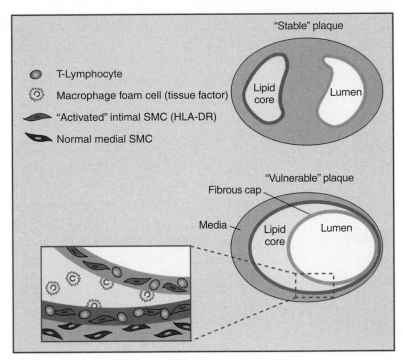

FIG. 15.3 Stable and vulnerable plaques. (From Aehlert, B. [2017]. *ACLS study guide* [5th ed.]. Mosby.)

Plaque Erosion and Rupture

A *thrombus* (blood clot) forms on the surface of the plaque after it erodes or in the plaque itself after the fibrous cap ruptures. The thrombus often extends into the arterial lumen. Generally, a plaque does not rupture until its core becomes highly saturated with lipids. Rupture of the fibrous cap is at least three times more common than is erosion of the plaque surface.

Erosion (wearing away) occurs when the endothelial layer covering the plaque has worn away, exposing the plaque itself. A platelet-rich thrombus immediately forms on the exposed surface of the plaque, increasing the size of the plaque.

Rupture (disruption) of the fibrous cap is most likely to occur at its leading edge, the area of the cap adjacent to the normal arterial wall. The cause of the rupture may be one or more of the following:

- Progressive weakening and/or thinning of the fibrous cap
- Sudden surges in blood pressure, heart rate, or blood flow (as seen with emotional stress or heavy physical exertion, particularly in sedentary people)
- Spasm of the coronary artery at the site of the plaque
- Repetitive flexion of the artery at the site of the plaque during the cardiac cycle

After the fibrous cap ruptures, blood enters the plaque and mixes with the atheromatous lipid gruel. This process appears to greatly enhance thrombus formation, immediately producing a thrombus rich in platelets and fibrin. Initially the thrombus may not extend beyond the plaque, causing no further occlusion. However, the thrombus often continues to grow, extending beyond the fibrous cap into the arterial lumen,

partially or completely occluding it. As the thrombus grows into the lumen, it becomes rich in fibrin. Sometimes clumps of platelets break off the distal end of the main thrombus and flow downstream, causing additional obstruction of smaller coronary arteries.

Once the thrombus has formed, it may partially or completely disintegrate spontaneously, in a process called *spontaneous thrombolysis*. Or it may undergo further thrombosis and enlarge. Sometimes the thrombus becomes organized by the deposition of connective tissue, evolving into a fibrotic lesion (scar).

THROMBUS FORMATION AND LYSIS

To understand the treatment of ACSs, you must understand how a thrombus forms when an arterial atherosclerotic plaque is damaged and how the thrombus is eventually lysed (broken down). The following are the principal components necessary for thrombus formation and lysis (Table 15.2).

Blood Components

PLATELETS

Platelets contain adhesive glycoprotein (GP) receptors that bind to various components of connective tissue and blood to form thrombi. The following are the main GP receptors and their functions:

- GP Ia binds the platelets directly to collagen fibers present in connective tissue.
- GP Ib binds the platelets to von Willebrand factor (a tissue component).

TABLE 15.2	Components of Thrombus Formation and Lysis	
Process	Component	Function
Thrombus formation	Blood (platelets)	
	Glycoprotein (GP) Ia	Binds platelets directly to collagen fibers
	GP Ib	Binds platelets to von Willebrand factor
	GP IIb/IIIa	Binds initially to von Willebrand factor, then to fibrinogen after platelet activation
	Adenosine (ADP), serotonin, thromboxane A$_2$ (TxA$_2$)	Stimulates platelet aggregation
	Prothrombin	Converts to thrombin when activated by tissue factor released from injured blood vessel walls; thrombin then converts fibrinogen to fibrin
	Fibrinogen	Converts to fibrin when exposed to thrombin
	Tissue	
	von Willebrand factor	Binds to platelets' GP Ib and GP IIb/IIIa and to collagen fibers
	Collagen fibers	Bind directly to platelets' GP Ia and to GP Ib and GP IIb/IIIa via von Willebrand factor
	Tissue factor	Initiates the conversion of prothrombin to thrombin
Thrombolysis	Blood (platelets)	
	Plasminogen	Converts to plasmin when activated by tissue plasminogen activator; plasmin then dissolves the fibrin (fibrinolysis), causing the thrombus to break apart (thrombolysis)
	Tissue	
	Tissue plasminogen activator (tPA)	Activates plasminogen to convert to plasmin

- GP IIb/IIIa binds the platelets to von Willebrand factor and, after the platelets are activated, to fibrinogen.

Platelets also contain several substances released after platelet activation that promote thrombus formation by stimulating platelet aggregation:
- Adenosine diphosphate (ADP)
- Serotonin
- Thromboxane A$_2$ (TxA$_2$)

PROTHROMBIN

Prothrombin is a plasma protein activated when blood is exposed to tissue factor, which is released from the damaged arterial wall. Prothrombin is converted to thrombin, which in turn converts fibrinogen to fibrin.

FIBRINOGEN

Fibrinogen is a plasma protein. When exposed to thrombin, it is converted to fibrin, an elastic, threadlike filament.

PLASMINOGEN

Plasminogen is a plasma GP that converts to an enzyme—plasmin—when activated by tissue plasminogen activator. This substance is normally present in the endothelium that lines the blood vessels. Plasmin, in turn, dissolves the fibrin strands by binding the platelets together within a thrombus. This process is called *fibrinolysis*. Plasminogen normally attaches itself to fibrin during thrombus formation, making it instantly available for conversion to plasmin when needed.

Tissue Components

VON WILLEBRAND FACTOR

Von Willebrand factor is a protein stored in the cells of the endothelium that lines the arteries. When exposed to blood after an injury to the endothelial cells, von Willebrand factor immediately binds to the platelets via GP Ib and GP IIb/IIIa receptors. It adheres the platelets to the collagen fibers located beneath the endothelium in the intima.

COLLAGEN FIBERS

Collagen is composed of white protein fibers. It is present within the intima of the arterial wall. After an injury and exposure to blood, the collagen fibers immediately and directly bind to the platelets via GP Ia. They also bind to them indirectly by means of von Willebrand factor via GP Ib and GP IIb/IIIa.

TISSUE FACTOR

Tissue factor is present in platelets and leukocytes—in fact, it's a component of all circulatory system tissue. When released after injury, it initiates the conversion of prothrombin to thrombin in order to heal injured vessels. Unfortunately, this healing creates a plaque that can rupture, creating a thrombus that can occlude the coronary artery.

TISSUE PLASMINOGEN ACTIVATOR

Tissue plasminogen activator (tPA) is a glycoprotein present primarily in the vascular endothelium that, when released into the plasma, activates plasminogen to convert to plasmin. Plasmin in turn dissolves fibrinogen and fibrin.

Phases of Thrombus Formation

Coronary artery thrombus formation occurs in four phases (Fig. 15.4), as described next.

PHASE 1: SUBENDOTHELIAL EXPOSURE AND VASOCONSTRICTION

When an atherosclerotic plaque becomes eroded or ruptures, the platelets are immediately exposed to collagen fibers and von Willebrand factor present within the cap of the atherosclerotic plaque. Platelets begin to fill the gap, and the vessel constricts in an attempt to minimize the rupture. This process is mediated by TxA$_2$.

PHASE 2: PLATELET ADHESION AND ACTIVATION

The GP Ia receptors on the platelets bind directly to the collagen fibers, and the GP Ib and GP IIb/IIIa receptors bind to von Willebrand factor, which in turn also binds to the collagen fibers. Consequently, the platelets adhere to the collagen fibers within the plaque, forming a layer of platelets overlying the damaged area.

Upon binding to the collagen fibers, the platelets are activated. Their shape changes from smooth ovals to tiny spheres as they release ADP, serotonin, and TxA$_2$. These substances stimulate platelet aggregation (clumping). Platelet activation is also stimulated by the lipid-rich gruel within the atherosclerotic plaque. At the same time, the GP IIb/IIIa receptors are prompted to bind to fibrinogen, and tissue factor is released from the tissue and platelets.

PHASE 3: PLATELET AGGREGATION

Once activated, the platelets bind to each other by means of fibrinogen, a cordlike structure that adheres to the GP IIb/IIIa receptors on the platelets. One strand of fibrinogen can bind to two platelets—one at each end. Stimulated by ADP and TxA$_2$, the binding of fibrinogen to the GP IIb/IIIa receptors is greatly enhanced, causing rapid growth of the platelet plug. By this time, tissue factor has converted the prothrombin in the area of the damaged plaque to thrombin.

PHASE 4: THROMBUS FORMATION

At first, the platelet plug is rather unstable. It becomes firmer as the fibrinogen between the platelets is replaced by stronger strands of fibrin. This occurs as tissue factor converts prothrombin to thrombin. Thrombin in turn converts fibrinogen to fibrin threads. Plasminogen usually becomes attached to the fibrin during its formation. As the thrombus grows, red blood cells and leukocytes (white blood cells) become entrapped in the platelet–fibrin mesh.

Phases of Thrombolysis

Thrombolysis, the breakdown of the thrombus, can be initiated by the intravenous injection of thrombolytic drugs, such as alteplase, reteplase, and tenecteplase. These agents work by interfering with TxA$_2$ activity.

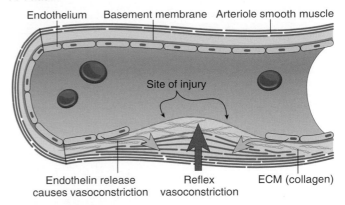

A Phase 1

Endothelium Basement membrane Arteriole smooth muscle

Site of injury

Endothelin release causes vasoconstriction Reflex vasoconstriction ECM (collagen)

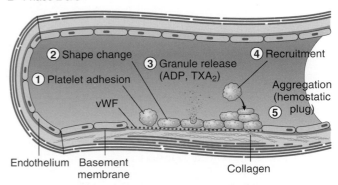

B Phase 2 & 3

② Shape change ④ Recruitment
③ Granule release (ADP, TXA$_2$)
① Platelet adhesion Aggregation (hemostatic plug) ⑤
vWF

Endothelium Basement membrane Collagen

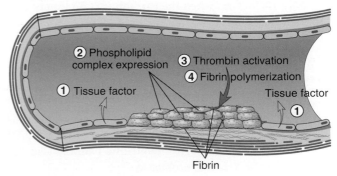

C Phase 4

② Phospholipid complex expression ③ Thrombin activation
④ Fibrin polymerization
① Tissue factor Tissue factor ①
Fibrin

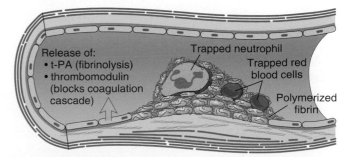

D Phase 5

Release of:
• t-PA (fibrinolysis)
• thrombomodulin (blocks coagulation cascade)

Trapped neutrophil
Trapped red blood cells
Polymerized fibrin

FIG. 15.4 Thrombus formation. (From Kumar, V., Abbas, A., Fausto, N., & Asteret, J. [2010]. *Robbins and Cotran pathologic basis for disease* [8th ed.]. Saunders.)

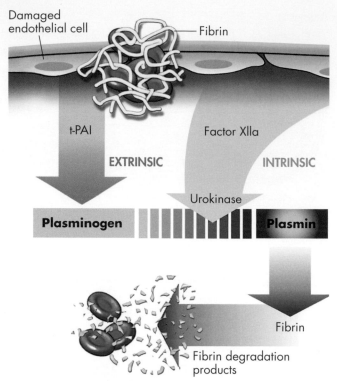

FIG. 15.5 Thrombolysis. (From Huether, S. [2012]. *Understanding pathophysiology* [5th ed.]. Mosby.)

Normally, however, the breakdown of a thrombus—*thrombolysis*—occurs when the thrombus is no longer needed to maintain the integrity of the blood vessel wall. Natural thrombolysis consists of three phases (Fig. 15.5).

PHASE 1: ACTIVATION OF INTRINSIC AND EXTRINSIC PATHWAYS

The central reaction is the conversion of plasminogen to the enzyme plasmin. Plasminogen is activated through the extrinsic pathway (Fig. 15.5, blue), initiated by the release of tPA from the endothelial cells, and through the intrinsic pathway (Fig. 15.5, gold) from factor XIIa and urokinase.

PHASE 2: PLASMIN FORMATION

Tissue plasminogen activator, factor XIIa, or urokinase activates plasminogen, converting it to plasmin.

PHASE 3: FIBRINOLYSIS

Plasmin breaks down the fibrin into soluble fragments, causing the platelets to separate from each other and the thrombus to break apart.

> **AUTHOR'S NOTE** There are multiple points at which the process of thrombus formation can be inhibited by administering pharmaceutical agents to augment the body's natural mechanisms. Additionally, thrombolysis can be aided by administering agents that promote fibrinolysis. Together, these options constitute the mainstay of noninvasive treatment of acute MI.

MYOCARDIAL ISCHEMIA, INJURY, AND INFARCTION

Ischemia

Myocardial ischemia is present the moment the supply of oxygen to the myocardium becomes insufficient to meet the demands of cellular metabolism. This leads to a deficiency of oxygen (hypoxia) within the cardiac cells. For a short time after the onset of hypoxia, certain reversible ischemic changes occur in the internal structure of the affected cells. These ischemic changes cause a delay in the depolarization and repolarization of the cells. The cells can tolerate mild to moderate hypoxia for a short period (usually a matter of several minutes), with no great effect on their function. The myocardial cells may partially lose their ability to contract, and the specialized cells of the electrical conduction system may become less efficient in generating or conducting electrical impulses. When adequate blood flow and oxygenation are restored, however, these cells usually return to a normal or near-normal condition.

Injury

If ischemia is severe or prolonged, the hypoxic cells sustain *myocardial injury* and stop functioning normally. They become unable to contract fully and to generate or conduct electrical impulses properly. At this stage, the damage to the cells still remains reversible, and the injured cells remain viable and salvageable for some time. As in ischemic cells, injured cells may also return to normal or nearly normal if adequate blood flow and oxygenation are restored. The degree to which they can withstand injury and the extent to which they return to normal depend on the length and severity of the ischemia and their condition before the period of deprivation.

Infarction

If severe myocardial ischemia continues because of a persistent absence of blood supply, the cells have no oxygen supply and eventually sustain irreversible injury and die, becoming electrically inert. At the moment of cellular death (necrosis), MI is said to have occurred. Necrotic cells *do not* return to normal upon revascularization or oxygenation.

> **AUTHOR'S NOTE** Myocardial ischemia and injury are reversible, whereas MI is not. The goals of therapy are to minimize the period or ischemia and, if that's not possible, to minimize the area of myocardium infarcted.

Categorization of Causes

Myocardial ischemia, injury, and infarction are caused by the failure of local coronary arteries to supply sufficient oxygenated blood to the myocardial tissue. This can have a variety of causes, which are categorized as follows.

TYPE 1

Type refers to an MI caused by the acute occlusion of a severely narrowed atherosclerotic coronary artery by a coronary thrombus after the rupture of an atherosclerotic plaque, with hemorrhage within the plaque extending into the arterial lumen. Coronary thrombosis after plaque rupture is the most common cause of MI, occurring in about 90% of patients with acute MI.

TYPE 2

Type 2 refers to an MI caused by increased oxygen demand or decreased oxygen delivery to the heart. This can occur from any of the following (in order of frequency):

- Respiratory failure: Decreased oxygen levels in the blood associated with hypoxia from conditions like chronic obstructive pulmonary disease (COPD), emphysema, pulmonary edema, and pneumonia (30%).
- Supraventricular and ventricular tachycardia (fast heart rhythms): These decrease the period of diastole and increase oxygen demand by the heart (30%).
- Anemia: Low hemoglobin levels decrease the delivery of oxygen to the heart (20%).
- Shock: Decreased coronary arterial blood flow for any reason other than coronary artery occlusion or spasm, such as a bradyarrhythmias (slow heart rhythms), pulmonary embolism, hypotension, or shock from any cause (10%).
- Multifactorial. A combination of these factors (10%).

> **AUTHOR'S NOTE** Coronary artery spasm, in the absence of plaque rupture, caused by the constriction of smooth muscle in the wall of the coronary artery, has been described in the literature and may be associated with the use of drugs such as cocaine. However, its contribution to the overall causes of MI is quite low.

TYPE 3

Type 3 refers to an MI associated with sudden cardiac death from lethal rhythm disturbance.

TYPES 4 AND 5

Types 4 and 5 refer to an MI associated with an operative procedure.

PATHOPHYSIOLOGY OF MYOCARDIAL INFARCTION

Typically, an MI at its height consists of a central area of dead, necrotic tissue, called the *zone of infarction (or necrosis)*; surrounded by a layer of injured myocardial tissue, called the *zone of injury*; and then by an outer layer of ischemic tissue, called the *zone of ischemia* (Fig. 15.6).

An MI may be either transmural or nontransmural. A *transmural infarction* is one in which the zone of infarction involves the entire thickness of the ventricular wall, from the endocardial (inner) to the epicardial (outer) layers of the myocardium. A *nontransmural infarction,* on the other hand, is one in which the zone of infarction only involves a part of the ventricular

wall, usually the subendocardial area of the myocardium. For that reason, the nontransmural infarction is referred to as a *subendocardial MI.*

As it relates to the ECG, MIs are categorized as either STEMI or NSTEMI. Generally speaking, transmural infarction causes a STEMI. Nontransmural infarction that involves a large enough area of the myocardium will lead to a STEMI, whereas one that involves a smaller area will lead to an NSTEMI.

Type 1 MI is most likely to present as STEMI, whereas type 2 more often presents as NSTEMI.

> **AUTHOR'S NOTE** Transmural MI often produces what is termed *pathologic Q waves,* a term that will be described later in the chapter. For that reason, a transmural MI is also referred to as a *Q-wave MI,* whereas a nontransmural MI is referred to as a *non–Q-wave* MI. Additionally, because the nontransmural infarction evolves from the subendocardium, it is referred to as a *subendocardial infarction.* Although this can be confusing, it is important to remember the various ways that infarctions are described by different texts and clinicians. To summarize the approach taken in this text, transmural infarction is often referred to as *Q-wave MI* and *STEMI,* and nontransmural infarction is referred to as *non–Q-wave MI* and *NSTEMI* or simply as a *subendocardial MI* (Fig. 15.7).

Phases of a Classic Type 1 ST-Segment-Elevation Myocardial Infarction

The evolution and resolution of a classical type 1 STEMI can be divided into four phases. It begins in the subendocardium, presumably because this area has the least supply of blood. The infarct then progresses outward until it involves the entire myocardium. While necrosis is progressing from the endocardium to the epicardium, the MI is said to be evolving.

PHASE 1

Within the first 2 hours after coronary artery occlusion, the following sequence of changes occurs in the myocardium supplied by the occluded artery (Fig. 15.8, *A*):

1. Within seconds of the coronary artery occlusion, extensive myocardial ischemia occurs.
2. During the first 20 to 40 minutes (on average, 30 minutes) of the onset of the MI, reversible myocardial injury appears in the subendocardium.
3. About 30 minutes after the interruption of blood flow, irreversible myocardial necrosis (infarction) occurs in the subendocardium as myocardial injury begins to spread outward toward the epicardium.
4. One hour after the onset, myocardial necrosis has spread through over one-third of the myocardium.
5. At 2 hours, myocardial necrosis has spread through about half of the myocardium.

PHASE 2

Between 2 and 24 hours after the occlusion, the evolution of the MI is completed in the following sequence (Fig. 15.8, *B*):

1. At 3 hours, about two-thirds of the myocardial cells within the affected myocardium become necrotic.

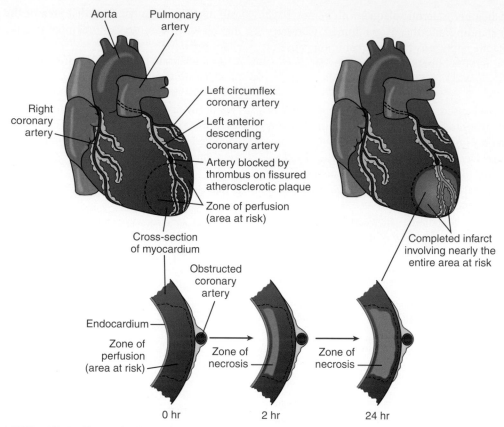

FIG. 15.6 Zone of infarction. (Modified from Mann, D. L., Zipes, D. Libby, P., & Bonow, R. [Eds.]. [2015]. *Braunwald's heart disease* [10th ed.]. Saunders.)

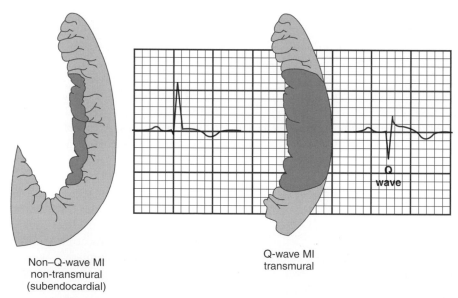

FIG. 15.7 Nontransmural versus transmural myocardial infarction.

2. By 6 hours, only a small percentage of the cells remain viable. For all practical purposes, the evolution of the transmural MI is complete.

3. Twenty-four hours after onset, the progression of myocardial necrosis to the epicardium is usually complete.

PHASE 3

After the first day and during the next 24 to 72 hours, little or no ischemic or injured myocardial cells remain because all cells have either died or recovered. Acute inflammation with edema and cellular infiltration begins within the necrotic tissue during this phase.

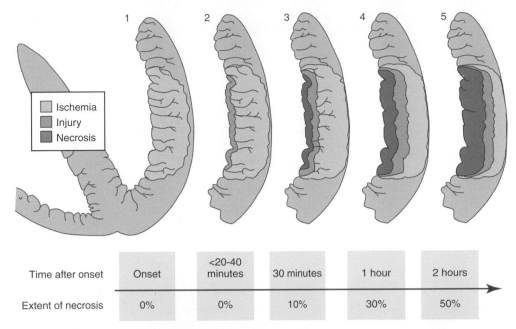

Ischemia
Injury
Necrosis

Time after onset	Onset	<20-40 minutes	30 minutes	1 hour	2 hours
Extent of necrosis	0%	0%	10%	30%	50%

A   Phase 1: Transmural MI (0-2 hours)

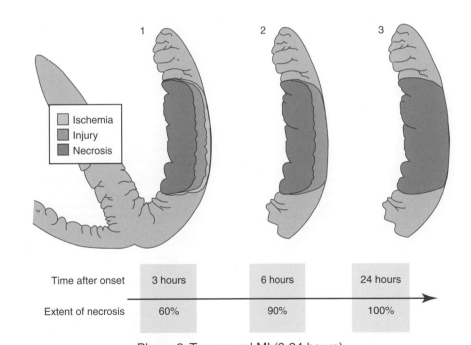

Ischemia
Injury
Necrosis

Time after onset	3 hours	6 hours	24 hours
Extent of necrosis	60%	90%	100%

B   Phase 2: Transmural MI (2-24 hours)

FIG. 15.8 The first two early phases of an acute myocardial infarction. (A) Phase 1. (B) Phase 2.

PHASE 4

During the second week, inflammation continues, followed by proliferation of connective tissue during the third week. Healing with replacement of the necrotic tissue with fibrous connective tissue is generally complete by the seventh week.

Table 15.3 summarizes the four phases of an evolving acute transmural MI.

Anatomic Locations of Myocardial Infarction

The site of the MI depends on which coronary artery is occluded (Fig. 15.9). Table 15.4 lists the locations of an MI relative to the sites of coronary artery occlusion.

ECG Changes in Myocardial Infarction

The ECG in an evolving MI, with its varying mix of myocardial ischemia, injury, and necrosis, is characterized by changes in

TABLE 15.3	Phases of Acute Transmural Myocardial Infarction (MI)	
Phase	**Time After Onset of Acute MI**	**Pathophysiology**
1	0–2 hr (first few hours)	Extensive myocardial ischemia and injury occur, with about 50% of the myocardium becoming necrotic
2	2–24 hr (first day)	The evolution of the MI is complete, with about two-thirds of the myocardium becoming necrotic by 3 hr and most of the rest becoming necrotic by 6 hr
3	24–72 hr (second to third day)	Little or no ischemic or injured myocardial cells remain because all cells have either died or recovered; acute inflammation begins within the necrotic tissue
4	2–8 wk	Fibrous tissue completely replaces the necrotic tissue

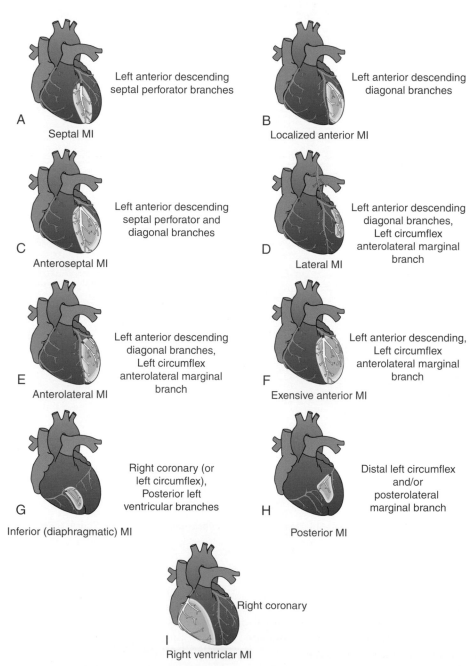

A   Septal MI — Left anterior descending septal perforator branches

B   Localized anterior MI — Left anterior descending diagonal branches

C   Anteroseptal MI — Left anterior descending septal perforator and diagonal branches

D   Lateral MI — Left anterior descending diagonal branches, Left circumflex anterolateral marginal branch

E   Anterolateral MI — Left anterior descending diagonal branches, Left circumflex anterolateral marginal branch

F   Exensive anterior MI — Left anterior descending, Left circumflex anterolateral marginal branch

G   Inferior (diaphragmatic) MI — Right coronary (or left circumflex), Posterior left ventricular branches

H   Posterior MI — Distal left circumflex and/or posterolateral marginal branch

I   Right ventriclar MI — Right coronary

FIG. 15.9 Location of myocardial infarction in relation to the coronary arteries occluded.

TABLE 15.4	Anatomic Locations of Myocardial Infarction Relative to Coronary Artery Occlusion
Location of Infarction	**Site of Occlusion**
Septal MI (Fig. 15.9, *A*)	LAD beyond the first diagonal branch, involving the septal perforator arteries
Anterior (localized) MI (Fig. 15.9, *B*)	Diagonal arteries of the LAD
Anteroseptal MI (Fig. 15.9, *C*)	LAD involving both the septal perforator and diagonal arteries
Lateral MI (Fig. 15.9, *D*)	Laterally located diagonal arteries of the LAD and/or the anterolateral marginal branch of the LCx
Anterolateral MI (Fig. 15.9, *E*)	Diagonal arteries of the LAD alone or in conjunction with the anterolateral marginal branch of the LCx
Extensive anterior MI (Fig. 15.9, *F*)	LAD alone or in conjunction with the anterolateral marginal branch of the LCx
Inferior (diaphragmatic) MI (Fig. 15.9, *G*)	(1) Posterior left ventricular branches of the RCA or, less commonly, the left circumflex coronary of the left coronary artery or (2) the RCA before the branching of the posterior descending, AV node, and posterior left ventricular arteries
Posterior MI (Fig. 15.9, *H*)	Distal LCx and/or posterolateral marginal branch of the LCx
Right ventricular MI with inferior (diaphragmatic) MI (Fig. 15.9, *I*)	RCA

MI, Myocardial infarction; *LAD,* left anterior descending coronary artery; *RCA,* right coronary artery; *LCx,* left circumflex coronary artery.

three components of the ECG—the T wave, ST segment, and QRS complex, specifically the Q wave. The changes, summarized in Table 15.5, include the following:

- *Myocardial ischemia:* T-wave changes and ST-segment elevation or depression
- *Myocardial injury:* ST-segment elevation or depression
- *Myocardial necrosis:* Pathologic Q wave

The nature of these ECG changes and the leads in which they appear will depend on (1) the anatomic location of the MI in the ventricles (anterior, posterior, inferior, or right ventricular) and (2) the extent of the involvement of the myocardial wall (transmural or nontransmural).

The changes in the QRS complex, ST segment, and T wave reflect the changes in the movement of the electrical impulse within the ischemic or infarcted region. The magnitude of these changes depends on the size and location of the affected region. The size and location of the affected region depend on the coronary artery involved.

> **AUTHOR'S NOTE** The ECG changes that occur in MI include T-wave changes associated with myocardial ischemia, ST-segment changes linked to myocardial injury, and Q-wave changes caused by myocardial infarction (necrosis).

As was discussed in earlier chapters, certain leads have specific views of the heart, which correspond to anatomic areas of coronary perfusion. The leads that record the electrical forces in a particular view of the area of the myocardium involved by myocardial ischemia, injury, and infarction are termed *facing leads.* The leads that record the electrical forces that view the involved myocardium directly opposite the area of ischemia, injury, or infarction are termed *reciprocal leads.* The ECG findings in the reciprocal lead are referred to as *reciprocal changes.* ECG leads that examine the same area of the heart are referred to as *contiguous.* For example, the precordial leads V_1 and V_2

both face the anterior wall of the left ventricle and therefore are contiguous. Finding abnormal changes in contiguous leads enhances the accuracy of ECG interpretation.

> **AUTHOR'S NOTE** *Facing* and *reciprocal leads* refer to the fact that the facing leads view the area of ischemia, injury, or infarction, whereas the reciprocal leads view the area from the opposite direction.

> **AUTHOR'S NOTE** Contiguous leads are leads facing the same area of the heart. ECG changes in two or more contiguous leads support the conclusion of ischemia and/or infarction occurring in the area of the heart that the leads view.

T WAVE

Changes to the T wave indicating myocardial ischemia usually appear within seconds of the onset of the MI. This is referred to as an *ischemic T wave.* Such waves appear over the zone of ischemia in the facing leads. They are the result of a delay or change in direction of myocardial repolarization (Fig. 15.10). They may be abnormally tall and peaked or deeply inverted. In addition, the QT interval associated with the ischemic T wave is usually prolonged.

Whether the ischemic T wave is upright or inverted depends on whether the ischemia is transmural or nontransmural, respectively. In normal hearts, repolarization begins at the epicardium and progresses toward the endocardium, producing a positive T wave.

In subendocardial (nontransmural) ischemia, repolarization of the subendocardial cells is delayed. Repolarization progresses in the normal direction, from the epicardium to the endocardium, but slows when it reaches the ischemic subendocardial area. This produces a prolonged QT interval and a symmetrically positive, tall, and peaked T wave.

TABLE 15.5	ECG Changes in Transmural Myocardial Infarction		
Stage	**Severity**	**Changes in Facing Leads**	**Changes in Reciprocal Leads**
Ischemia	Reversible	Tall, peaked (a) or inverted (b) T wave	Inverted (a) or tall, peaked (b) T wave
Ischemia, injury	Reversible	Elevated ST segment	Depressed ST segment
Necrosis	Irreversible	Pathologic Q wave and QS complex	Tall R wave

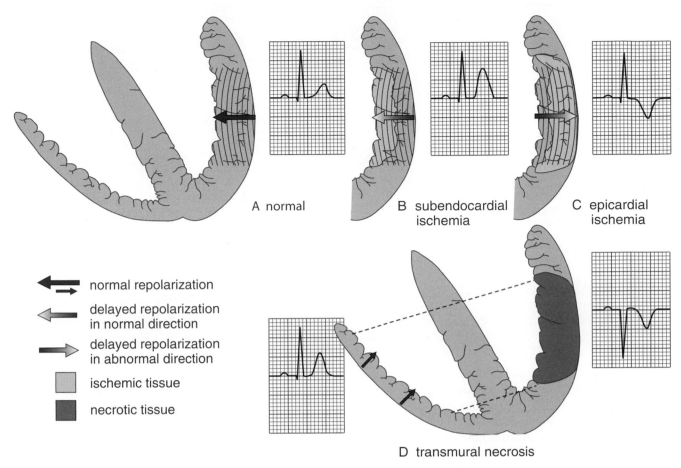

A normal

B subendocardial ischemia

C epicardial ischemia

→ normal repolarization

→ delayed repolarization in normal direction

→ delayed repolarization in abnormal direction

ischemic tissue

necrotic tissue

D transmural necrosis

FIG. 15.10 Mechanism of ischemic T waves.

In transmural ischemia, on the other hand, repolarization of the subepicardial cells is delayed. Consequently, repolarization begins at the endocardium. It progresses in a reverse direction, from the endocardium to the epicardium, slowing when it reaches the ischemic subepicardial area. This produces a prolonged QT interval and a symmetrically inverted, deep T wave.

An ischemic T wave is often accompanied by depression or elevation of the ST segment, another manifestation of myocardial ischemia. Ischemic T waves and associated ST-segment changes revert to normal quickly after an anginal attack.

Deeply inverted T waves also appear in association with pathologic Q waves over the zone of necrosis in the later phases of acute MI. These T waves are deeply inverted, mirror images of the upright T waves normally generated in the opposite ventricular wall, being produced the same way as pathologic Q waves, which will be described later.

In a typical transmural MI, in the leads that normally (in the absence of an MI) show an upright T wave, the ischemic T wave is initially prolonged, abnormally tall, symmetrical, and peaked. Occasionally, the wave becomes extremely tall—the *hyperacute T wave*—appearing for only a short time at the onset of ischemia. Almost immediately after the onset of ischemia, the ST segment becomes elevated, causing the ST-T complex elevation typical of a transmural infarction. This ST-T complex pattern continues through the injury phase into the necrosis phase, at which time a pathologic Q wave begins to appear.

In a typical subendocardial MI, the T wave that follows the onset of infarction appears isoelectric, biphasic, or inverted. It is usually associated with a depressed ST segment resembling that seen in angina. Unlike the ST-T wave complex associated with angina, however, which quickly reverts to normal after an anginal attack, this abnormal ST-T complex returns to normal more gradually as healing proceeds. It often does not resolve completely.

ST SEGMENT

ST-segment changes occur in MI, indicating myocardial ischemia and injury. The ST segment can also be affected by noninfarction conditions such as pericarditis, hyperkalemia, ventricular hypertrophy, bundle-branch block, drug effects, and early repolarization. These conditions were reviewed in Chapter 14. The ST-segment changes are characterized as either elevation or depression.

ST Elevation

ST-segment elevation is an ECG sign of severe, extensive, transmural, myocardial ischemia and injury in the evolution of a Q-wave MI. It may also be seen less often in the evolution of

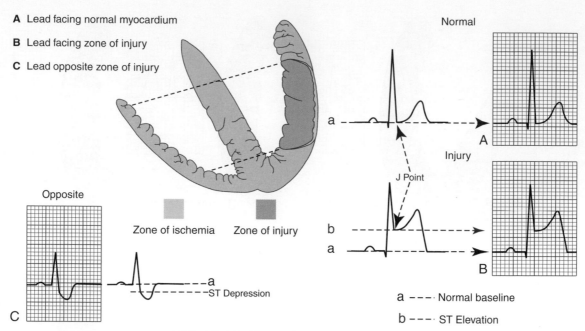

A Lead facing normal myocardium

B Lead facing zone of injury

C Lead opposite zone of injury

Zone of ischemia   Zone of injury

Opposite

Normal

Injury

J Point

a - - - - ST Depression

a - - - - Normal baseline

b - - - - ST Elevation

FIG. 15.11 The mechanism of ST elevation.

a non–Q-wave MI. An ST segment is considered elevated when it is 1 mm (0.1 mV) above the baseline, measured 0.04 second (1 small square) after the J point of the QRS complex (Fig. 15.11).

ST elevation usually appears within minutes after the onset of infarction, initially indicating extensive myocardial ischemia and foreshadowing a progression first to myocardial injury within 20 to 40 minutes (average, 30 minutes) and then to significant myocardial necrosis in about 2 hours. The ST segment is elevated in the leads facing the zone of ischemia and injury and is depressed in the reciprocal leads. ST-segment elevation may be accompanied by an increase in the size of the R wave, but as the ischemia continues, the R wave becomes smaller.

The cause of ST-segment elevation in acute MI is the "current of injury," an electrical manifestation of the inability of cardiac cells injured by severe ischemia to maintain a normal resting membrane potential during phase 4 of the cardiac action potential (see Chapter 1).

After the ischemic and injury phases, as the MI progresses, the injured myocardial tissue turns necrotic, and the current of injury disappears as the tissue becomes electrically silent. The ST segment becomes less elevated in the facing leads and finally returns to the baseline.

ST Depression

ST-segment depression is an ECG sign of subendocardial ischemia and injury. Similar to the criteria for ST elevation, an ST segment is considered depressed when it is 1 mm (0.1 mV) below the baseline, measured 0.04 second (1 small square) after the J point of the QRS complex.

ST depression usually appears within minutes after the onset of a subendocardial non–Q-wave MI and during an anginal attack. ST depression may also be seen, but less often, in a Q-wave MI. The ST-segment depression is usually seen in multiple leads

and cannot be used reliably to localize the area of ischemia.

The ST-segment depression of subendocardial ischemia and injury has been classified as to the shape of the segment, such as downsloping, horizontal, and upsloping (Fig. 15.12). The downsloping of an ST segment is most specific for subendocardial ischemia and injury. Horizontal sloping is of intermediate specificity, and upsloping is the least specific. Regardless of the slope, a depressed ST segment associated with an ischemic T wave is a reliable manifestation of myocardial ischemia.

ST-segment depression quickly reverts to normal after an anginal attack as the ischemia resolves and usually returns to normal after MI.

> **AUTHOR'S NOTE** The definitions used for ST-segment elevation and depression presented in this text are considered the simplest way of interpreting their cause. Other texts use more complex reasoning, and the reader should be aware that the exact mechanism for these ECG changes is debatable.

Q WAVE

The Q wave is the first negative deflection of the QRS complex. It may be normal (physiologic) or abnormal (pathologic) (Fig. 15.13).

Physiologic Q Wave

A physiologic Q wave is the result of the normal depolarization of the interventricular septum from left to right. For this reason, the small normal q waves are referred to as *septal q waves*. These relatively small electrical impulses are the first step in depolarization of the ventricles. The electrical forces responsible for the normal Q wave are negative because they travel away from the leads in which they appear. They move in the direction opposite

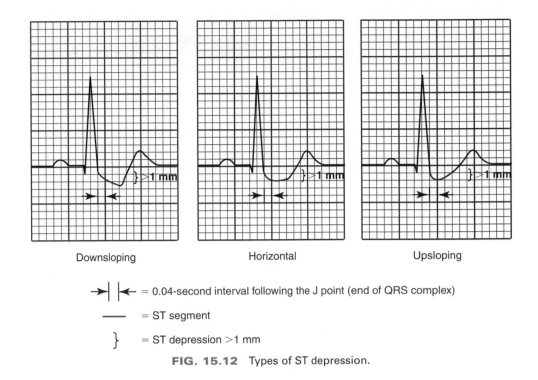

Downsloping   Horizontal   Upsloping

➤| |◄— = 0.04-second interval following the J point (end of QRS complex)

——— = ST segment

} = ST depression >1 mm

FIG. 15.12 Types of ST depression.

the positive electrical impulses producing the R wave. Because the interventricular septum is thin, the electrical forces are small and of short duration. The resultant septal q wave is less than 0.04 second wide. Its depth is less than 25% of the height of the following R wave. This small, normal q wave is usually present in leads I, II, III, aVL, aVF, V_5, and V_6.

Pathologic Q Wave

A Q wave produced by irreversible myocardial necrosis after an MI is referred to as a *pathologic Q wave*. It is defined as a Q wave of at least 0.04 second in duration and having a depth of at least 25% of the height of the following R wave. In the precordial leads, the Q wave may be so deep that it only returns to the baseline as the S wave. In this case there is no R wave at all, and the complex is referred to as a *QS wave*. Despite the absence of an R wave, the Q wave is pathologic because in the normal condition, an R wave would be present. For example, the normal R wave begins small in V_1 and V_2 and becomes progressively larger across the remaining precordial leads to V_6. This is referred to as *R-wave progression*.

A pathologic Q wave appears in less than 50% of patients with MI. When it does appear, it does so within 8 to 12 hours of the onset of the MI. It reaches its maximum size within 24 to 48 hours. It typically appears in the facing leads directly over necrotic, infarcted myocardial tissue—the zone of infarction. A pathologic Q wave may persist indefinitely or disappear in a few months or years. An MI with a pathologic Q wave is called a *Q-wave MI*.

The cause of a pathologic Q wave differs from that of a normal Q wave. A popular concept is referred to as the *window theory*. It proposes that because the infarcted myocardium does not depolarize or repolarize, no electrical impulses are generated,

producing an electrically silent area. This electrically silent area can be visualized as a window through which the facing leads actually view the endocardium of the opposite ventricular wall. Because depolarization progresses from the endocardium outward, the electrical impulses generated by the wall opposite the infarct will be traveling away from the leads facing the infarct. Therefore these leads will detect the electrical impulses generated by the opposite ventricular wall as large negative Q waves.

The presence and size of the pathologic Q wave and the number of leads in which it occurs depend on the size of the infarct. The larger the infarct, the larger the window. Consequently, the larger the Q wave is and the greater the number of contiguous leads in which it appears.

In contrast, the smaller the infarct, the smaller is the Q wave in both width and depth, and the fewer the facing leads with a Q wave. If the infarct is relatively small, involving only the subendocardial region, a pathologic Q wave may be absent, producing a non–Q-wave MI. Occasionally, a transmural MI, if small enough, will not generate a pathologic Q wave.

A large Q wave may be present in certain leads without being considered pathologic. A Q wave is usually ignored in the following leads, especially if it occurs under certain circumstances. Table 15.6 lists the leads and conditions under which such a Q wave may be considered clinically irrelevant.

AUTHOR'S NOTE Although it is true that the ST elevation refers to injury, its presence in contiguous leads is used to determine the location of the infarction because the goal of treatment is to limit the degree of damage and necrosis. Because Q waves don't appear until after the damage, they are not a reliable means of locating the infarction in the emergent situation.

Normal

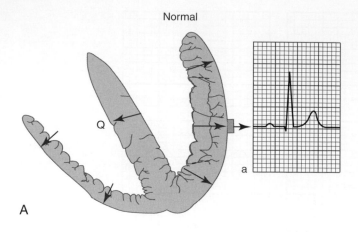

A

Transmural MI

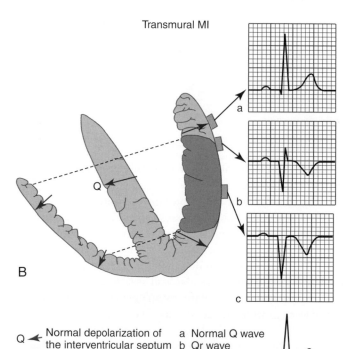

B

Q ←── Normal depolarization of
     the interventricular septum
▨ Necrotic tissue

a Normal Q wave
b Qr wave
c QS wave

FIG. 15.13 Physiologic and pathologic Q waves.

TABLE 15.6	Conditions Under Which a Q Wave May Be Considered Clinically Irrelevant
Lead	**Interpretation**
aVR	Q wave usually ignored because the QRS complex in this lead normally consists of a large S wave.
aVL	QS or QR wave in lead aVL alone in which the QRS axis is greater than 60° (that is, an electrically vertical heart) is usually ignored.
aVF	QS or QR wave alone is considered insignificant unless accompanied by a significant Q wave, ST-segment elevation, and abnormal T-wave changes in one or both of the other inferior leads (II and III).
III	Q wave by itself is considered insignificant unless both of the following are true: 1. It is accompanied by significant Q wave, ST-segment elevation, and abnormal T-wave changes in the other inferior leads (lead II or aVF or both). 2. The Q wave in lead III is wider and deeper than those in leads II and aVF.
V_1	Q wave by itself is considered insignificant unless it is accompanied by ST-segment elevation and abnormal T-wave changes in the other precordial leads (leads V_2–V_6).

Other considerations

- Q waves in the presence of left bundle-branch block and left anterior and posterior fascicular blocks are usually not considered significant.
- The presence of right bundle-branch block does not affect the significance of Q waves.
- Left ventricular hypertrophy may or may not affect the significance of Q waves.

present. Because there are no facing leads in a posterior MI, there are no diagnostic ST-segment elevations or pathologic Q waves present in the ECG leads. A posterior MI is diagnosed if reciprocal ECG changes of ST-segment depression and tall R waves are present in leads V_1 to V_4. This topic will be discussed in detail in the next chapter.

TAKE-HOME POINTS

- The myocardium is perfused by the left and right coronary arteries, which branch and feed specific areas of the heart with oxygen. Interruption of blood supply to specific coronary arteries causes myocardial ischemia and infarction of predictable areas of the heart.
- Atheromatous plaques form in the coronary arteries because of coronary artery disease. By a combination of erosion or disruption, such a plaque can occlude the coronary artery.
- When coronary artery perfusion is diminished from any cause, an ACS can be the result. The three recognized syndromes are unstable angina, NSTEMI, and STEMI.
- Once a plaque ruptures, thrombus formation begins. The phases of thrombosis involve multiple blood and tissue components, the action of which may be inhibited by administering pharmacologic agents.

Tables 15.7 and 15.8 summarize the ECG changes that occur during the four phases of transmural and nontransmural MIs, respectively.

Determining the Site of a Q-Wave Myocardial Infarction

The location of an acute Q-wave MI is determined by the facing leads in which ST-segment elevation and pathologic Q wave appear (Table 15.9 and Fig. 15.14). To reliably identify the anatomic location of the infarction, the ECG changes must be present in two or more contiguous leads—that is, two or more leads that face and view the same area of the heart. For example, if ST-segment elevation and/or pathologic Q waves appear in any V_1 to V_6, the MI is in the anterior wall of the left ventricle and is referred to as an *anterior MI*. If ST-segment elevation and/or pathologic Q waves appear in leads II, III, and aVF, the MI is said to be *inferior*. If, in an inferior infarction, the ST segment in V_{4R} also becomes elevated, a so-called right ventricular MI is

TABLE 15.7	ECG Changes in the Facing Leads During Transmural Myocardial Infarction				
Phase of Infarction	**Q Wave**	**R Wave**	**ST Segment**	**T Wave**	**ECG**
Phase 1 (0–2 hr) Onset of extensive ischemia occurs immediately, subendocardial injury occurs within 20–40 min, and subendocardial necrosis occurs in about 30 min; necrosis extends to about half of the myocardial wall by 2 hr	Unchanged	Unchanged or abnormally all	Onset of elevation	Amplitude increases; peaking may occur	
Phase 2 (2–24 hr) Transmural infarction is considered complete by 6 hr as necrosis involves about 90% of the myocardial wall; the rest of the necrosis occurs by the end of phase 2	Width and depth begin to increase	Amplitude begins to decrease	Maximum elevation	Amplitude and peaking lessen; T wave still positive	
Phase 3 (24–72 hr) Little or no ischemia or injury remains as healing begins	Reaches maximum size	Absent	Returns to baseline	Become maximally inverted	
Phase 4 (2–8 wk) Replacement of the necrotic tissue by fibrous tissue	Q wave persists	May return partially	Usually normal	Slight inversion	

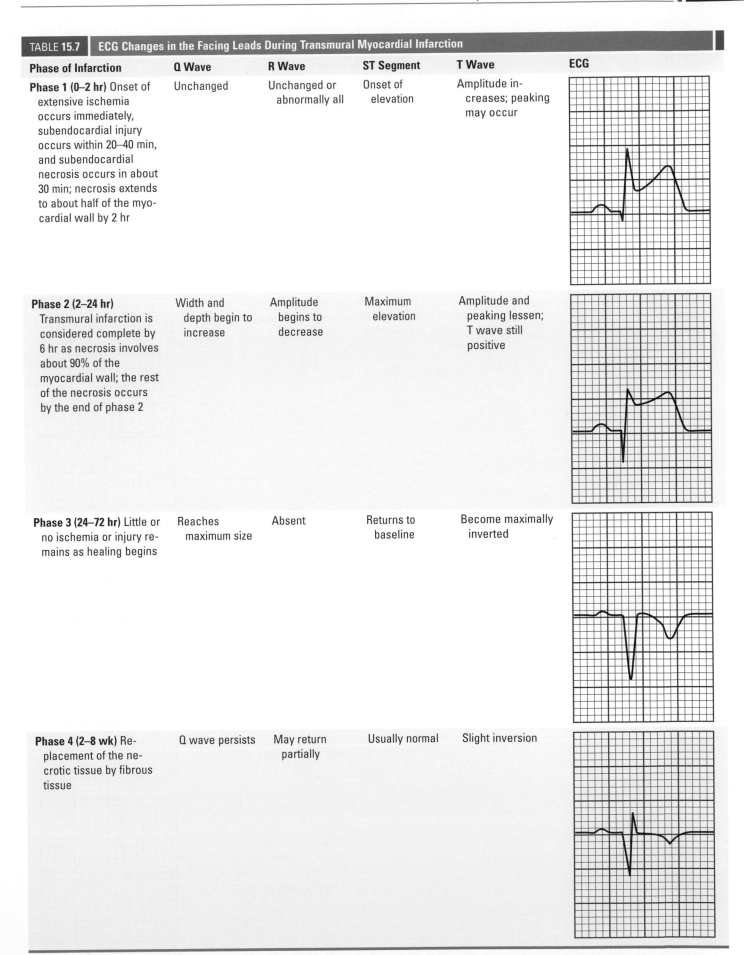

TABLE 15.8	ECG Changes in the Facing Leads During Nontransmural Myocardial Infarction				
Phase of Infarction	**Q Wave**	**R Wave**	**ST Segment**	**T Wave**	**ECG**
Phase 1 (0–2 hr) Onset of localized ischemia occurs immediately; subendocardial injury occurs within 20–40 min, and subendocardial necrosis occurs in about 30 min	Unchanged	Unchanged	Onset of depression	Amplitude may or may not increase slightly	
Phase 2 (2–24 hr) Subendocardial infarction is considered complete by 6 hr; generally, the necrosis involves only the inner parts of the myocardium (usually the subendocardial area), without extending to the epicardial surface	Unchanged	Amplitude may begin to decrease somewhat	Maximal level of depression	Inversion may occur	
Phase 3 (24–72 hr) Little or no ischemia or injury remains as healing begins	Unchanged	Unchanged	Usually returns to normal	Inversion may occur	
Phase 4 (2–8 wk) Infarcted tissue is replaced by fibrous tissue	Unchanged	Unchanged	Usually returns to normal	Usually returns to normal	

TABLE 15.9	Leads Relative to the Site of Myocardial Infarction	
Site of Infarction	**Facing Leads**	**Reciprocal Leads**
Septal (interventricular septum)	V_1–V_2	None
Anterior wall (localized)	V_3–V_4	None
Anteroseptal (anterior wall and septum)	V_1–V_4	None
Lateral wall	I, aVL, and V_5 or V_6	II, III, and aVF
Anterolateral wall	I, aVL, and V_3–V_6	II, III, and aVF
Extensive infarct of anterior wall	I, aVL, and V_1–V_6	II, III, and aVF
Inferior wall	II, III, and aVF	I and aVL
Posterior wall	None	V_1–V_4
Right ventricle	II, III, aVF, and V_{4R}	I and aVL

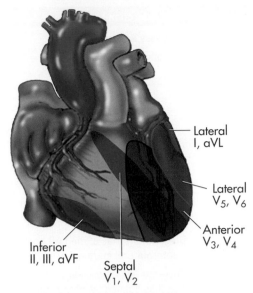

Lateral
I, aVL

Lateral
V_5, V_6

Anterior
V_3, V_4

Inferior
II, III, aVF

Septal
V_1, V_2

FIG. 15.14 Site of infarction associated with each ECG lead.

- Likewise, thrombolysis involves multiple steps and may be augmented by drug therapy.
- The specific ECG changes associated with ACSs include ischemic T waves, ST-segment elevation and depression, and pathologic Q waves.
- The presence of these ECG changes in specific leads correlates with the anatomic location of the ischemia, injury, and/or infarction.
- Facing leads are those in which the positive electrode directly views the area of injury or ischemia, whereas reciprocal leads view the area of injury or ischemia from the opposite direction.
- Two or more leads that view the same area of the heart are called *contiguous leads*.

- T-wave changes are associated with myocardial ischemia, ST elevation is associated with injury, and pathologic Q waves are associated with MI.
- ST elevation is an indicator of a transmural MI, whereas ST depression is an indicator of a subendocardial MI.
- A transmural MI results in Q-wave formation if sufficient myocardium is infarcted, whereas a subendocardial MI does not result in Q-wave formation.
- Table 15.10 details the relationship between the location of the infarction, the coronary arteries occluded, the facing ECG leads, and the complications that may occur.

TABLE 15.10	Myocardial Infarction Location and Associated Coronary Circulation, Facing ECG Leads, and Complications		
Type	**Coronary Arteries Involved**	**Facing Leads**	**Complications**
Septal MI	Septal perforator arteries of the LAD	V_1–V_2 (ST)	AV block: Second-degree type II AV block[a] Second-degree 2:1 and advanced AV block[a] Third-degree AV block[a] Bundle-branch block: RBBB LBBB LAFB LPFB[b]
Anterior (localized) MI	Diagonal arteries of the LAD	V_3–V_4 (ST)	LV dysfunction: CHF Cardiogenic shock
Lateral MI	Diagonal arteries of the LAD and/or the anterolateral marginal artery of the LCx	I, aVL, V_5–V_6 (ST)	LV dysfunction: CHF (moderate)
Inferior MI	Posterior left ventricular arteries of the RCA or, less commonly, of the LCx. The posterior descending coronary artery and the AV node artery may also be involved.	II, III, aVF (ST)	LV dysfunction: CHF (mild, if any) AV block: First-degree AV block[c] Second-degree type I AV block[c] Second-degree 2:1 and advanced AV block[c] Third-degree AV block[c] Bundle-branch block: LPFB[d]
Posterior MI	Distal LCx and/or posterolateral marginal artery of the LCx	None Opposite leads: V_1–V_4 (STg)	LV dysfunction: CHF (mild, if any)
Right ventricular MI	RCA, including the SA node and AV node arteries, the posterior descending coronary artery, and the posterior left ventricular arteries	II, III, aVF, V_{4R} (ST)	RV dysfunction: Right heart failure Rhythms: Sinus arrest Sinus bradycardia Atrial premature beats Atrial flutter Atrial fibrillation AV blocks: First-degree AV block[c] Second-degree type I AV block[c] Second-degree 2:1 and advanced AV block[c] Third-degree AV block[c] Bundle-branch blocks: LPFB[d]

g, ST-segment depression; *AV,* atrioventricular; *CHF,* congestive heart failure; *LAD,* left anterior descending coronary artery; *LAFB,* left anterior fascicular block; *LBBB,* left bundle branch block; *LCx,* left circumflex artery; *LPFB,* left posterior fascicular block; *LV,* left ventricular; *MI,* myocardial infarction; *RBBB,* right bundle branch block; *RCA,* right coronary artery; *RV,* right ventricular; *SA,* sinoatrial.

[a] With an abnormally wide QRS complex.

[b] In conjunction with right ventricular or inferior infarction.

c With a normal QRS complex.

[d] In conjunction with septal infarction.

CHAPTER REVIEW QUESTIONS

1. Which artery arises from the left main coronary artery at an obtuse angle and runs posteriorly along the left atrioventricular groove, ending over the posterior wall of the left ventricle?
   A. Left anterior descending coronary artery
   B. Left circumflex coronary artery
   C. Right ventricular artery
   D. Septal perforator artery

2. Which artery most often supplies the SA node with blood?
   A. The conus artery
   B. The left anterior descending coronary artery
   C. The left circumflex coronary
   D. The RCA

3. What is the most common cause of MI?
   A. Cocaine toxicity
   B. Coronary artery spasm
   C. Increased myocardial workload
   D. Occlusion of an atherosclerotic coronary artery

4. What is the most common cause of acute MI?
   A. Air embolism
   B. Coronary artery spasm
   C. Coronary thrombosis
   D. Hypertension

5. What happens when necrotic cells are supplied with blood and oxygen?
   A. They do not return to normal function.
   B. They return to normal or near-normal function.
   C. They revert to a previous state of injury.
   D. They usually return to normal in about 24 hours.

6. Which term describes an MI in which the zone of infarction involves the entire full thickness of the ventricular wall, from the endocardium to the epicardial surface?
   A. Necrotic infarction
   B. Nontransmural infarction
   C. Subendocardial infarction
   D. Transmural infarction

7. The window theory best describes the mechanism for the presence of which of the following?
   A. Inverted T waves
   B. Pathologic Q wave
   C. ST-segment elevation
   D. ST-segment depression

8. The appearance of inverted or tall, peaked T waves in a facing lead during the early phase of an acute MI indicates what?
   A. Infarct
   B. Injury
   C. Ischemia
   D. Necrosis

9. The most likely cause of an inferior MI is an occlusion of which artery?
   A. Anterolateral marginal artery
   B. Left anterior descending coronary artery
   C. Posterior descending coronary artery
   D. RCA

10. Which of the following represents the primary ECG finding in a transmural MI?
    A. ST-segment depression
    B. Q waves
    C. T-wave inversion
    D. Hyperacute R waves

16

ECG Diagnosis of Myocardial Infarction

Myocardial infarction (MI) evolves through several stages. At the onset of ischemia and injury, the MI is referred to as *acute*. ECG changes are specific to the area of the heart involved in the MI. During acute MI, ST-segment and T-wave changes are predominant. If quickly treated, the ECG can return to normal after acute MI.

acute MI

The initial 24 hours after the onset of an MI.

In most cases, however, a sufficient amount of muscle dies to promote the development of late ECG changes. Late ECG changes, which occur over the next 24 to 72 hours, generally manifest as pathologic Q waves. Therefore the presence of a Q wave indicates that the patient had an MI in the area reflected by the ECG.

late ECG changes

Pathologic Q waves or other changes that occur 24 to 72 hours after the onset of MI, indicating the area of infarction.

AUTHOR'S NOTE The ECG changes presented for each specific MI are based on typical first-time infarcts. They may not represent actual changes in a particular patient's ECG. Variations can occur for many reasons: individual differences in the size of the heart and its position and rotation within the chest, distribution of the coronary artery circulation, the presence of a bundle-branch block or ventricular hypertrophy, history of MI, and coexisting ECG changes attributable to drugs or electrolyte imbalances.

SEPTAL MYOCARDIAL INFARCTION

Coronary Arteries Involved and Site of Occlusion

Left coronary artery, specifically the left anterior descending (LAD) beyond the first diagonal branch, involving the septal perforator arteries (Fig. 16.1).

Location of Infarct

The anterior wall of the left ventricle overlying the interventricular septum and the anterior two-thirds of the interventricular septum.

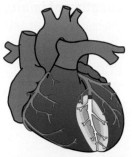

Infarct-related arteries

Left anterior descending septal perforator branches

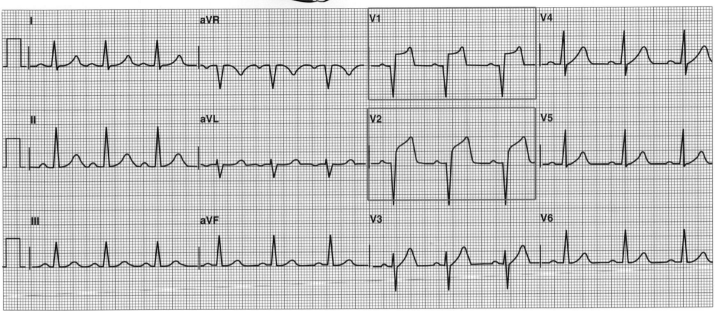

FIG. 16.1   Septal myocardial infarction.

TABLE 16.1	ECG Changes in Septal Myocardial Infarction			
	Q Wave	**R Wave**	**ST Segment**	**T Wave**
Acute	Absent septal q wave in I, II, III, aVF, and V_4–V_6 QS wave in V_1–V_2	Absent septal r wave in V_1–V_2	Elevated in V_1–V_2	Sometimes abnormally tall, with peaking in V_1–V_2
Late	QS complex in V_1–V_2	Same as in phase 1	Return of ST segment to baseline throughout	T-wave inversion in V_1–V_2

ECG Changes

In acute MI, there is an absence of the small r wave that normally appears in the right precordial leads V_1 to V_2, producing a QS wave in these leads. Because this r wave indicates depolarization of the interventricular septum, it is referred to as a *septal r wave*. The small septal q wave that normally appears in leads I, II, III, aVF, and V_4 to V_6 is also absent. Other ECG changes associated with a septal MI are summarized in Table 16.1.

AUTHOR'S NOTE Applying the electrodes for the precordial leads can result in the septal r waves appearing smaller than normal or not being present at all. To avoid this, you should ensure that the electrodes for V_1 to V_2 are applied in the correct position (on both sides of sternum at the fourth intercostal space).

ANTERIOR MYOCARDIAL INFARCTION

Coronary Arteries Involved

The left coronary artery, specifically the diagonal arteries of the LAD (Fig. 16.2).

Location of Infarct

The anterior wall of the left ventricle immediately to the left of the interventricular septum.

ECG Changes

Table 16.2 summarizes the ECG changes associated with an anterior MI.

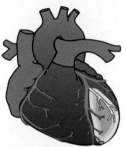

Infarct-related arteries
Left anterior descending diagonal branches

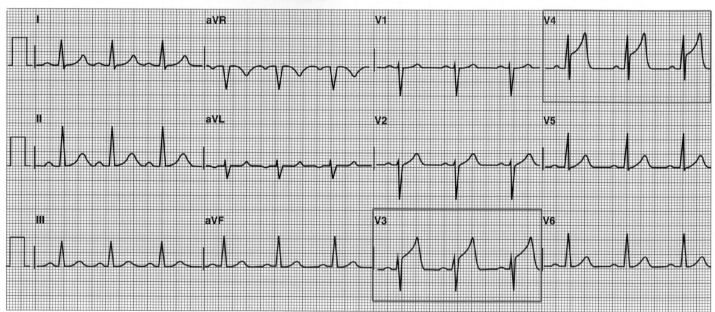

FIG. 16.2 Anterior (localized) myocardial infarction.

TABLE 16.2	ECG Changes in Anterior Myocardial Infarction			
	Q Wave	**R Wave**	**ST Segment**	**T Wave**
Acute	Normal Q wave	Normal or abnormally tall R wave in V_3–V_4	Elevated in V_3–V_4	Sometimes abnormally tall, with peaking in V_3–V_4
Late	QS complex in V_3–V_4	Absent in V_3–V_4	Return of ST segment to baseline throughout	T-wave inversion in V_3–V_4

ANTEROSEPTAL MYOCARDIAL INFARCTION

Coronary Arteries Involved

The left coronary artery, specifically the LAD, involving both the septal perforator and diagonal arteries (Fig. 16.3).

Location of Infarct

The anterior wall of the left ventricle overlying the interventricular septum and immediately to its left, along with the anterior two-thirds of the interventricular septum.

ECG Changes

Table 16.3 summarizes the ECG changes in an anteroseptal MI.

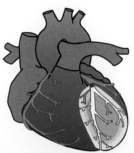

Infarct-related arteries

Left anterior descending
septal perforator branches
diagonal branches

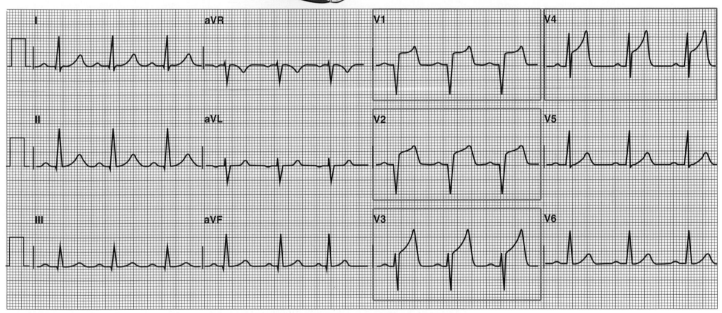

FIG. 16.3 Anteroseptal myocardial infarction.

TABLE 16.3	ECG Changes in Anteroseptal Myocardial Infarction			
	Q Wave	**R Wave**	**ST Segment**	**T Wave**
Acute	Absent septal q wave where normally present in I, II, III, aVF, and V_4–V_6 QS wave in V_1–V_2	Absent septal r wave in V_1–V_2 Normal or abnormally tall R wave in V_3–V_4	Elevated in V_1–V_4	Sometimes abnormally tall, with peaking in V_1–V_4
Late	Absence of normal septal r waves produces QS complex in V_1–V_4	Absent in V_1–V_4	Return of the ST segments to the baseline throughout	T-wave inversion in V_1–V_4

▌LATERAL MYOCARDIAL INFARCTION

Coronary Arteries Involved

The left coronary artery is affected. More specifically, the diagonal arteries of the LAD and/or the anterolateral marginal artery of the left circumflex coronary artery (LCx) (Fig. 16.4).

Location of Infarct

The lateral wall of the left ventricle.

ECG Changes

Table 16.4 summarizes the ECG changes that occur in a lateral MI.

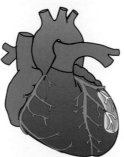

Infarct-related arteries

Left anterior descending
septal perforator branches
diagonal branches

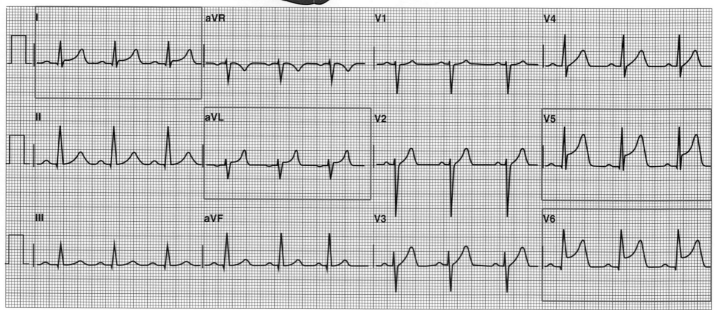

FIG. 16.4 Lateral myocardial infarction.

TABLE 16.4	ECG Changes in Lateral MI			
	Q Wave	**R Wave**	**ST Segment**	**T Wave**
Acute	Minimally abnormal in I, aVL, and V$_5$ or V$_6$ or both	Normal or abnormally tall R wave in I, aVL, and V$_5$ or V$_6$ or both	Elevated in I, aVL, and V$_5$ or V$_6$ or both Depressed in II, III, and aVF	Sometimes abnormally tall, with peaking in I, aVL, and V$_5$ or V$_6$ or both
Late	Significantly abnormal in I and aVL QS wave or complex in V$_5$ or V$_6$ or both	Decreased or absent in V$_5$ or V$_6$ or both Small R wave in I and aVL	Return of ST segment to baseline throughout	T-wave inversion in I, aVL, and V$_5$ or V$_6$ or both Tall T wave in II, III, and aVF

ANTEROLATERAL MYOCARDIAL INFARCTION

Coronary Arteries Involved

The major artery involved is the left coronary artery, specifically the diagonal arteries of the LAD, either alone or with the anterolateral marginal artery of the LCx (Fig. 16.5).

Location of Infarct

The anterior and lateral walls of the left ventricle.

ECG Changes

Table 16.5 summarizes the ECG changes in an anterolateral MI.

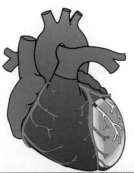

Infarct-related arteries

Left anterior descending diagonal branches

Left circumflex anterolateral marginal branch

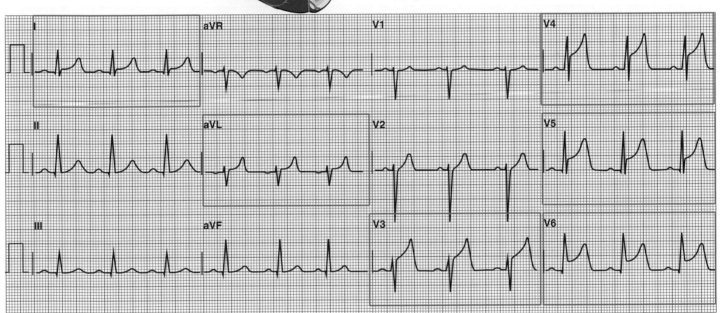

FIG. 16.5 Anterolateral myocardial infarction.

TABLE 16.5	ECG Changes in Anterolateral Myocardial Infarction			
	Q Wave	**R Wave**	**ST Segment**	**T Wave**
Acute	Minimally abnormal in I, aVL, and V_3–V_5	Normal or abnormally tall R wave in I, aVL, and V_3–V_6	Elevated in I, aVL, and V_3–V_6 Depressed in II, III, and aVF	Sometimes abnormally tall, with peaking in I, aVL, and V_3–V_6
Late	Significantly abnormal in I and aVL QS wave or complex in V_3–V_6	Decreased or absent in V_3–V_6 Small R wave in I and aVL	Return of ST segment to baseline throughout	T-wave inversion in I, aVL, and V_3–V_6 Tall T wave in II, III, and aVF

EXTENSIVE ANTERIOR MYOCARDIAL INFARCTION

Coronary Arteries Involved

The left coronary artery, specifically the LAD, either alone or with the anterolateral marginal artery of the LCx (Fig. 16.6).

Location of Infarct

The entire anterior and lateral walls of the left ventricle and the anterior two-thirds of the interventricular septum.

ECG Changes

A combination of all changes seen in anteroseptal, anterior, and anterolateral MIs is seen on ECG in an extensive anterior MI. Table 16.6 summarizes those changes.

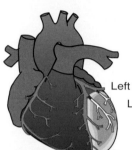

Infarct-related arteries

Left anterior descending septal perforator branches diagonal branches

Left circumflex anterolateral marginal branch

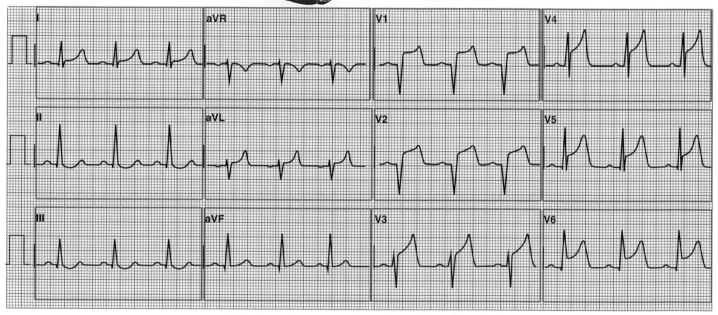

FIG. 16.6   Extensive anterior myocardial infarction.

TABLE 16.6	ECG Changes in Extensive Anterior Myocardial Infarction			
	Q Wave	**R Wave**	**ST Segment**	**T Wave**
Acute	Absent septal q wave in leads I, II, III, aVR, and V_4–V_6 QS wave in V_1–V_2	Absent septal r wave in V_1–V_2 Normal or abnormally tall R wave in I, aVL, and V_3–V_6	Elevated in I, aVL, and V_1–V_6 Depressed in II, III, and aVF	Sometimes abnormally tall, with peaking in I, aVL, and V_1–V_6
Late	Significantly abnormal in I and aVL QS wave or complex in V_1–V_6	Absent in V_1–V_2 Decreased or absent in V_3–V_6 Small R wave in I and aVL	Return of ST segment to baseline throughout	T-wave inversion in I and aVL; absent in V_1–V_6 Tall T wave in II, III, and aVF

INFERIOR MYOCARDIAL INFARCTION

Coronary Arteries Involved

The posterior left ventricular arteries of the right coronary artery (RCA) or, less often, the LCx of the left coronary artery. The posterior descending coronary artery (PDA) and the atrioventricular (AV)-node artery may also be involved (Fig. 16.7).

Location of Infarct

The inferior wall of the left ventricle that rests on the diaphragm. If the LCx is occluded, the infarction extends somewhat into the lateral wall of the left ventricle, causing an inferolateral MI. If the PDA and the AV-node artery are involved, the MI extends into the posterior third of the interventricular septum and the AV node as well.

ECG Changes

Table 16.7 summarizes the ECG changes characteristic of an inferior MI.

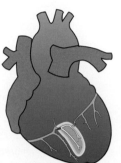

Infarct-related arteries

Right coronary (or left circumflex)
posterior left ventricular branches

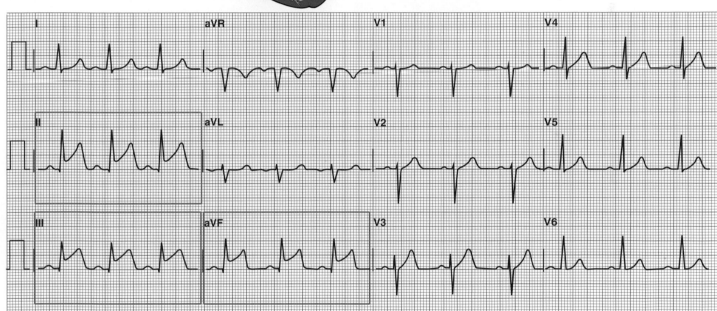

FIG. 16.7 Inferior myocardial infarction.

TABLE 16.7	ECG Changes in Inferior Myocardial Infarction			
	Q Wave	R Wave	ST Segment	T Wave
Acute	Normal Q wave	Normal or abnormally tall R wave in II, III, and aVF	Elevated in II, III, aVF Depressed in I and aVL	Sometimes abnormally tall, with peaking in II, III, and aVF
Late	QS wave or complex in II, III, and aVF	Decreased or absent in II, III, and aVF	Return of ST segment to baseline throughout	T wave inversion in II, III, and aVF Tall T wave in I and aVL

POSTERIOR MYOCARDIAL INFARCTION

Coronary Arteries Involved

The distal LCx and/or posterolateral marginal artery of the LCx (Fig. 16.8).

Location of Infarct

The posterior wall of the left ventricle, located just below the posterior left AV groove and extending to the inferior wall of the left ventricle.

ECG Changes

In a posterior MI, there are no facing leads. Changes that occur in the other leads are summarized in Table 16.8.

RIGHT VENTRICULAR MYOCARDIAL INFARCTION

Coronary Arteries Involved

The RCA with its distal branches—the posterior left ventricular arteries, the PDA, and the AV-node artery (Fig. 16.9).

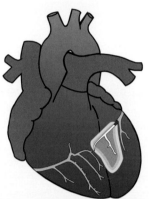

Infarct-related arteries

Distal left circumflex
and/or posterolateral
marginal branch

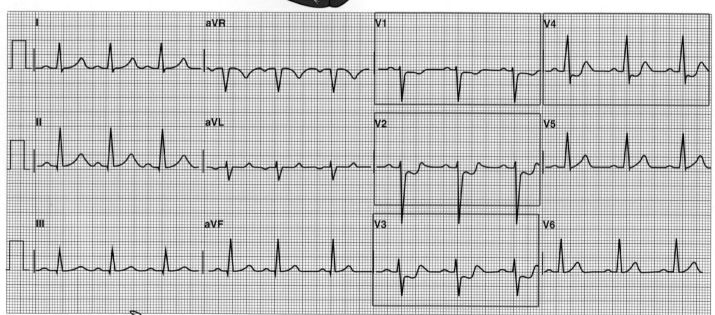

FIG. 16.8 Posterior myocardial infarction.

TABLE 16.8	ECG Changes in Posterior Myocardial Infarction				
	Q Wave	**R Wave**		**ST Segment**	**T Wave**
Acute	Normal Q wave	Normal R wave		Depressed in V_1–V_4	Inverted in V_1 and sometimes in V_2
Late	Same as in phase 1	Large R wave in V_1–V_4, with slurring and notching in V_1 S wave decreased in V_1, resulting in an R/S ratio of 1 in V_1		Return of ST segment to baseline throughout	Tall T wave in V_1–V_4

Location of Infarct

The anterior, posterior, inferior, and lateral walls of the right ventricle; the posterior third of the interventricular septum; the inferior wall of the left ventricle; and the AV node.

ECG Changes

Table 16.9 summarizes the ECG changes in a right ventricular MI.

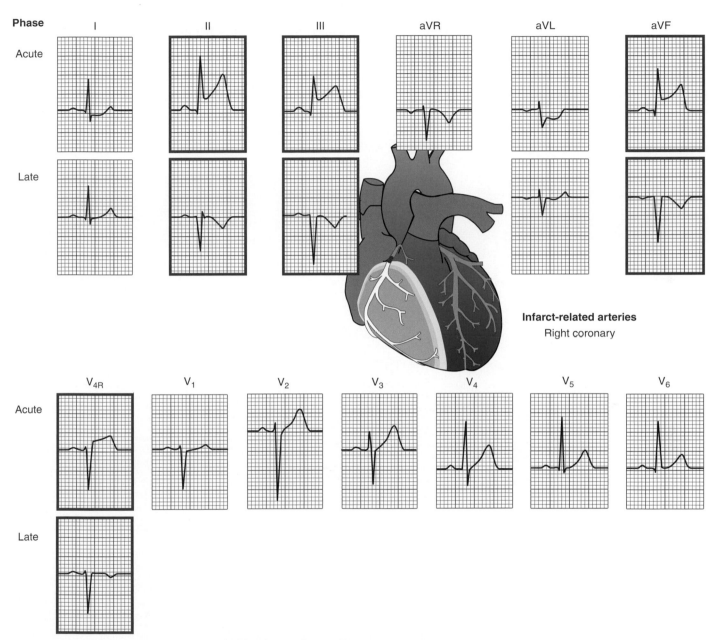

FIG. 16.9 Right ventricular myocardial infarction.

TABLE 16.9	ECG Changes in Right Ventricular Myocardial Infarction			
	Q Wave	**R Wave**	**ST Segment**	**T Wave**
Acute	Normal Q wave	Normal or abnormally tall R wave in II, III, and aVF	Elevated in II, III, aVF, and V_{4R} Depressed in I and aVL	Sometimes abnormally tall, with peaking in II, III, and aVF
Late	QS wave or complex in II, III, and aVF	Decreased or absent in II, III, and aVF	Return of ST segment to baseline throughout	T-wave inversion in II, III, aVF, and V_{4R} Tall T wave in I and aVL

DIAGNOSING MI IN THE PRESENCE OF BUNDLE-BRANCH BLOCK

Bundle-branch blocks result in significant widening of the QRS complex (greater than 120 ms). This can cause the terminal (final) portion of the QRS to slur into the ST segment, resulting in an ST segment that appears to be elevated or depressed compared with an ST segment following a normal and narrow QRS complex.

Right Bundle-Branch Block and MI

The QRS complex associated with a right bundle-branch block (RBBB) is generally positive (majority of the complex is upright) and returns normally to the baseline (Fig. 16.10). An

MI in the presence of RBBB is detected by the same criteria used in the 12-lead ECG without a bundle-branch block—that is, 1 mm or more of ST-segment elevation in the two or more contiguous precordial leads (Fig. 16.11) or 2 mm or more of ST-segment elevation in two or more contiguous limb leads (Fig. 16.12).

Left Bundle-Branch Block and MI

Detecting MI in the presence of a left bundle-branch block (LBBB) requires you to remember that the T wave is normally discordant (deflected in the opposite direction) to the terminal (final) portion of the QRS complex (Fig. 16.13). That is, the T wave deflects downward in the leads where the QRS complex is predominantly positive and upward in the leads where the QRS complex is predominantly negative. Some have proposed

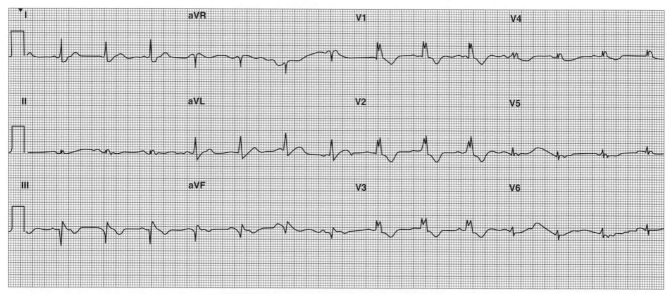

FIG. 16.10   Right bundle-branch block.

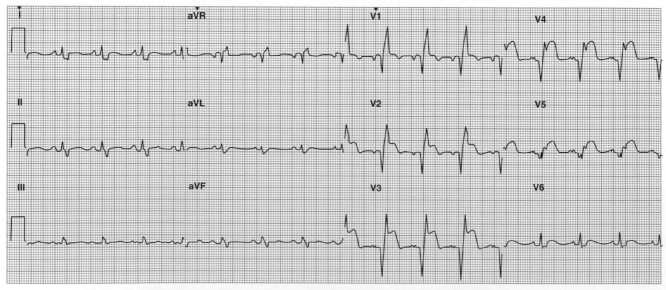

FIG. 16.11   Anterior myocardial infarction and right bundle-branch block.

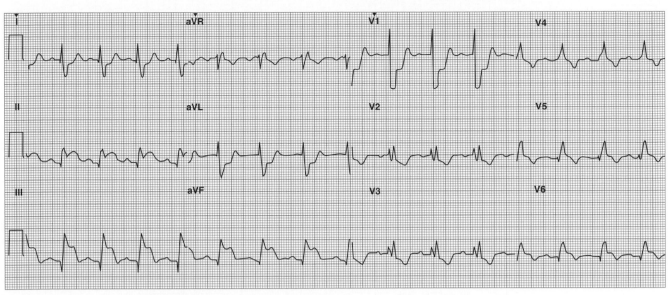

FIG. 16.12 Inferior myocardial infarction and right bundle-branch block.

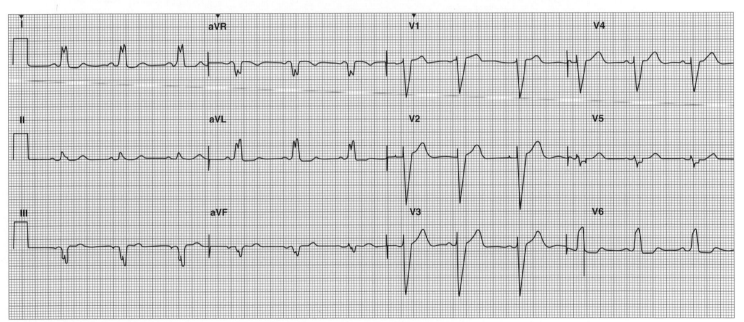

FIG. 16.13 Left bundle-branch block.

that the presence of a new LBBB in the context of a patient with acute coronary syndrome (ACS) signs and symptoms should be considered diagnostic for MI. However, this has resulted in a high false-positive rate, sending patients unnecessarily to the catheterization lab.

The *Sgarbossa* criteria (Fig. 16.14) have emerged to assist in the detection of MI (Figs. 16.15 and 16.16) in the presence of LBBB. They include the following;

1. Concordant ST elevation greater than 1 mm in leads with a positive QRS complex
2. Concordant ST depression greater than 1 mm in V_1 to V_3

3. Excessively discordant ST elevation greater than 5 mm in leads with a negative QRS complex

Additionally, the Sgarbossa criteria can be used in patients with an internal pacemaker. Remember that the QRS complex associated with a pacemaker is identical to that with a bundle-branch block.

AUTHOR'S NOTE The Sgarbossa criteria are very specific to the presence of an MI. However, they are not very sensitive, meaning that they are not always present in a patient with LBBB and MI.

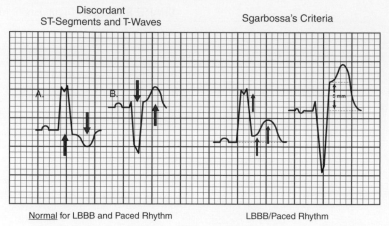

Discordant ST-Segments and T-Waves   Sgarbossa's Criteria

A.   B.

Normal for LBBB and Paced Rhythm   LBBB/Paced Rhythm

FIG. 16.14 Sgarbossa criteria and left bundle-branch block.

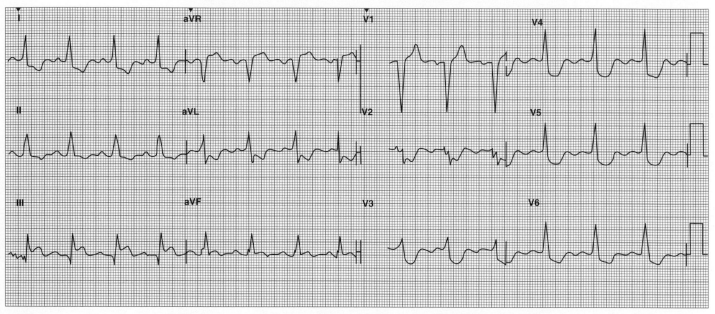

FIG. 16.15 Anterior myocardial infarction and left bundle-branch block.

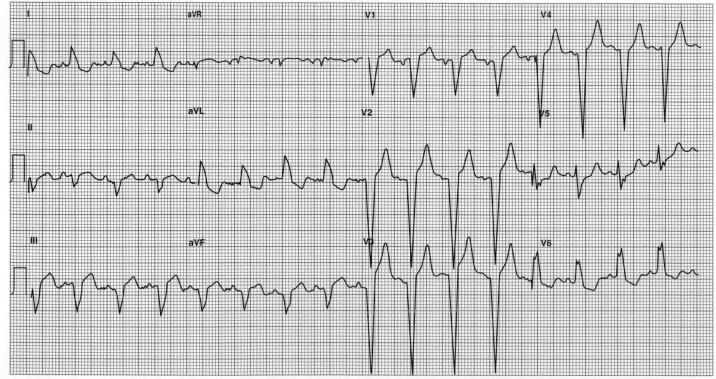

FIG. 16.16 Inferior myocardial infarction and left bundle-branch block.

DIAGNOSING MI IN THE PRESENCE OF LEFT VENTRICULAR HYPERTROPHY

Left ventricular hypertrophy (LVH) results in QRS complexes that are excessively tall. This is a result of the depolarization of an increased mass of myocardial tissue. Consequently, the repolarization is also altered, resulting in what appears to be ST elevation consistent with MI. This is particularly true in the precordial leads. Therefore, making the diagnosis of MI in the presence of LVH can be extremely difficult. The following approaches may be used to increase the likelihood that the ST-segment changes are a result of myocardial ischemia:

1. ST segment is greater than 2 mm in the inferior leads (Fig. 16.17).
2. ST-segment elevation in the precordial leads exceeds 25% of the depth or height of the RS wave (Fig. 16.18).

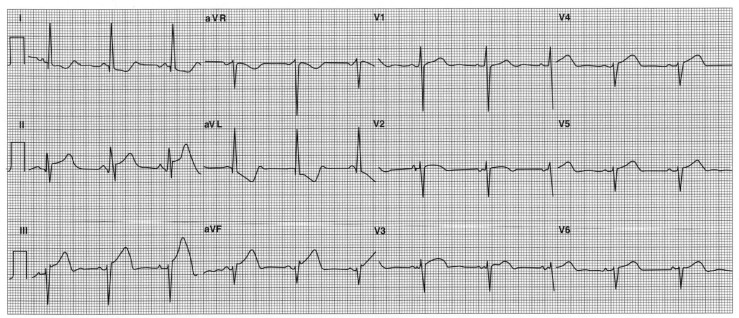

FIG. 16.17 Inferior myocardial infarction and left ventricular hypertrophy.

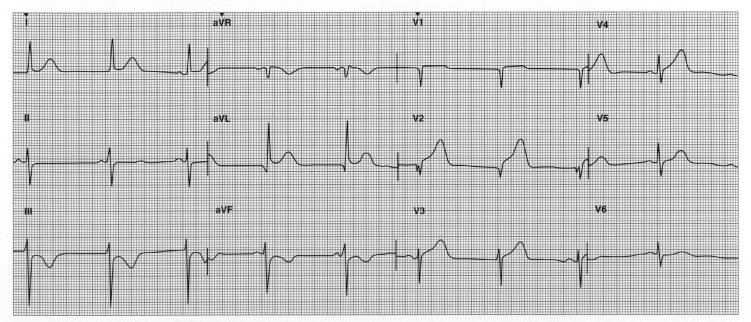

FIG. 16.18 Anterior myocardial infarction and left ventricular hypertrophy.

DISTINGUISHING PERICARDITIS FROM MYOCARDIAL INFARCTION

As described in Chapter 14, pericarditis is an inflammation of the pericardial sac, which envelops the heart. The ECG findings in pericarditis include ST-segment elevation and PR-segment depression in almost every lead except aVR and V_1 (Fig. 16.19). If only two or three contiguous leads are examined, you may misinterpret the ECG as being diagnostic of an MI. To avoid this, be sure to systematically examine every lead. Additionally, pericarditis can be localized to one area of the pericardium, leading to localized ST-segment elevation that also mimics ST-segment-elevation myocardial infarction (STEMI). The following findings support the diagnosis of STEMI versus pericarditis:

1. ST depression in any leads other than aVR or V_1
2. Convex or horizontal ST elevation
3. ST-segment elevation is greater in lead III than in lead II.

   Serial ECGs and cardiac biomarker levels may improve the diagnosis. However, if the patient's history and physical are consistent with ACS and there is any question that the ECG may represent STEMI, it is prudent to involve a cardiologist early and consider angiography.

TAKE-HOME POINTS

- Because the 12-lead ECG views the heart from different angles, the presence of ECG changes during an MI permits you to determine which part of the heart is involved.
- Knowing the coronary circulation allows you to predict which coronary artery is occluded.
- The ECG changes are either acute, occurring during the active ischemia and injury of the MI, or late, indicating that the MI has already occurred.
- Acute ECG changes in MI include ST-segment elevation and/or depression and T-wave inversion.
- Pathologic Q waves are the hallmark of late ECG findings as a result of MI.
- LBBB, LVH, and pericarditis are three of the most common conditions that make the ECG diagnosis of STEMI more difficult.
- The presence of the Sgarbossa criteria indicates an increased likelihood that a STEMI is present, whereas their absence does not eliminate the diagnosis of STEMI.
- LVH often causes nondiagnostic ST elevation that can be confused with STEMI.
- Pericarditis can be differentiated from STEMI in most cases. However, when the diagnosis is unclear, early angiography is indicated.

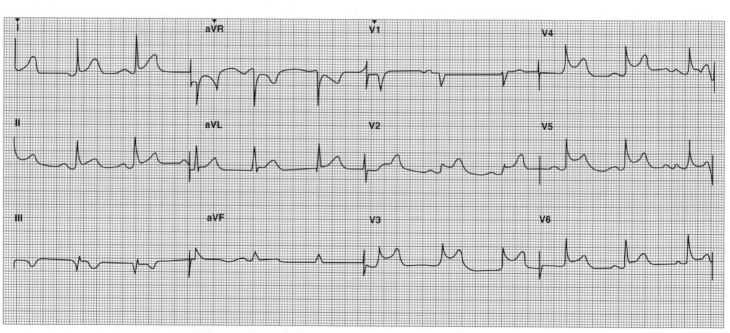

FIG. 16.19 Anterior myocardial infarction mimicking pericarditis.

CHAPTER REVIEW QUESTIONS

1. Which type of MI presents with ST-segment elevation, tall T waves, and taller-than-normal R waves in leads V_3 and V_4 and late with QS complexes and T-wave inversion in those leads?
   A. Anterior (localized) MI
   B. Anteroseptal MI
   C. Lateral MI
   D. Septal MI

2. Which of these MIs presents with ST-segment elevation, tall T waves, and taller-than-normal R waves in leads I, aVL, V_5, and/or V_6 in addition to ST-segment depression in leads II, III, and aVF?
   A. Anterior (localized)
   B. Anteroseptal
   C. Lateral
   D. Septal

3. Which type of MI presents late with QS complexes and T-wave inversion in leads V_1 to V_2 and absent normal septal q waves in leads II, III, and aVF?
   A. Anterior (localized)
   B. Anteroseptal
   C. Lateral
   D. Septal

4. Which type of MI presents acutely with ST-segment elevation, tall T waves, and taller-than-normal R waves in leads I, aVL, and V_3 to V_6 and ST-segment depression in leads II, III, and aVF?
   A. Anterior (localized) MI
   B. Anterolateral MI
   C. Lateral MI
   D. Septal MI

5. Which type of MI involves the posterior left ventricular arteries of the RCA or the LCx of the left coronary artery?
   A. Anteroseptal MI
   B. Inferior MI
   C. Left ventricular MI
   D. Posterior MI

6. Which type of MI presents acutely with ST-segment elevation, tall T waves, and taller-than-normal R waves in

leads II, III, and aVF and ST-segment depression in leads I and aVL?
   A. Anteroseptal MI
   B. Inferior MI
   C. Lateral MI
   D. Posterior MI

7. Which type of MI presents late with large R waves and tall T waves in leads V_1 to V_4, an R wave of 0. 04 second in width with slurring and notching in V_1, and an R/S ratio of 1 in V_1?
   A. Anteroseptal MI
   B. Inferior MI
   C. Posterior MI
   D. Right ventricular MI

8. The Sgarbossa criteria include each of the following except which one?
   A. Concordant ST elevation greater than 1 mm in leads with a positive QRS complex
   B. Discordant ST depression in two or more contiguous leads
   C. Concordant ST depression greater than 1 mm in V_1 to V_3
   D. Excessively discordant ST elevation greater than 5 mm in leads with a negative QRS complex

9. The diagnosis of STEMI in the presence of LVH is
   A. impossible.
   B. supported by the presence of ST-segment elevation or depression that is more than 25% the height of the RS wave.
   C. supported by the presence of discordant ST-segment depression only in lead aVR.
   D. excluded by the presence of ST-segment elevation of greater than 2 mm in the inferior leads II, III, and aVF.

10. The ECG findings that support the diagnosis of STEMI over pericarditis include all of the following except which one?
    A. ST depression in any leads other than aVR or V_1
    B. Convex or horizontal ST elevation
    C. ST-segment elevation that is greater in lead III than II
    D. ST depression only in leads aVR or V_1

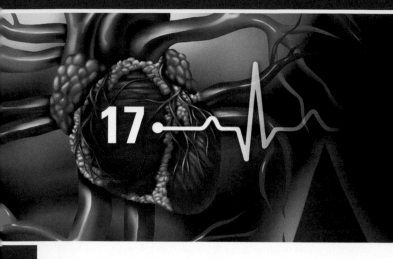

17 Diagnosis and Treatment of Acute Coronary Syndrome

Acute coronary syndrome (ACS) is so named because it represents a constellation of signs and symptoms, along with characteristic ECG findings, cardiac biomarkers, and risk factors for coronary heart disease. To make an accurate and efficient diagnosis, the first step is to recognize these signs and symptoms; perform a rapid assessment of the patient's risk; and obtain a diagnostic 12-lead ECG, proper lab tests, and appropriate consultations.

In the prehospital arena, it's vital to develop a standard strategy or approach to the patient with chest pain. This will help you determine quickly if the patient is having an ST-segment-elevation myocardial infarction (STEMI). If so, he or she must be rapidly delivered to a facility capable of performing reperfusion therapy. A reliable standard approach begins with a detailed history and physical examination, paying particular attention to the signs and symptoms of ACS.

Obtaining an accurate history remains crucial in diagnosing ACS. On the other hand, an inaccurate history can result in misinterpretation of the patient's ECG findings—a leading cause of malpractice suits from patients with unrecognized myocardial infarction (MI).

AUTHOR'S NOTE Maintaining a high index of suspicion for ACS when examining any patient with chest pain is vital to avoid failing to diagnose an MI. Three groups of patients at risk of unrecognized MI are women, the elderly, and people with diabetes.

PRESENTATION OF MYOCARDIAL INFARCTION

Sex- and Age-Related Differences

Studies show that women have STEMI at an older age than men. Although some variation exists, when large databases of MI patients are examined, the symptoms of STEMI are generally more alike than different in men and women. Older adults with STEMI are significantly less likely than younger patients to complain of chest discomfort. Older patients are more likely to report shortness of breath and other atypical symptoms, such as syncope, generalized weakness, and unexplained nausea.

Diabetes Mellitus

Patients with diabetes may have an impaired ability to recognize chest pain (angina). This is especially true if the patient has neuropathy involving the autonomic nervous system. A diabetic patient may misinterpret dyspnea, nausea, vomiting, fatigue, or diaphoresis as disturbances of glucose regulation. Up to 50% of people who have type 2 diabetes for longer than 10 years will have autonomic nervous system dysfunction manifested as impaired heart rate variability.

HISTORY TAKING IN SUSPECTED ACUTE CORONARY SYNDROME

History taking in patients with suspected ACS must be methodical, sufficiently thorough, and detailed, yet concise enough

There are three primary questions to be addressed:
1. Are signs and symptoms consistent with ACS?
2. Does the patient have risk factors for ACS?
3. If ST-segment-elevation myocardial infarction (STEMI) is present on the ECG, is the patient a candidate for reperfusion?

To expedite the interview, ask patients to describe their primary concern in their own words. Address those concerns, and then proceed with the following set of questions:
- Do you have any chest pain or discomfort?
  - If so, when did it start?
  - Rate it on a scale from 0 to 10, with 10 being the worst pain you've experienced and 0 being no pain at all.
  - Is it sharp or dull?
  - Does it radiate?
  - Does anything make it better or worse?
  - Have you taken anything for it? Did it help?
- Are you having any difficulty breathing, or are you feeling fatigued?
- Do you feel dizzy or light-headed, as if you might faint?
- Do you feel any numbness or tingling in your hands, feet, or limbs?
- Do you feel nauseated or have any other symptoms I should be aware of?

not to delay the initiation of reperfusion therapy if the patient is a suitable candidate. The questions to be addressed are listed in ECG Keys Box 17.1.

Chief Complaint

The most common physical complaint a patient with ACS has is chest discomfort or pain. The severity varies. It is usually rated on a scale of 0 to 10, with 10 being the most severe pain/discomfort and 0 being no pain/discomfort. It is important to keep in mind that many patients will not admit to having chest pain but will acknowledge feeling chest discomfort, pressure, or heaviness. Discomfort should be considered the same as pain. Chest discomfort is often described as a crushing, vicelike constriction. The patient may say that it feels like an elephant is sitting on their chest. Some patients describe the pain as heartburn or indigestion that is occasionally relieved by belching or burping.

The discomfort is usually substernal (beneath the breastbone). However, it may originate in or radiate to areas such as the neck, jaw, upper extremities, epigastrium (over the stomach), or the area between the shoulder blades. The discomfort of ACS usually lasts longer than 30 minutes. It may come and go or be constant.

> **AUTHOR'S NOTE** To obtain an accurate history, be sure to ask about "discomfort," not just chest pain.

Ask when the discomfort began, how long it lasted; what seemed to happen before it started; and what, if anything, made

it better or worse. For the patient with a history of stable angina, ask the patient whether the current discomfort represents a change in the pattern or severity of the discomfort. If the patient took his or her own nitroglycerin before the examination began, it is important to determine its effect and consider whether the medication may have been outdated or simply ineffective.

Despite the quality or severity of the discomfort, the most important feature to determine is the time of its onset. Determining whether the patient will benefit from reperfusion therapy depends on knowing as accurately as possible when the ischemia began.

It is important to ask about associated symptoms, such as shortness of breath, fatigue, nausea, sweating, dizziness, and paresthesias. In the absence of typical angina, such symptoms are referred to as *anginal equivalents*. They are more often seen in patients with unstable angina and non–ST-segment-elevation myocardial infarction (NSTEMI).

anginal equivalent

Symptoms such as dyspnea, diaphoresis, profuse vomiting, and arm or jaw pain that are caused by ACS in the absence of chest pain. These symptoms are most common in the elderly and in those with diabetes.

Past Medical History

The past medical history of a patient with suspected ACS should focus on cardiac issues. Determine whether the patient has had prior episodes of myocardial ischemia, such as stable or unstable angina, MI, coronary bypass surgery, or angioplasty. Ask the patient whether he or she has diabetes mellitus. Consider the possibility of aortic dissection, the risk of bleeding, and the potential for cerebrovascular disease.

HYPERTENSION

Assess for hypertension. Chronic, severe, poorly controlled hypertension and severe uncontrolled hypertension on presentation are relative contraindications to fibrinolytic therapy.

POSSIBILITY OF AORTIC DISSECTION

Aortic dissection occurs most often in older adults with hypertension. It is characterized by severe, tearing pain that radiates directly to the back. It is associated with dyspnea or syncope. Appropriate studies must be quickly undertaken. Keep in mind that the dissection may extend to the pericardial sac and produce cardiac tamponade or disrupt the origin of a coronary artery. If perfusion of a coronary artery is interrupted, the ECG may be consistent with a STEMI, potentially supporting the administration of fibrinolytic drugs, which could prove fatal, instead of pursuing definitive care with surgery.

RISK OF BLEEDING

Patients should be asked about previous bleeding problems, such as bleeding during surgery or dental procedures, history of gastrointestinal bleeding, cerebrovascular accidents, unexplained anemia, and melena (stool stained with dark blood).

Administering an antiplatelet, antithrombin, or fibrinolytic agent as part of the treatment for STEMI will increase any underlying bleeding risk. The patient with ACS often has medical conditions that place him or her at risk of both MI and stroke, so look for evidence of prior episodes of cerebrovascular disease. In addition, ask the patient whether he or she has ever had an ischemic stroke, intracerebral hemorrhage (ICH), or subarachnoid hemorrhage. Finally, ask about any recent trauma and/or surgery.

SIGNS AND SYMPTOMS OF ACUTE CORONARY SYNDROME

The signs and symptoms of ACS generally reflect the extent of myocardial ischemia, injury, and infarction. They also indicate the severity of the complications that may be present, which can include dangerous heart rhythms, heart failure, or shock. Although pain is the most common symptom in ACS, it is important to note that many of the following signs and symptoms can be present even in the absence of pain. This is referred to as *anginal equivalents.*

Symptoms

Early recognition of ACS symptoms by patients or friends or family is often the first step in encouraging patients to seek medical attention. Despite public awareness of the signs and symptoms of MI, such as chest pain, many are unaware of other common associated symptoms, such as arm, shoulder, neck, and jaw pain, or less common symptoms, such as shortness of breath and clammy skin or sweating.

Patients wait an average of 2 hours before seeking medical attention, often thinking the symptoms will go away. The reasons for these delays include fear that they may, in fact, be having a heart attack, denial of the severity of the symptoms, and misinterpreting the symptoms as something else, such as indigestion.

GENERAL AND NEUROLOGIC SYMPTOMS

General and neurologic symptoms of ACS include the following, in varying degrees:

- Anxiety and apprehension
- Restlessness and agitation, with a fear of impending death or a sense of doom
- Extreme fatigue and weakness
- Light-headedness
- Confusion, disorientation, or drowsiness
- Fainting or loss of consciousness (syncope)

When first seen, the patient with ACS may appear fully alert and oriented. However, heart failure, myocardial rupture, or an abnormal rhythm may decrease cardiac output. If cardiac output is inadequate, shock or hypoxia and symptoms of cerebral hypoperfusion (reduced blood flow) will rapidly occur. These symptoms often include marked anxiety and apprehension, restlessness, and agitation, with a fear of imminent death or

impending doom. Extreme fatigue or weakness and light-headedness are usually present if the cardiac output is inadequate.

These vague symptoms of weakness are more common in patients with less typical presentations of ACS. This is particularly true of the elderly and those with diabetes. Additionally, patients who have had a heart transplant, who have surgically lost their vagal nerve attachments to the heart, may be pain-free and only present with complaints of weakness, fatigue, and shortness of breath.

CARDIOVASCULAR SYMPTOMS

Angina

Angina is the discomfort—often chest pain—associated with ACS and is the most conspicuous symptom of ACS. It appears in 70% to 80% of patients with acute MI. The pain usually manifests as a substernal or retrosternal constriction or crushing sensation. The pain may be atypical or absent in the remaining 20% to 30% of patients, particularly in older adults, people with diabetes, and those who are having their first attack. When pain is absent, the MI is said to be *silent.* Nevertheless, acute MI is usually indicated by other signs and symptoms.

The pain of ACS is a result of the decreased supply of oxygen to the myocardium and the accumulation of carbon dioxide and lactic acid in myocardial tissue. It is important to recognize that this anginal pain is produced by the ischemic myocardium and not by the portion of the heart that is already infarcted. Infarcted myocardium is dead and therefore produces no pain. The zone of ischemia surrounding the infarct is responsible for the pain. Therefore, as long as the pain continues, there is ongoing ischemia and thus the potential for further infarction.

The pain of stable and unstable angina is often similar. They can be differentiated from each other, however, by an accurate and detailed history. Unlike the pain of stable angina, which usually occurs after physical activity, the unstable anginal pain often begins while the patient is at rest. Some patients are awakened by the pain, usually during the early-morning hours. Often, patients with their first acute MI (about 50%) have experienced recurrent warning attacks of anginal pain (preinfarction or prodromal angina) for hours or days before the attack.

The pain is usually constant after a crescendolike appearance. It sometimes varies in intensity. It does not move, nor does coughing, breathing, or changing body position alter or alleviate it. In localizing the pain, the patient may place a clenched fist against his or her sternum. This is referred to as the *Levine sign,* after Dr. Samuel Levine.

Although the pain of ACS sometimes lasts only a few minutes and disappears spontaneously, it generally lasts longer than 30 minutes. Usually it persists for an hour or longer. In most cases, it can be relieved only by medication, such as nitroglycerin or an opiate, such as fentanyl or morphine sulfate. There is evidence that fentanyl is superior to morphine in the treatment of angina. Morphine is more likely to result in hypotension, nausea, and vomiting. Fentanyl is faster in onset and shorter in duration than morphine and can be more easily titrated. Administering nitroglycerin, as outlined in ECG Keys Box 17.2,

BOX 17.2 ECG KEYS	Nitroglycerin Administration in Acute Coronary Syndrome

- Administer nitroglycerin 0.4 mg:
  - If the patient's systolic blood pressure is 100 mm Hg or greater, administer by sublingual tablet or lingual aerosol.
  - Administer with the patient sitting or lying down.
  - If hypotension does not occur, repeat approximately every 5 minutes as necessary, for a total dose of three tablets or three lingual aerosol applications.
- If nitroglycerin is not effective after the third dose or the pain is severe:
  - Administer fentanyl 1 mcg/kg IV slowly over 1 to 2 minutes and repeat in 5 to 10 minutes as necessary.

AND

  - Start an IV infusion of nitroglycerin at a rate of 5 mg/min, and increase the rate of infusion by 5 mg/min every 5 to 10 minutes until one of the following occurs, at which time, stop increasing the infusion rate and continue it at its current rate:
    - The chest pain is relieved.
    - The mean arterial blood pressure drops by 10% in a patient with normal pressure.
    - The mean arterial blood pressure drops by 30% in a hypertensive patient.
- If at any time the mean arterial blood pressure drops below 80 mm Hg or the systolic blood pressure drops below 90 mm Hg:
  - Slow or temporarily stop the IV infusion of nitroglycerin.
- If the patient is apprehensive and anxious but has little or no pain, consider an anxiolytic agent:
  - Administer diazepam 2.5 to 5 mg IV slowly or lorazepam 0.5 to 1 mg IV slowly.
- If nausea or vomiting is present:
  - Administer ondansetron 4 mg IV or prochlorperazine 2.5 to 10 mg IV.

BOX 17.3 ECG KEYS	Differentiation of Acute Coronary Syndrome (ACS) and Non-ACS Chest Pain

Characteristics of ACS Chest Pain
- Location of the pain—substernal, diffuse, poorly localized
- Description of the pain—crushing, pressure, squeezing, heaviness
- Radiation of the pain—shoulder(s), left arm/elbow/wrist, neck, jaw, teeth
- Relationship to body movement—not positional, not reproducible with palpation
- Duration of the pain—usually 20 minutes or longer
- Associated emotional and psychological manifestations
- Unresponsiveness to rest and/or nitroglycerin

Characteristics of Non-ACS Chest Pain
- Location of the pain—pinpoint, well localized
- Description of the pain—sharp, stabbing
- Radiation of the pain—lower abdomen, pelvis
- Relationship to body movement—pleuritic, painful to touch
- Duration of the pain—seconds to less than a few minutes
- Pain alleviated with physical activity

BOX 17.4 ECG KEYS	Chest Pain That Can Mimic That of ACS

- **Myocarditis or pericarditis.** Pain associated with acute myocarditis and pericarditis tends to be more sharp and stabbing and is worsened when the patient leans forward. The pain lasts seconds to minutes, and the condition is associated with other signs and symptoms not consistent with ACS.
- **Aortic dissection.** Pain is said to be excruciating. Patients may describe a tearing sensation in the back. One or more major pulses may be absent.
- **Spontaneous pneumothorax.** Pain occurs when the parietal and visceral pleura of the lung separate, leading to a collapse of the affected lung. The pain associated with a spontaneous pneumothorax is usually pleuritic, being worsened with inspiration. It is generally well localized.
- **Pulmonary embolus.** A pulmonary embolism occurs when thrombi lodge in distal pulmonary arteries, leading to infarction of the affected lung tissue. Pain from pulmonary embolism tends to be well localized and is generally located in the lateral chest wall, with little, if any, radiation.

may ease the pain of ACS. However, this is not diagnostic, nor does it mean that no further workup is needed. For example, if the pain of ACS is associated with exertion, it can be confused with stable angina. If the pain is unresponsive to rest or three nitroglycerin tablets during the first 15 minutes after its onset, it is more likely caused by acute MI. However, if the pain is relieved but not completely resolved after a single nitroglycerin tablet, the patient should seek medical attention immediately because he or she may have a partially obstructed lesion causing ischemia and infarction.

AUTHOR'S NOTE A nitroglycerin infusion should be administered by infusion pump to control dosing and avoid accidental overdose, which can cause hypotension.

A patient with chest pain matching one or more of the characteristics listed in ECG Keys Box 17.3 should, until proven otherwise, be considered to be having ACS and be managed accordingly, regardless of age. Several conditions do, however, present with pain mimicking that of ACS (ECG Keys Box 17.4).

Stable Angina

Angina induced by exertion that characteristically remains unchanged from episode to episode (after the same amount of exertion) and that is relieved promptly with rest is considered *stable angina*. It is attributable to a stable atherosclerotic plaque that causes significant coronary artery stenosis.

Unstable Angina

Unstable angina is considered to be present if one or more of the following occurs:
- A new onset of exertional angina
- Preexisting angina that becomes more frequent, lasts longer, or begins at a lower threshold of exertion

- The occurrence of angina at rest (usually lasting 20 minutes or longer)

The most common cause of unstable angina is disruption of an atherosclerotic plaque as a result of inflammation. This is followed by plaque expansion, erosion or rupture, and thrombus formation. Then spontaneous thrombolysis occurs, and blood flow is restored. First-time partial occlusion of the coronary artery causes a new onset of exertional angina. Worsening of an existing stenosis causes an increase in the preexisting anginal pattern. Temporary total obstruction causes angina at rest.

If an imbalance between oxygen demand and supply suddenly arises, unstable angina can occur even if there is no increase in the size of the stenotic lesion within the atherosclerotic coronary artery.

Palpitations. A regular heartbeat interrupted by one or more premature contractions is a common cardiac irregularity present in most patients with acute MI. In addition, such heartbeat irregularities are often experienced by people under stress. This sensation occurs under the left breast, or substernally. Patients describe it as "palpitations" or the sensation of "skipping a beat." It is difficult to assess the significance of palpitations in asymptomatic people. In those with ACS symptoms, however, palpitations may indicate the presence of a serious rhythm disturbance that could lead to cardiac arrest. The most common cause of a grossly irregular pulse is atrial fibrillation, which is often chronic and usually a result of MI. Other causes include premature atrial or ventricular contractions. The latter, particularly if multiform and frequent, is commonly seen with myocardial ischemia.

RESPIRATORY SYMPTOMS

Dyspnea. Dyspnea—that is, shortness of breath or difficulty breathing—is often seen in ACS. It may appear gradually or suddenly. It is the primary symptom of left ventricular failure resulting in pulmonary edema. It is characterized by rapid, shallow, and labored respiration. Dyspnea is always accompanied by an awareness of discomfort and, when it is severe, by extreme apprehension and agitation. The patient may have a sensation of suffocation or a tight, constricting sensation in the chest and possibly pain on breathing. It may assume one of several forms, including *dyspnea on exertion* (DOE), *orthopnea,* or *paroxysmal nocturnal dyspnea.*

- DOE is usually the first noticeable symptom of left-heart failure. It first appears after exercise or physical effort, such as climbing a flight of stairs or walking a distance that previously did not produce shortness of breath.
- *Orthopnea* is dyspnea that occurs when lying down and is relieved only if the patient stands up or assumes a sitting or semireclining position.
- *Paroxysmal nocturnal dyspnea* is characterized by sudden attacks of severe dyspnea at night. The patient may be asymptomatic during the day. It is caused by the gradual redistribution of blood and body fluids from the lower extremities to the lungs after the patient has been lying in bed for several hours. The left heart cannot cope with the increased volume of fluid presented to it. Left-heart failure

and pulmonary edema occur as a result, forcing the patient to sit up in bed or use extra pillows to breathe comfortably.

Cough. Cough accompanied by clear or blood-tinged sputum, a productive cough, is a symptom in patients with pulmonary edema associated with left-heart failure. It is caused by excessive bronchial secretions arising from congested mucous membranes. The cough can be spasmodic and productive of copious, frothy sputum. Hemorrhaging from congested bronchial mucosa makes the sputum pink or blood tinged (hemoptysis).

Wheezing. Wheezing may accompany a patient's cough. This is particularly true in those with a coexisting history of chronic obstructive pulmonary disease (COPD), especially emphysema. Even in the absence of lung disease, the aforementioned bronchial secretions can cause the patient to wheeze, worsening the perception of dyspnea.

GASTROINTESTINAL SYMPTOMS

Gastrointestinal (GI) symptoms of ACS include the following:

- **Loss of appetite (anorexia).** Loss of appetite (anorexia) and nausea, with or without vomiting, are common in ACS.
- **Nausea and vomiting.** The patient may misinterpret these gastrointestinal symptoms as indigestion and ignore them, especially if the pain radiates from the chest into the epigastric region. Patients with inferior wall MI are more likely to have nausea and other GI symptoms than infarctions in other areas of the heart. This is attributable to the Bezold–Jarisch reflex, a response initiated by increased stimulation of the parasympathetic nervous system.
- **Thirst.** The patient with ACS usually has increased sympathetic tone because of the combination of pain and fear. This causes predictable symptoms, such as dry mouth and thirst.

Signs

GENERAL APPEARANCE AND NEUROLOGIC SIGNS

The patient with acute MI may be alert and oriented but may also exhibit the following general neurologic signs and symptoms of ACS:

- Fright
- Anxiety and apprehension
- Restlessness and agitation
- Disorientation and drowsiness
- Restlessness or agitation
- Decreased level of consciousness or even unconsciousness

If hypotension or shock occurs, the patient becomes confused and disoriented, then drowsy and unresponsive. A patient who has severe pulmonary congestion and edema is typically sitting up, struggling to breathe.

VITAL SIGNS

Vital signs are pulse, respiration, and blood pressure. In patients with ACS, they vary with the site and extent of myocardial damage and the degree of autonomic nervous system imbalance.

Pulse rate. The pulse rate is usually normal (60–100 beats/min) but may be rapid (>100 beats/min [tachycardia]) because of the predominance of sympathetic nervous system activity. It may also be slow (less than 60 beats/min [bradycardia]) if the parasympathetic nervous system activity predominates. Patients with an acute inferior wall MI are more prone to developing bradycardia as a result of increased vagal stimulation and/or the appearance of atrioventricular (AV) block.

Pulse rhythm. The rhythm of the pulse may be regular or irregular. In a small percentage of patients, an irregular pulse caused by numerous premature ventricular complexes (PVCs) or ventricular bigeminy may indicate a life-threatening rhythm and impending cardiac arrest.

Respiration. Respiration in ACS may vary, depending on the presence or absence of anxiety, heart failure, hypoxia, hypotension, and shock. The respiratory rate may be slow, less than 12 per minute; normal, 12 to 20 per minute at rest (eupnea); or rapid, greater than 20 per minute (tachypnea). The rhythm of breathing may be regular or irregular. The depth of respiration may be normal, shallow, or deep. Respiration may appear quiet, labored and noisy, or gasping. Usually, the respiratory rate is greater than 20 per minute (tachypnea) and shallow. In heart failure, respiration is typically rapid and shallow and is often labored and noisy. In addition, use of the accessory muscles of respiration may be prominent during labored breathing.

APPEARANCE OF THE SKIN

The skin in ACS may have the following characteristics:
- Pale, cold, sweaty, and clammy
- Cyanotic (bluish)

The skin is usually pale, cold, and clammy in a patient with ACS because of increased sympathetic nervous system activity or because of hypotension and shock. Both constrict superficial blood vessels and stimulate sweat glands. The vasoconstriction causes the skin to feel cool to the touch, and the sweating gives it a clammy feel. The stimulation of sweat glands can lead to profuse sweating that can be so severe as to make it difficult to keep the ECG electrodes attached to the skin by their adhesive pads.

If cyanosis (caused by decreased oxygenation of arterial blood) of the skin, fingernail beds, and mucous membranes is present, pulmonary congestion and edema may be present, causing hypoxemia. In the presence of both severe shock and cyanosis, the skin assumes a mottled, bluish-red appearance. The lips may be normal, pale, or cyanotic.

APPEARANCE OF THE VEINS

The neck veins may be normal, distended, pulsating, or collapsed. Generally, the patient's neck veins are assessed with the patient in a supine, semireclining position, propped up at a 45-degree angle. Normally, when lying flat, the jugular neck veins are moderately distended. They are flat, however, when sitting up. Coughing or grunting while sitting or reclining will usually distend the jugular veins in the patient with no evidence of heart failure. Distention of the neck veins typically occurs in right-heart failure when the venous pressure significantly increases. The degree of distention depends on the severity of the failure. In mild right-heart failure, the neck veins are only slightly to moderately distended. When the failure is severe, the jugular veins become markedly distended and pulsate, even when the patient is sitting upright. The neck veins may also be slightly distended in left-heart failure because of the increased pressure in the right ventricle and atrium, which reflects the increased pressure in the left atrium via the pulmonary circulation.

In hypotension and shock, by contrast, the neck veins are usually collapsed when the patient is sitting or propped up at a 45-degree angle. If right-heart failure is also present in hypotension and shock, however, the neck veins may be distended and pulsating.

CARDIOVASCULAR SIGNS

The first heart sound (S_1) correlates to the closure of the AV valves. The second heart sound (S_2) is caused by premature closing of the aortic valve, before the pulmonary valve closes. A third heart sound (S_3) occurs in patients with STEMI. It usually indicates severe left ventricular dysfunction and particularly elevated ventricular filling pressure. It is caused by blood flowing across the mitral valve and decelerating rapidly as it strikes the poorly functioning left ventricular wall. It is especially likely to occur in patients with large infarctions. This sound is best detected at the apex of the heart with the patient in the left lateral recumbent position. A third heart sound may be caused not only by left ventricular failure but also by increased flow into the left ventricle, as occurs when mitral regurgitation or ventricular septal defect complicates STEMI.

These heart sounds are often muffled and are occasionally inaudible during the early phases of MI. Their intensity returns to normal during recovery. A soft first heart sound may also indicate prolongation of the PR interval. Pericardial friction rub is the sound of the myocardium rubbing against the pericardial sac. This sound is caused by inflammation of the affected epicardium. Pericardial friction rub may be heard in patients with STEMI, especially those sustaining a large transmural infarction. Rubs are probably more common than reported. They can be heard within 24 hours or as late as 2 weeks after the onset of infarction. Most often, however, they are noted on the second or third day. Occasionally, in patients with extensive infarction, a loud rub can be heard for many days.

Patients with STEMI and a pericardial friction rub may have pericardial effusion, a collection of fluid within the pericardial sac. Pericardial effusion can be detected on ECG by the presence of electrical alternans. Delayed onset of the rub and the associated discomfort of pericarditis (as late as 3 months after infarction) are characteristic of the (now rare) post-MI (Dressler) syndrome. Pericardial friction rubs are most readily audible along the left sternal border or just inside the point of maximal impulse at the apex of the heart. Loud rubs may be audible over the entire thorax and even over the back.

Breath Sounds. The breath sounds produced by the flow of air through the air passages may be normal, labored and noisy, decreased, or absent. In pulmonary congestion and edema, the breath sounds on auscultation are usually slightly diminished or even absent at one or both bases of the lungs posteriorly. This is attributable to the decrease or absence of airflow through partially or completely obstructed air passages in the congested and edematous parts of the lungs.

Rales, Rhonchi, and Wheezes. The passage of air through bronchi and bronchioles narrowed by edema and spasm and filled with fluid and foam produces abnormal respiratory sounds called *rales, rhonchi,* and *wheezes.* They vary in sound texture and intensity, depending on the size of the air passages involved and the degree of fluid accumulation. Rales may be fine or coarse according to their site of origin. They are very fine (crepitant, crackling, or bubbling) when originating in the very small air passages, such as the alveoli and terminal bronchioles, and coarse (gurgling) when originating in larger bronchioles. Rales have a moist sound to them. The most common source of rales is from fluid collecting in the alveoli. They are worse in the lower lung fields, where pulmonary congestion occurs first and progresses upward as heart failure worsens. Rales are the most common sign in pulmonary edema attributable to left-heart failure and are the cause of dyspnea.

Rhonchi are generally louder, rougher, and coarser sounds than rales. They usually originate in the larger air passages (that is, the trachea and larger bronchi), most often because of increased secretion from mucous membranes. Rhonchi may occur in pulmonary edema but are more common in bronchitis and pneumonia. Dry, coarse rattling in the throat may also be present. Rhonchi clear with coughing and then return over a period of time as the secretions accumulate, whereas rales do not.

The patient may appear to be choking or coughing spasmodically, with expectoration of frothy sputum, often pink or blood tinged (hemoptysis). This occurs in fulminant cases of heart failure when an excessive amount of fluid has traversed the pulmonary vasculature, draining into the bronchial tree. Wheezing occurs when there is a narrowing of the bronchi and bronchioles. This is often associated with asthma and emphysema but can be heard with heart failure. Patients with emphysema and heart failure may present with both wheezes and rales as the fluid precipitates narrowing of the terminal bronchioles. This has been termed *cardiac asthma,* but unlike the typical exacerbation of emphysema, the underlying cause is pulmonary edema rather than the collapse or spasm of terminal bronchioles. Rales, rhonchi, and wheezes are heard best by auscultation. If they are loud enough, however, they can be heard without a stethoscope. In patients with early left-heart failure, fine, crepitant rales and wheezes are often heard at both bases of the lungs posteriorly and sometimes as high up as the shoulder blades. These sounds may be present at one or both bases of the lungs only, or up to the shoulder blades posteriorly, or throughout the lungs and anteriorly as well. Rales can be elicited by having the patient breathe deeply and forcefully through a wide-open mouth. These sounds are best heard during inspiration, especially toward the end of a deep breath. Rhonchi can be heard during both exhalation and late inspiration over the bronchi and trachea.

Consolidation and Pleural Effusion. When a segment of the lung becomes completely filled with fluid, preventing air from entering, consolidation is present. Breath sounds and rales that were present initially now disappear. The breath sounds may also be markedly decreased or even absent over one or both bases of the lungs posteriorly because of fluid in the pleural space (pleural effusion) caused by right-heart failure. This is primarily because the lungs are compressed by the effusion. The areas of the lungs where the breath sounds decrease or disappear because of consolidation or pleural effusion lose their resonance. Thus dullness to percussion may be present over one or both lungs, particularly at the bases of the lungs posteriorly.

APPEARANCE OF BODY TISSUES

Edema. Edema is the accumulation of serous fluid in body tissue. It may be confined to one or more areas, or it can exist throughout the body. When generalized, it is known as *anasarca.*

Some degree of edema is always present in right-heart failure. Early in the course of fluid retention, weight gain is the only sign of increased body fluid. As heart failure worsens, however, more fluid accumulates. This produces noticeable swelling of the legs, especially in the anterior lower leg in front of the tibia (pretibial edema) and in the feet and ankles (pedal edema), the lower part of the back over the spine (presacral edema), and in the abdominal wall. The skin usually becomes taut and shiny over the edematous tissue. When pressure is applied with a finger, a dent appears that does not disappear immediately when the pressure is withdrawn. This sign of peripheral edema is called *pitting edema.* By contrast, *nonpitting edema* is caused by tissue swelling as a result of trauma or inflammation. Table 17.1 summarizes the signs and symptoms of ACS.

MANAGEMENT OF ACUTE CORONARY SYNDROME

The following management strategies are based on the current literature and endorsed by the author. However, state, regional, and local protocol may vary. Therefore all management strategies should be modified based on the applicable scope of practice and in consultation with medical specialists and professional organizations.

Additionally, although protocols and strategies may be presented in a linear format, it is reasonable to assume that several steps will occur simultaneously. The sequence should be viewed as a general outline, not necessarily a step-by-step process.

GOALS OF MANAGEMENT

The primary goal of ACS management is to correct the ischemia and stop the progression or at least limit the damage of the infarction by reperfusing the ischemic tissue (Fig. 17.1). Reperfusion can occur either by administering fibrinolytic drugs to dissolve the occlusion or by performing percutaneous coronary intervention (PCI). Each of these goals is time critical. With each passing minute, more myocardial damage occurs, and the potential benefit of treatment diminishes. Therefore time limits have been set (Fig. 17.2). The goal is to limit ischemia to 120 minutes or less and to have a door-to-needle time of

TABLE 17.1	Acute Coronary Syndrome Signs and Symptoms	
	Sign	**Symptom**
General and neurologic	• Alert and oriented • Restless • Anxious • Apprehensive	• Anxiety • Apprehension • Extreme fatigue and weakness • Restlessness and agitation, with a fear of impending death (or a sense of impending doom) are common.
Cardiovascular	• Distant heart sounds • A third heart sound (S_3) early in diastole (left ventricular dysfunction) • A fourth heart sound (S_4) late in diastole (nondiagnostic) • A pericardial friction rub	• Chest pain • Frequent palpitations
Respiratory	• Normal or labored • Rapid and shallow • Rales (fluid in alveoli) • Rhonchi (secretions in bronchioles) • Wheezing—"cardiac asthma" • Dullness to percussion (pleural effusion)	• Dyspnea • Choking • Cough
Gastrointestinal	• Vomiting	• Nausea • Loss of appetite (anorexia)
Vital Signs		
Pulse	• Usually normal, but may be >100/min (tachycardia) or >60/min (bradycardia). • The rhythm may be regular or irregular. • The force of the pulse may be normal, strong, and full, or if hypotension or shock is present, it may be weak and thready.	
Respiration	• Typically >20/min (tachypnea) and shallow, but may be 12–20/min (normal, eupnea) or less • May be regular or irregular • Depth may be normal, shallow, or deep • Labored and noisy or gasping • Accessory muscles use may be prominent if severe pulmonary congestion and edema are present.	
Blood pressure	• May be normal, elevated (>140 mm Hg), or low (>90 mm Hg) if hypotension or shock is present	
Skin	• Pale • Clammy • Sweating (diaphoresis) • Cyanosis • Delayed capillary refill	
Veins	• Normal • Moderately distended (in left-heart failure and mild right-heart failure) • Markedly distended and pulsating (in severe right-heart failure) • Collapsed (in hypotension or shock)	
Body tissue	• Pitting edema tibia (pretibial edema) • Lower part of the back over the spine (presacral edema) • Abdominal wall • Entire body (anasarca)	

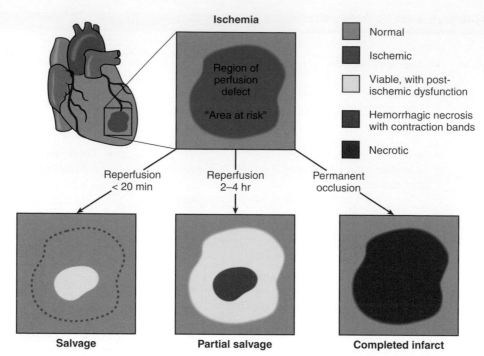

FIG. 17.1 Myocardial salvage from reperfusion. (From Mann, D. L., Zipes, D., Libby, P., & Bonow, R. [Eds.]. [2015]. *Braunwald*'s heart disease [10th ed.]. Saunders.)

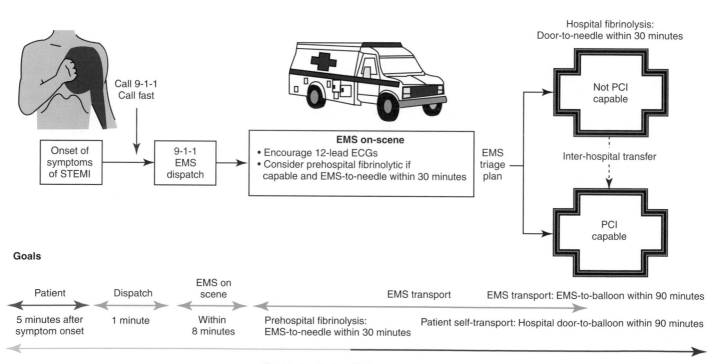

FIG. 17.2 Reperfusion treatment goals. (From Antman, E. M., Hand, M., Armstrong, P. W., Bates, E. R., Green, L. A., Halasyamani, L. K., Hochman, J. S., Krumholz, H. M., Lamas, G. A., Mullany, C. J., Pearle, D. L., Sloan, M. A., Smith, C. A., Jr., & 2004 Writing Committee Members. [2008]. 2007 focused update of the ACC/AHA 2004 guidelines for the management of patients with ST elevation myocardial infarction. *Circulation, 117*[2], 296–329.)

30 minutes or less. It has been proposed that the clock should start at the moment the first diagnostic ECG is acquired.

Initial Assessment and Management of Chest Pain (Fig. 17.3)

Initial assessment and management of chest pain are performed by prehospital/emergency department personnel as follows:

1. Administer oxygen 4 L/min nasal cannula or 100% nonrebreather mask if patient shows signs of respiratory distress or oxygen saturation dips to 94% or lower. Titrate oxygen to maintain oxygen saturation between 94% and 98%. Avoid inducing 100% oxygen saturation.
2. Quickly assess the patient's circulatory status while obtaining the vital signs, including level of consciousness. Repeat as the situation requires and circumstances permit.
3. Begin monitoring the ECG for significant rhythms.

4. Start an intravenous (IV) line with either normal saline (NS) or 5% dextrose in water (D_5W) to keep the vein open (TKO) to administer medications.
5. While performing steps 1 to 4, obtain a brief history and physical examination to determine the cause of the chest pain.

AND

6. Obtain a 12-lead ECG (plus lead V_{4R}, if indicated), using an ECG monitor with or without computerized ECG interpretation. If appropriate, transmit the 12-lead ECG and/or the computerized ECG interpretation to the base hospital for physician interpretation.

Determine the following:
A. ST depression is evident.
B. STEMI is evident (criterion A or B).
C. ECG is nondiagnostic.

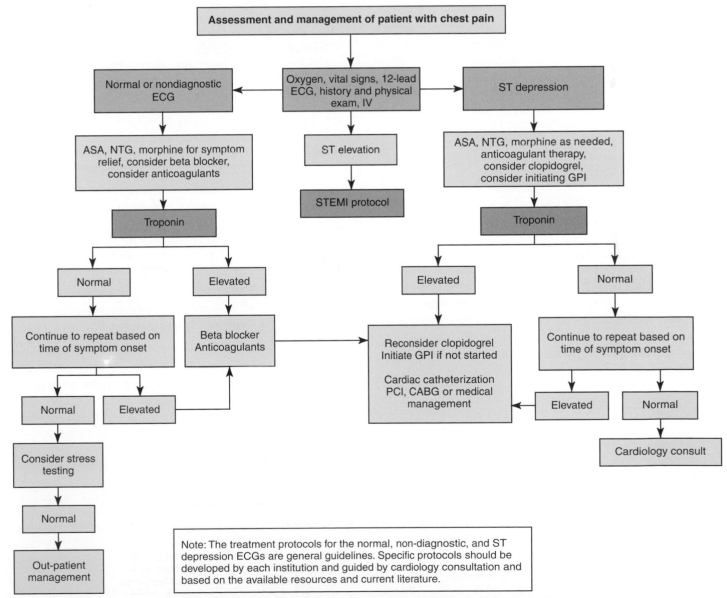

FIG. 17.3 Initial assessment and management of patient with chest pain.

Note that "Normal ECG" is not listed as an option. That's because in the setting of an ACS evaluation, there is no such thing as a "normal ECG." Instead, the ECG without ST changes should be considered nondiagnostic.

> **AUTHOR'S NOTE** Research has shown that the administration of oxygen resulting in an oxygen saturation of 100% results in the formation of what is referred to as *free radicals*. They are composed of free oxygen atoms instead of the oxygen molecule that is composed of two oxygen atoms. Free radicals injure the hypoxic myocardial cells and increase the likelihood of irreversible injury.

Prehospital Emergency Medical Service Management

The earlier the patient with STEMI is identified, the earlier management can be instituted. Current ECG monitor/defibrillators have built-in algorithms to detect ST changes indicative of myocardial ischemia and injury. Research has shown that paramedics can accurately interpret 12-lead ECGs and appropriately triage patients. Combining these capabilities with cellular technology allows emergency medical services (EMS) to transmit the ECG to the receiving hospital for additional interpretation if the diagnosis is unclear. Typical prehospital STEMI programs function by acquiring an ECG and applying the following criteria (systems may use either criterion A or B):

- Criterion A: Two or more contiguous leads with 1 mm or more ST elevation in the inferior leads or 1 mm or more ST elevation in the precordial leads
- Criterion B: Two or more contiguous leads with 1 mm or more ST elevation in the inferior leads or 2 mm or more ST elevation in the precordial leads

> **AUTHOR'S NOTE** Criterion A is more sensitive than criterion B because it would activate the STEMI system with less ST elevation in the precordial leads. However, there is evidence that 1 mm of ST elevation in the precordial leads may be a result of other conditions besides STEMI. Therefore applying this criterion would result in a higher rate of false-positive activations (patients without an actual MI). Regardless, with proper quality improvement and oversight, either criterion may be used in a prehospital STEMI-detection protocol.

If criteria are met, then transport the patient to the nearest appropriate facility (PCI-capable facility preferred). ECG Keys Box 17.5 outlines the criteria for determining the appropriate reperfusion therapy, PCI or fibrinolytic:

- If the facility is PCI capable, notify the facility as soon as possible to mobilize the catheterization team and interventional cardiologist. Patients with STEMI should be transported to PCI-capable hospitals when the time from EMS transport to balloon procedure can be accomplished within 90 minutes.
- If the facility is non–PCI capable, notify the facility as soon as possible to ensure that the emergency department (ED) is prepared to receive patient and begin fibrinolytic therapy quickly. Patients with STEMI should be transported to

---

BOX 17.5 ECG KEYS | **Determination of Appropriate Reperfusion Therapy**

Step 1: Assess Time and Risk
- Time since onset of symptoms
- Degree of certainty of ST-segment-elevation myocardial infarction (STEMI)
- Eligibility for fibrinolytic therapy (see ECG Keys Boxes 17.6 and 17.7)
- Time required to transport patient to skilled percutaneous coronary intervention (PCI) facility

Step 2: Determine Whether Fibrinolysis or PCI Is Preferred
Primary percutaneous coronary interventional therapy is generally preferred in the following situations:
- A skilled PCI facility is available and a door-to-device time of 90 minutes or less can be attained.
- Patient has a high risk of STEMI.
- Patient is in cardiogenic shock.
- Patient has a contraindication to fibrinolytic therapy, including increased bleeding risk and intracerebral hemorrhage.
- Patient presented late for treatment (symptoms began 3 hours ago or longer).
- Diagnosis of STEMI is in doubt.
  Fibrinolysis is generally preferred in the following situations:
- The catheterization lab is occupied or otherwise unavailable, resulting in a door-to-device time of longer than 120 minutes.
- Vascular access may be difficult.
- A skilled PCI facility is inaccessible.
- Time to transport to skilled PCI facility would result in the first medical contact-to-device time being longer than 120 minutes.

---

non–PCI-capable hospitals only if door-to-needle time (time to fibrinolytic administration) is within 30 minutes. Once there, perform the following:

- Determine the patient's eligibility for fibrinolytic therapy (ECG Keys Box 17.6).
- Determine whether any absolute contraindications for fibrinolytic therapy exist (ECG Keys Box 17.7).
- Proceed to fibrinolytic administration.

Emergency Department Management

RISK ASSESSMENT

Once the history and physical examination are completed, the clinician should be able to determine fairly accurately the likelihood that symptoms are consistent with ACS. It is important to perform this risk assessment at this point before relying solely on the ECG and cardiac enzymes, for the following reasons:
1. The ECG may be nondiagnostic.
2. The cardiac enzymes may not be available, or the patient may need to be transferred to definitive care.

Table 17.2 provides a method of assessing the likelihood that the patient's presentation is consistent with ACS. At this point, a diagnostic 12-lead ECG should be performed and the presence of STEMI and NSTEMI determined.

DIAGNOSIS

12-Lead ECG. Patients whose complaints suggest ACS should be taken immediately into an examining room for

BOX 17.6 ECG KEYS | **Eligibility for Thrombolytic Therapy**

Initial Patient Assessment

Yes	No	
		Pain lasting >15 minutes but <12 hours
		Hypertension: systolic blood pressure <180 mm Hg
		Diastolic blood pressure <110 mm Hg
		Right vs. left arm systolic blood pressure difference <15 mm Hg (suspect aortic aneurysm)
		Signs and symptoms of congestive heart failure
		Signs and symptoms of cardiogenic shock
		12-lead ECG with significant ST-segment and T-wave changes
		Estimated time of arrival at emergency department _____

History

Yes	No	
		Recent (within 6 weeks) major surgery (for example, intracranial or intraspinal surgery), obstetric delivery, organ biopsy, or previous puncture of noncompressible blood vessels
		Significant head or facial trauma within previous 6 months
		Pregnant female
		Hemostatic defects, including those secondary to severe hepatic or renal disease, and anticoagulants
		Cardiopulmonary resuscitation >10 minutes
		Any other condition in which bleeding may occur, especially if its management would be particularly difficult because of its location
		Cerebrovascular disease, including cerebrovascular accident (CVA), seizure, cerebral aneurysm, intracranial neoplasm, or arteriovenous (AV) malformation
		Suspected aortic dissection or known aneurysm

BOX 17.7 ECG KEYS | **Contraindications and Cautions for the Use of Fibrinolytic Agents in Acute Myocardial Infarction**

Absolute Contraindications
- Active internal bleeding (for example, gastrointestinal or genitourinary), excluding menses
- Any prior intracerebral hemorrhage
- Significant closed-head or facial trauma within 3 months
- Ischemic stroke within 3 months
- Recent intracranial or intraspinal surgery or trauma
- Known intracranial neoplasm, arteriovenous malformation, or cerebral aneurysm
- Suspected aortic dissection

Relative Contraindications
- Recent puncture of noncompressible blood vessels
- Known bleeding diathesis
- For streptokinase/anistreplase: prior exposure (more than 5 days ago) or prior allergic reaction to these agents
- Traumatic or prolonged (>10 minutes) cardiopulmonary resuscitation
- Major surgery (<3 weeks)
- Current use of oral anticoagulants (for example, warfarin sodium) with international normalized ratio >2–3
- History of recent (within 2–4 weeks) gastrointestinal, genitourinary, or other internal bleeding
- Active peptic ulcer
- History of chronic, severe, poorly controlled hypertension
- Severe uncontrolled hypertension on presentation (systolic blood pressure >180 mm Hg or diastolic blood pressure >110 mm Hg)
- History of prior ischemic cerebrovascular accident <3 months, dementia, or known intracranial pathology not covered in contraindications
- Pregnancy

TABLE 17.2	Factors Indicating the Likelihood of Acute Coronary Syndrome		
	High Likelihood	**Intermediate Likelihood**	**Low Likelihood**
History	• Chest or left arm pain or discomfort as chief symptom reproducing prior documented angina • Known history of CHD, including MI	• Chest or left arm pain or discomfort as chief symptom • Age greater than 70 years • Male • Diabetes	• Probable ischemic symptoms in the absence of any of the intermediate likelihood characteristics
Examination	• Temporary mitral regurgitation murmur, hypotension, diaphoresis, pulmonary edema, or rales	• Extracardiac vascular disease	• Chest discomfort reproduced by palpation
ECG	• New, or presumably new, temporary ST-segment elevation (1 mm or greater) or T-wave inversion in multiple precordial leads	• Fixed Q waves • ST depression of 0.5–1 mm or T-wave inversion of 1 mm	• T-wave flattening or inversion less than 1 mm in leads with dominant R waves • Normal ECG
Cardiac markers	• Elevated cardiac TnI, TnT, or CK-MB	• Normal	• Normal

CHD, Coronary heart disease; *CK-MB*, creatine kinase MB isoenzyme; *MI*, myocardial infarction; *TnI*, troponin I; *TnT*, troponin T.
Modified from Braunwald, E., Jones, R. H., Mark, D. B., Brown, J., Brown, L., Cheitlin, M. D., Concannon, C. A., Cowan, M., Edwards, C., & Fuster, V. (1994). *Unstable angina: Diagnosis and management* (AHCPR Publication No. 94-0602). U.S. Dept of Health and Human Services.

evaluation. The goal is to obtain a 12-lead ECG within 10 minutes of arrival at the ED.

Once obtained, the 12-lead ECG should be evaluated by a qualified provider as soon as possible, with a goal of less than 10 minutes. The patient should then be evaluated to determine whether he or she is a candidate for reperfusion therapy.

If the ECG shows diagnostic ST elevation in contiguous leads, as discussed in Chapter 16, then the diagnosis of STEMI is made. If ST depression and T-wave inversion are present, then NSTEMI is more likely; however, a posterior wall MI must be considered if the ST-segment depression is in V_1 to V_4. In the absence of ST-segment changes, the working diagnosis is unstable angina. Until the levels of the cardiac markers are known, the patient is now in the unstable angina/NSTEMI category.

The diagnosis of MI is confirmed with cardiac markers in more than 90% of patients with ST-segment elevation. Up to 25% of patients without ST-segment elevation have elevated creatine kinase MB isoenzyme (CK-MB) and develop a Q-wave MI. The remaining 75% have non–Q-wave MI. Between 1% and 6% of patients with a completely normal ECG and chest pain are eventually diagnosed with NSTEMI, and at least 4% will have unstable angina.

In the event the initial ECG is nondiagnostic, obtaining serial 12-lead ECGs or monitoring the patient with continuous ST-segment deviation monitoring allows you to detect subtle changes in the ECG, which can confirm the diagnosis and appropriately alter the therapy. Obtaining a 12-lead ECG when the patient is symptomatic is significantly more accurate in detecting ST changes if the pain is associated with ACS.

Cardiac Biomarkers. Upon admission to the ED, blood studies are routinely performed to determine whether certain proteins and enzymes (cardiac biomarkers) released from damaged or necrotic myocardial tissue are abnormally elevated. Another reason to obtain the cardiac markers is that almost 50% of patients with chest pain suggestive of ACS have a nondiagnostic ECG and are later found to have had an MI. This can only be confirmed by measuring cardiac biomarkers. Among patients admitted to the hospital with chest pain, less than 20% are subsequently diagnosed as having had an MI. In most patients, clinicians must obtain serum cardiac marker measurements at periodic intervals to either establish or exclude the diagnosis of MI.

The cardiac biomarkers currently used include creatinine kinase and troponin.

Creatinine Kinase

- *CK-MB.* CK-MB is an enzyme specific to the heart muscle. Its level increases primarily after myocardial necrosis (tissue death). Three isoenzymes of CK exist (MM, BB, and MB):
  - Brain and kidney tissue contain mostly the BB isoenzyme.
  - Skeletal muscle contains principally MM but does contain some MB (1%–3%).
  - Cardiac muscle contains both MM and MB isoenzymes. Levels of CK-MB may increase in certain situations:
- Strenuous exercise, particularly in trained long-distance runners or professional athletes, can elevate both total CK and CK-MB.
- Trauma or surgery involving the brain, kidneys, heart, or skeletal muscle can elevate CK-MB.
- Small quantities of CK-MB isoenzyme occur in tissues other than the heart.

Nevertheless, unless the patient is an elite athlete or has had recent surgery that might offer an alternative explanation, elevated levels of CK-MB can be considered to have been caused by MI. Provided the sample has been accurately tested and was drawn within 4 hours of the onset of STEMI, the CK-MB level may be used to diagnose MI.

After 4 hours, however, the heart may have sustained significant damage. Thereafter, the CK-MB level cannot be relied on to diagnosis acute MI or to determine whether reperfusion therapy is appropriate. One notable exception is reinfarction within a matter of days following an acute MI.

Cardiac Troponin T and Troponin I

The troponins, like CK-MB, are also specific to the myocardium. They increase not only after myocardial necrosis but also after myocardial injury. The troponin complex consists of three subunits that regulate the calcium-mediated contractile process of striated muscle:

1. Troponin C, which binds calcium
2. Troponin I (TnI), which binds to actin and inhibits actin–myosin interactions
3. Troponin T (TnT), which binds to tropomyosin, thereby attaching the troponin complex to the thin filament

Because cardiac-specific troponins I and T (cTnI and cTnT) accurately distinguish skeletal muscle damage from cardiac muscle damage, the troponins are now considered the preferred cardiac marker for diagnosing MI. However, because troponins remain elevated for 5 to 14 days or even longer, a sudden rise in the CK-MB level may be the only usable cardiac marker to indicate reinfarction.

As shown in Fig. 17.4, myoglobin is the first serum marker to become elevated after an acute MI; however, this biomarker is rarely measured today because of its low specificity to cardiac tissue. Myoglobin elevation is followed by the troponins and CK-MB. Each clinical laboratory will have a predetermined diagnostic level for ACS based on the type of testing performed. Therefore when interpreting the results, it's helpful to become as familiar as possible with the test used and be aware of the diagnostic value set by the laboratory at which the test is performed. Because diagnostic levels of these serum enzymes may not appear in the blood until 20 minutes after an acute MI, testing the level of these markers may not be helpful during the early phase of acute MI. However, bedside point-of-care testing for cardiac markers continues to improve in both speed and accuracy.

> **AUTHOR'S NOTE** The diagnostic level of each cardiac marker is determined by the clinical laboratory performing the test, and therefore there is no "standard" value for any of the cardiac markers.

DETERMINATION OF APPROPRIATE THERAPY

The choice of which reperfusion therapy to use will, in most cases, be based on the capability of the facility. This should be established by existing policies developed by a multidisciplinary group of physicians and hospital policymakers. Such policies allow preapproved orders and procedures, thereby limiting delays. Multidisciplinary review of STEMI cases provides continuous quality improvement of the process. The goal is to ensure that management practices are kept current and address issues that prevent the facility from meeting time-critical goals. Once the patient has been identified as a candidate for reperfusion therapy, he or she must be moved to definitive care as quickly as possible. From the onset of pain, the clock begins to tick. The decision as to which reperfusion therapy is most appropriate

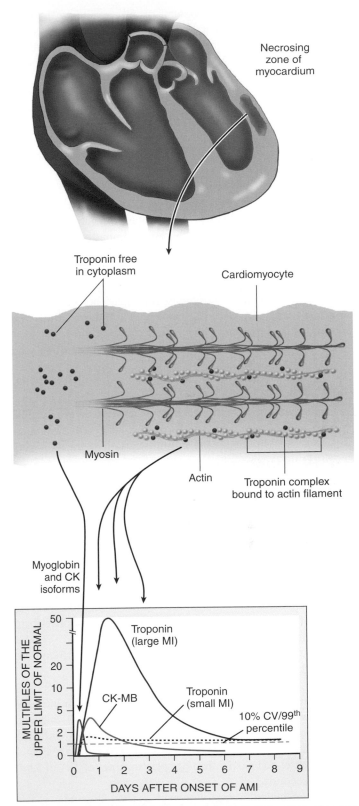

FIG. 17.4 Time of appearance and degree of elevation of serum markers after the onset of acute myocardial infarction. (Modified from Antman, E. M. [2002]. Decision making with cardiac troponin tests. *New England Journal of Medicine, 346*[26], 2079–2082; and Jaffe, A. S., Babiun, L., & Apple, F. S. (2006). Biomarkers in acute cardiac disease: The present and the future. *Journal of the American College of Cardiology, 48*[1], 1–11.)

will depend on local and regional resources. Follow the steps outlined in ECG Keys Box 17.5 to make the determination. If fibrinolytics are considered, follow the steps outlined in ECG Keys Boxes 17.6 and 17.7 to determine whether the patient is a suitable candidate.

MANAGEMENT OF SPECIFIC CONDITIONS

ST-Elevation Myocardial Infarction

Once the 12-lead ECG is obtained and meets STEMI criteria, a decision must be made as to the most appropriate reperfusion therapy. The primary goals in the management of acute MI are to stop the formation of the thrombus, dissolve the thrombus already formed, and open up the occluded coronary artery. These steps should occur as soon as possible after admission to the ED, ideally within 90 minutes. If PCI can be accomplished within 90 minutes, proceed to primary PCI. If dysrhythmias are present initially or at any time, refer to Chapter 11.

The STEMI protocol for reperfusion therapy is outlined next (Fig. 17.5).

STEP ONE

Step one is to prevent the further expansion of the original thrombus and/or prevent the formation of a new thrombus. This is accomplished by the administration of the following drugs (Table 17.3):

- An **antiplatelet agent**, such as aspirin, that inhibits thromboxane (TxA_2) formation and its release from the platelets, thus partially impeding platelet aggregation. Administer a chewable aspirin, 162 to 325 mg.
- An **anticoagulant**, such as enoxaparin (Lovenox), a low-molecular-weight (LMW) heparin, or unfractionated heparin, blocks the conversion of prothrombin to thrombin and inhibits the action of thrombin on fibrinogen, thus preventing the conversion of fibrinogen to fibrin threads. Heparin does not, however, interfere with the adhesion of platelets to the collagen fibers in the arterial wall.
  - Administer enoxaparin 30 mg IV followed in 15 minutes by 1 mg/kg enoxaparin subcutaneously.

OR

  - Administer a 60-U/kg bolus of unfractionated heparin IV (maximum 4000-U bolus for patients >70 kg), followed by a 12-U/kg/hr unfractionated heparin IV infusion (maximum 1000 U/hr for patients >70 kg), to maintain an activated partial thromboplastin time (aPTT) of 50 to 70 seconds.
  - A prostaglandin inhibitor, such as the following:
  - Clopidogrel (Plavix) 600 mg orally
  - Prasugrel (Effient) 60 mg orally
  - Ticagrelor (Brilinta) 180 mg orally
- A *platelet glycoprotein (GP) IIb/IIIa receptor inhibitor (GPI)*, such as abciximab (ReoPro) or eptifibatide (Integrilin), blocks the GP IIb/IIIa receptors on activated platelets from binding to fibrinogen, thus inhibiting platelet adhesion and aggregation and further thrombus formation. Consider the administration of a GP IIb/IIIa receptor inhibitor for patients younger than 75 with extensive anterior MIs and minimal risk of bleeding.
  - Administer abciximab 0.25 mg/kg IV.

AND

  - Start an abciximab infusion at 0.125 mcg/kg/min.

OR

  - Administer eptifibatide 180 mcg/kg IV.

AND

  - Start an eptifibatide infusion at 2 mcg/kg/min.

AND

  - Move rapidly to catheterization lab.

CAUTION: After administering any of these drugs, closely monitor the patient for bleeding.

> **AUTHOR'S NOTE** If a GP IIb/IIa receptor inhibitor is administered in combination with a fibrinolytic agent, the dosage of the fibrinolytic agent should be reduced to approximately half of that indicated earlier (for example, a 5-U bolus of reteplase IV initially; a 15- to 25-mg bolus of tenecteplase IV).

STEP TWO

Option 1

Dissolve or lyse the existing thrombus using a fibrinolytic agent, such as alteplase (tPA), reteplase (rPA), or tenecteplase (TNK-tPA), which converts plasminogen, normally present in the blood, to plasmin, an enzyme that dissolves fibrin (fibrinolysis) within the thrombus, helping break apart the thrombus (thrombolysis).

If acute MI is confirmed and no contraindications to fibrinolytic therapy are present:

- Administer reteplase 10 U IV over 2 minutes and repeat in 30 minutes.

OR

- Administer tenecteplase 30 to 50 mg IV over 5 seconds based on the patient's weight, as indicated in Table 17.4.

Option 2

Enlarge the lumen of the occluded section of the affected coronary artery mechanically by means of one or more of the following catheter-based PCIs:

- **Percutaneous coronary angioplasty** (PCA; Fig. 17.6). The insertion of a balloon-tipped catheter into the occluded or narrowed coronary artery, followed by the inflation of the balloon, thus fracturing the atherosclerotic plaque and dilating the arterial lumen. This procedure, also referred to as *balloon angioplasty,* is the most commonly performed invasive treatment for coronary artery occlusion. It is often followed by the insertion of a coronary artery stent.
- **Coronary artery stenting** (Fig. 17.7). The insertion of a cylindrical wire sheath into the occluded or narrowed coronary artery, followed by the expansion of the sheath to fit snugly within the dilated lumen of the coronary artery.

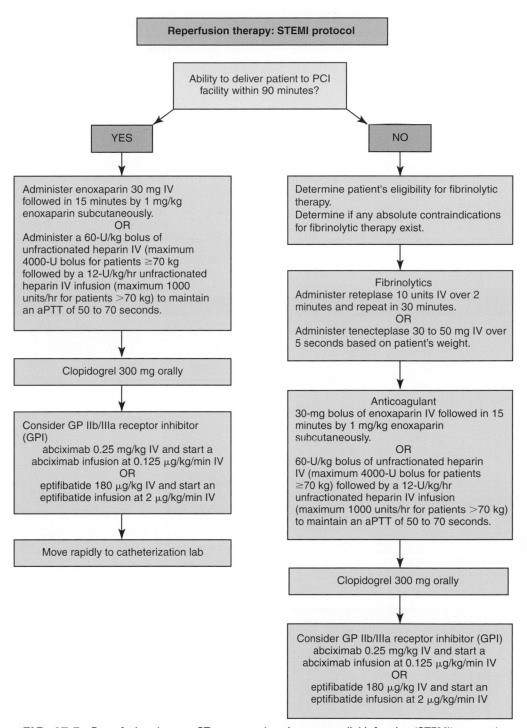

FIG. 17.5 Reperfusion therapy: ST-segment-elevation myocardial infarction (STEMI) protocol.

Stents may be used alone as a primary procedure or after balloon angioplasty. Often these stents are coated with agents to prevent restenosis (drug-eluting stents).

- **Directional coronary atherectomy (DCA).** The mechanical removal of a noncalcified thrombus through a catheter inserted in the occluded or narrowed coronary artery.
- **Rotational atherectomy.** The use of a rotational, drill-like device to remove a calcified thrombus.

Emergency coronary artery bypass grafting (CABG) should be considered under the following conditions if still within 4 to 6 hours of the onset of symptoms of acute MI:

- Reperfusion of the occluded coronary artery fails using the previous PCIs and the patient is hemodynamically unstable (that is, in cardiogenic shock) or continues to have persistent chest pain.
- The PCIs listed earlier are contraindicated.
- Multivessel coronary artery disease is present.

TABLE 17.3	Antithrombus Drugs Used in the Management of Acute Myocardial Infarction	
Drug Category	**Action**	**Drug**
Antiplatelet agent	Inhibits thromboxane A_2 (TxA_2) formation and release from platelets, thereby inhibiting platelet aggregation	Aspirin Clopidogrel (Plavix) Prasugrel (Effient) Ticagrelor (Brilinta)
Anticoagulant	Blocks conversion of fibrinogen to fibrin by inhibiting the action of thrombin on fibrinogen	Low-molecular-weight heparin such as enoxaparin (Lovenox) or unfractionated heparin
GP IIb/IIIa receptor inhibitor	Inhibits platelet adhesion and aggregation by blocking the platelets' glycoprotein (GP) IIb/IIIa receptors	Abciximab (ReoPro) Eptifibatide (Integrilin)
Thrombolytic agent	Converts plasminogen to plasmin, which in turn dissolves the fibrin binding the platelets together	Alteplase (Activase) (tPA) Reteplase (Retavase) (rPA) Tenecteplase (TNKase) (TNK-tPA)

TABLE 17.4	Tenecteplase Dosage Table				
Patient's weight	<60 kg	60 to <70 kg	70 to <80 kg	80 to <90 kg	≥90 kg
TNK-tPA (mg)	30 mg	35 mg	40 mg	45 mg	50 mg
Volume (mL)	(6 mL)	(7 mL)	(8 mL)	(9 mL)	(10 mL)

TNK-tPA, Tenecteplase

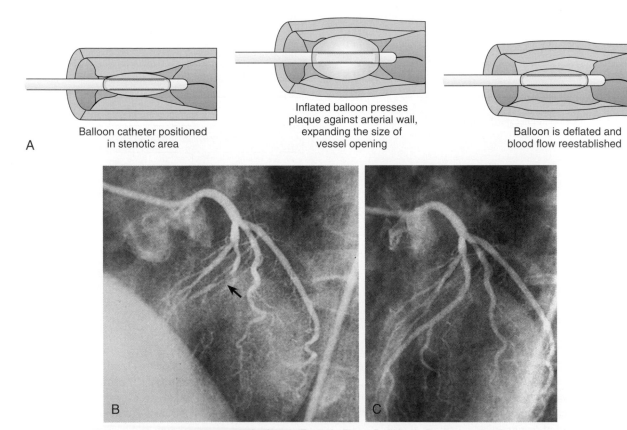

A   Balloon catheter positioned in stenotic area

Inflated balloon presses plaque against arterial wall, expanding the size of vessel opening

Balloon is deflated and blood flow reestablished

B   C

FIG. 17.6 Percutaneous angioplasty. (From LaFleur, B. [2014]. *Exploring medical language: A student-directed approach* [9th ed.]. Mosby.)

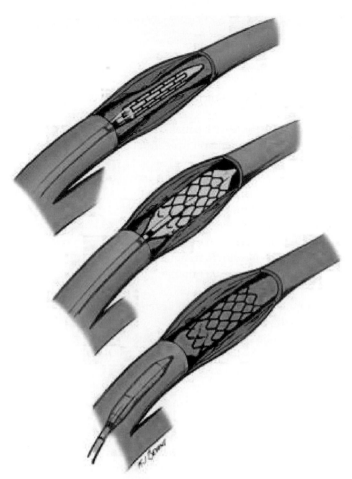

FIG. 17.7 Stent placement. (From Bevans, M., & McLimore, E. (1992). Intracoronary stents: A new approach to coronary artery dilatation. *Journal of Cardiovascular Nursing, 7*(1), 34–49.)

TAKE-HOME POINTS

- A patient's history includes information about his or her symptoms and any previous illness. It includes the chief complaint, history of present illness, and past medical history. The *chief complaint* is a short statement of the patient's major symptom(s) requiring emergency medical care. The history of present illness is a more detailed description of the patient's chief complaint and includes the symptoms, onset, severity, duration, and relationship to precipitating causes, such as exercise, emotion, body position, and so forth.
- *Past cardiac history* is a brief review of previous cardiovascular diseases and their treatment. This includes any history of previous MIs, angina, heart failure, dysrhythmias, syncope,

hypertension, and so forth; previous hospitalizations; medications currently being taken; and any known allergies.

- Once an appropriate history is obtained, or even while questioning the patient, a physical examination is performed to determine whether the physical signs, including vital signs, are consistent with ACS. These signs, in conjunction with the patient's history and the presence of abnormal ECG changes (ST-segment elevation or depression and T-wave changes) will help indicate the correct diagnosis and determine appropriate management.
- ACS manifests with significant signs and symptoms. The symptoms and signs in ACS vary, depending on the location and extent of the heart damage and degree of autonomic nervous system activity (sympathetic or parasympathetic) present.
- A *symptom* is defined as an abnormal feeling of distress or an awareness of disturbances in bodily function experienced by the patient. Symptoms are subjective expressions of what the patient is experiencing. The symptoms are obtained during the taking of the patient's history. Examples of symptoms of ACS are marked apprehension, chest pain, dyspnea, palpitations, and nausea.
- *Signs* are abnormalities of the patient's body structure and function that are detected by initial inspection of the patient and by the physical examination. Signs are objective findings that can be physically seen or monitored. Some examples of signs of ACS include tachycardia, distention of the neck veins, edema, and cyanosis.
- The patient presenting with chest pain represents a significant clinical challenge. To avoid missing the diagnosis, it's important to use a methodical approach to the history and physical examination and to recognize the signs and symptoms of ACS (see Table 17.1).
- Understanding the role and limitations of the 12-lead ECG, as well as the timing of the release of cardiac markers from the myocardium, helps you accurately determine the patient's risk of ACS.
- To promote the greatest benefit in caring for a patient with ACS, time-sensitive goals have been established. The overall goal is to limit the amount of time the myocardium is ischemic to less than 120 minutes.
- Early performance of ECG and initiation of reperfusion strategies are vital in meeting the time-sensitive goals for the treatment of MI.
- STEMI management is directed at stopping the formation of the thrombus, dissolving the thrombus, and opening the occluded coronary artery.
- The decision to choose PCI over fibrinolytic therapy is based on the availability of resources and the condition of the patient.

CHAPTER REVIEW QUESTIONS

1. Which of the following plays the greatest role in recognizing MI?
   A. Accurate interpretation of the ECG
   B. Early administration of nitroglycerin
   C. Rapid availability of cardiac markers
   D. Recognizing the signs and symptoms of ACS

2. The patient with ACS who presents without chest pain but with other signs and symptoms consistent with ACS has what?
   A. Anginal equivalents
   B. A silent MI
   C. Not had a heart attack
   D. Unstable angina

3. How is the chest pain of ACS most often described?
   A. A heavy pressure
   B. Lasting less than a minute
   C. Painful to the touch
   D. Worse with breathing

4. An agitated patient presents with dyspnea on exertion, wheezing, and a cough producing blood-tinged sputum. Vital signs are as follows: pulse is 104 and regular, respiration is 24 and shallow, and blood pressure is 160/90 mm Hg. Neck veins are distended, and an S_3 heart murmur is noted. This patient is most likely suffering from what?
   A. Cardiogenic shock
   B. Left-heart failure
   C. Right-heart failure
   D. Uncomplicated acute MI

5. In NSTEMI, the 12-lead ECG is nondiagnostic, and the diagnosis is based on what?
   A. Cardiac biomarkers
   B. Serial ECG changes
   C. The history
   D. The history in combination with elevated cardiac markers

6. The ultimate goal in treating the patient with MI is to do what?
   A. Administer aspirin to all patients with chest pain.
   B. Administer nitroglycerin as soon as possible.
   C. Identify the at-risk patient as quickly as possible.
   D. Limit the amount of myocardial damage.

7. The time-critical goal of patient arrival to administration of fibrinolytics is referred to as the _____ time, and it should be within _____.
   A. ECG-to-needle; 30 minutes
   B. door-to-device; 30 minutes
   C. door-to-needle; 30 minutes
   D. door-to-device; 90 minutes

8. Antiplatelet agents are administered to do what?
   A. Destroy the thrombus
   B. Maintain the patency of the vessel
   C. Prevent the formation of additional thrombi
   D. Thin the blood to promote bleeding

9. LMW heparin, warfarin, and abciximab exert their effect on the thrombus by which mechanism?
   A. Inhibition of platelet aggregation
   B. Inhibition of thromboxane A_1 release
   C. Promotion of healing of the ruptured plaque
   D. Promotion of destruction of fibrin

10. Which process entails inserting a balloon-tipped catheter into an occluded artery to fracture an atherosclerotic plaque and dilate the arterial lumen?
    A. Coronary artery stenting
    B. Directional coronary atherectomy
    C. Percutaneous coronary angioplasty
    D. Rotational atherectomy

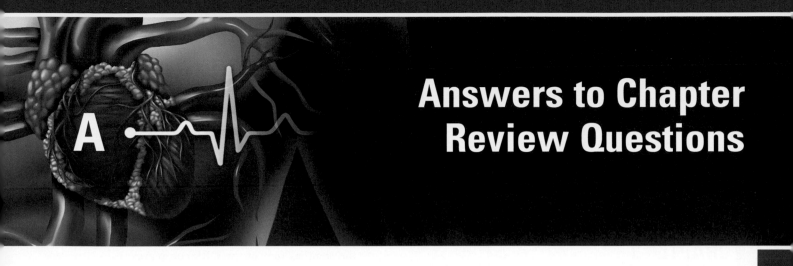

CHAPTER 1

1. (B) The inner layer of the serous pericardium is called the *visceral pericardium* or **epicardium.**
2. (C) The **right** heart pumps blood into the **pulmonary** circulation (the blood vessels within the lungs and those carrying blood to and from the lungs). The **left** heart pumps blood into the **systemic** circulation (the blood vessels in the rest of the body and those carrying blood to and from the body).
3. (C) The right ventricle pumps unoxygenated blood through the **pulmonary** valve and into the lungs through the **pulmonary** artery. In the lungs, the blood picks up oxygen and releases excess carbon dioxide.
4. (C) The period of relaxation and filling of the ventricles with blood is called **ventricular diastole.**
5. (C) The electrical conduction system of the heart is composed of the following structures: the sinoatrial (SA) node, internodal atrial conduction tracts, the atrioventricular (AV) junction, **left and right bundle branches,** and the Purkinje network. The coronary sinus, atrial septa, and vagus nerve are not components of the electrical conduction system.
6. (A) **Automaticity** is the ability of cardiac cells to spontaneously depolarize.
7. (D) When a myocardial cell is in the resting state, a high concentration of **positively** charged **sodium** ions (Na1) (cations) is present outside the cell.
8. (A) Cardiac cells cannot be stimulated to depolarize during the **absolute refractory period** because they have not sufficiently repolarized.
9. (D) The **SA node** is normally the dominant and primary pacemaker of the heart because it possesses the highest level of automaticity.
10. (A) The **firing** of the vagus nerve will cause a slowing of the heart.
11. See Fig. 1.1 for answers.

CHAPTER 2

1. (A) The ECG is a record of the electrical activity (electric current) generated by the **depolarization and repolarization of the atria and ventricles.** The electrical impulses responsible for initiating depolarization of the atria and ventricles are too small to be detected by the ECG electrodes, and the mechanical contraction and relaxation of the atria and ventricles do not generate electrical activity.
2. (D) Dark vertical lines are **0.20 second** (5 mm) apart, whereas light vertical lines are **0.04 second** (1 mm) apart.
3. (B) The sensitivity of the ECG machine is calibrated so that a **1-millivolt** electrical signal produces a **10-mm** deflection on the ECG, equivalent to two large squares on the ECG paper.
4. (B) Atrial depolarization is recorded as the P wave, **ventricular depolarization as the QRS complex,** atrial repolarization as the atrial T wave, and ventricular repolarization as the T wave.
5. (D) Atrial depolarization is recorded as the P wave, ventricular depolarization as the QRS complex, atrial repolarization as the atrial T wave, and **ventricular repolarization as the T wave.**
6. (C) Muscle tremors, poor electrode contact, external chest compressions, and turning the gain up can all cause artifacts on an ECG tracing. However, the **most common cause of artifact is poor electrode contact with the skin,** usually as a result of diaphoresis or hair.
7. (D) An EGG lead composed of a single positive electrode and a zero reference point (the central terminal) is called a *unipolar lead*.
8. (C) Monitoring lead II is obtained by attaching the negative electrode to the **right arm** and the positive electrode to the **left leg.**

9. (D) If the positive ECG electrode is attached to the left leg or lower left anterior chest, all of the electric impulses generated in the heart that flow toward the positive electrode will be recorded as **positive (upright)** deflections. The impulses flowing away from the positive electrode will be recorded as negative (inverted) deflections.

10. (D) Monitoring lead MCL₁ is obtained by attaching the positive **electrode to the right side of the anterior chest in the fourth intercostal space just right of the sternum.**

CHAPTER 3

1. (B) Increased left atrial pressure resulting in left atrial dilatation and hypertrophy is found in hypertension, **mitral and aortic valvular disease,** and acute myocardial infarction. Pulmonary edema secondary to left heart failure may also cause wide, notched P waves.

2. (D) The normal PR interval is between **0.12 and 0.20 second.**

3. (D) An ectopic P wave represents atrial depolarization occurring in an **abnormal direction** or **sequence** or both.

4. (B) A normal QRS complex represents normal **depolarization of the ventricles.**

5. (D) The time from the onset of the QRS complex to the peak of the R wave is the **ventricular activation time** (VAT). The VAT represents the time taken for depolarization of the interventricular septum plus depolarization of the ventricle from the endocardium to the epicardium under the facing lead.

6. (B) The **atrio–His fibers** form an accessory conduction pathway that connects the atria with the lowest part of the atrioventricular (AV) node near the bundle of His and not with the ventricles directly, as do the other accessory conduction pathways. For this reason, they do not cause ventricular preexcitation (that is, atrio–His preexcitation). Delta waves are absent.

7. (C) Abnormal ventricular repolarization (the **T wave**) may result from myocardial ischemia, acute myocardial infarction (MI), myocarditis, pericarditis, ventricular enlargement (hypertrophy), electrolyte imbalance (for example, excess serum potassium), or administration of certain cardiac drugs (for example, quinidine, procainamide).

8. (C) An abnormally tall U wave may be present in **hypokalemia, cardiomyopathy,** and left ventricular hypertrophy and may follow the administration of digitalis, quinidine, and procainamide.

9. (C) A **prolonged PR interval** (one that is greater in duration than 0.20 second) indicates that a delay of progression of the electrical impulse through the AV node, bundle of His, or rarely, the bundle branches is present.

10. (C) An abnormal ST segment indicates **abnormal ventricular repolarization,** a common consequence of myocardial ischemia and acute myocardial infarction (MI). It is also present in ventricular fibrosis or aneurysm, pericarditis, left ventricular enlargement (hypertrophy), and administration of digitalis.

CHAPTER 4

1. (B) The **heart-rate calculator ruler** is most accurate if the rhythm is regular.

2. (A) The 6-second count method can be used when the rhythm is either regular or **irregular.**

3. (B) The heart rate is **75 beats/min**. Provided the ECG has a regular rate, one method to determine the rate is to count the large squares (0.20-second squares) between the peaks of two consecutive R waves and divide this number into 300.

4. (D) The rate of the normally conducted P waves is usually the **same as that of the QRS complexes.** If an atrioventricular (AV) block is present, it may be **greater.**

5. (A) If QRS complexes are present but do not regularly precede or follow the P waves, a **complete atrioventricular (AV) block (third-degree AV block) is present.** Another term used to describe the condition when QRS complexes occur totally unrelated to the P, P′, or F waves is *AV dissociation.*

6. (B) If atrial flutter or fibrillation waves are present, the electrical impulses responsible for them have originated in the **atria.**

7. (B) If the P waves are inverted in lead II, the electrical impulses responsible for the P waves most likely have originated in the **lower atria.**

8. (D) A PR interval of less than 0.12 second is usually present in an atrial arrhythmia arising in the atria near the atrioventricular (AV) junction and in a junctional arrhythmia. It is also present in ventricular preexcitation and atrio–His preexcitation.

9. (A) If the QRS complexes are 0.12 second or less in duration, the electrical impulses responsible for the QRS complexes most likely have originated in the **sinoatrial (SA) node,** atria, or atrioventricular (AV) junction.

10. (D) A QRS originating in the Purkinje network will travel through slower and abnormal pathways; it will have a **bizarre shape** and duration **longer than 0.12 second.**

CHAPTER 5

1. (C) Typically, the heart rate **increases** during inspiration and **decreases** during expiration.

2. (B) The most common type of sinus arrhythmia, the one related to respiration, is a normal phenomenon commonly seen in children, young adults, and elderly individuals. It is caused by the **inhibitory vagal effect** of respiration on the sinoatrial (SA) node.

3. (C) Another, less common type of sinus arrhythmia is not related to respiration. It may occur in healthy individuals but is more commonly found in adult patients with **heart disease or acute myocardial infarction (MI)** and in those **on digitalis** or morphine.

4. (C) A dysrhythmia originating in the sinoatrial (SA) node with a regular rate of less than 60 beats/min is called *sinus bradycardia.*

5. (A) Sinus bradycardia may be caused by **excessive inhibitory vagal tone on the sinoatrial (SA) node, a decrease in sympathetic tone on the SA node,** and **hypothermia,** among other things.

6. (C) A mild sinus bradycardia has a heartbeat of **50 to 59 beats/min.**

7. (B) A patient with marked sinus bradycardia who is symptomatic will likely have **hypotension and decreased cerebral perfusion.**

8. (A) Symptomatic sinus tachycardia is best treated by **addressing the underlying cause.**

9. (C) **Sinus arrest** is an arrhythmia caused by episodes of failure in the automaticity of the sinoatrial (SA) node, resulting in bradycardia or asystole.

10. (B) **Digitalis** is the most common cause of sinoatrial (SA) exit block. Beta blockers and quinidine may also cause this condition.

CHAPTER 6

1. (D) A dysrhythmia originating in pacemakers that shifts back and forth between the sinoatrial (SA) node and an ectopic pacemaker in the atria or atrioventricular (AV) junction is called a *wandering atrial pacemaker.* It is characterized by P waves of varying size, shape, and direction in any given lead.

2. (D) The dysrhythmia described in question 1 may normally be seen in the **very young,** the elderly, and athletes.

3. (A) An extra atrial complex consisting of a positive P wave in lead II followed by a normal or abnormal QRS complex occurring earlier than the next beat of the underlying rhythm is called a *premature atrial complex.* It is followed by a noncompensatory pause.

4. (B) A nonconducted or blocked premature atrial complex (PAC) is a **P′ wave that is not followed by a QRS complex.**

5. (D) The QRS complex of a premature atrial complex (PAC) usually resembles that of the **underlying rhythm.**

6. (B) Two premature atrial complexes (PACs) in a row are called a *couplet.*

7. (B) An arrhythmia originating in an ectopic pacemaker in the atrial node with an atrial rate between 160 and 240 beats/min is called *atrial tachycardia.*

8. (D) The **reduction in cardiac output** accompanying atrial tachycardia can cause syncope, light-headedness, and dizziness. In patients with coronary artery disease, it can also cause angina, congestive heart failure, or an acute myocardial infarction (MI).

9. (D) Atrial flutter is characterized by **flutter waves with a sawtooth appearance** occurring at a rate of 240 to 360 per minute.

10. (A) **Atrial fibrillation** is characterized by multiple dissimilar, small atrial f waves occurring at a rate of 350 to 600 per minute.

CHAPTER 7

1. (A) Absent P′ waves in a junctional dysrhythmia indicate that **atrial depolarizations have not occurred because of a retrograde atrioventricular (AV) block** between the ectopic pacemaker site in the AV junction and the atria and/or they occurred during the QRS complex.

2. (C) If the ectopic pacemaker in the AV junction discharges too soon after the preceding QRS complex, the **premature P′ wave may not be followed by a QRS complex.**

3. (B) An extra QRS that originates from an ectopic pacemaker in the atrioventricular (AV) junction, occurring before the next expected beat of the underlying rhythm, is called a *premature junctional complex,* or **PJC.**

4. (D) The QRS complex of a premature junctional complex (PJC) usually resembles that of the underlying rhythm, being 0.10 second or less in duration. The QRS complex, however, may be 0.12 second or longer in duration and resemble that of a **premature ventricular contraction if aberrant ventricular conduction is present.** The QRS complex may precede or follow the P′ wave with which it is associated.

5. (C) The pause after the premature junctional complex (PJC) is **compensatory,** unlike that after the premature atrial complex (PAC), because the retrograde P′ of the PJC does not depolarize the sinoatrial (SA) node. The next QRS complex occurs sooner than expected because the SA node has **not been reset.**

6. (C) More than four to six premature junctional complexes (PJCs) per minute may indicate an **enhanced automaticity** or a **reentry mechanism** in the atrioventricular (**AV**) **junction** and that more serious **junctional arrhythmias may occur,** but this is **not a normal variant.**

7. (B) A dysrhythmia originating in an escape pacemaker in the atrioventricular (AV) junction with a regular rate of greater than 100 beats/min is called a *junctional tachycardia.*

8. (A) By definition, any dysrhythmia that originates above the ventricles and has a rate greater than 150 beats/min is termed *supraventricular tachycardia* (SVT). **Paroxysmal supraventricular tachycardia** (PSVT) is more clinically significant because of the abrupt onset and significant symptomatology.

9. (C) Paroxysmal supraventricular tachycardia (PSVT) is characterized by a heart rate between 160 and 240 beats/min and an **abrupt onset and termination.** The electrophysiologic mechanism responsible for PSVT is a reentry mechanism involving the atrioventricular (AV) node.

10. (D) When the rate of supraventricular tachycardia (SVT) is high and when there are ventricular conduction delays, SVT is difficult to distinguish from **ventricular tachycardia.**

CHAPTER 8

1. (D) An unexpected abnormally wide and bizarre QRS complex originating in an ectopic site in the ventricles is called a **premature ventricular complex (PVC).**

2. (D) Premature ventricular complexes (PVCs) that originate from a single ectopic pacemaker site are called *unifocal*.

3. (D) A premature ventricular complex (PVC) may **trigger ventricular fibrillation if it occurs on the T wave** or depolarizes the sinoatrial (SA) node, momentarily suppressing it, so that the next P wave of the underlying rhythm appears **later** than expected. A PVC occurring simultaneously with a normal QRS forms a **fusion beat**.

4. (B) A noncompensatory pause is **two** times the preceding R-R interval.

5. (D) A QRS that has characteristics of both a premature ventricular complex (PVC) and a QRS complex of the underlying rhythm is called a **fusion beat**.

6. (C) Groups of two premature ventricular complexes (PVCs) are called *couplets.* Three PVCs in a row is a **run of ventricular tachycardia (V-tach)**.

7. (C) A form of ventricular tachycardia characterized by QRS complexes that gradually change back and forth from one shape, size, and direction to another over a series of beats is called *torsades de pointes*.

8. (C) Ventricular fibrillation is a life-threatening arrhythmia requiring immediate defibrillation, which is most successful when the **fibrillatory waves are large or coarse**.

9. (A) Asymptomatic accelerated idioventricular rhythm is characterized by a ventricular rate of between 40 and 100 beats/min. It is often seen in **acute myocardial infarction**.

10. (D) A ventricular rhythm with a rate of less than 40 beats/min is a **ventricular escape rhythm**.

CHAPTER 9

1. (A) A dysrhythmia that occurs commonly in acute inferior myocardial infarction (MI) because of the effect of an increase in vagal tone and ischemia on the atrioventricular (AV) node is called a *first-degree AV block*.

2. (B) A dysrhythmia in which there is a progressive lengthening delay after each P wave in the conduction of electrical impulses through the AV node until the conduction of the electrical impulses is completely blocked is called a **second-degree type I AV block** or Wenckebach block.

3. (A) A second-degree type I atrioventricular (AV) block is usually transient, reversible, and asymptomatic, yet the patient should be monitored and observed because **it can progress to a higher-degree AV block.** It is more commonly associated with an acute **inferior** wall myocardial infarction (MI).

4. (C) A dysrhythmia in which a complete block of conduction of electrical impulses occurs in one bundle branch and an intermittent block in the other is called a **second-degree type II AV block.**

5. (D) **Temporary cardiac pacing** is indicated immediately in a symptomatic second-degree type II atrioventricular (AV) block that occurs after an acute anteroseptal myocardial infarction (MI).

6. (C) A second-degree advanced atrioventricular (AV) block has an AV conduction **ratio of 3:1 or greater** (that is, 3:1, 4:1, 6:1, 8:1, or greater).

7. (C) The absence of conduction of electrical impulses through the atrioventricular (AV) node, bundle of His, or bundle branches, characterized by independent beating of the atria and ventricles, is called a **third-degree AV block.**

8. (D) An escape pacemaker in the atrioventricular (AV) junction has an inherent firing rate of **40 to 60 beats/min.**

9. (A) If an atrioventricular (AV) junctional or ventricular escape pacemaker does not take over after a sudden onset of third-degree AV block, asystole will occur. No pulse is generated, and **cardiac arrest** occurs.

10. (B) The clinical significance of atrioventricular (AV) blocks is primarily attributable to their resultant effect on heart rate, which is that of the **ventricular response** from the escape pacemaker.

CHAPTER 10

1. (C) **Symptomatic bradydysrhythmias,** such as third-degree atrioventricular (AV) block and advanced AV block, are indications for permanent pacemaker insertion. Digitalis toxicity and complications related to acute myocardial infarction are usually treated with temporary pacemakers. Pacemakers are not indicated in the treatment of premature ventricular complexes (PVCs).

2. (A) As scar tissue builds up around the pacemaker tip of the electrode, it affects the ability of the electrode to **sense** the electrical activity of the heart.

3. (A) **Demand pacemakers** fire when the intrinsic heart rate falls below the lower set limit. Fixed-rate pacemakers fire at a preset rate, regardless of the underlying heart rate.

4. (B) **Left bundle-branch block (LBBB) appearance** occurs because the electrode lies within the right ventricle, resulting in a delay to reach the left bundle branch. The QRS duration will exceed 0.12 second, and there is no normal P wave generated by a pacemaker QRS complex.

5. (B) The code **DDD** indicates a pacemaker that paces and senses both the atria and ventricles and is inhibited by electrical activity in either. The first letter (D = dual) indicates that it paces both atria and ventricles. The second letter (D = dual) indicates that it senses both the atria and the ventricles. The third letter (D = dual) indicates that it is inhibited by electrical discharge from either the atria or/and ventricle.

6. (D) The **ventricular refractory** period is that time after the discharge of a ventricular pacer spike during which the pacemaker will not fire again. The lower limit is the maximum time the pacemaker will allow between consecutive R waves before discharging the pacemaker. *Absolute* and *relative refractory period* are terms that relate to normal repolarization of the ventricles and are unrelated to pacemakers.

7. (B) The application of the insulated circular magnet **causes the pacemaker to go into default fixed-rate mode,** which should allow visualization of pacer spikes on the ECG if the pacemaker battery and lead are functioning.

8. (C) Implantable cardioverter-defibrillators (ICDs) are indicated for nonreversible causes of ventricular tachycardia (VT).

Digitalis toxicity can be treated by withholding the drug and administering Digibind if indicated.

9. (A) **Implantable cardioverter-defibrillators (ICDs) and pacemakers can be interrogated by an external device,** which can download the generator's internal parameters, such as sensing and pacing rate, along with the energy that will be used for cardioversion/defibrillation. Only ICDs can cardiovert and overdrive pace. The electrode of the ICD is different from that of the pacemaker because it has a larger surface area to allow it to pass the higher current to the endocardium.

10. (C) An abrupt increase in implantable cardioverter-defibrillator (ICD) firing can occur for a host of reasons, which include lead fracture, oversensing of T waves, tachy-dysrhythmias, and actual ventricular tachycardia. A dead battery would result in a lack of firing. Bradycardia would result in a pacing activity, which would not be as noticeable as ICD firing. Regardless, the **patient must be placed on cardiac monitoring** to determine the underlying cardiac activity. The patient would not necessarily have to suffer cardiac arrest for the ICD to fire.

CHAPTER 11

1. (D) In a patient with symptomatic bradycardia and an ECG showing a second-degree type II atrioventricular (AV) block, you should administer oxygen, start an intravenous (IV) line, and begin **transcutaneous pacing (TCP).** Administration of atropine would be reasonable if TPC was not immediately available. There is no role for a vasopressor at this point, and an antiarrhythmic would not be indicated.

2. (A) Patients with symptomatic sinus tachycardia should be treated with the **appropriate treatment for the underlying cause of the tachycardia** (that is, anxiety, exercise, pain, fever, congestive heart failure, hypoxemia, hypovolemia, hypotension, or shock).

3. (D) If a patient is stable with an ECG showing paroxysmal supraventricular tachycardia (PSVT) after administering oxygen and starting an intravenous (IV) line, you should **attempt vagal maneuvers.** Make sure to verify the absence of known carotid artery disease or carotid bruits before attempting carotid sinus massage.

4. (B) Your patient presents with chest pain and signs and symptoms of an acute myocardial infarction (MI). The ECG shows atrial tachycardia without a block. After administering oxygen and starting an intravenous (IV) line, you should immediately **consider a loading dose of amiodarone.**

5. (A) Adenosine may slow the rate of an unknown narrow-complex QRS tachycardia thought initially to be supraventricular tachycardia (SVT), only to reveal an underlying rhythm of atrial tachycardia, atrial fibrillation, or atrial flutter. It should be administered as fast as possible, followed by a bolus of saline to ensure it reaches the heart. It may not always convert the rhythm, thus requiring other agents or electrical therapy to be considered.

6. (C) A patient with atrial fibrillation of less than 48 hours in duration who is hemodynamically unstable and hypotensive should be **immediately cardioverted and receive a loading dose of amiodarone.**

7. (B) Your patient is conscious and hemodynamically stable, with a pulse and an ECG showing monomorphic ventricular tachycardia. After administering oxygen and starting an intravenous (IV) line, you should perform the following: **administer a 150-mg loading dose of amiodarone IV.**

8. (D) If your patient in question 7 begins to complain of chest pain and then becomes pulseless, you should immediately deliver **defibrillation** of 360 joules.

9. (D) Treatment with atrioventricular (AV) nodal blocking drugs, such as adenosine, calcium-channel blockers, and beta blockers, may increase conduction via the accessory pathway, with a resultant increase in ventricular rate and possible degeneration into ventricular tachycardia (VT) or ventricular fibrillation (VF). In a hemodynamically unstable patient with Wolff–Parkinson–White (WPW), urgent cardioversion is required. Medical treatment options in a stable patient include procainamide or amiodarone.

10. (B) Patients with atrial fibrillation for longer than 48 hours are at risk for developing a mural thrombus that can result in an embolic stroke if the rhythm is converted before placing the patient on anticoagulants. Immediate conversion of atrial flutter is only undertaken if the patient is hemodynamically unstable.

CHAPTER 12

1. (A) A **bipolar** lead represents the difference in electrical potential between two electrodes.

2. (D) The "a" in aVR, aVL, and aVF stands for **augmented.**

3. (B) The electrical impulses of **lead I + lead III = lead II** is called *Einthoven's law.*

4. (B) Lead aVL is obtained by measuring the electric current between the positive electrode attached to the **left arm** and the central terminal formed by the electrodes attached to the **right arm and left leg.**

5. (B) A **precordial** lead measures the difference in electrical potential between a chest electrode and the central terminal.

6. (D) The placement of the positive chest electrode is as follows:
   V_1: right side of the sternum in the fourth intercostal space
   V_2: left side of the sternum in the fourth intercostal space
   V_3: midway between V_2 and V_4
   V_4: left **midclavicular line in the fifth intercostal space**
   V_5: left anterior axillary line at the same level as V_4
   V_6: left midaxillary line at the same level as V_4

7. (D) An electric impulse flowing toward the positive pole produces **a positive deflection** on the ECG.

8. (A) The more parallel the electric impulse is to the axis of the lead, the **larger** the deflection. The more perpendicular, the smaller the deflection.

9. (B) A predominantly negative QRS complex indicates that the **positive** pole of the vector of the QRS axis lies somewhere on the **negative** side of the perpendicular axis.

10. (B) This indicates a QRS complex with a normal axis between **0° and +90°.**

CHAPTER 13

1. (D) The time from the onset of the QRS complex to the peak of the R wave in the QRS complex is called the *ventricular activation time* (VAT).
2. (B) The anterior portion of the interventricular septum is supplied with blood from the **left anterior descending coronary artery.**
3. (D) The main blood supply of the atrioventricular (AV) node and proximal part of the bundle of His is the AV-node artery, which arises from the **right coronary artery** in 85% to 90% of the hearts. In the rest of the hearts, the AV-node artery arises from the left circumflex coronary artery.
4. (B) Common causes of bundle-branch and fascicular blocks are cardiomyopathy, **ischemic heart disease,** idiopathic degenerative disease of the electrical conduction system, severe left ventricular hypertrophy, and of course, acute myocardial infarction (MI).
5. (A) In the setting of an acute myocardial infarction (MI), a right bundle-branch block occurs primarily in an **anteroseptal MI** and, rarely, in an inferior MI.
6. (B) In patients with an acute myocardial infarction (MI) complicated by a bundle-branch block, the **incidence of pump failure and ventricular arrhythmias is much higher** than in those not so complicated.
7. (C) Common causes of chronic right bundle-branch blocks include **myocarditis, cardiomyopathy, and cardiac surgery.**
8. (B) In a right bundle-branch block, the QRS complex in lead V_1 is **wide, with a classic triphasic rSR′ pattern**.
9. (B) When the electrical impulses are prevented from directly entering the anterior and lateral walls of the left ventricle, the condition is called a *left anterior fascicular block*.
10. (A) The most common bifascicular block is a **right bundle-branch block (RBBB) with** a **left anterior fascicular block.**

CHAPTER 14

1. (C) A chronic condition of the heart characterized by an increase in the thickness of a chamber's myocardial wall secondary to the increase in the size of the muscle fibers is called *hypertrophy*. *Dilatation* is enlargement of the chamber, and atrophy is thinning of the muscle wall. *Stenosis* refers to stiffening or scarring, which usually affects the valves.
2. (A) A patient with mitral valve insufficiency or left-heart failure may develop **left atrial and ventricular enlargement.**
3. (C) Left ventricular hypertrophy, a condition usually caused by increased pressure or volume in the left ventricle, is often found in **systemic hypertension, acute myocardial infarction (MI),** mitral insufficiency, hypertrophic cardiomyopathy, and aortic stenosis or insufficiency. The other listed answers are associated with right ventricular hypertrophy.
4. (D) **Pericarditis** is an inflammatory disease directly involving the epicardium, with deposition of inflammatory cells and a variable amount of serous, fibrous, purulent, or hemorrhagic exudate within the sac surrounding the heart.
5. (A) In diffuse pericarditis, the ST segment is elevated in **all leads except aVR and V_1.**
6. (C) **Hyperkalemia** is an excess of serum potassium above the normal levels of 3.5 to 5.0 mEq/L.
7. (D) The ECG changes that occur at various levels of excess serum potassium are as follows: **the QRS complexes widen, and the T waves become tall**; the ST segments disappear, and the T waves become peaked; the PR intervals become prolonged, and a "sine wave" QRS-ST-T pattern appears.
8. (A) A medication normally prescribed to heart patients that, when taken in excess, causes depression of myocardial contractility, atrioventricular (AV) block, ventricular asystole, premature ventricular complexes (PVCs), and ventricular tachycardia and fibrillation is **digitalis.**
9. (A) The ECG changes in acute pulmonary embolism include a **QRS axis of greater than** +90°.
10. (B) The Osborn wave is a sign of **hypothermia.**

CHAPTER 15

1. (B) The artery that arises from the left main coronary artery at an obtuse angle and runs posteriorly along the left atrioventricular (AV) groove to end in the back of the left ventricle is called the *left circumflex* coronary artery. This is the case in 85% to 90% of hearts. In the remaining percentage, the left circumflex coronary artery continues along the AV groove to become the posterior descending coronary artery while giving rise to the posterior left ventricular arteries and the AV-node artery.
2. (D) The sinoatrial (SA) node is supplied with blood by the SA-node artery, which arises from either the left circumflex coronary artery (in 40%–50% of hearts) or the **right coronary artery** (in 50%–60% of hearts).
3. (D) The most common cause of myocardial ischemia or infarction is an **occlusion of an atherosclerotic coronary artery.** Other causes include coronary artery spasm, increased myocardial workload, toxic exposure to cocaine or ethanol, decreased level of oxygen in the blood delivered to the myocardium, and decreased coronary artery blood flow from whatever cause.
4. (C) Atherosclerosis results in the development of vulnerable plaques, which can rupture and result in a thrombus that occludes the coronary artery. Hypertension is a cardiac risk factor but is not the primary cause of a myocardial infarction (MI). Coronary spasm may result in an MI but is very rare, as is the potential for a coronary air embolus.
5. (A) The necrotic myocardial cell is dead and will never return to any level of functioning, even after reestablishing perfusion and oxygenation.
6. (D) A myocardial infarction in which the zone of infarction involves the entire full thickness of the ventricular wall, from the endocardium to the epicardial surface, is called a *transmural infarction*.
7. (B) The "window" theory provides an explanation for the appearance of **pathologic Q waves** through which the facing lead views the Q wave of the normal myocardium on the opposite side of the infarction.

8. (C) Inverted or tall peaked T waves in the facing leads during the early phase of an acute myocardial infarction (MI) are an indication of **ischemia.** Necrosis and infarction are signified by the presence of pathologic Q waves and injury by ST-segment elevation.

9. (D) The most likely cause of an inferior myocardial infarction (MI) is an occlusion of the posterior left ventricular arteries, which, in the majority of persons, branch from the **right coronary artery.**

10. (B) ST-segment depression and T-wave inversion represent ECG evidence of ischemia. A Q wave indicates that there was a transmural myocardial infarction (MI).

CHAPTER 16

1. (A) A **localized anterior myocardial infarction** presents early with ST-segment elevation, with tall T waves and taller-than-normal R waves in the midprecordial leads V_3 and V_4, and it presents late with QS complexes with T-wave inversion in leads V_3 and V_4.

2. (C) A **lateral myocardial infarction** presents early with ST-segment depression in leads II, III, and aVF and ST-segment elevation, tall T waves, and taller-than-normal R waves in leads I, aVL, and the left precordial lead V_5 or V_6 or both.

3. (D) A **septal myocardial infarction** presents late with QS complexes with T-wave inversions in leads V_1 to V_2 and absent normal "septal" q waves in leads II, III, and aVF.

4. (B) An **anterolateral myocardial infarction** presents early with ST-segment elevation, tall T waves, and taller-than-normal R waves in leads I and aVL and the precordial leads V_3 to V_6 and ST-segment depression in leads II, III, and aVF.

5. (B) An **inferior myocardial infarction** involves the posterior left ventricular arteries arising from the right coronary artery or the left circumflex coronary artery of the left coronary artery.

6. (A) An **inferior myocardial infarction** is noted by the presence of ST-segment elevation, tall T waves, and taller-than-normal R waves in leads II, III, and aVF; ST-segment elevation in V_{4R}; and ST-segment depression in leads I and aVL.

7. (C) A **posterior myocardial infarction** presents late with large R waves and tall T waves in leads V_1 to V_4; an R wave ≥ 0.04 second in width, with slurring and notching in V_1; and an R/S ratio of ≥ 1 in V_1.

8. (B) The Sgarbossa criteria consist of the following:
   - Concordant ST elevation of greater than 1 mm in leads with a positive QRS complex
   - Concordant ST depression of greater than 1 mm in V_1 to V_3
   - Excessively discordant ST elevation of greater than 5 mm in leads with a negative QRS complex

9. (B) The criteria for detecting ST-segment-elevation myocardial infarction (STEMI) in the presence of left ventricular hypertrophy (LVH) are an ST segment of greater than 2 mm in the inferior leads and/or ST-segment elevation in the precordial leads exceeding 25% of the depth or height of the RS wave.

10. (D) The following findings support the diagnosis of ST-segment-elevation myocardial infarction (STEMI) versus pericarditis:
    - ST depression in any leads other than aVR or V_1
    - Convex or horizontal ST elevation
    - ST-segment elevation that is greater in lead III than II

CHAPTER 17

1. (D) **Recognizing the signs and symptoms of acute coronary syndrome (ACS)** is the single most important factor both for the patient and clinician in avoiding unrecognized myocardial infarctions.

2. (A) **Anginal equivalents** are symptoms other than typical chest pain that are consistent with acute coronary syndrome (ACS). They occur more commonly in the elderly, in patients with diabetes, and in women. A silent myocardial infarction (MI) is one in which an MI occurs but the patient had no symptoms.

3. (A) The typical ACS chest pain is a crushing, **heavy pressure** of substernal pain that lasts more than 5 minutes and is not associated with breathing or movement.

4. (C) In the early phases of left-heart failure, pulmonary edema causes **dyspnea with exertion.** As it progresses, the dyspnea worsens and occurs while at rest and lying down. Chest pain and cough are not specific to the condition.

5. (D) The patient with a nondiagnostic 12-lead ECG must have a risk stratification performed. This will include **a combination of history and cardiac markers** to make the diagnosis of non–ST-segment-elevation myocardial infarction (NSTEMI). Neither one alone is sufficient to make the diagnosis, and serial ECGs will not result in changes.

6. (D) When caring for a patient experiencing a myocardial infarction, all treatment is designed to **limit the amount of myocardial damage.** This is accomplished by rapid identification and early administration of nitroglycerin, antiplatelets, and reperfusion therapy.

7. (C) The goal for administering fibrinolytics is referred to as *door-to-needle* time and should occur within **30 minutes.**

8. (C) Antiplatelet agents **stop the formation of additional thrombi** by blocking substances such as thromboxane. Fibrinolytics lyse the thrombus, and only percutaneous transluminal coronary angioplasty (PTCA) mechanically opens the vessels. The goal is *not* to thin the blood but only to stop additional thrombus formation.

9. (A) Low-molecular-weight (LMW) heparin, warfarin, and abciximab exert their effect on the thrombus by **inhibiting platelet aggregation.** Aspirin exerts its effect by inhibiting thromboxane A_1 release, and reteplase exerts its effect by promoting lysis of fibrin.

10. (C) **Percutaneous coronary angioplasty** (PCA) is a procedure in which a balloon-tipped catheter is inserted into an occluded artery, and then the balloon is inflated, thereby fracturing the atherosclerotic plaque and dilating the arterial lumen. This procedure is also referred to as *balloon angioplasty.*

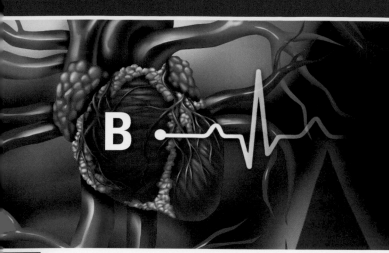

I. DYSRHYTHMIAS

1.

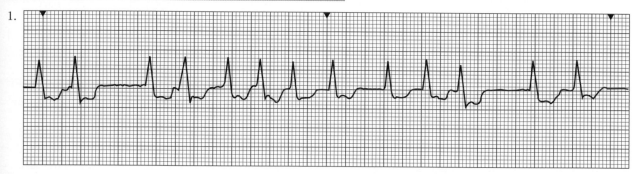

Rate: _____   PR Interval (PRI): _____
Rhythm: _____   QRS: _____
P Waves: _____ Interpretation (Interp): _____

2.

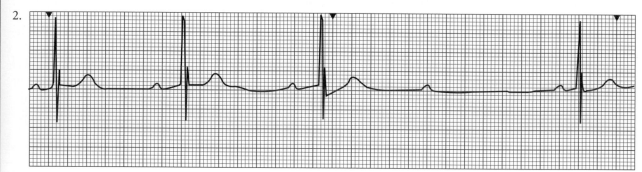

Rate: _____   PRI: _____
Rhythm: _____   QRS: _____
P Waves: _____ Interp: _____

3.

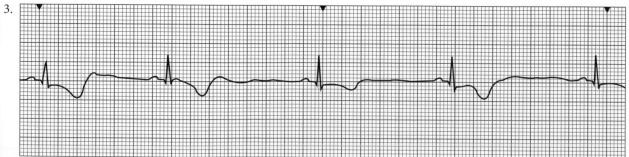

Rate: _____   PRI: _____
Rhythm: _____   QRS: _____
P Waves: _____ Interp: _____

4.

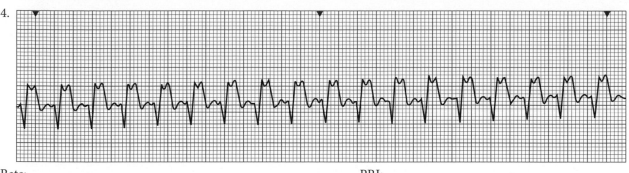

Rate: _____ PRI: _____

Rhythm: _____ QRS: _____

P Waves: _____ Interp: _____

5.

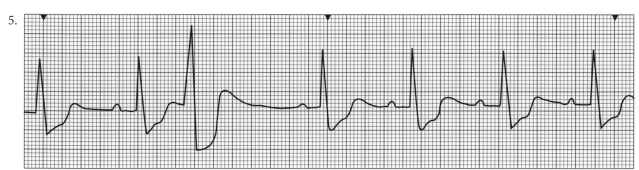

Rate: _____ PRI: _____

Rhythm: _____ QRS: _____

P Waves: _____ Interp: _____

6.

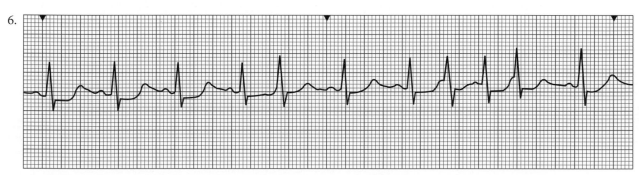

Rate: _____ PRI: _____

Rhythm: _____ QRS: _____

P Waves: _____ Interp: _____

7.

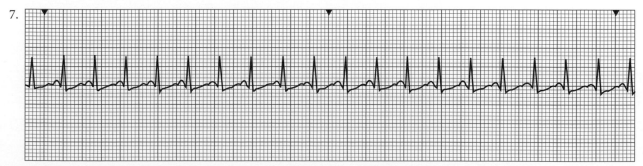

Rate: _____ PRI: _____

Rhythm: _____ QRS: _____

P Waves: _____ Interp: _____

8.

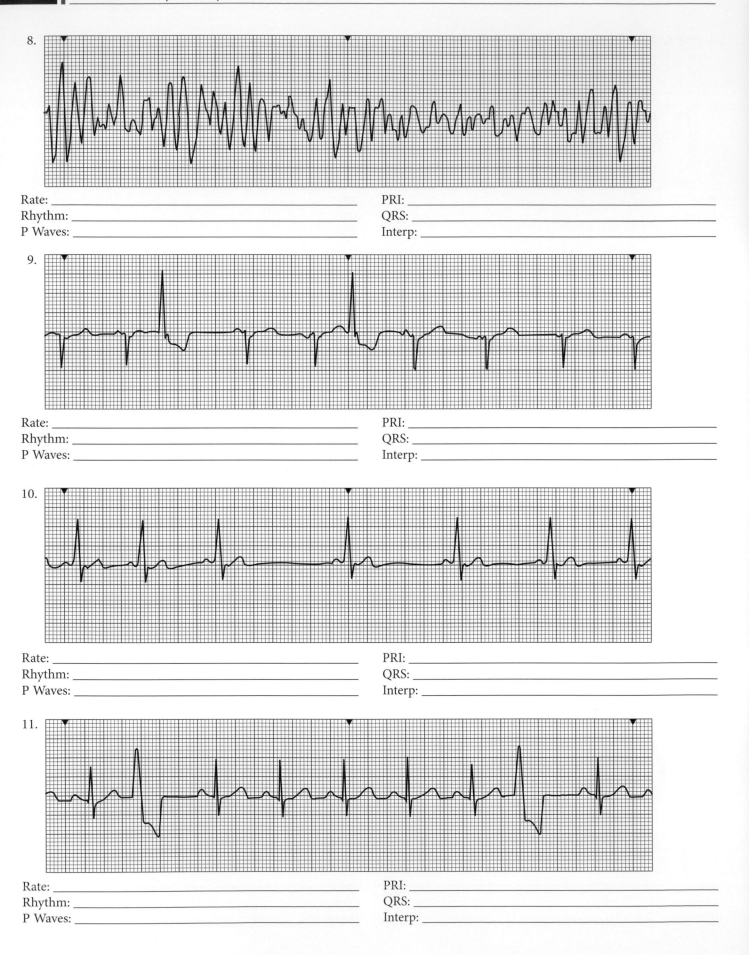

Rate: _____

Rhythm: _____

P Waves: _____

PRI: _____

QRS: _____

Interp: _____

9.

Rate: _____

Rhythm: _____

P Waves: _____

PRI: _____

QRS: _____

Interp: _____

10.

Rate: _____

Rhythm: _____

P Waves: _____

PRI: _____

QRS: _____

Interp: _____

11.

Rate: _____

Rhythm: _____

P Waves: _____

PRI: _____

QRS: _____

Interp: _____

12.

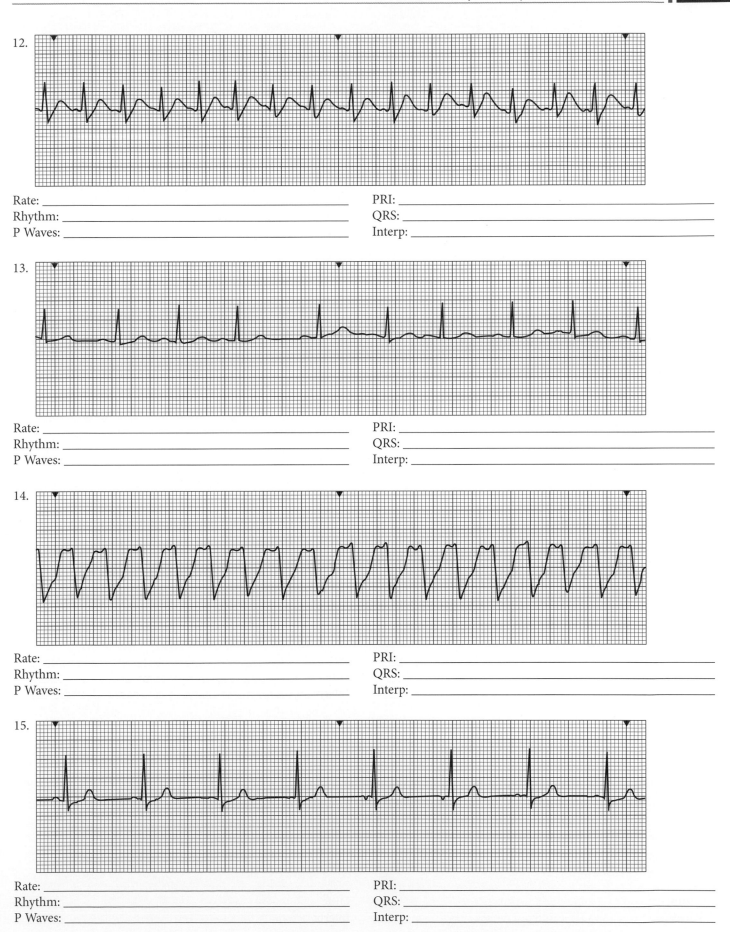

Rate: _____   PRI: _____
Rhythm: _____   QRS: _____
P Waves: _____   Interp: _____

13.

Rate: _____   PRI: _____
Rhythm: _____   QRS: _____
P Waves: _____   Interp: _____

14.

Rate: _____   PRI: _____
Rhythm: _____   QRS: _____
P Waves: _____   Interp: _____

15.

Rate: _____   PRI: _____
Rhythm: _____   QRS: _____
P Waves: _____   Interp: _____

16.

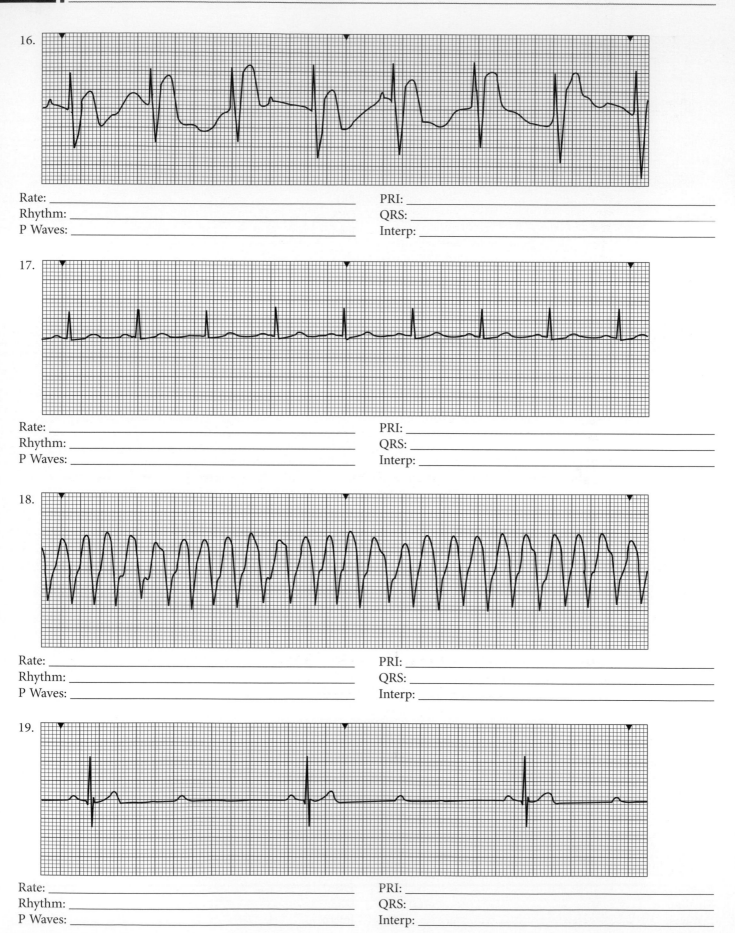

Rate: _____   PRI: _____
Rhythm: _____   QRS: _____
P Waves: _____   Interp: _____

17.

Rate: _____   PRI: _____
Rhythm: _____   QRS: _____
P Waves: _____   Interp: _____

18.

Rate: _____   PRI: _____
Rhythm: _____   QRS: _____
P Waves: _____   Interp: _____

19.

Rate: _____   PRI: _____
Rhythm: _____   QRS: _____
P Waves: _____   Interp: _____

20.

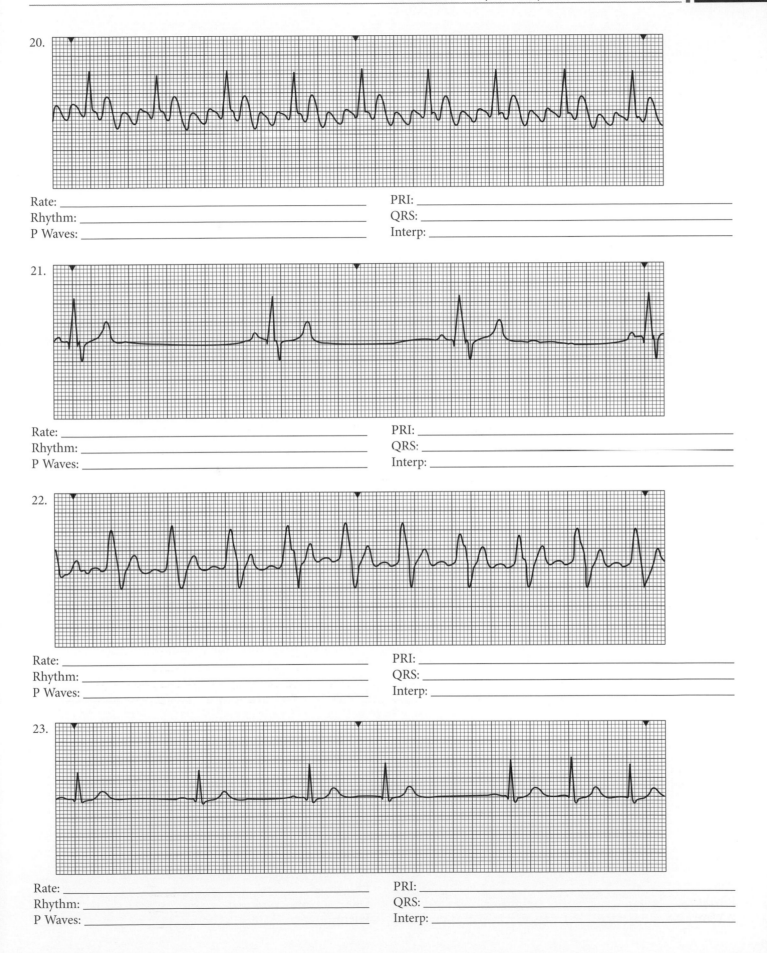

Rate: _____   PRI: _____
Rhythm: _____   QRS: _____
P Waves: _____   Interp: _____

21.

Rate: _____   PRI: _____
Rhythm: _____   QRS: _____
P Waves: _____   Interp: _____

22.

Rate: _____   PRI: _____
Rhythm: _____   QRS: _____
P Waves: _____   Interp: _____

23.

Rate: _____   PRI: _____
Rhythm: _____   QRS: _____
P Waves: _____   Interp: _____

24.

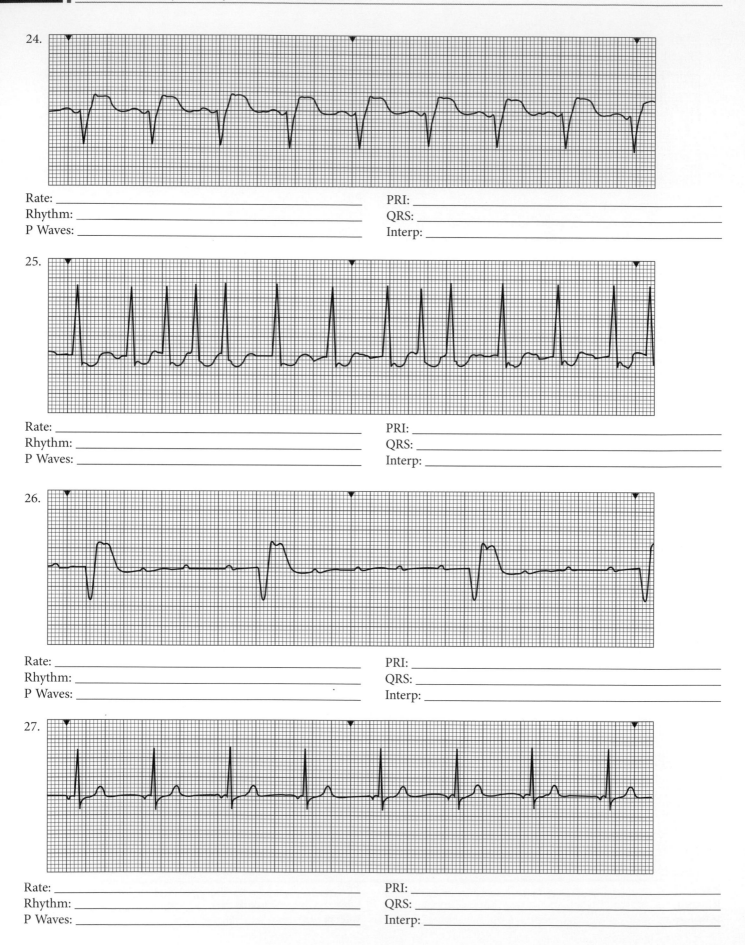

Rate: _____ PRI: _____
Rhythm: _____ QRS: _____
P Waves: _____ Interp: _____

25.

Rate: _____ PRI: _____
Rhythm: _____ QRS: _____
P Waves: _____ Interp: _____

26.

Rate: _____ PRI: _____
Rhythm: _____ QRS: _____
P Waves: _____ Interp: _____

27.

Rate: _____ PRI: _____
Rhythm: _____ QRS: _____
P Waves: _____ Interp: _____

28.

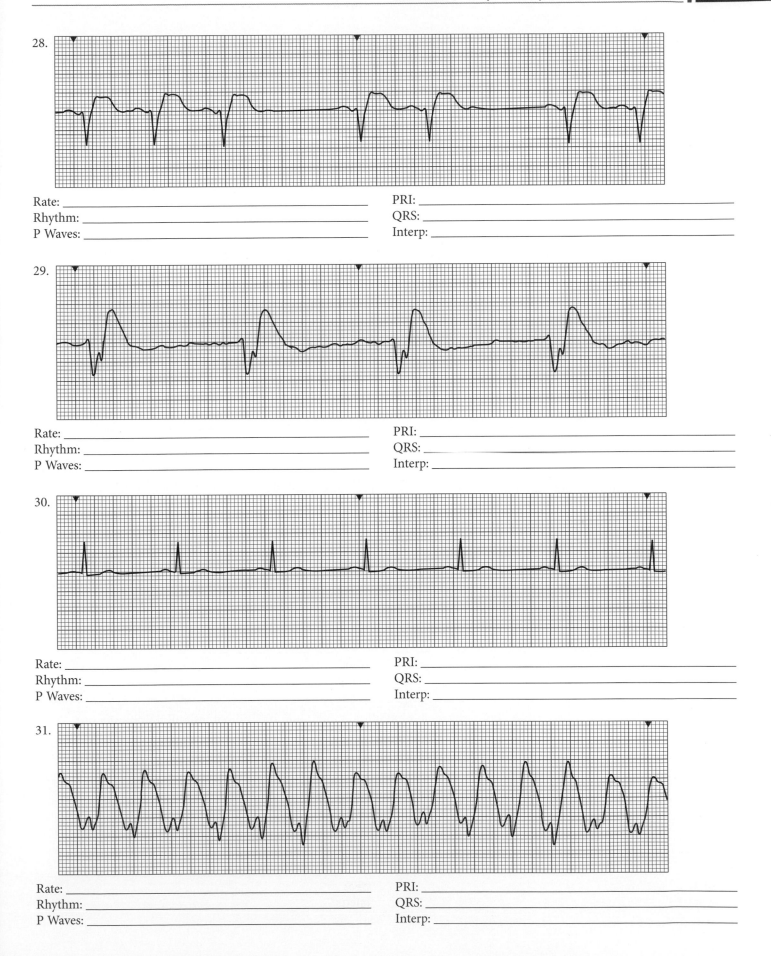

Rate: _____ PRI: _____
Rhythm: _____ QRS: _____
P Waves: _____ Interp: _____

29.

Rate: _____ PRI: _____
Rhythm: _____ QRS: _____
P Waves: _____ Interp: _____

30.

Rate: _____ PRI: _____
Rhythm: _____ QRS: _____
P Waves: _____ Interp: _____

31.

Rate: _____ PRI: _____
Rhythm: _____ QRS: _____
P Waves: _____ Interp: _____

32.

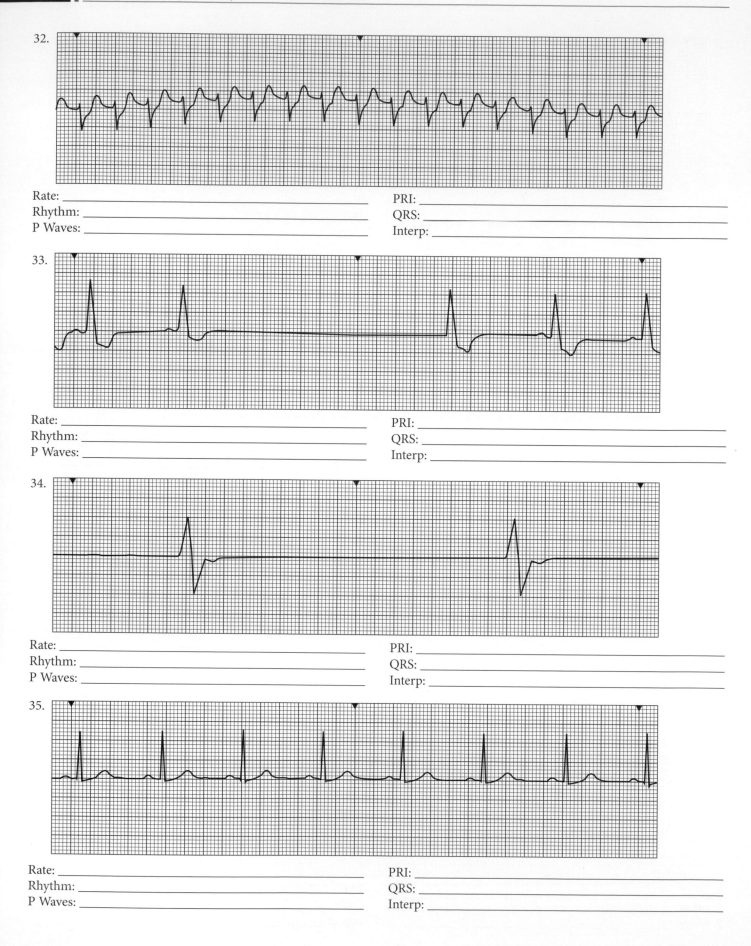

Rate: _____   PRI: _____
Rhythm: _____   QRS: _____
P Waves: _____   Interp: _____

33.

Rate: _____   PRI: _____
Rhythm: _____   QRS: _____
P Waves: _____   Interp: _____

34.

Rate: _____   PRI: _____
Rhythm: _____   QRS: _____
P Waves: _____   Interp: _____

35.

Rate: _____   PRI: _____
Rhythm: _____   QRS: _____
P Waves: _____   Interp: _____

36.

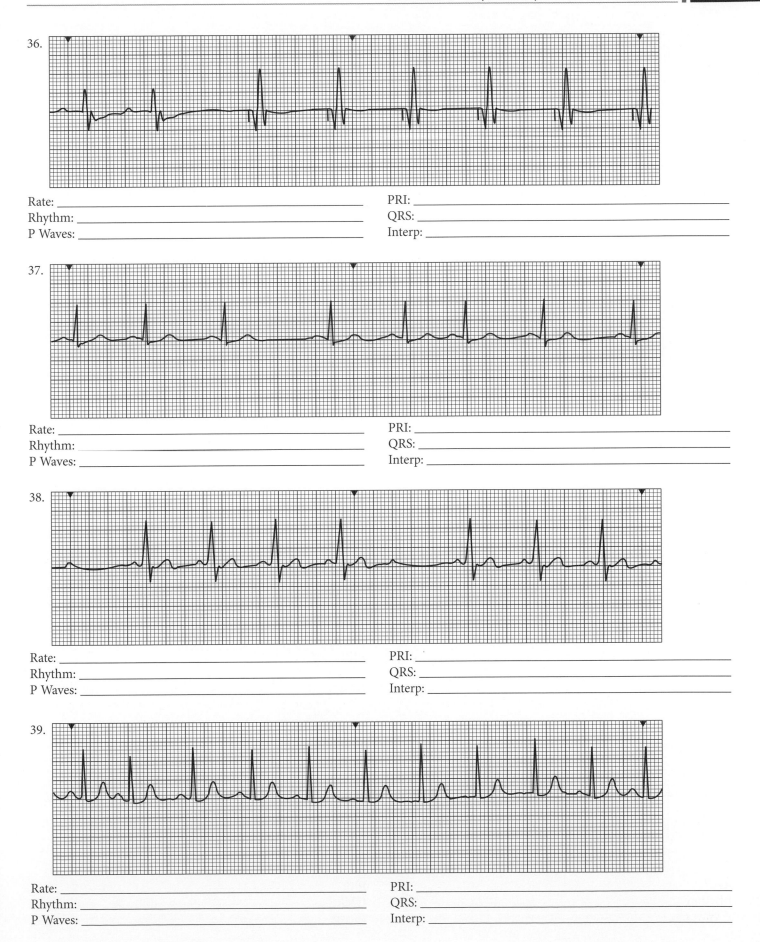

Rate: _____

Rhythm: _____

P Waves: _____

PRI: _____

QRS: _____

Interp: _____

37.

Rate: _____

Rhythm: _____

P Waves: _____

PRI: _____

QRS: _____

Interp: _____

38.

Rate: _____

Rhythm: _____

P Waves: _____

PRI: _____

QRS: _____

Interp: _____

39.

Rate: _____

Rhythm: _____

P Waves: _____

PRI: _____

QRS: _____

Interp: _____

40.

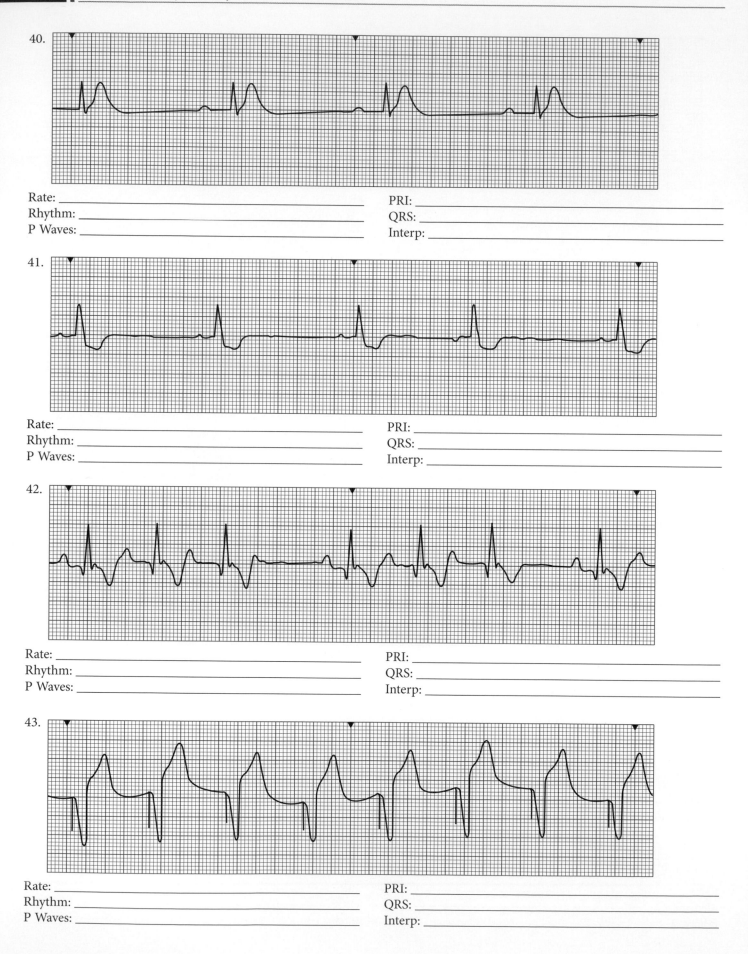

Rate: _____ PRI: _____
Rhythm: _____ QRS: _____
P Waves: _____ Interp: _____

41.

Rate: _____ PRI: _____
Rhythm: _____ QRS: _____
P Waves: _____ Interp: _____

42.

Rate: _____ PRI: _____
Rhythm: _____ QRS: _____
P Waves: _____ Interp: _____

43.

Rate: _____ PRI: _____
Rhythm: _____ QRS: _____
P Waves: _____ Interp: _____

44.

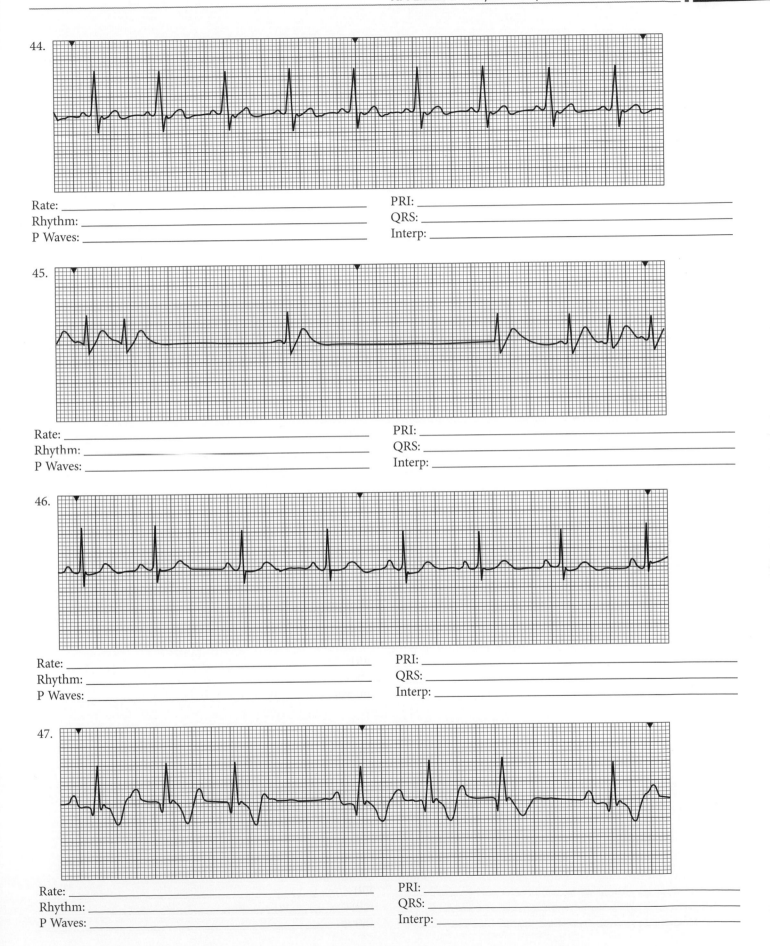

Rate: _____   PRI: _____
Rhythm: _____   QRS: _____
P Waves: _____   Interp: _____

45.

Rate: _____   PRI: _____
Rhythm: _____   QRS: _____
P Waves: _____   Interp: _____

46.

Rate: _____   PRI: _____
Rhythm: _____   QRS: _____
P Waves: _____   Interp: _____

47.

Rate: _____   PRI: _____
Rhythm: _____   QRS: _____
P Waves: _____   Interp: _____

48.

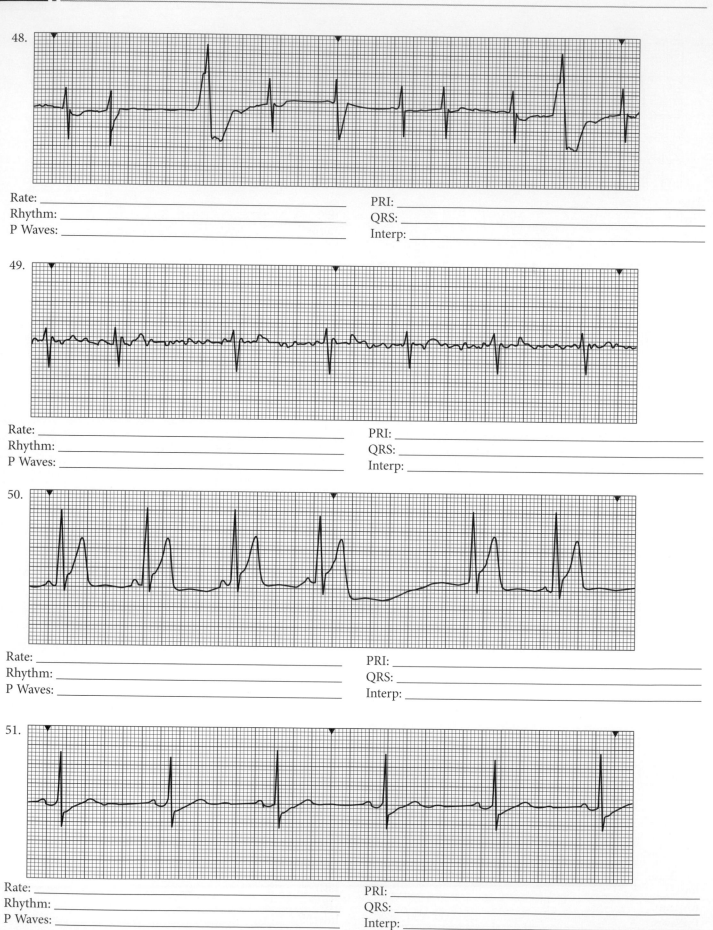

Rate: _____ PRI: _____
Rhythm: _____ QRS: _____
P Waves: _____ Interp: _____

49.

Rate: _____ PRI: _____
Rhythm: _____ QRS: _____
P Waves: _____ Interp: _____

50.

Rate: _____ PRI: _____
Rhythm: _____ QRS: _____
P Waves: _____ Interp: _____

51.

Rate: _____ PRI: _____
Rhythm: _____ QRS: _____
P Waves: _____ Interp: _____

52.

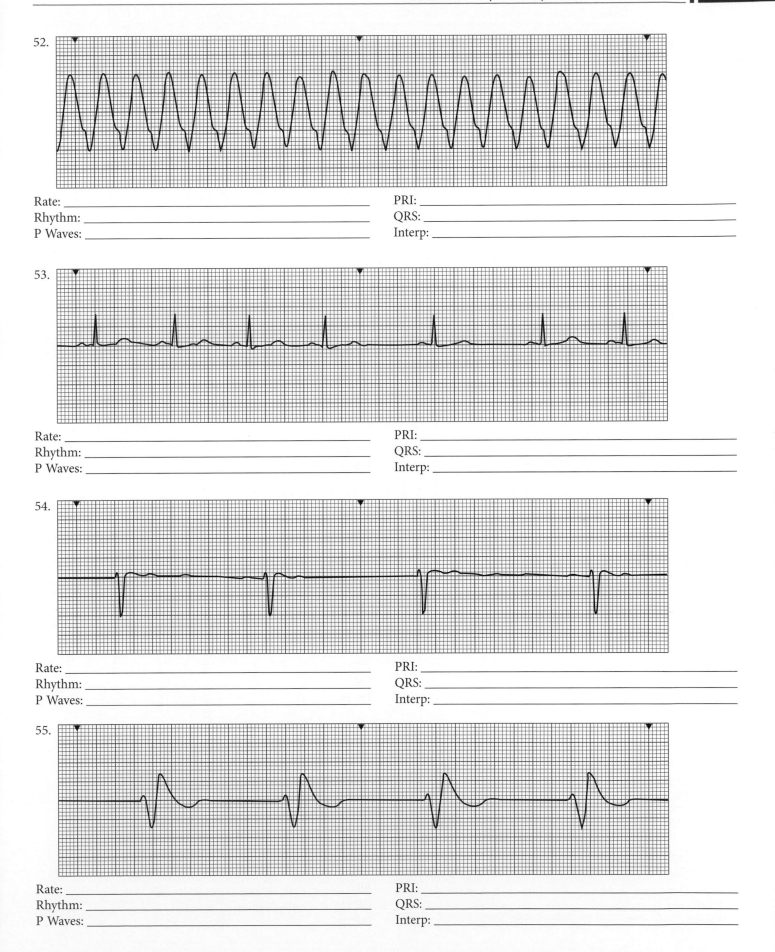

Rate: _____

Rhythm: _____

P Waves: _____

PRI: _____

QRS: _____

Interp: _____

53.

Rate: _____

Rhythm: _____

P Waves: _____

PRI: _____

QRS: _____

Interp: _____

54.

Rate: _____

Rhythm: _____

P Waves: _____

PRI: _____

QRS: _____

Interp: _____

55.

Rate: _____

Rhythm: _____

P Waves: _____

PRI: _____

QRS: _____

Interp: _____

56.

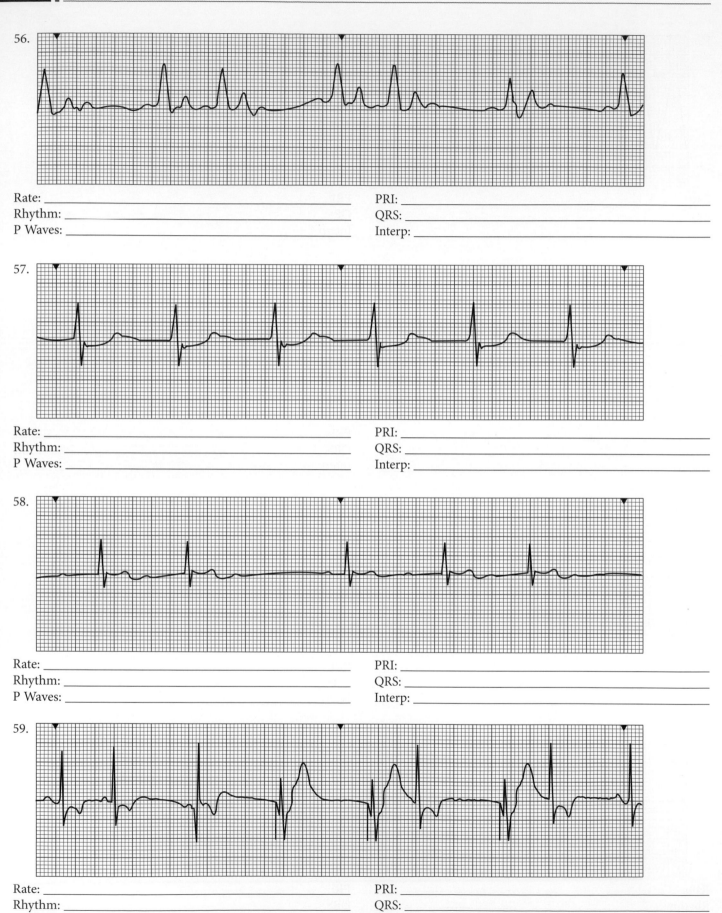

Rate: _____ PRI: _____
Rhythm: _____ QRS: _____
P Waves: _____ Interp: _____

57.

Rate: _____ PRI: _____
Rhythm: _____ QRS: _____
P Waves: _____ Interp: _____

58.

Rate: _____ PRI: _____
Rhythm: _____ QRS: _____
P Waves: _____ Interp: _____

59.

Rate: _____ PRI: _____
Rhythm: _____ QRS: _____
P Waves: _____ Interp: _____

60.

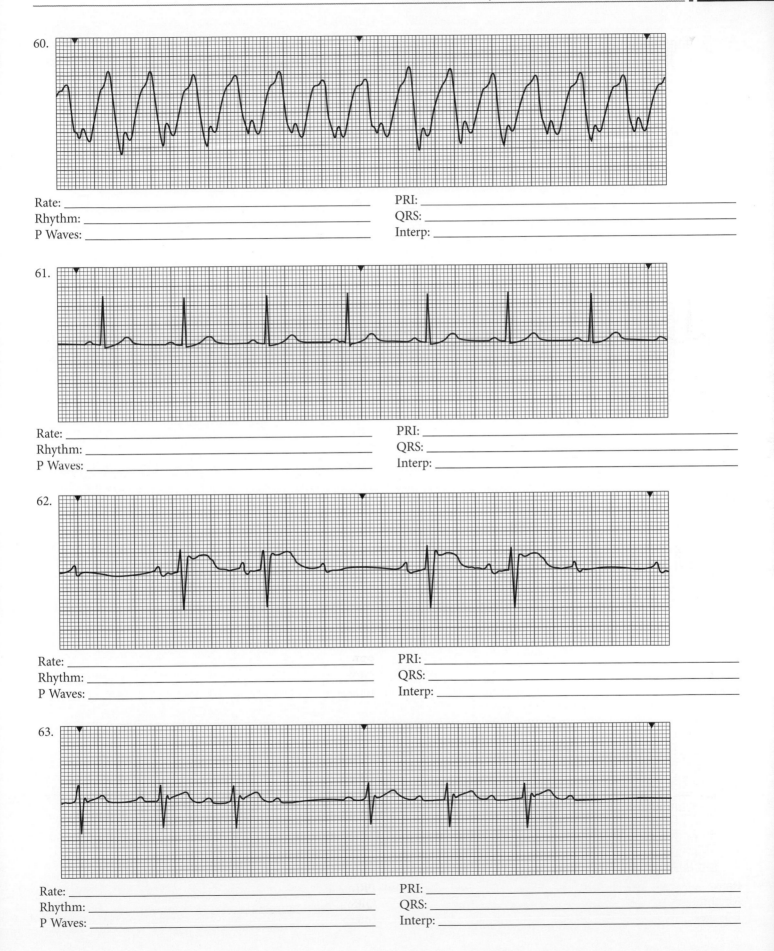

Rate: _____ PRI: _____
Rhythm: _____ QRS: _____
P Waves: _____ Interp: _____

61.

Rate: _____ PRI: _____
Rhythm: _____ QRS: _____
P Waves: _____ Interp: _____

62.

Rate: _____ PRI: _____
Rhythm: _____ QRS: _____
P Waves: _____ Interp: _____

63.

Rate: _____ PRI: _____
Rhythm: _____ QRS: _____
P Waves: _____ Interp: _____

64.

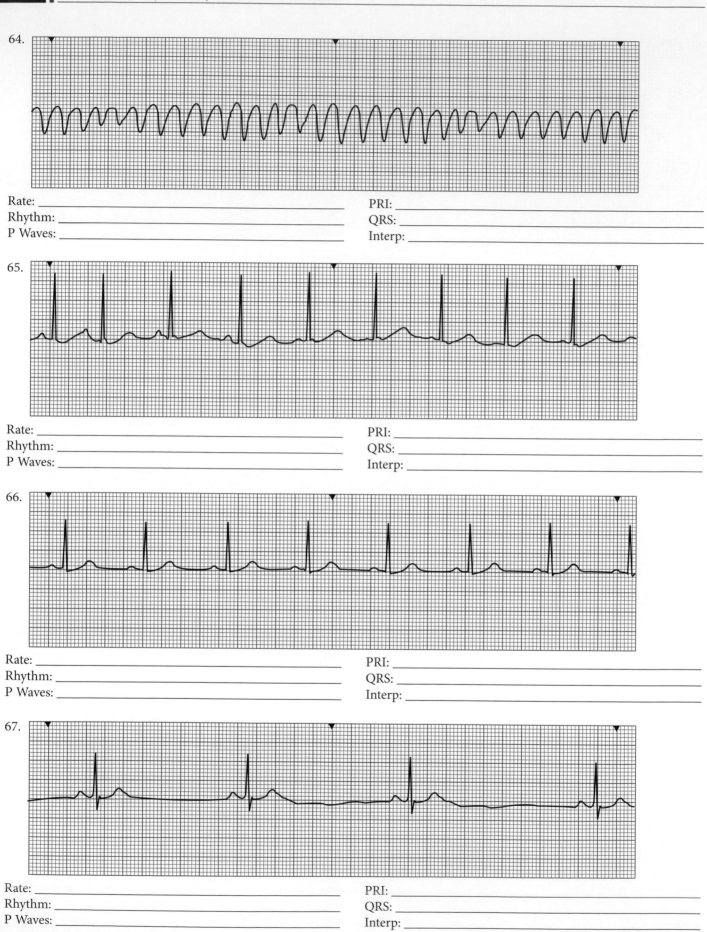

Rate: _____ PRI: _____
Rhythm: _____ QRS: _____
P Waves: _____ Interp: _____

65.

Rate: _____ PRI: _____
Rhythm: _____ QRS: _____
P Waves: _____ Interp: _____

66.

Rate: _____ PRI: _____
Rhythm: _____ QRS: _____
P Waves: _____ Interp: _____

67.

Rate: _____ PRI: _____
Rhythm: _____ QRS: _____
P Waves: _____ Interp: _____

68.

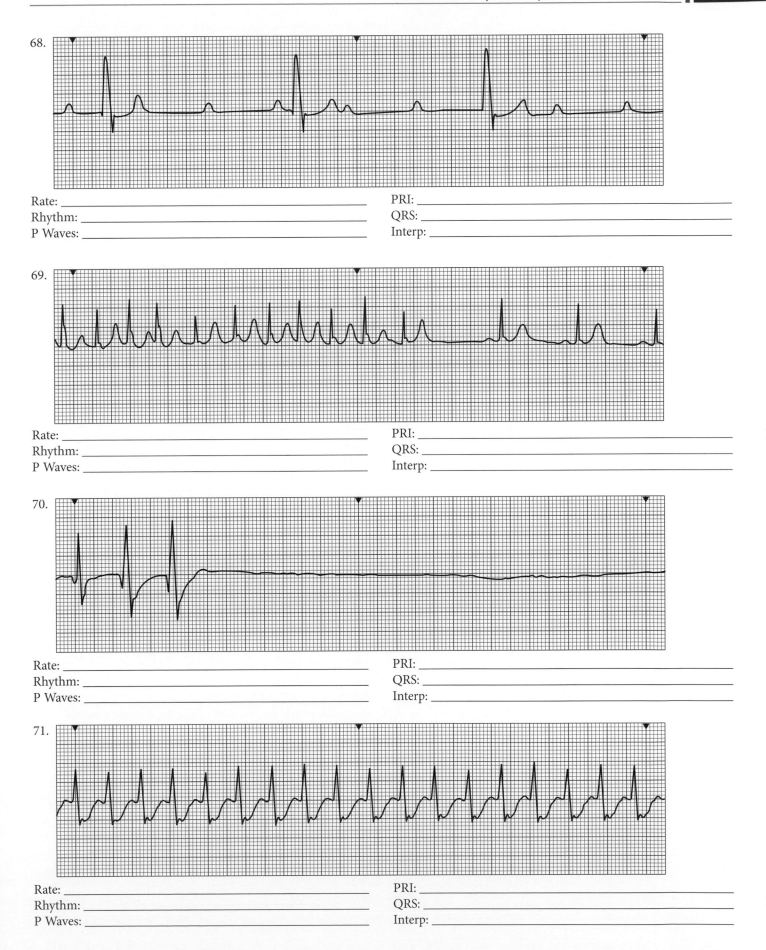

Rate: _____   PRI: _____

Rhythm: _____   QRS: _____

P Waves: _____   Interp: _____

69.

Rate: _____   PRI: _____

Rhythm: _____   QRS: _____

P Waves: _____   Interp: _____

70.

Rate: _____   PRI: _____

Rhythm: _____   QRS: _____

P Waves: _____   Interp: _____

71.

Rate: _____   PRI: _____

Rhythm: _____   QRS: _____

P Waves: _____   Interp: _____

72.

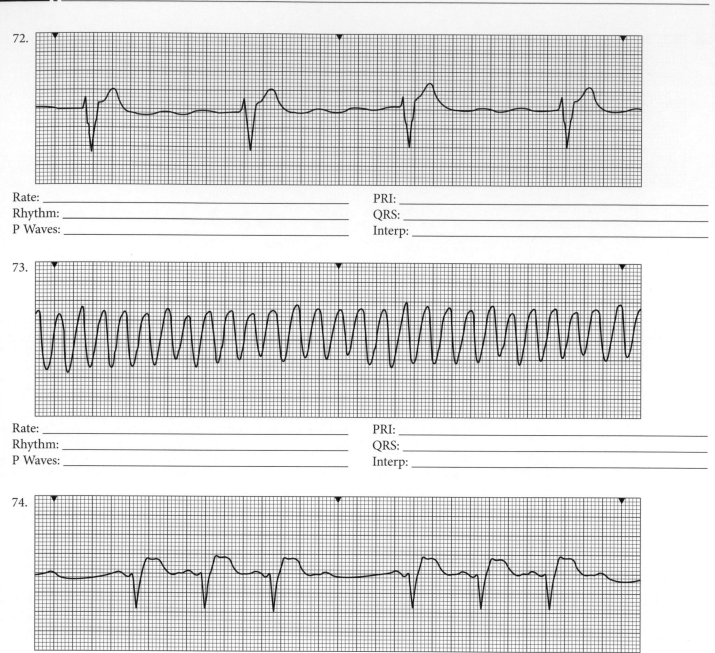

Rate: _____ PRI: _____
Rhythm: _____ QRS: _____
P Waves: _____ Interp: _____

73.

Rate: _____ PRI: _____
Rhythm: _____ QRS: _____
P Waves: _____ Interp: _____

74.

Rate: _____ PRI: _____
Rhythm: _____ QRS: _____
P Waves: _____ Interp: _____

75.

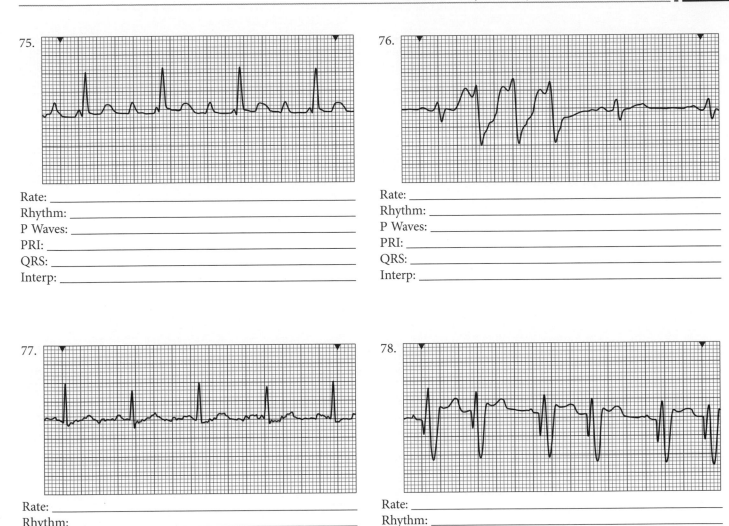

Rate: _____

Rhythm: _____

P Waves: _____

PRI: _____

QRS: _____

Interp: _____

76.

Rate: _____

Rhythm: _____

P Waves: _____

PRI: _____

QRS: _____

Interp: _____

77.

Rate: _____

Rhythm: _____

P Waves: _____

PRI: _____

QRS: _____

Interp: _____

78.

Rate: _____

Rhythm: _____

P Waves: _____

PRI: _____

QRS: _____

Interp: _____

79.

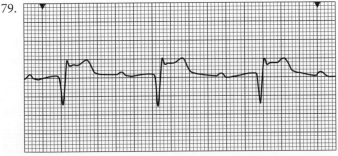

Rate: _____

Rhythm: _____

P Waves: _____

PRI: _____

QRS: _____

Interp: _____

80.

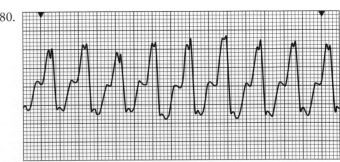

Rate: _____

Rhythm: _____

P Waves: _____

PRI: _____

QRS: _____

Interp: _____

81.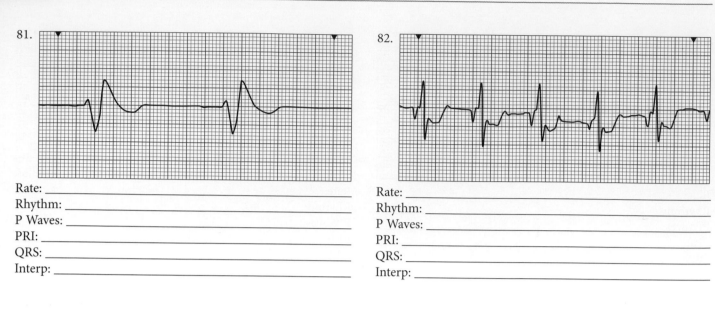

Rate: _____

Rhythm: _____

P Waves: _____

PRI: _____

QRS: _____

Interp: _____

82.

Rate: _____

Rhythm: _____

P Waves: _____

PRI: _____

QRS: _____

Interp: _____

83.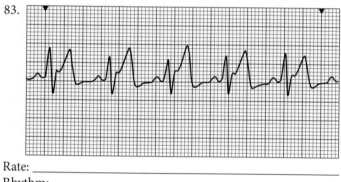

Rate: _____

Rhythm: _____

P Waves: _____

PRI: _____

QRS: _____

Interp: _____

84.

Rate: _____

Rhythm: _____

P Waves: _____

PRI: _____

QRS: _____

Interp: _____

85.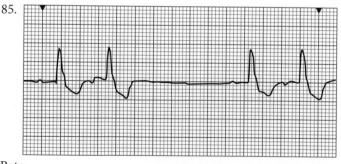

Rate: _____

Rhythm: _____

P Waves: _____

PRI: _____

QRS: _____

Interp: _____

86.

Rate: _____

Rhythm: _____

P Waves: _____

PRI: _____

QRS: _____

Interp: _____

87.

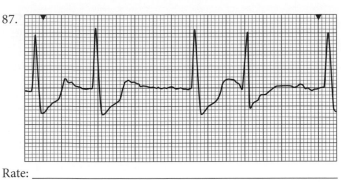

Rate: _____
Rhythm: _____
P Waves: _____
PRI: _____
QRS: _____
Interp: _____

88.

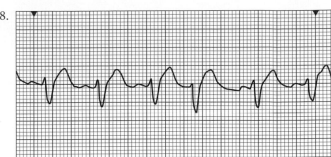

Rate: _____
Rhythm: _____
P Waves: _____
PRI: _____
QRS: _____
Interp: _____

89.

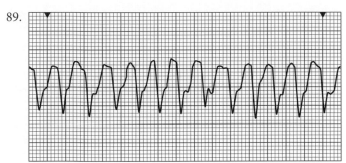

Rate: _____
Rhythm: _____
P Waves: _____
PRI: _____
QRS: _____
Interp: _____

90.

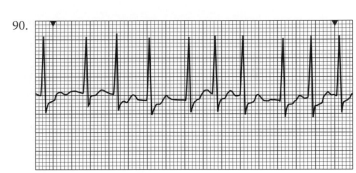

Rate: _____
Rhythm: _____
P Waves: _____
PRI: _____
QRS: _____
Interp: _____

91.

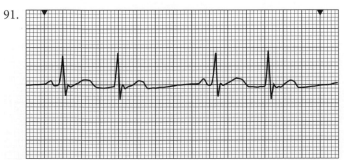

Rate: _____
Rhythm: _____
P Waves: _____
PRI: _____
QRS: _____
Interp: _____

92.

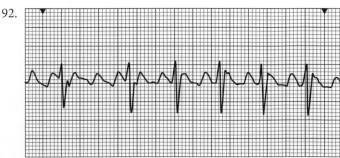

Rate: _____
Rhythm: _____
P Waves: _____
PRI: _____
QRS: _____
Interp: _____

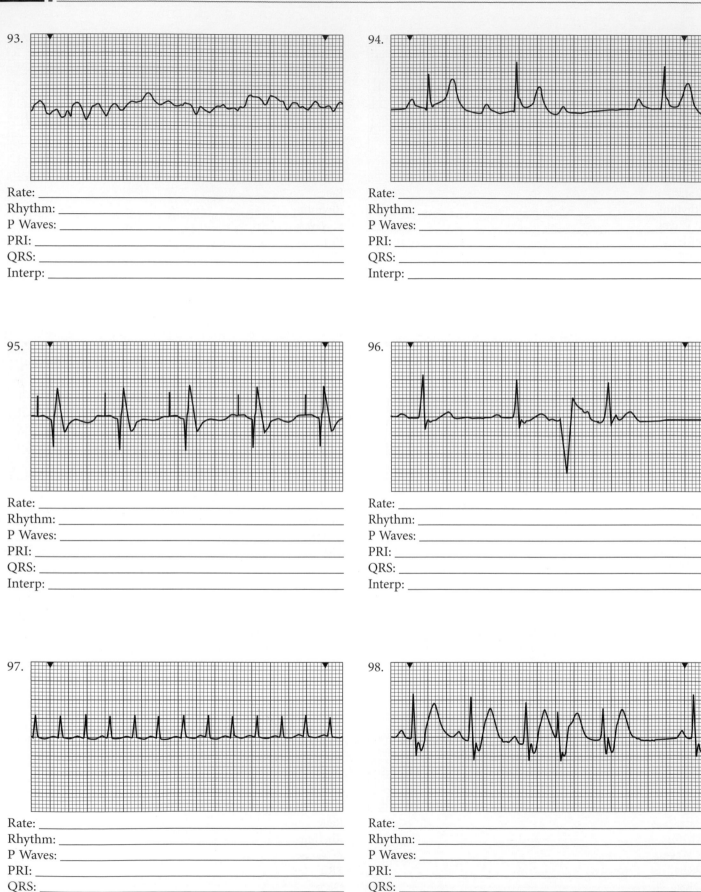

93.

Rate: _____

Rhythm: _____

P Waves: _____

PRI: _____

QRS: _____

Interp: _____

94.

Rate: _____

Rhythm: _____

P Waves: _____

PRI: _____

QRS: _____

Interp: _____

95.

Rate: _____

Rhythm: _____

P Waves: _____

PRI: _____

QRS: _____

Interp: _____

96.

Rate: _____

Rhythm: _____

P Waves: _____

PRI: _____

QRS: _____

Interp: _____

97.

Rate: _____

Rhythm: _____

P Waves: _____

PRI: _____

QRS: _____

Interp: _____

98.

Rate: _____

Rhythm: _____

P Waves: _____

PRI: _____

QRS: _____

Interp: _____

99.

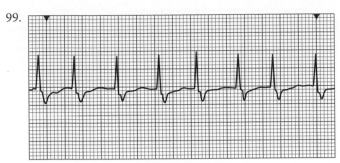

Rate: _____

Rhythm: _____

P Waves: _____

PRI: _____

QRS: _____

Interp: _____

100.

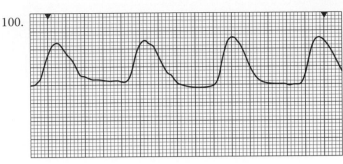

Rate: _____

Rhythm: _____

P Waves: _____

PRI: _____

QRS: _____

Interp: _____

101.

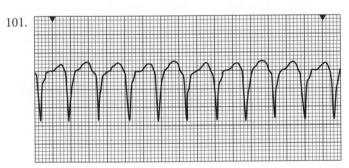

Rate: _____

Rhythm: _____

P Waves: _____

PRI: _____

QRS: _____

Interp: _____

102.

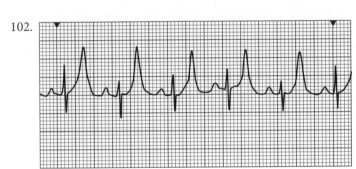

Rate: _____

Rhythm: _____

P Waves: _____

PRI: _____

QRS: _____

Interp: _____

103.

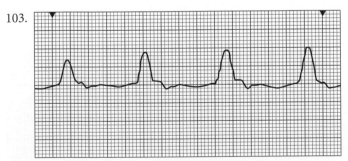

Rate: _____

Rhythm: _____

P Waves: _____

PRI: _____

QRS: _____

Interp: _____

104.

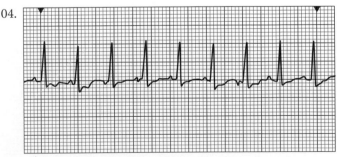

Rate: _____

Rhythm: _____

P Waves: _____

PRI: _____

QRS: _____

Interp: _____

105.

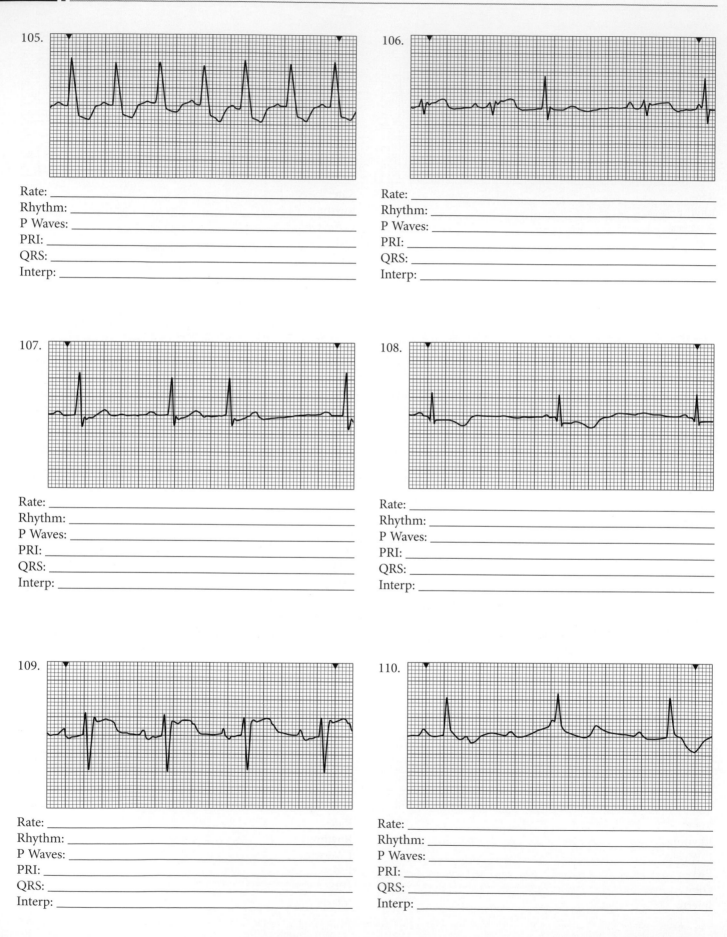

Rate: _____

Rhythm: _____

P Waves: _____

PRI: _____

QRS: _____

Interp: _____

106.

Rate: _____

Rhythm: _____

P Waves: _____

PRI: _____

QRS: _____

Interp: _____

107.

Rate: _____

Rhythm: _____

P Waves: _____

PRI: _____

QRS: _____

Interp: _____

108.

Rate: _____

Rhythm: _____

P Waves: _____

PRI: _____

QRS: _____

Interp: _____

109.

Rate: _____

Rhythm: _____

P Waves: _____

PRI: _____

QRS: _____

Interp: _____

110.

Rate: _____

Rhythm: _____

P Waves: _____

PRI: _____

QRS: _____

Interp: _____

111.

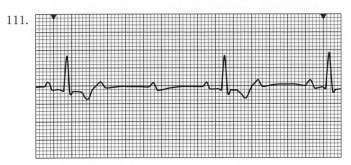

Rate: _____

Rhythm: _____

P Waves: _____

PRI: _____

QRS: _____

Interp: _____

112.

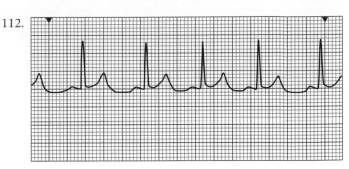

Rate: _____

Rhythm: _____

P Waves: _____

PRI: _____

QRS: _____

Interp: _____

113.

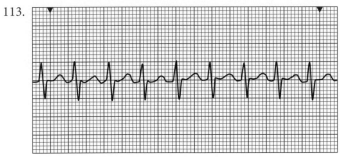

Rate: _____

Rhythm: _____

P Waves: _____

PRI: _____

QRS: _____

Interp: _____

114.

Rate: _____

Rhythm: _____

P Waves: _____

PRI: _____

QRS: _____

Interp: _____

115.

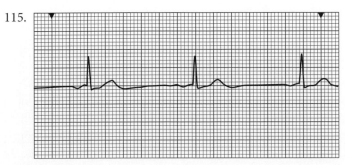

Rate: _____

Rhythm: _____

P Waves: _____

PRI: _____

QRS: _____

Interp: _____

116.

Rate: _____

Rhythm: _____

P Waves: _____

PRI: _____

QRS: _____

Interp: _____

117.

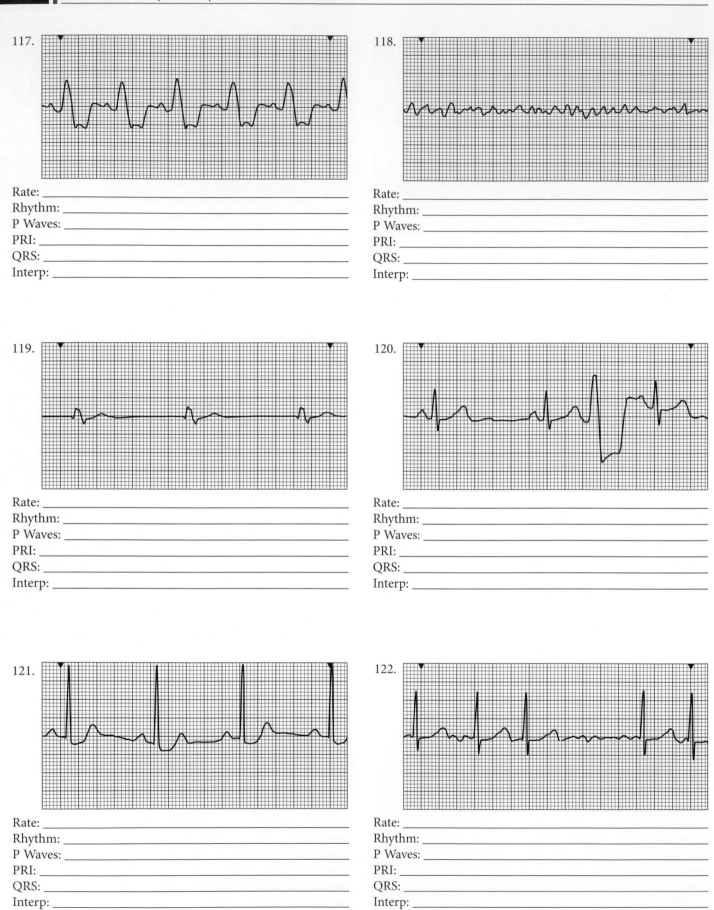

Rate: _____

Rhythm: _____

P Waves: _____

PRI: _____

QRS: _____

Interp: _____

118.

Rate: _____

Rhythm: _____

P Waves: _____

PRI: _____

QRS: _____

Interp: _____

119.

Rate: _____

Rhythm: _____

P Waves: _____

PRI: _____

QRS: _____

Interp: _____

120.

Rate: _____

Rhythm: _____

P Waves: _____

PRI: _____

QRS: _____

Interp: _____

121.

Rate: _____

Rhythm: _____

P Waves: _____

PRI: _____

QRS: _____

Interp: _____

122.

Rate: _____

Rhythm: _____

P Waves: _____

PRI: _____

QRS: _____

Interp: _____

123.

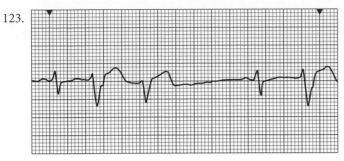

Rate: _____
Rhythm: _____
P Waves: _____
PRI: _____
QRS: _____
Interp: _____

124.

Rate: _____
Rhythm: _____
P Waves: _____
PRI: _____
QRS: _____
Interp: _____

125.

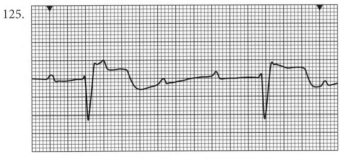

Rate: _____
Rhythm: _____
P Waves: _____
PRI: _____
QRS: _____
Interp: _____

126.

Rate: _____
Rhythm: _____
P Waves: _____
PRI: _____
QRS: _____
Interp: _____

127.

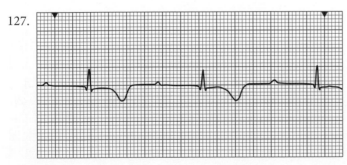

Rate: _____
Rhythm: _____
P Waves: _____
PRI: _____
QRS: _____
Interp: _____

128.

Rate: _____
Rhythm: _____
P Waves: _____
PRI: _____
QRS: _____
Interp: _____

129.

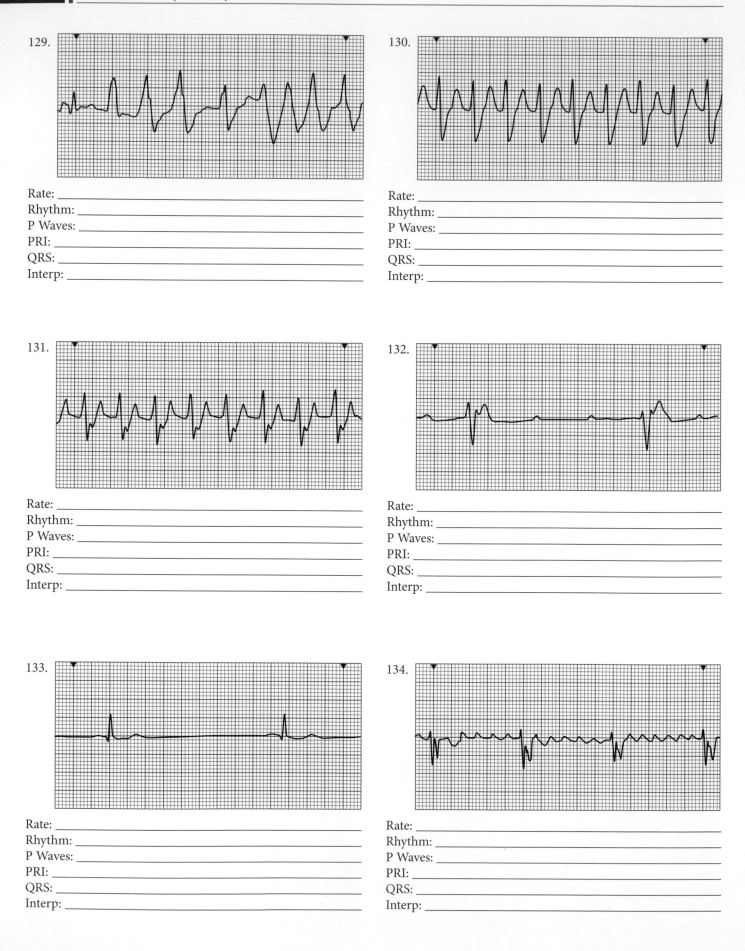

Rate: _____

Rhythm: _____

P Waves: _____

PRI: _____

QRS: _____

Interp: _____

130.

Rate: _____

Rhythm: _____

P Waves: _____

PRI: _____

QRS: _____

Interp: _____

131.

Rate: _____

Rhythm: _____

P Waves: _____

PRI: _____

QRS: _____

Interp: _____

132.

Rate: _____

Rhythm: _____

P Waves: _____

PRI: _____

QRS: _____

Interp: _____

133.

Rate: _____

Rhythm: _____

P Waves: _____

PRI: _____

QRS: _____

Interp: _____

134.

Rate: _____

Rhythm: _____

P Waves: _____

PRI: _____

QRS: _____

Interp: _____

135.

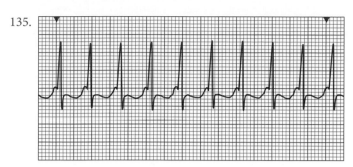

Rate: _____

Rhythm: _____

P Waves: _____

PRI: _____

QRS: _____

Interp: _____

136.

Rate: _____

Rhythm: _____

P Waves: _____

PRI: _____

QRS: _____

Interp: _____

137.

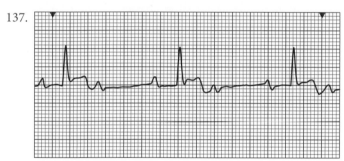

Rate: _____

Rhythm: _____

P Waves: _____

PRI: _____

QRS: _____

Interp: _____

138.

Rate: _____

Rhythm: _____

P Waves: _____

PRI: _____

QRS: _____

Interp: _____

139.

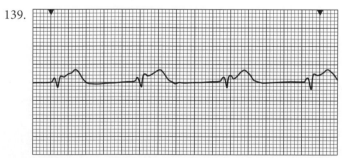

Rate: _____

Rhythm: _____

P Waves: _____

PRI: _____

QRS: _____

Interp: _____

140.

Rate: _____

Rhythm: _____

P Waves: _____

PRI: _____

QRS: _____

Interp: _____

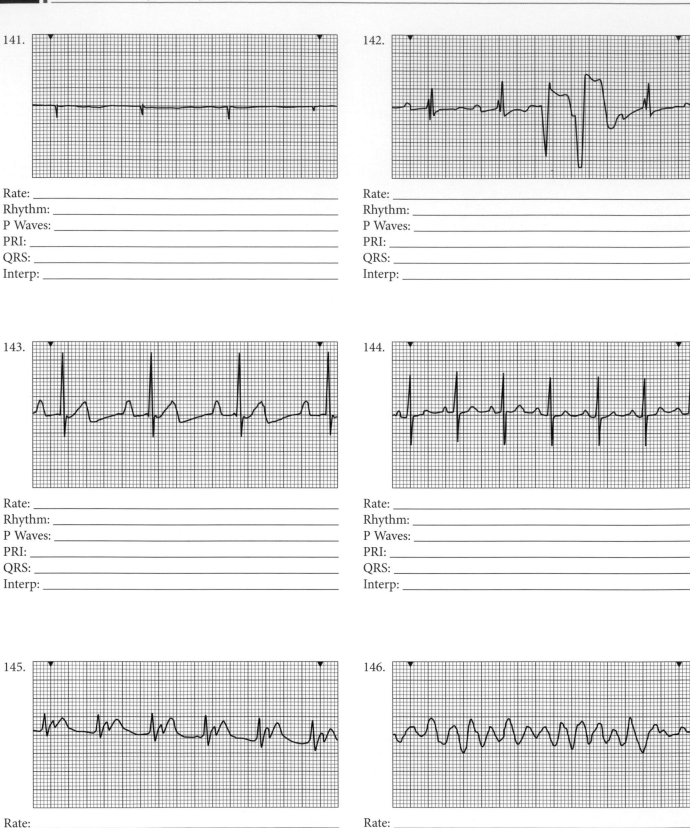

141.

Rate: _____

Rhythm: _____

P Waves: _____

PRI: _____

QRS: _____

Interp: _____

142.

Rate: _____

Rhythm: _____

P Waves: _____

PRI: _____

QRS: _____

Interp: _____

143.

Rate: _____

Rhythm: _____

P Waves: _____

PRI: _____

QRS: _____

Interp: _____

144.

Rate: _____

Rhythm: _____

P Waves: _____

PRI: _____

QRS: _____

Interp: _____

145.

Rate: _____

Rhythm: _____

P Waves: _____

PRI: _____

QRS: _____

Interp: _____

146.

Rate: _____

Rhythm: _____

P Waves: _____

PRI: _____

QRS: _____

Interp: _____

147.

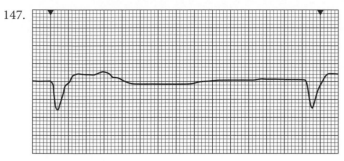

Rate: _____

Rhythm: _____

P Waves: _____

PRI: _____

QRS: _____

Interp: _____

148.

Rate: _____

Rhythm: _____

P Waves: _____

PRI: _____

QRS: _____

Interp: _____

149.

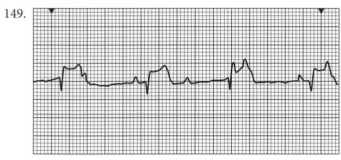

Rate: _____

Rhythm: _____

P Waves: _____

PRI: _____

QRS: _____

Interp: _____

150.

Rate: _____

Rhythm: _____

P Waves: _____

PRI: _____

QRS: _____

Interp: _____

151.

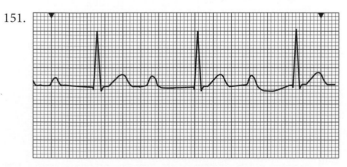

Rate: _____

Rhythm: _____

P Waves: _____

PRI: _____

QRS: _____

Interp: _____

152.

Rate: _____

Rhythm: _____

P Waves: _____

PRI: _____

QRS: _____

Interp: _____

153.

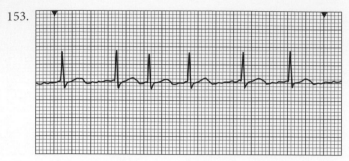

Rate: _____

Rhythm: _____

P Waves: _____

PRI: _____

QRS: _____

Interp: _____

154.

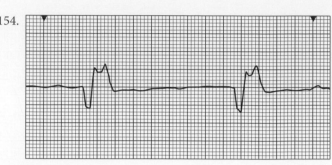

Rate: _____

Rhythm: _____

P Waves: _____

PRI: _____

QRS: _____

Interp: _____

155.

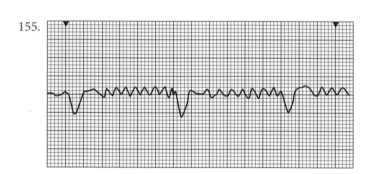

Rate: _____

Rhythm: _____

P Waves: _____

PRI: _____

QRS: _____

Interp: _____

156.

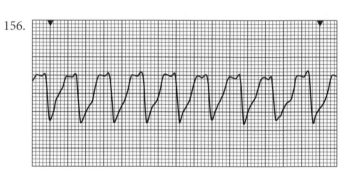

Rate: _____

Rhythm: _____

P Waves: _____

PRI: _____

QRS: _____

Interp: _____

157.

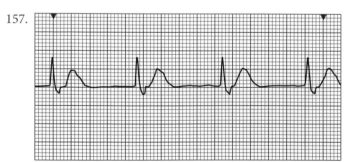

Rate: _____

Rhythm: _____

P Waves: _____

PRI: _____

QRS: _____

Interp: _____

158.

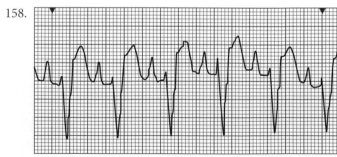

Rate: _____

Rhythm: _____

P Waves: _____

PRI: _____

QRS: _____

Interp: _____

159.

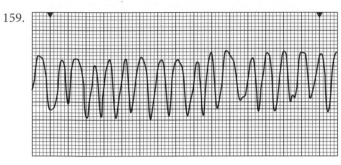

Rate: _____

Rhythm: _____

P Waves: _____

PRI: _____

QRS: _____

Interp: _____

160.

Rate: _____

Rhythm: _____

P Waves: _____

PRI: _____

QRS: _____

Interp: _____

161.

Rate: _____

Rhythm: _____

P Waves: _____

PRI: _____

QRS: _____

Interp: _____

162.

Rate: _____

Rhythm: _____

P Waves: _____

PRI: _____

QRS: _____

Interp: _____

163.

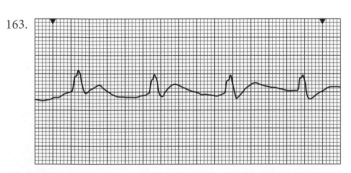

Rate: _____

Rhythm: _____

P Waves: _____

PRI: _____

QRS: _____

Interp: _____

164.

Rate: _____

Rhythm: _____

P Waves: _____

PRI: _____

QRS: _____

Interp: _____

165.

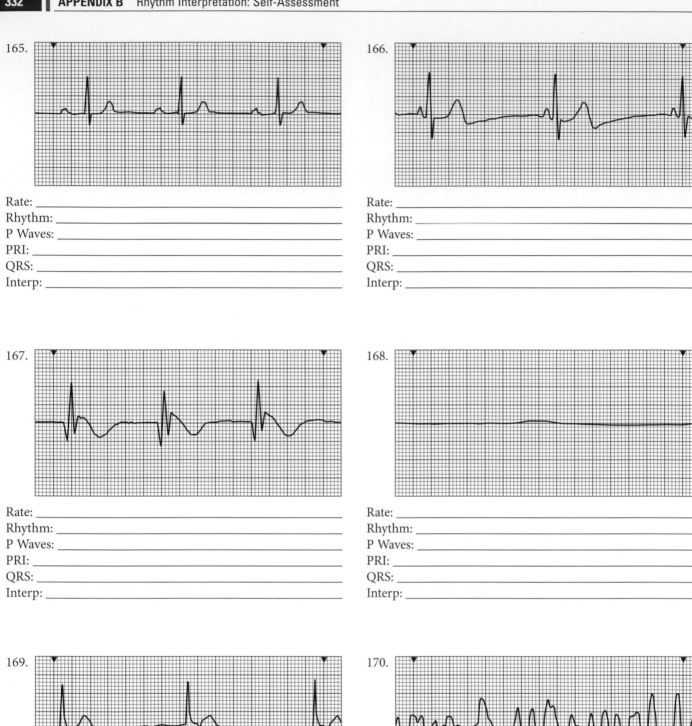

Rate: _____
Rhythm: _____
P Waves: _____
PRI: _____
QRS: _____
Interp: _____

166.

Rate: _____
Rhythm: _____
P Waves: _____
PRI: _____
QRS: _____
Interp: _____

167.

Rate: _____
Rhythm: _____
P Waves: _____
PRI: _____
QRS: _____
Interp: _____

168.

Rate: _____
Rhythm: _____
P Waves: _____
PRI: _____
QRS: _____
Interp: _____

169.

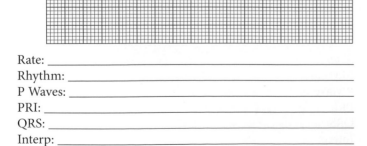

Rate: _____
Rhythm: _____
P Waves: _____
PRI: _____
QRS: _____
Interp: _____

170.

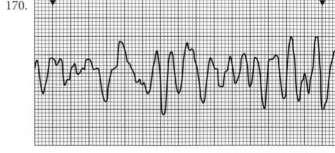

Rate: _____
Rhythm: _____
P Waves: _____
PRI: _____
QRS: _____
Interp: _____

171.

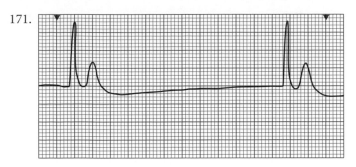

Rate: _____
Rhythm: _____
P Waves: _____
PRI: _____
QRS: _____
Interp: _____

172.

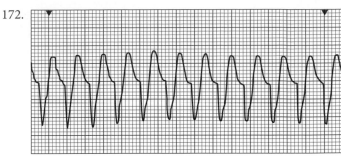

Rate: _____
Rhythm: _____
P Waves: _____
PRI: _____
QRS: _____
Interp: _____

173.

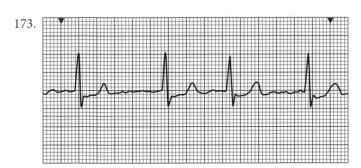

Rate: _____
Rhythm: _____
P Waves: _____
PRI: _____
QRS: _____
Interp: _____

174.

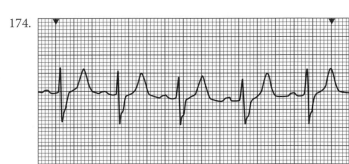

Rate: _____
Rhythm: _____
P Waves: _____
PRI: _____
QRS: _____
Interp: _____

175.

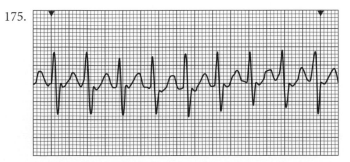

Rate: _____
Rhythm: _____
P Waves: _____
PRI: _____
QRS: _____
Interp: _____

176.

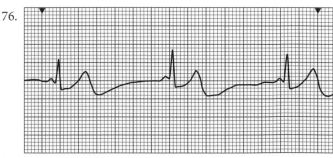

Rate: _____
Rhythm: _____
P Waves: _____
PRI: _____
QRS: _____
Interp: _____

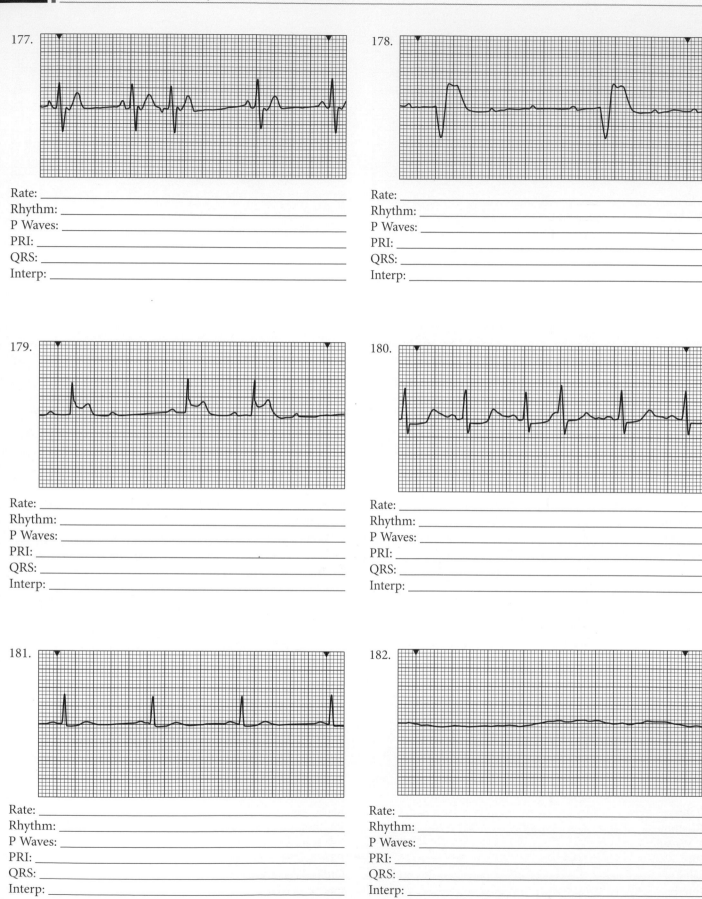

177.

Rate: _____

Rhythm: _____

P Waves: _____

PRI: _____

QRS: _____

Interp: _____

178.

Rate: _____

Rhythm: _____

P Waves: _____

PRI: _____

QRS: _____

Interp: _____

179.

Rate: _____

Rhythm: _____

P Waves: _____

PRI: _____

QRS: _____

Interp: _____

180.

Rate: _____

Rhythm: _____

P Waves: _____

PRI: _____

QRS: _____

Interp: _____

181.

Rate: _____

Rhythm: _____

P Waves: _____

PRI: _____

QRS: _____

Interp: _____

182.

Rate: _____

Rhythm: _____

P Waves: _____

PRI: _____

QRS: _____

Interp: _____

183.

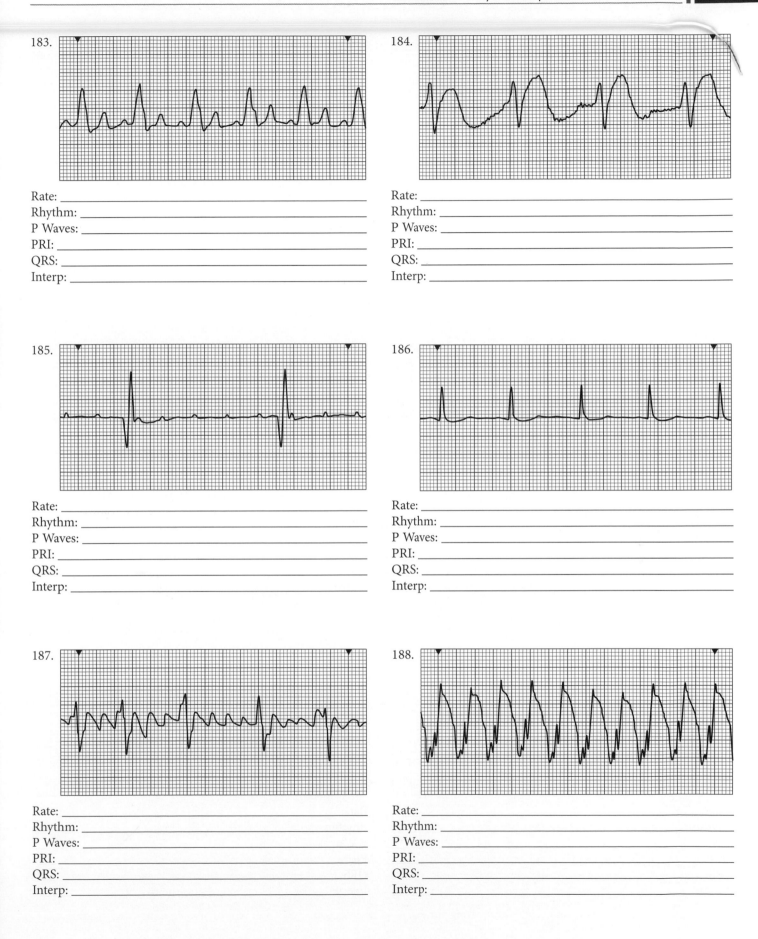

Rate: _____

Rhythm: _____

P Waves: _____

PRI: _____

QRS: _____

Interp: _____

184.

Rate: _____

Rhythm: _____

P Waves: _____

PRI: _____

QRS: _____

Interp: _____

185.

Rate: _____

Rhythm: _____

P Waves: _____

PRI: _____

QRS: _____

Interp: _____

186.

Rate: _____

Rhythm: _____

P Waves: _____

PRI: _____

QRS: _____

Interp: _____

187.

Rate: _____

Rhythm: _____

P Waves: _____

PRI: _____

QRS: _____

Interp: _____

188.

Rate: _____

Rhythm: _____

P Waves: _____

PRI: _____

QRS: _____

Interp: _____

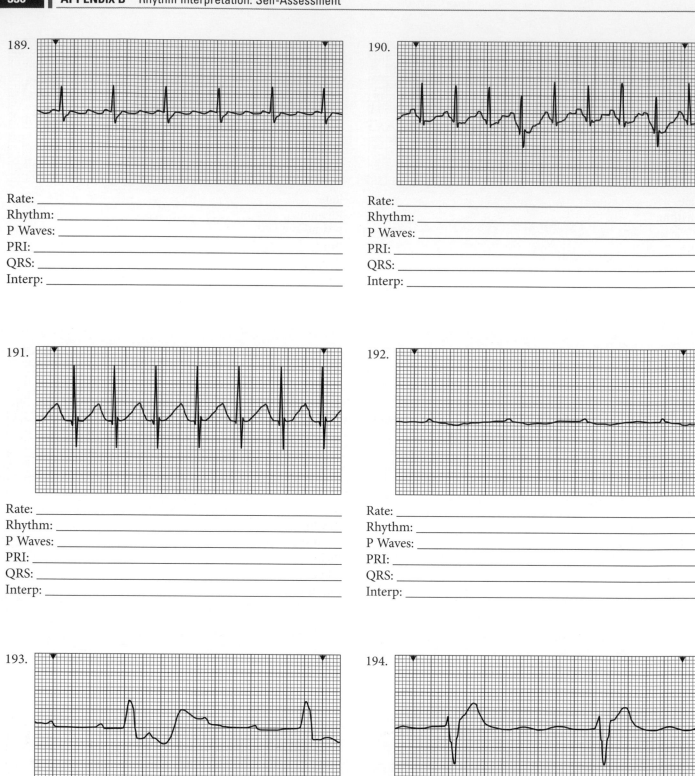

189.

Rate: _____

Rhythm: _____

P Waves: _____

PRI: _____

QRS: _____

Interp: _____

190.

Rate: _____

Rhythm: _____

P Waves: _____

PRI: _____

QRS: _____

Interp: _____

191.

Rate: _____

Rhythm: _____

P Waves: _____

PRI: _____

QRS: _____

Interp: _____

192.

Rate: _____

Rhythm: _____

P Waves: _____

PRI: _____

QRS: _____

Interp: _____

193.

Rate: _____

Rhythm: _____

P Waves: _____

PRI: _____

QRS: _____

Interp: _____

194.

Rate: _____

Rhythm: _____

P Waves: _____

PRI: _____

QRS: _____

Interp: _____

195.

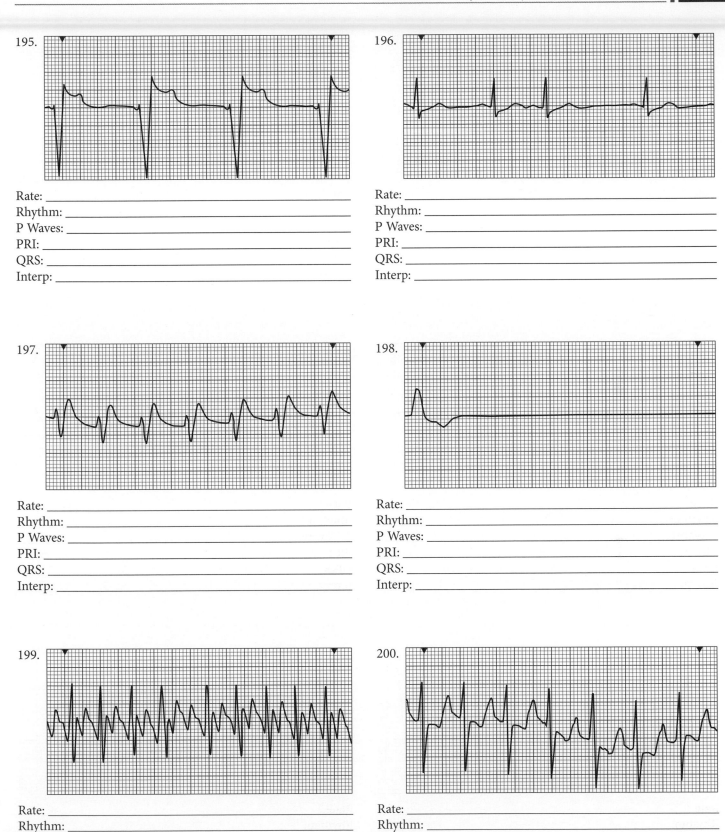

Rate: _____

Rhythm: _____

P Waves: _____

PRI: _____

QRS: _____

Interp: _____

196.

Rate: _____

Rhythm: _____

P Waves: _____

PRI: _____

QRS: _____

Interp: _____

197.

Rate: _____

Rhythm: _____

P Waves: _____

PRI: _____

QRS: _____

Interp: _____

198.

Rate: _____

Rhythm: _____

P Waves: _____

PRI: _____

QRS: _____

Interp: _____

199.

Rate: _____

Rhythm: _____

P Waves: _____

PRI: _____

QRS: _____

Interp: _____

200.

Rate: _____

Rhythm: _____

P Waves: _____

PRI: _____

QRS: _____

Interp: _____

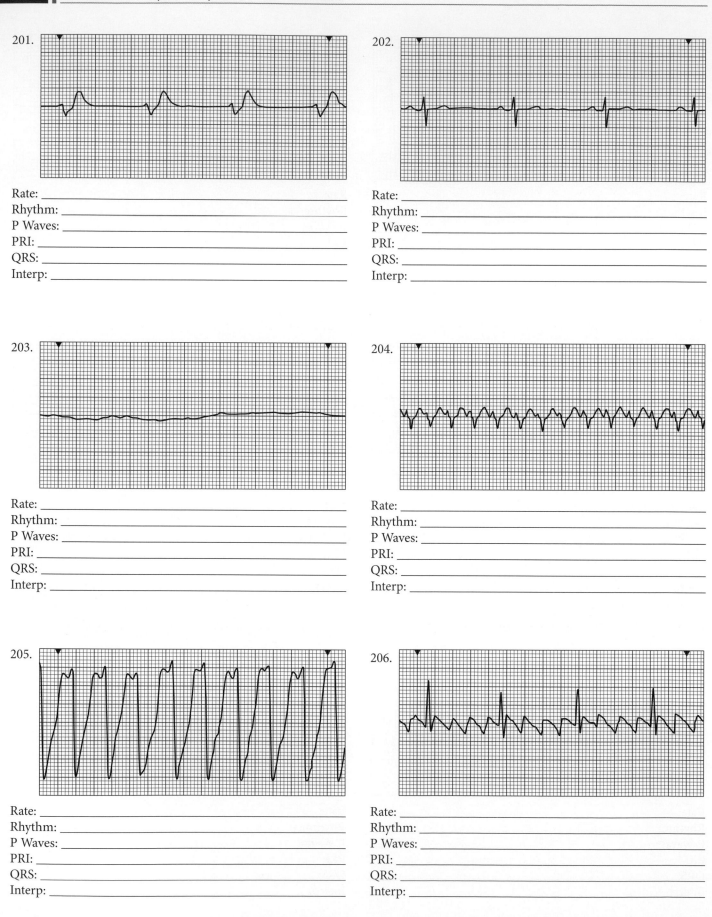

201.

Rate: _____
Rhythm: _____
P Waves: _____
PRI: _____
QRS: _____
Interp: _____

202.

Rate: _____
Rhythm: _____
P Waves: _____
PRI: _____
QRS: _____
Interp: _____

203.

Rate: _____
Rhythm: _____
P Waves: _____
PRI: _____
QRS: _____
Interp: _____

204.

Rate: _____
Rhythm: _____
P Waves: _____
PRI: _____
QRS: _____
Interp: _____

205.

Rate: _____
Rhythm: _____
P Waves: _____
PRI: _____
QRS: _____
Interp: _____

206.

Rate: _____
Rhythm: _____
P Waves: _____
PRI: _____
QRS: _____
Interp: _____

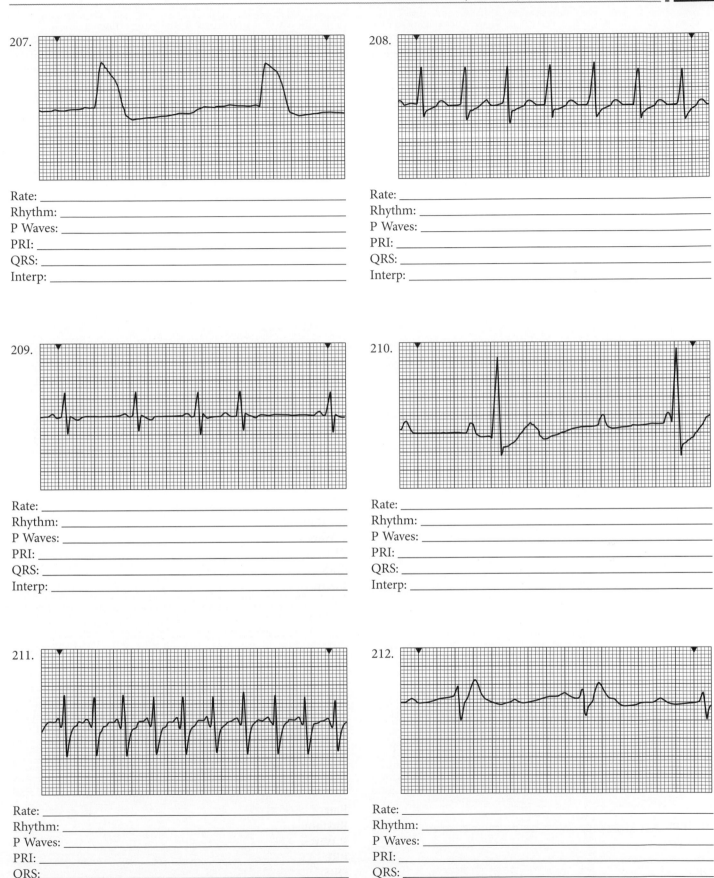

207.

Rate: _____
Rhythm: _____
P Waves: _____
PRI: _____
QRS: _____
Interp: _____

208.

Rate: _____
Rhythm: _____
P Waves: _____
PRI: _____
QRS: _____
Interp: _____

209.

Rate: _____
Rhythm: _____
P Waves: _____
PRI: _____
QRS: _____
Interp: _____

210.

Rate: _____
Rhythm: _____
P Waves: _____
PRI: _____
QRS: _____
Interp: _____

211.

Rate: _____
Rhythm: _____
P Waves: _____
PRI: _____
QRS: _____
Interp: _____

212.

Rate: _____
Rhythm: _____
P Waves: _____
PRI: _____
QRS: _____
Interp: _____

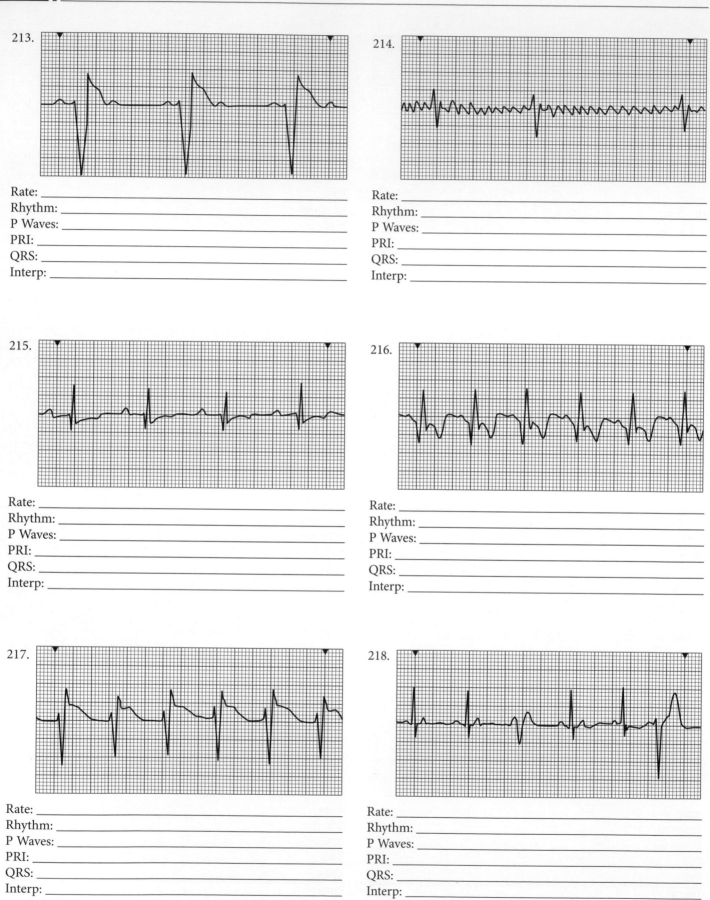

213.

Rate: _____
Rhythm: _____
P Waves: _____
PRI: _____
QRS: _____
Interp: _____

214.

Rate: _____
Rhythm: _____
P Waves: _____
PRI: _____
QRS: _____
Interp: _____

215.

Rate: _____
Rhythm: _____
P Waves: _____
PRI: _____
QRS: _____
Interp: _____

216.

Rate: _____
Rhythm: _____
P Waves: _____
PRI: _____
QRS: _____
Interp: _____

217.

Rate: _____
Rhythm: _____
P Waves: _____
PRI: _____
QRS: _____
Interp: _____

218.

Rate: _____
Rhythm: _____
P Waves: _____
PRI: _____
QRS: _____
Interp: _____

219.

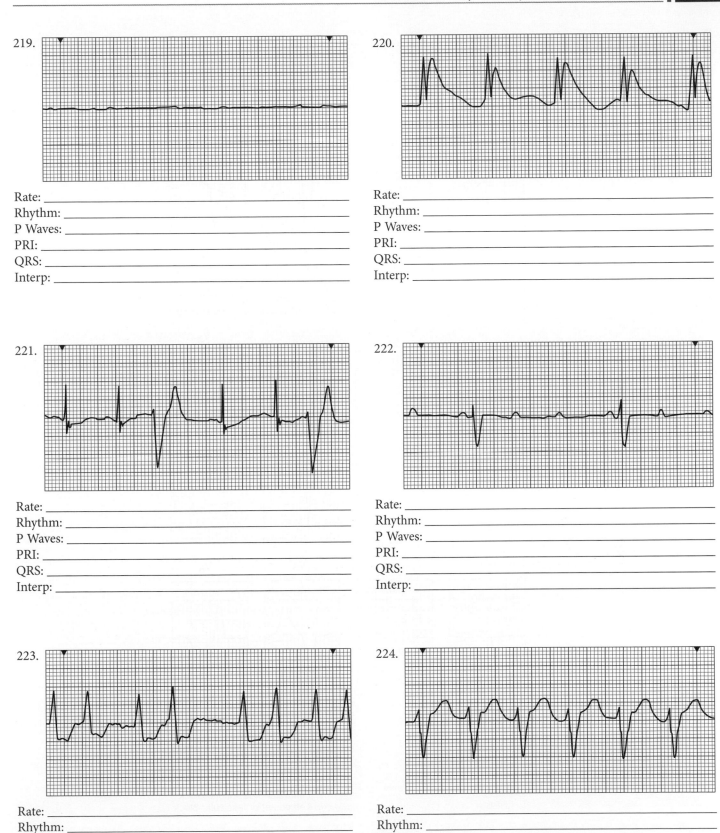

Rate: _____

Rhythm: _____

P Waves: _____

PRI: _____

QRS: _____

Interp: _____

220.

Rate: _____

Rhythm: _____

P Waves: _____

PRI: _____

QRS: _____

Interp: _____

221.

Rate: _____

Rhythm: _____

P Waves: _____

PRI: _____

QRS: _____

Interp: _____

222.

Rate: _____

Rhythm: _____

P Waves: _____

PRI: _____

QRS: _____

Interp: _____

223.

Rate: _____

Rhythm: _____

P Waves: _____

PRI: _____

QRS: _____

Interp: _____

224.

Rate: _____

Rhythm: _____

P Waves: _____

PRI: _____

QRS: _____

Interp: _____

II. BUNDLE-BRANCH AND FASCICULAR BLOCKS

225.

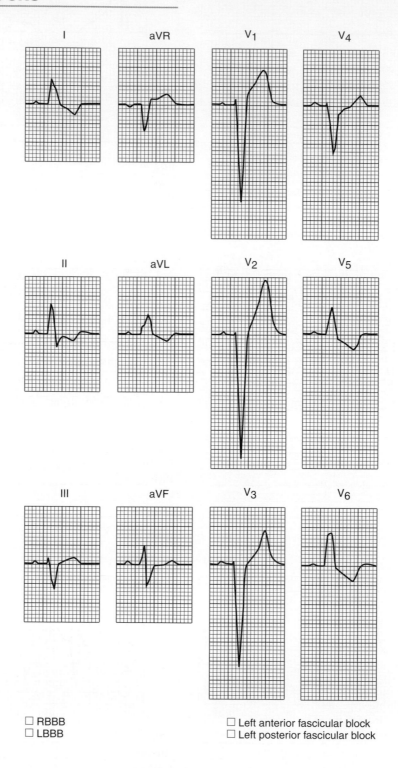

☐ RBBB
☐ LBBB

☐ Left anterior fascicular block
☐ Left posterior fascicular block

226.

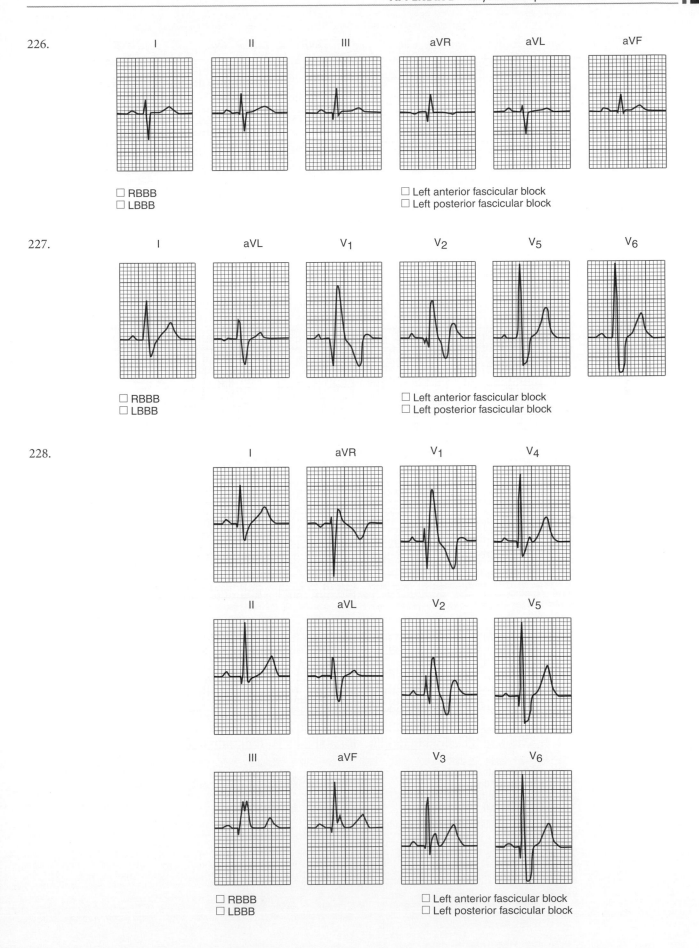

I   II   III   aVR   aVL   aVF

☐ RBBB   ☐ Left anterior fascicular block
☐ LBBB   ☐ Left posterior fascicular block

227.

I   aVL   V1   V2   V5   V6

☐ RBBB   ☐ Left anterior fascicular block
☐ LBBB   ☐ Left posterior fascicular block

228.

I   aVR   V1   V4

II   aVL   V2   V5

III   aVF   V3   V6

☐ RBBB   ☐ Left anterior fascicular block
☐ LBBB   ☐ Left posterior fascicular block

229.

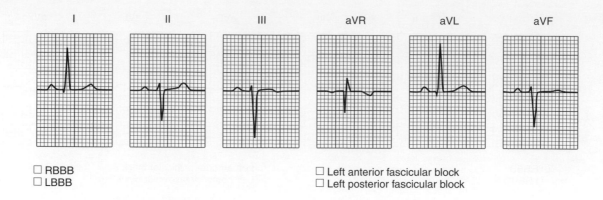

I   II   III   aVR   aVL   aVF

☐ RBBB   ☐ Left anterior fascicular block
☐ LBBB   ☐ Left posterior fascicular block

III. MYOCARDIAL INFARCTIONS

230.

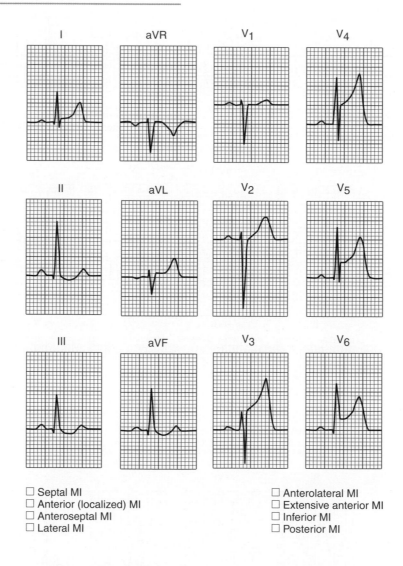

I   aVR V_1 V_4

II   aVL V_2 V_5

III   aVF V_3 V_6

☐ Septal MI   ☐ Anterolateral MI
☐ Anterior (localized) MI   ☐ Extensive anterior MI
☐ Anteroseptal MI   ☐ Inferior MI
☐ Lateral MI   ☐ Posterior MI

231.

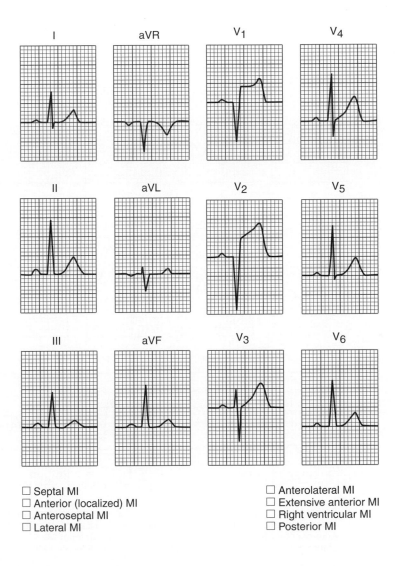

☐ Septal MI
☐ Anterior (localized) MI
☐ Anteroseptal MI
☐ Lateral MI

☐ Anterolateral MI
☐ Extensive anterior MI
☐ Right ventricular MI
☐ Posterior MI

232.

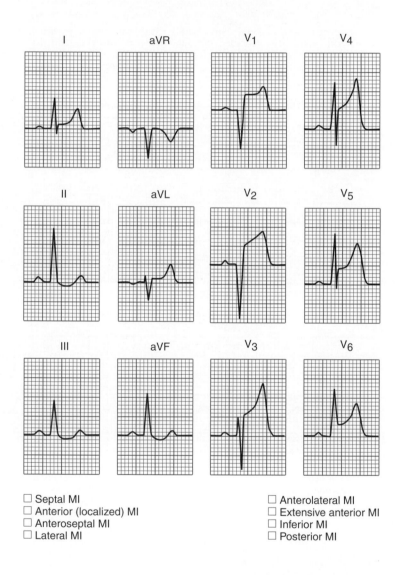

☐ Septal MI
☐ Anterior (localized) MI
☐ Anteroseptal MI
☐ Lateral MI

☐ Anterolateral MI
☐ Extensive anterior MI
☐ Inferior MI
☐ Posterior MI

233.

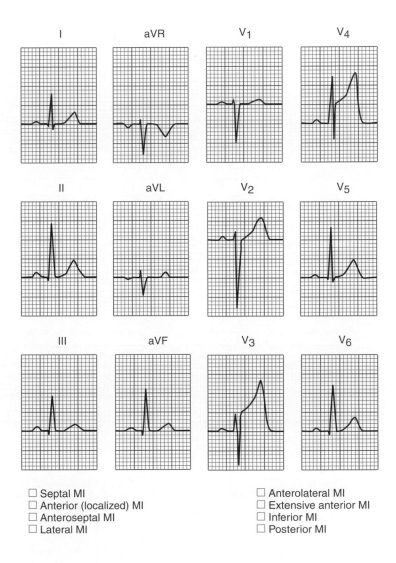

☐ Septal MI
☐ Anterior (localized) MI
☐ Anteroseptal MI
☐ Lateral MI

☐ Anterolateral MI
☐ Extensive anterior MI
☐ Inferior MI
☐ Posterior MI

234.

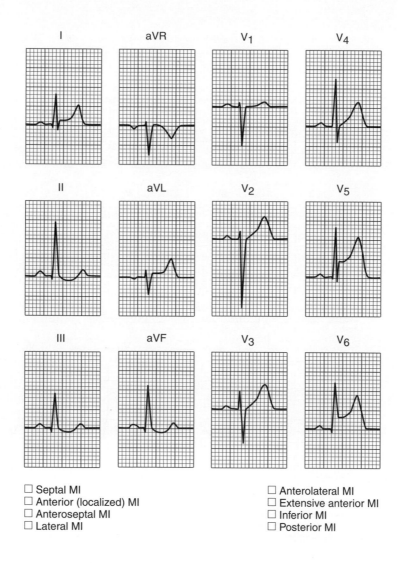

☐ Septal MI
☐ Anterior (localized) MI
☐ Anteroseptal MI
☐ Lateral MI

☐ Anterolateral MI
☐ Extensive anterior MI
☐ Inferior MI
☐ Posterior MI

235.

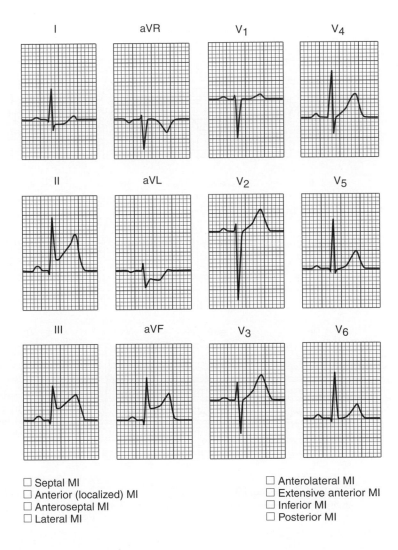

I   aVR   V₁   V₄

II   aVL   V₂   V₅

III   aVF   V₃   V₆

☐ Septal MI
☐ Anterior (localized) MI
☐ Anteroseptal MI
☐ Lateral MI

☐ Anterolateral MI
☐ Extensive anterior MI
☐ Inferior MI
☐ Posterior MI

236.

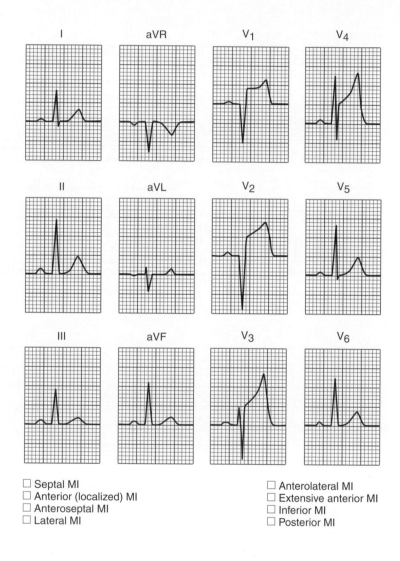

☐ Septal MI
☐ Anterior (localized) MI
☐ Anteroseptal MI
☐ Lateral MI

☐ Anterolateral MI
☐ Extensive anterior MI
☐ Inferior MI
☐ Posterior MI

237.

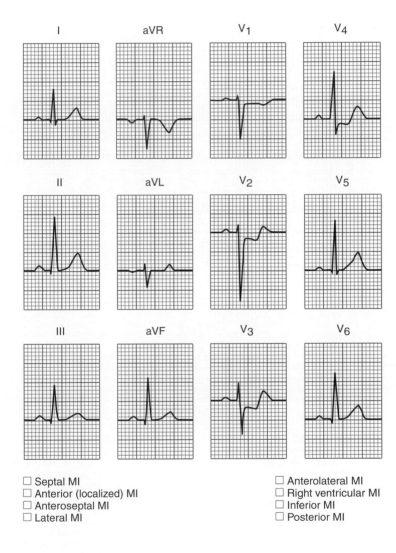

☐ Septal MI
☐ Anterior (localized) MI
☐ Anteroseptal MI
☐ Lateral MI

☐ Anterolateral MI
☐ Right ventricular MI
☐ Inferior MI
☐ Posterior MI

238.

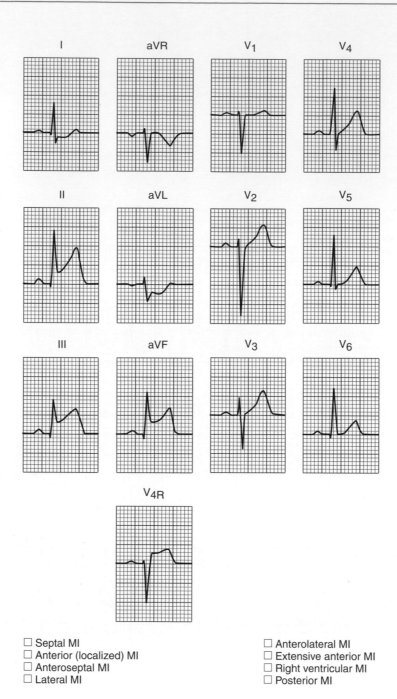

I aVR V₁ V₄

II aVL V₂ V₅

III aVF V₃ V₆

V₄R

☐ Septal MI
☐ Anterior (localized) MI
☐ Anteroseptal MI
☐ Lateral MI

☐ Anterolateral MI
☐ Extensive anterior MI
☐ Right ventricular MI
☐ Posterior MI

IV. QRS AXES

239.
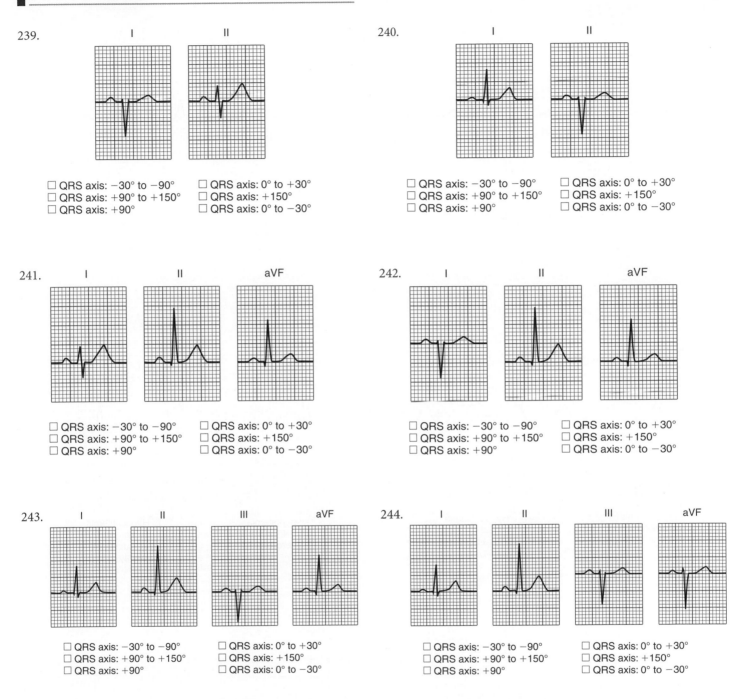

□ QRS axis: −30° to −90°   □ QRS axis: 0° to +30°
□ QRS axis: +90° to +150° □ QRS axis: +150°
□ QRS axis: +90°   □ QRS axis: 0° to −30°

240.

□ QRS axis: −30° to −90°   □ QRS axis: 0° to +30°
□ QRS axis: +90° to +150° □ QRS axis: +150°
□ QRS axis: +90°   □ QRS axis: 0° to −30°

241.

□ QRS axis: −30° to −90°   □ QRS axis: 0° to +30°
□ QRS axis: +90° to +150° □ QRS axis: +150°
□ QRS axis: +90°   □ QRS axis: 0° to −30°

242.

□ QRS axis: −30° to −90°   □ QRS axis: 0° to +30°
□ QRS axis: +90° to +150° □ QRS axis: +150°
□ QRS axis: +90°   □ QRS axis: 0° to −30°

243.

□ QRS axis: −30° to −90°   □ QRS axis: 0° to +30°
□ QRS axis: +90° to +150° □ QRS axis: +150°
□ QRS axis: +90°   □ QRS axis: 0° to −30°

244.

□ QRS axis: −30° to −90°   □ QRS axis: 0° to +30°
□ QRS axis: +90° to +150° □ QRS axis: +150°
□ QRS axis: +90°   □ QRS axis: 0° to −30°

V. ECG CHANGES: DRUG AND ELECTROLYTE

245.

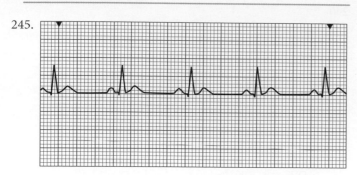

☐ Hyperkalemia   ☐ Hypocalcemia
☐ Hypokalemia   ☐ Digitalis effect
☐ Hypercalcemia   ☐ Procainamide/quinidine toxicity

246.

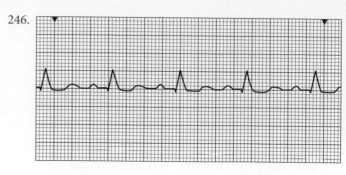

☐ Hyperkalemia   ☐ Hypocalcemia
☐ Hypokalemia   ☐ Digitalis effect
☐ Hypercalcemia   ☐ Procainamide/quinidine toxicity

247.

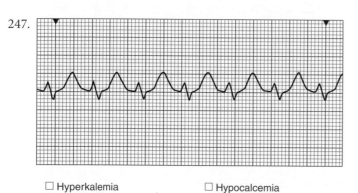

☐ Hyperkalemia   ☐ Hypocalcemia
☐ Hypokalemia   ☐ Digitalis effect
☐ Hypercalcemia   ☐ Procainamide/quinidine toxicity

248.

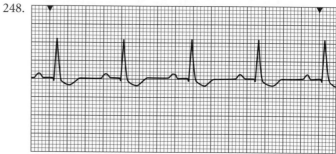

☐ Hyperkalemia   ☐ Hypocalcemia
☐ Hypokalemia   ☐ Digitalis effect
☐ Hypercalcemia   ☐ Procainamide/quinidine toxicity

249.

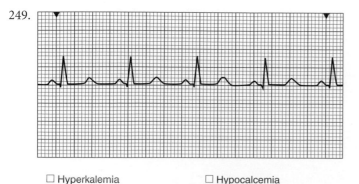

☐ Hyperkalemia   ☐ Hypocalcemia
☐ Hypokalemia   ☐ Digitalis effect
☐ Hypercalcemia   ☐ Procainamide/quinidine toxicity

250.

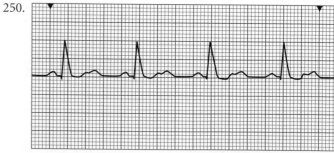

☐ Hyperkalemia   ☐ Hypocalcemia
☐ Hypokalemia   ☐ Digitalis effect
☐ Hypercalcemia   ☐ Procainamide/quinidine toxicity

VI. ECG CHANGES: MISCELLANEOUS

251.

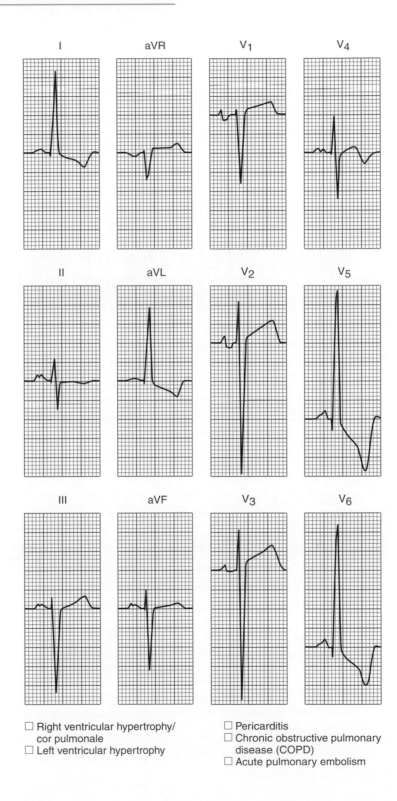

I	aVR	V₁	V₄
II	aVL	V₂	V₅
III	aVF	V₃	V₆

☐ Right ventricular hypertrophy/
cor pulmonale

☐ Left ventricular hypertrophy

☐ Pericarditis

☐ Chronic obstructive pulmonary
disease (COPD)

☐ Acute pulmonary embolism

252.

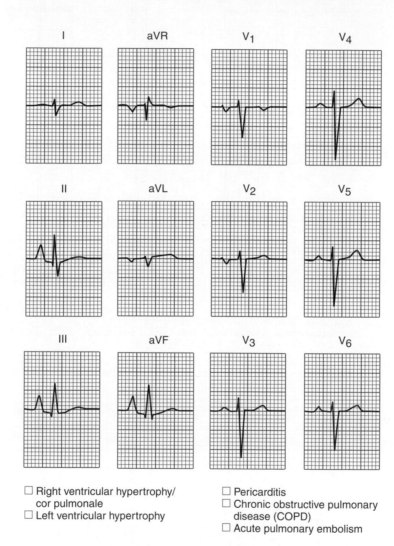

I	aVR	V₁	V₄
II	aVL	V₂	V₅
III	aVF	V₃	V₆

☐ Right ventricular hypertrophy/
   cor pulmonale
☐ Left ventricular hypertrophy

☐ Pericarditis
☐ Chronic obstructive pulmonary
   disease (COPD)
☐ Acute pulmonary embolism

253.

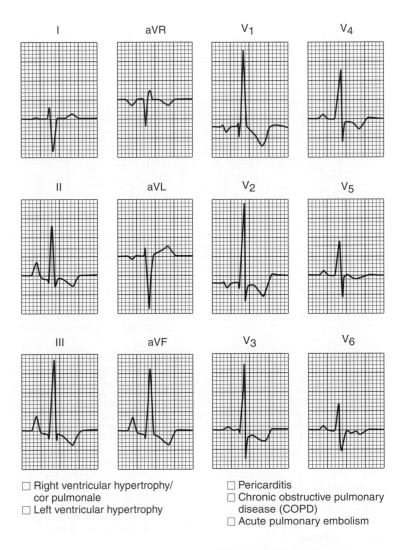

I aVR V₁ V₄

II aVL V₂ V₅

III aVF V₃ V₆

☐ Right ventricular hypertrophy/
   cor pulmonale
☐ Left ventricular hypertrophy

☐ Pericarditis
☐ Chronic obstructive pulmonary
   disease (COPD)
☐ Acute pulmonary embolism

254.

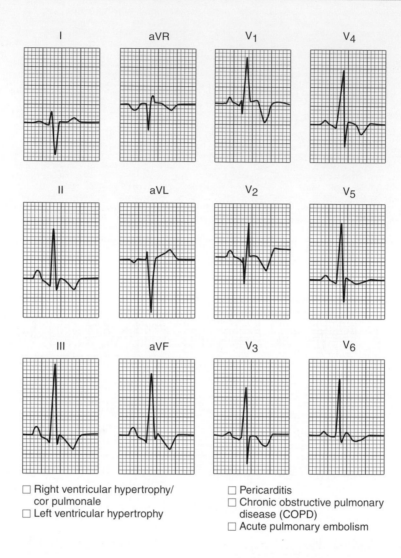

I   aVR   V₁   V₄

II   aVL   V₂   V₅

III   aVF   V₃   V₆

☐ Right ventricular hypertrophy/ cor pulmonale
☐ Left ventricular hypertrophy

☐ Pericarditis
☐ Chronic obstructive pulmonary disease (COPD)
☐ Acute pulmonary embolism

255.

I   II   III

☐ Right ventricular hypertrophy/ cor pulmonale
☐ Left ventricular hypertrophy

☐ Pericarditis
☐ Chronic obstructive pulmonary disease (COPD)
☐ Acute pulmonary embolism

256.

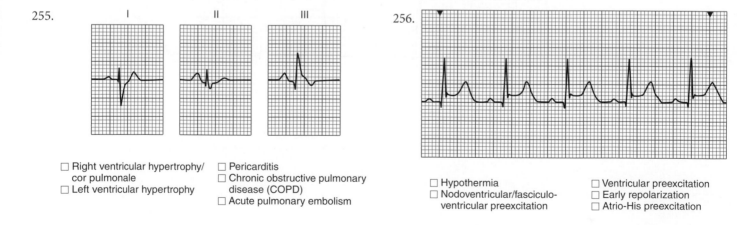

☐ Hypothermia
☐ Nodoventricular/fasciculo-ventricular preexcitation

☐ Ventricular preexcitation
☐ Early repolarization
☐ Atrio-His preexcitation

257.

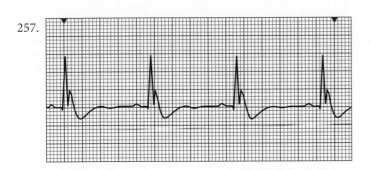

- ☐ Hypothermia
- ☐ Nodoventricular/fasciculo-
  ventricular preexcitation
- ☐ Ventricular preexcitation
- ☐ Early repolarization
- ☐ Atrio-His preexcitation

258.

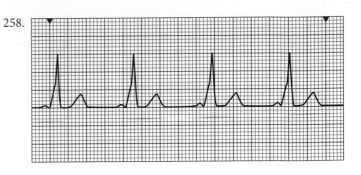

- ☐ Hypothermia
- ☐ Nodoventricular/fasciculo-
  ventricular preexcitation
- ☐ Ventricular preexcitation
- ☐ Early repolarization
- ☐ Atrio-His preexcitation

259.

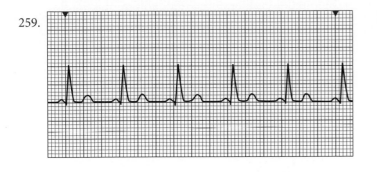

- ☐ Hypothermia
- ☐ Nodoventricular/fasciculo-
  ventricular preexcitation
- ☐ Ventricular preexcitation
- ☐ Early repolarization
- ☐ Atrio-His preexcitation

260.

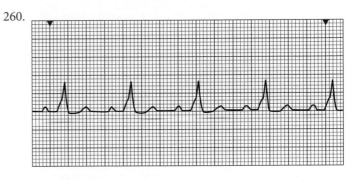

- ☐ Hypothermia
- ☐ Nodoventricular/fasciculo-
  ventricular preexcitation
- ☐ Ventricular preexcitation
- ☐ Early repolarization
- ☐ Atrio-His preexcitation

VII. SCENARIOS

Scenario 1

The ambulance is dispatched to a local shopping center for a female who has "fainted." On arrival, you find a 62-year-old female who is alert and oriented. She is sitting on a chair, accompanied by her daughter. She states she just completed her home peritoneal dialysis when she decided to go shopping. The patient states she has a history of renal failure and congestive heart failure (CHF) and takes "a water pill, potassium, and a baby aspirin." She denies any allergies. On examination, you find the patient's skin warm, pink, and moist. Lungs are clear bilaterally. Blood pressure is 104/60, pulse is 62 and regular, respiratory rate is 24, and O_2 saturation is 95%. You apply the cardiac monitor and see the following rhythm:

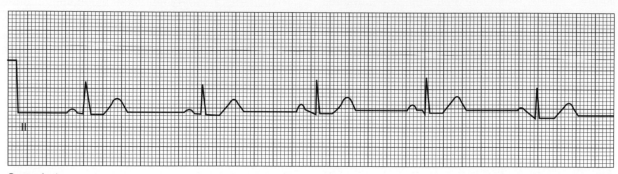

Scenario 1

261. The monitor reveals
   A. normal sinus rhythm.
   B. sinus arrhythmia.
   C. sinus bradycardia.
   D. wandering atrial pacemaker.

Because of the syncopal episode, you elect to obtain a 12-lead ECG.

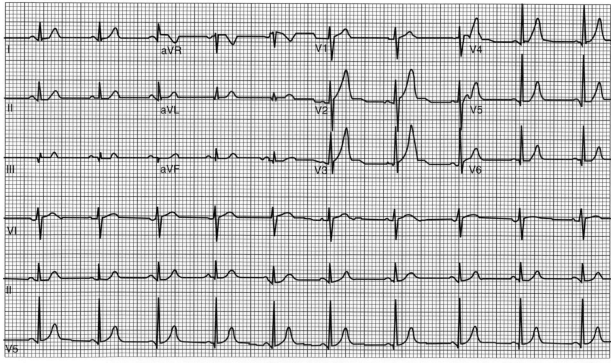

Scenario 1

262. The most striking finding on this patient's 12-lead ECG is
    A. anterior wall ST elevation.
    B. peaked T waves in the precordial leads.
    C. poor R-wave progression across the precordial leads.
    D. prolonged QT interval.
263. The changes noted in question 262 are caused by
    A. coronary artery occlusion.
    B. hyperkalemia.
    C. hypocalcemia.
    D. hypothermia.

Scenario 2

A 33-year-old female comes to the emergency room with complaints of "sudden onset of heart pounding and missing beats." She states she has had this before once or twice, but this is the worst one. She denies chest pain but does say she feels weak. She has a history of insulin-dependent diabetes but is very compliant with her testing and medications. She states she does not take any other medicines and is allergic to penicillin (PCN). She is alert and oriented (A&O) ×4; skin is warm, pink, and dry. Blood pressure is 110/70, pulse is weak and rapid, and respiratory rate is 24. After applying the monitor, you see the following:

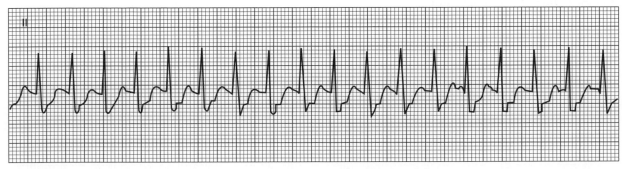

Scenario 2

264. The dysrhythmia is most likely
    A. atrial flutter with 1:1 conduction.
    B. atrial tachycardia.
    C. paroxysmal supraventricular tachycardia.
    D. sinus tachycardia.
265. If the patient was stable but the QRS was wide, what step would assist in differentiating this rhythm from ventricular tachycardia?
    A. 12-lead ECG
    B. Administration of 6 mg adenosine IV
    C. Administration of 150 mg amiodarone IV
    D. Vagal maneuvers

266. This dysrhythmia is caused by
    A. early repolarization of the atrioventricular (AV) node.
    B. ectopic focus in the atria firing rapidly.
    C. partial block of conduction through the AV node.
    D. reentry mechanism from the AV node into the accessory pathways between the sinoatrial (SA) and AV node.

Scenario 3

An 82-year-old man comes to the emergency department (ED) complaining of flulike symptoms. He is concerned because he has not been able to get the immunization and was instructed to do so by his physician. He complains of nausea, some slight difficulty breathing, chills, and chest tightness. His skin is pale, cool, and clammy. Blood pressure is 94/64; pulse is 50, weak and regular; and respiratory rate is 20. He does not remember his medications, but his son is bringing them in. He needs assistance getting onto the ED cart. Once the patient is on the monitor, you find the following:

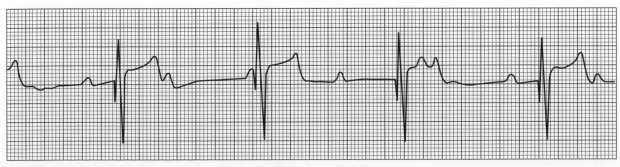

Scenario 3

267. The rhythm on the monitor is
 A. first-degree atrioventricular (AV) block (AVB).
 B. second-degree AVB type I.
 C. second-degree AVB type II.
 D. third-degree AVB
268. The QRS most likely originates from the
 A. AV node.
 B. bundle of His.
 C. Purkinje network.
 D. sinoatrial (SA) node.
269. The most appropriate initial therapy for this condition is
 A. administration of 1 mg atropine.
 B. administration of 1 mg epinephrine.
 C. initiation of transcutaneous pacing.
 D. placing the patient in a supine position, administering oxygen, and establishing vascular access.

Scenario 4

You are called to an office building for a 57-year-old man with dizziness. His secretary states that the patient came in all week with a cold. Today when he got up to go to a meeting, he fell to the floor but did not lose consciousness. You find him sitting on a chair. He seems a little confused but states he is "perfectly healthy" other than this "sinus thing." He has been taking over-the-counter decongestants and Tylenol but takes no other medication. His skin is pale, cool, and clammy. Blood pressure is 80/56, pulse is absent at the wrist, respiratory rate is 18, and O_2 saturation is 96%. You see the following rhythm on the monitor:

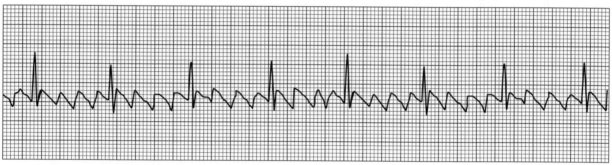

Scenario 4

270. The rhythm on the monitor is
 A. atrial fibrillation/flutter with rapid ventricular response.
 B. multiatrial tachycardia.
 C. paroxysmal supraventricular tachycardia.
 D. sinus tachycardia with premature atrial complexes.
271. The regularity of this rhythm is referred to as
 A. regular.
 B. patterned irregularity.
 C. unpatterned irregularity.
 D. grossly or irregularly irregular.

272. The most likely cause for the dysrhythmia in this patient is
 A. acute myocardial infarction.
 B. adrenergic stimulation from decongestants.
 C. dehydration.
 D. reentrant mechanism in the atrioventricular (AV) node.

Scenario 5

You have responded to a cardiac arrest. After 2 minutes of cardiopulmonary resuscitation (CPR), the monitor shows ventricular fibrillation, and you defibrillate at 360 joules and resume CPR for another 2 minutes. At this point, vascular access has been obtained, and you stop CPR to analyze the rhythm and check for a pulse. You note no pulse and see the following on the monitor:

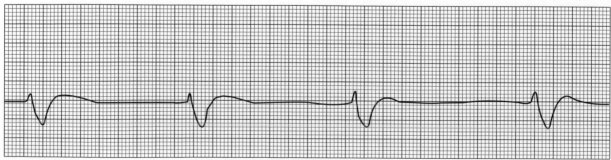

Scenario 5

273. The rhythm is
    A. asystole.
    B. pulseless electrical activity.
    C. ventricular escape rhythm.
    D. ventricular fibrillation.
274. The next steps in resuscitation include which of the following?
    A. Check for signs of life, and if prolonged "downtime," consider discontinuing efforts.
    B. Continue CPR; administer 1 mg atropine, 1 mg epinephrine, and 150 mg amiodarone; and recheck rhythm in 2 minutes.
    C. Continue CPR, administer 40 units vasopressin, and recheck rhythm in 2 minutes.
    D. Immediately defibrillate with 360 joules.

275. The goal of defibrillation in cardiac arrest resuscitation is to
    A. electrically obliterate the source of myocardial ischemia.
    B. repolarize the entire myocardium simultaneously.
    C. stimulate the pacemaker cells to fire.
    D. terminate ventricular fibrillation/ventricular tachycardia.

Scenario 6

The ambulance is dispatched for a 36-year-old business executive who became ill during a board meeting. He complains of a dull aching pain in his left shoulder and chest, with radiation to his upper back. He states he has had some nausea and heartburn all week, so he has been taking antacids. He noticed some discomfort in his shoulder yesterday but attributed it to a pulled muscle. He takes nonsteroidal antiinflammatory drugs (NSAIDs) for routine pain but has nothing prescribed. He smokes one pack of cigarettes a day. Blood pressure is 158/90, pulse is 88, and respiratory rate is 18. His cardiac rhythm shows the following, and a 12-lead ECG is taken.

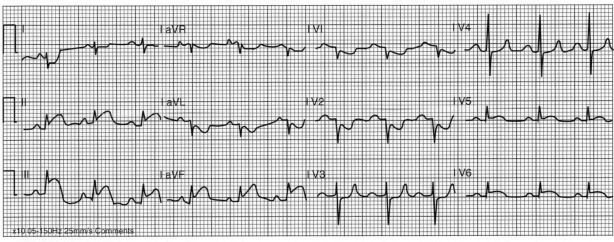

Scenario 6

276. The 12-lead ECG is diagnostic of
    A. acute anterior wall myocardial infarction.
    B. acute inferior wall myocardial infarction.
    C. acute inferior-lateral wall myocardial infarction with posterior extension.
    D. unstable angina.
277. The most likely coronary artery involved is the
    A. distal left circumflex.
    B. left anterior descending.
    C. left main coronary artery.
    D. right coronary artery.
278. Initial care for this patient should include
    A. a rapid assessment for percutaneous coronary intervention (PCI) candidacy.
    B. administration of beta blockers.
    C. administration of heparin.
    D. administration of morphine sulfate for pain.

Scenario 7

Emergency medical services (EMS) are called to the nursing home for a 92-year-old female who has had a fever for 4 days and appears to have become less responsive. Staff states that the patient had a couple of episodes of vomiting with the fever. The patient is normally not oriented but is pleasant and converses. Today she appears agitated, does not socialize, and pushed her granddaughter when she came to visit. She has a history of congestive heart failure (CHF), emphysema, and dementia. Her skin is pale, warm, and dry. Blood pressure is 178/80, pulse is 45, respiratory rate is 26, and oxygen saturation is 97% on 2 L of O₂ via nasal cannula. Your monitor shows the following:

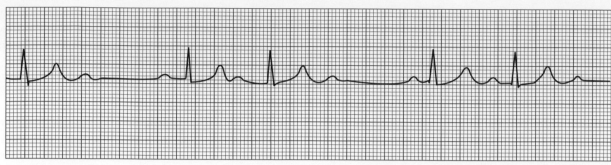

Scenario 7

279. The rhythm on the monitor is
   A. sinus rhythm with sinus arrest.
   B. second-degree atrioventricular (AV) block (AVB) type I (Wenckebach).
   C. second-degree AVB type II.
   D. advanced second-degree AVB.

280. The conduction ratio of this dysrhythmia is
   A. 1:2.
   B. 2:1.
   C. 2:3.
   D. 3:2.

281. The most likely cause of the dysrhythmia in this patient is
   A. conduction defect not associated with any acute cause.
   B. dehydration.
   C. digitalis toxicity.
   D. hypoxia.

Scenario 8

A 50-year-old male presents to triage in the emergency department (ED) with vague complaints of not feeling well. He becomes unresponsive but has a pulse. The code team arrives and places the defibrillator patches on the patient, and the following rhythm is present:

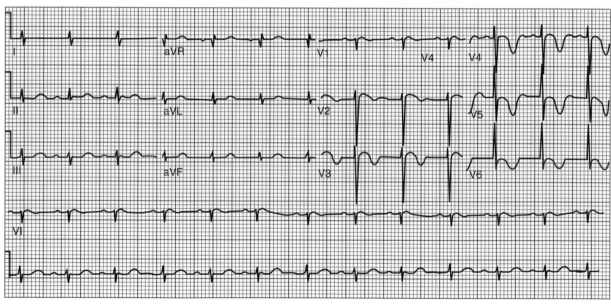

Scenario 8

282. The rhythm is most likely
   A. supraventricular tachycardia.
   B. torsades de pointes.
   C. ventricular fibrillation.
   D. ventricular tachycardia.

283. The most appropriate initial step in this patient's resuscitation is
   A. applying high-flow oxygen and assisting ventilation if necessary.
   B. establishing vascular access and administering 150 mg amiodarone.
   C. immediately defibrillating the patient with 360 joules.
   D. performing synchronized cardioversion at 100 joules.

Following the procedure performed in question 283, a 12-lead ECG is obtained and reveals the following:

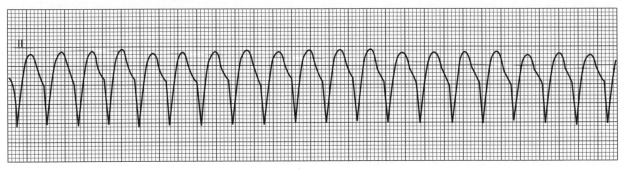

Scenario 8

284. Which of the following best describes the 12-lead ECG findings?
    A. Acute anterior wall myocardial infarction
    B. Acute anteroseptal wall myocardial infarction
    C. Acute inferior wall myocardial infarction
    D. Anterolateral wall ischemia

Scenario 9

A 63-year-old male complains of chest pain for the past 2 days. He states he has no medical problems. He also states he has had some nausea and vomiting. When it didn't resolve, he became concerned and came to the doctor's office. He appears to be in good health. He states that he still works full time as an accountant and denies undue stress or lifestyle changes. Blood pressure is 158/78, pulse is 75, respiratory rate is 18, and O$_2$ saturation is 98%.

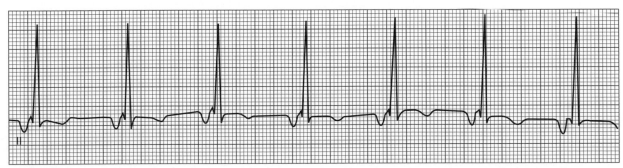

Scenario 9

285. The monitor reveals
    A. junctional tachycardia.
    B. junctional escape rhythm.
    C. multiatrial tachycardia.
    D. wandering atrial pacemaker.
286. In this patient, the most likely cause of the dysrhythmia is
    A. decongestant abuse.
    B. inferior wall myocardial infarction.
    C. pericarditis.
    D. rheumatic heart disease.

287. This dysrhythmia is a result of the disruption of normal conduction in the
    A. atrioventricular (AV) node.
    B. bundle of His.
    C. interatrial bundles.
    D. Purkinje network.

Scenario 10

A family brings a 76-year-old female to the emergency department. They state that she has been unusually tired and seems more short of breath than normal. They report her history of a myocardial infarction (MI) about 6 years ago and advise that she had a pacemaker placed at that time. They report that she has been healthy since that time. Her medications include nitroglycerin, digoxin, and Lasix for some ankle swelling and shortness of breath, which came after the heart attack. Blood pressure is 96/40, pulse is 45, and respiratory rate is 18. On the monitor, you see the following:

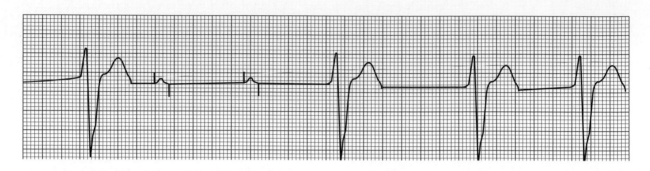

288. What type of pacemaker does the patient have?
    A. AAI
    B. DDI
    C. VDD
    D. VVI

289. The condition exhibited by the pacemaker malfunction is called
    A. automatic demand mode.
    B. failure to sense.
    C. failure to capture.
    D. failure to sense and capture.

290. Which of the following would not be indicated in the initial care of this patient?
    A. Administration of supplemental oxygen
    B. Initiation of transcutaneous pacing
    C. Large-volume fluid resuscitation for shock
    D. Obtaining STAT cardiology consult for evaluation of her pacemaker

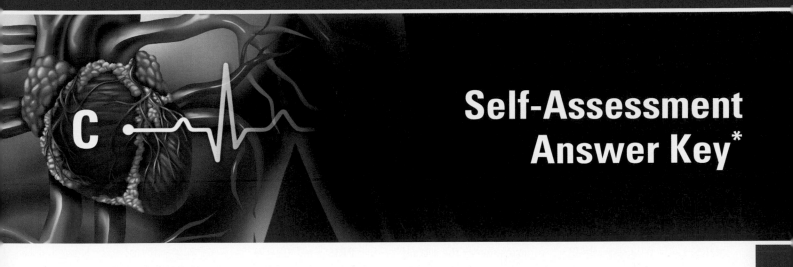

I. DYSRHYTHMIAS

1. **Rate:** 126 beats/min†
   Rhythm: Irregular
   P Waves: None; fine atrial fibrillation waves are present.
   PR Interval (PRI): None
   QRS: 0.10 sec
   Interpretation (Interp): Atrial fibrillation (fine)

2. **Rate:** 33 beats/min
   Rhythm: Irregular
   P Waves: Present; the first, second, third, and fifth P waves are followed by QRS complexes.
   PRI: 0.22–0.36 sec. The PR intervals progressively increase until a QRS complex fails to follow the P wave.
   QRS: 0.10 sec.
   Interp: Sinus rhythm with second-degree, type I atrioventricular (AV) block (Wenckebach)

3. **Rate:** 41 beats/min
   Rhythm: Irregular
   P Waves: Present; precede each QRS complex
   PRI: 0.16 sec
   QRS: 0.08 sec
   Interp: Sinus bradycardia with sinus arrhythmia

4. **Rate:** 170 beats/min
   Rhythm: Regular
   P Waves: Present; precede each QRS complex
   PRI: 0.12 sec
   QRS: About 0.12 sec
   Interp: Atrial tachycardia with wide QRS complexes

5. **Rate:** 62 beats/min
   Rhythm: Irregular
   P Waves: Present; precede the second, fourth, fifth, sixth, and seventh QRS complexes. The P waves are abnormal (0.16 sec in duration and notched).
   PRI: 0.26 sec
   QRS: 0.12 sec (all QRS complexes except the third QRS complex); 0.14 sec (third QRS complex)
   Interp: Sinus rhythm with first-degree atrioventricular (AV) block, bundle-branch block, and an isolated premature ventricular complex

6. **Rate:** 107 beats/min
   Rhythm: Irregular
   P Waves: Present; precede all QRS complexes except the fifth, eighth, ninth, and tenth QRS complexes
   PRI: 0.16 sec
   QRS: 0.09–0.10 sec
   Interp: Normal sinus rhythm with premature junctional complexes (fifth, eighth, ninth, and tenth QRS complexes) occurring singly and in group beats; the latter may be considered a short episode of junctional tachycardia.

7. **Rate:** 182 beats/min
   Rhythm: Regular
   P Waves: Present; precede each QRS complex
   PRI: 0.08 sec
   QRS: 0.09 sec
   Interp: Atrial tachycardia

8. **Rate:** Unmeasurable
   Rhythm: Irregular
   P Waves: None; coarse ventricular fibrillation waves are present.
   PRI: None
   QRS: None
   Interp: Ventricular fibrillation (coarse)

9. **Rate:** 89 beats/min
   Rhythm: Irregular
   P Waves: Present; precede all except the third and sixth QRS complexes. The shape and direction of the P waves vary from positive to negative.
   PRI: 0.6–0.12 sec
   QRS: 0.10 sec (all QRS complexes except the third and sixth QRS complexes); 0.12 sec (third and sixth QRS complexes)
   Interp: Wandering atrial pacemaker with unifocal (uniform) premature ventricular complexes

---

*Because of the possible distortion of the ECGs during printing, the measurement of the ECG components may vary slightly.
†The heart rates were calculated using R-R interval method 3.

10. **Rate:** 61 beats/min
    Rhythm: Irregular
    P Waves: Present; precede each QRS complex
    PRI: 0.12 sec
    QRS: 0.14 sec
    Interp: Sinus arrhythmia
11. **Rate:** 89 beats/min
    Rhythm: Irregular
    P Waves: Present; precede all QRS complexes except the second and eighth QRS complexes
    PRI: About 0.16 sec
    QRS: 0.08 sec (all QRS complexes except the second and eighth QRS complexes); 0.12 sec (second and eighth QRS complexes)
    Interp: Normal sinus rhythm with isolated unifocal (uniform) premature ventricular complexes
12. **Rate:** 145 beats/min
    Rhythm: Regular
    P Waves: Present; precede each QRS complex
    PRI: About 0.10 sec
    QRS: 0.08 sec
    Interp: Sinus tachycardia
13. **Rate:** 87 beats/min
    Rhythm: Irregular
    P Waves: Present; precede each QRS complex
    PRI: 0.18 sec
    QRS: 0.06 sec
    Interp: Sinus arrhythmia
14. **Rate:** 164 beats/min
    Rhythm: Regular
    P Waves: None
    PRI: None
    QRS: 0.12 sec
    Interp: Ventricular tachycardia
15. **Rate:** 74 beats/min
    Rhythm: Regular
    P Waves: Present; precede each QRS complex; shape and direction vary from positive to negative.
    PRI: 0.08–0.12 sec
    QRS: 0.08 sec
    Interp: Wandering atrial pacemaker
16. **Rate:** 70 beats/min (atrial rate: 52 beats/min)
    Rhythm: Regular
    P Waves: Present, but have no set relation to the QRS complexes
    PRI: None
    QRS: 0.14 sec
    Interp: Accelerated idioventricular rhythm with atrioventricular (AV) dissociation
17. **Rate:** 83 beats/min
    Rhythm: Regular
    P Waves: Present; precede each QRS complex
    PRI: 0.16 sec
    QRS: 0.06 sec
    Interp: Normal sinus rhythm

18. **Rate:** 229 beats/min
    Rhythm: Regular
    P Waves: None
    PRI: None
    QRS: 0.12 sec
    Interp: Ventricular tachycardia
19. **Rate:** 26 beats/min
    Rhythm: Regular
    P Waves: Present; the first, third, and fifth P waves are followed by QRS complexes. Atrioventricular (AV) conduction ratio is 2:1.
    PRI: 0.19 sec
    QRS: 0.10 sec
    Interp: Sinus rhythm with second-shape, 2:1 AV block
20. **Rate:** 84 beats/min
    Rhythm: Regular
    P Waves: None; atrial flutter waves are present.
    PRI: None
    QRS: 0.10 sec
    Interp: Atrial flutter
21. **Rate:** 30 beats/min
    Rhythm: Regular
    P Waves: Present; precede each QRS complex
    PRI: 0.17–0.18 sec
    QRS: 0.14 sec
    Interp: Sinus bradycardia with bundle-branch block
22. **Rate:** 98 beats/min
    Rhythm: Regular
    P Waves: Present; precede each QRS complex
    PRI: About 0.16 sec
    QRS: About 0.19 sec
    Interp: Normal sinus rhythm with bundle-branch block
23. **Rate:** 62 beats/min
    Rhythm: Irregular
    P Waves: Present; precede the first, second, third, and fifth QRS complexes
    PRI: 0.18 sec
    QRS: 0.12 sec
    Interp: Normal sinus rhythm with premature junctional complexes
24. **Rate:** 82 beats/min
    Rhythm: Regular
    P Waves: Present; precede each QRS complex. The P waves are abnormally wide.
    PRI: 0.16 sec
    QRS: 0.16 sec
    Interp: Normal sinus rhythm with bundle-branch block
25. **Rate:** 129 beats/min
    Rhythm: Irregular
    P Waves: None; fine atrial fibrillation waves are present.
    PRI: None
    QRS: About 0.10 sec
    Interp: Atrial fibrillation (fine)

26. **Rate:**   31 beats/min
    Rhythm: Irregular
    P Waves: Present; a QRS complex follows the first, fifth, and tenth P waves. Atrioventricular (AV) conduction ratios are 4:1 and 5:1.
    PRI: 0.34 sec
    QRS: 0.16 sec
    Interp: Sinus rhythm with second-degree advanced AV block and bundle-branch block

27. **Rate:**   75 beats/min
    Rhythm: Regular
    P Waves: Present; negative P waves precede each QRS complex
    PRI: 0.08 sec
    QRS: 0.08 sec
    Interp: Accelerated junctional rhythm

28. **Rate:**   62 beats/min
    Rhythm: Irregular. The R-R intervals between the third and fourth QRS complexes and the fifth and sixth QRS complexes are twice the R-R interval of the underlying sinus rhythm.
    P Waves: Present; precede each QRS complex
    PRI: 0.18 sec
    QRS: 0.18 sec
    Interp: Sinus rhythm with sinoatrial (SA) exit block and bundle-branch block

29. **Rate:**   37 beats/min
    Rhythm: Regular
    P Waves: None; atrial fibrillation waves are present.
    PRI: None
    QRS: About 0.24 sec
    Interp: Atrial fibrillation (fine) with ventricular escape rhythm

30. **Rate:**   60 beats/min
    Rhythm: Regular
    P Waves: Present; precede each QRS complex
    PRI: 0.16 sec
    QRS: 0.06 sec
    Interp: Normal sinus rhythm

31. **Rate:**   135 beats/min
    Rhythm: Regular
    P Waves: None
    PRI: None
    QRS: 0.26 sec
    Interp: Ventricular tachycardia

32. **Rate:**   163 beats/min
    Rhythm: Regular
    P Waves: None
    PRI: None
    QRS: 0.10 sec
    Interp: Junctional tachycardia

33. **Rate:**   41 beats/min
    Rhythm: Irregular

    P Waves: Present; precede the first, second, fourth, and fifth QRS complexes. The R-R interval between the second and fourth QRS complexes is four times the R-R interval of the underlying sinus rhythm.
    PRI: 0.14 sec
    QRS: 0.12 sec
    Interp: Sinus rhythm with sinoatrial (SA) exit block and an isolated junctional escape beat (third QRS complex)

34. **Rate:**   17 beats/min
    Rhythm: Undeterminable
    P Waves: None
    PRI: None
    QRS: 0.16 sec
    Interp: Ventricular escape rhythm

35. **Rate:**   70 beats/min
    Rhythm: Regular
    P Waves: Present; precede each QRS complex
    PRI: 0.16 sec
    QRS: 0.06 sec
    Interp: Normal sinus rhythm

36. **Rate:**   64 beats/min
    Rhythm: Irregular
    P Waves: Present; precede the first and second QRS complexes. Pacemaker spikes precede the rest of the QRS complexes.
    PRI: 0.26 sec
    QRS: 0.08 sec (first and second QRS complexes); 0.12 sec (third, fourth, fifth, sixth, and seventh QRS complexes)
    Interp: Sinus rhythm with first-degree atrioventricular (AV) block, followed by ventricular asystole and a ventricular demand pacemaker rhythm

37. **Rate:**   72 beats/min
    Rhythm: Irregular
    P Waves: Present; precede each QRS complex
    PRI: 0.16 sec
    QRS: 0.08 sec
    Interp: Sinus arrhythmia

38. **Rate:**   75 beats/min
    Rhythm: Irregular
    P Waves: Present; all but the first and sixth P waves are followed by QRS complexes. Atrioventricular (AV) conduction ratio is 5:4.
    PRI: 0.12–0.14 sec
    QRS: 0.12 sec
    Interp: Sinus rhythm with second-degree type II AV block

39. **Rate:**   101 beats/min
    Rhythm: Irregular
    P Waves: Present; precede each QRS complex. The shape and direction of the P waves vary from positive to negative.
    PRI: 0.12–0.18 sec

	QRS:	0.06 sec
	Interp:	Wandering atrial pacemaker
40.	**Rate:**	37 beats/min
	Rhythm:	Regular
	P Waves:	Present; precede each QRS complex
	PRI:	0.34 sec
	QRS:	0.08 sec
	Interp:	Sinus bradycardia with first-degree atrioventricular (AV) block
41.	**Rate:**	42 beats/min
	Rhythm:	Irregular
	P Waves:	Present; precede each QRS complex. The fourth P wave is negative; the rest are positive.
	PRI:	0.18–0.20 sec
	QRS:	0.16 sec
	Interp:	Sinus bradycardia with bundle-branch block and an isolated premature atrial complex
42.	**Rate:**	66 beats/min
	Rhythm:	Irregular
	P Waves:	Present; all the P waves except the fourth and eighth P waves are followed by QRS complexes.
	PRI:	0.22–0.40 sec. The PR intervals progressively increase until a QRS complex fails to follow the P wave.
	QRS:	0.16 sec
	Interp:	Sinus rhythm with second-degree type I atrioventricular (AV) block (Wenckebach) and bundle-branch block
43.	**Rate:**	74 beats/min
	Rhythm:	Regular
	P Waves:	None
	PRI:	None
	QRS:	0.12 sec
	Interp:	Pacemaker rhythm (ventricular pacemaker)
44.	**Rate:**	88 beats/min
	Rhythm:	Regular
	P Waves:	Present; precede each QRS complex
	PRI:	0.12 sec
	QRS:	0.14 sec
	Interp:	Normal sinus rhythm with bundle-branch block
45.	**Rate:**	61 beats/min
	Rhythm:	Irregular
	P Waves:	Present; precede all but the fourth QRS complex
	PRI:	0.12 sec
	QRS:	0.08 sec
	Interp:	Sinus rhythm with sinus arrest and a premature junctional complex
46.	**Rate:**	71 beats/min
	Rhythm:	**Slightly** irregular
	P Waves:	Present; precede each QRS complex
	PRI:	0.18 sec
	QRS:	About 0.10 sec
	Interp:	Sinus arrhythmia

47.	**Rate:**	66 beats/min
	Rhythm:	Irregular
	P Waves:	Present; all but the fourth and eighth P waves are followed by QRS complexes.
	PRI:	0.22–0.40 sec. The PR intervals progressively increase until a QRS complex fails to follow the P wave.
	QRS:	About 0.15 sec
	Interp:	Sinus rhythm with second-degree type I atrioventricular (AV) block (Wenckebach) and bundle-branch block
48.	**Rate:**	102 beats/min
	Rhythm:	Irregular
	P Waves:	None; fine atrial fibrillation waves are present.
	PRI:	None
	QRS:	About 0.10 sec (first, fifth, seventh, eighth, ninth, and tenth QRS complexes); 0.12–0.16 sec (second, third, fourth, sixth, and tenth QRS complexes). The shape and direction of the second, third, and fourth QRS complexes differ from each other. The second QRS complex is similar to the sixth QRS complex; the fourth QRS complex is similar to the tenth QRS complex.
	Interp:	Atrial fibrillation (fine) with third-degree atrioventricular (AV) block, accelerated junctional rhythm, multifocal (multiform) premature ventricular complexes (PVCs; group beats), and a short burst of ventricular tachycardia. AV dissociation is present.
49.	**Rate:**	63 beats/min
	Rhythm:	Irregular
	P Waves:	None; coarse atrial fibrillation waves are present.
	PRI:	None
	QRS:	0.13 sec
	Interp:	Atrial fibrillation (coarse) with bundle-branch block
50.	**Rate:**	57 beats/min.
	Rhythm:	Irregular. The R-R interval between the fourth and fifth QRS complexes is less than twice the R-R interval of the underlying sinus rhythm.
	P Waves:	Present; precede all but the fifth QRS complex
	PRI:	0.12 sec
	QRS:	About 0.12 sec
	Interp:	Sinus rhythm with sinus arrest and an isolated junctional escape beat
51.	**Rate:**	52 beats/min
	Rhythm:	Regular
	P Waves:	Present; precede each QRS complex
	PRI:	0.20 sec
	QRS:	0.08 sec
	Interp:	Normal sinus rhythm
52.	**Rate:**	183 beats/min
	Rhythm:	Regular
	P Waves:	None
	PRI:	None
	QRS:	0.16 sec

Interp: Ventricular tachycardia

53. **Rate:** 65 beats/min
    Rhythm: Irregular
    P Waves: Present; precede each QRS complex
    PRI: 0.16 sec
    QRS: 0.08 sec
    Interp: Sinus arrhythmia

54. **Rate:** 36 beats/min
    Rhythm: Regular
    P Waves: None
    PRI: None
    QRS: 0.12 sec
    Interp: Junctional escape rhythm

55. **Rate:** 40 beats/min
    Rhythm: Regular
    P Waves: None
    PRI: None
    QRS: 0.16 sec
    Interp: Ventricular escape rhythm

56. **Rate:** 59 beats/min
    Rhythm: Irregular
    P Waves: Present; the second, third, fifth, sixth, eighth, and tenth P waves are followed by QRS complexes. Atrioventricular (AV) conduction ratios are 3:2 and 2:1.
    PRI: About 0.16 sec
    QRS: About 0.16 sec
    Interp: Sinus rhythm with second-degree, type II 3:2 AV block and 2:1 AV block and bundle-branch block

57. **Rate:** 58 beats/min
    Rhythm: Regular
    P Waves: Present; negative P waves follow each QRS complex.
    PRI: None
    QRS: 0.16 sec
    Interp: Junctional escape rhythm with bundle-branch block

58. **Rate:** 53 beats/min
    Rhythm: Irregular
    P Waves: Present; the first, second, fourth, fifth, and sixth P waves are followed by QRS complexes
    PRI: 0.22–0.46 sec. The PR intervals progressively increase until a QRS complex fails to follow the P wave.
    QRS: 0.08 sec
    Interp: Sinus rhythm with second-degree type I atrioventricular (AV) block (Wenckebach)

59. **Rate:** 80 beats/min
    Rhythm: Irregular
    P Waves: Present; precede the first, second, third, sixth, eighth, and ninth QRS complexes. The third P wave is negative; the fifth wave is buried in the preceding T wave. Pacemaker spikes precede the third, fourth, fifth, and seventh QRS complexes.
    PRI: 0.12–0.18 sec

QRS: 0.07 sec (first, second, sixth, eighth, and ninth QRS complexes); 0.16 sec (fourth, fifth, and seventh QRS complexes). The third QRS complex is a fusion beat—a combination of the normally conducted QRS complex and the pacemaker induced ventricular QRS complex.
Interp: Sinus rhythm with episodes of ventricular demand pacemaker rhythm

60. **Rate:** 135 beats/min
    Rhythm: Regular
    P Waves: None
    PRI: None
    QRS: About 0.32–0.36 sec
    Interp: Ventricular tachycardia

61. **Rate:** 70 beats/min
    Rhythm: Regular
    P Waves: Present; precede each QRS complex
    PRI: 0.16 sec
    QRS: 0.06 sec
    Interp: Normal sinus rhythm

62. **Rate:** 52 beats/min
    Rhythm: Irregular
    P Waves: Present; the second, third, fifth, and sixth P waves are followed by QRS complexes. The atrioventricular (AV) conduction ratio is 3:2.
    PRI: 0.24–0.26 sec
    QRS: 0.16 sec
    Interp: Sinus rhythm with second-degree type II AV block and bundle-branch block

63. **Rate:** 64 beats/min
    Rhythm: Irregular
    P Waves: Present; the first, second, fourth, fifth, and sixth P waves are followed by QRS complexes.
    PRI: 0.24–0.36 sec. The PR intervals progressively increase until a QRS complex fails to follow the P wave.
    QRS: 0.12 sec
    Interp: Sinus rhythm with second-degree type I atrioventricular (AV) block (Wenckebach)

64. **Rate:** 284 beats/min
    Rhythm: Regular
    P Waves: None
    PRI: None
    QRS: About 0.20 sec
    Interp: Ventricular tachycardia

65. **Rate:** 87 beats/min
    Rhythm: Irregular
    P Waves: Present; precede each QRS complex
    PRI: 0.12–0.16 sec
    QRS: 0.04 sec
    Interp: Wandering atrial pacemaker

66. **Rate:** 70 beats/min
    Rhythm: Regular
    P Waves: Present; precede each QRS complex
    PRI: 0.16 sec
    QRS: 0.07 sec
    Interp: Normal sinus rhythm

67. **Rate:**   37 beats/min
    Rhythm: Regular
    P Waves: Present; precede each QRS complex
    PRI: 0.20 sec
    QRS: 0.12 sec
    Interp: Sinus bradycardia
68. **Rate:**   30 beats/min (atrial rate: 82 beats/min)
    Rhythm: Regular
    P Waves: Present, but have no set relation to the QRS complexes
    PRI: None
    QRS: 0.14 sec
    Interp: Third-degree atrioventricular (AV) block with wide QRS complexes
69. **Rate:**   125 beats/min (average); 165 beats/min (first part); 79 beats/min (second part)
    Rhythm: Irregular
    P Waves: Present; precede each QRS complex. In the first part, the P waves are superimposed on the preceding T waves.
    PRI: 0.16 sec
    QRS: About 0.08 sec
    Interp: Paroxysmal supraventricular tachycardia (PSVT) with reversion to normal sinus rhythm
70. **Rate:**   120 beats/min (three beats)
    Rhythm: Regular (three beats)
    P Waves: None
    PRI: None
    QRS: 0.14 sec
    Interp: Supraventricular tachycardia with wide QRS complexes or ventricular tachycardia followed by asystole
71. **Rate:**   174 beats/min
    Rhythm: Regular
    P Waves: None
    PRI: None
    QRS: 0.12 sec
    Interp: Supraventricular tachycardia
72. **Rate:**   36 beats/min
    Rhythm: Regular
    P Waves: None
    PRI: None
    QRS: 0.18 sec
    Interp: Junctional escape rhythm with bundle-branch block or ventricular escape rhythm
73. **Rate:**   263 beats/min
    Rhythm: Regular
    P Waves: None
    PRI: None
    QRS: About 0.20 sec
    Interp: Ventricular tachycardia
74. **Rate:**   69 beats/min
    Rhythm: Irregular
    P Waves: Present; the second, third, fourth, sixth, seventh, and eighth P waves are followed by QRS complexes. Atrioventricular (AV) conduction ratio is 4:3.

    PRI: 0.16 sec
    QRS: 0.20 sec
    Interp: Sinus rhythm with second-degree type II AV block and bundle-branch block
75. **Rate:**   72 beats/min
    Rhythm: Regular
    P Waves: P waves are present. A QRS complex follows every third P wave.
    PRI: 0.32 sec
    QRS: 0.08 sec
    Interp: Sinus rhythm with first-degree atrioventricular (AV) block
76. **Rate:**   104 beats/min
    Rhythm: Irregular
    P Waves: Present; precede the first, fifth, and sixth QRS complex
    PRI: 0.18 sec
    QRS: 0.12 sec (first, fifth, and sixth complexes); about 0.16 sec (second, third, and fourth QRS complex)
    Interp: Sinus rhythm with and unifocal (uniform) premature ventricular complexes occurring in a burst of three (ventricular tachycardia); R-on-T phenomenon
77. **Rate:**   82 beats/min
    Rhythm: Regular
    P Waves: Present; precede each QRS complex
    PRI: About 0.16 sec
    QRS: 0.08 sec
    Interp: Normal sinus rhythm with motion artifact
78. **Rate:**   100 beats/min
    Rhythm: Irregular
    P Waves: Present; precede QRS complexes 1, 3, and 5
    PRI: 0.12 sec
    QRS: About 0.20 sec
    Interp: Sinus rhythm with bundle-branch block and premature junctional complexes
79. **Rate:**   56 beats/min
    Rhythm: Regular
    P Waves: Present; precede each QRS complex
    PRI: 0.36–0.42 sec. The PR intervals progressively increase.
    QRS: About 0.12 sec
    Interp: Sinus rhythm with second-degree atrioventricular (AV) block (type undeterminable, probably type I AV block [Wenckebach])
80. **Rate:**   181 beats/min
    Rhythm: Regular
    P Waves: None
    PRI: None
    QRS: About 0.18 sec
    Interp: Supraventricular tachycardia with wide QRS complexes or ventricular tachycardia
81. **Rate:**   40 beats/min
    Rhythm: Undeterminable
    P Waves: None
    PRI: None.

QRS: About 0.20 sec
Interp: Ventricular escape rhythm

82. **Rate:** 94 beats/min
    Rhythm: Regular
    P Waves: Present; negative P waves precede each QRS complex.
    PRI: 0.08 sec
    QRS: 0.10 sec
    Interp: Accelerated junctional rhythm

83. **Rate:** 94 beats/min
    Rhythm: Regular
    P Waves: Present; precede each QRS complex
    PRI: 0.12 sec
    QRS: 0.12 sec
    Interp: Normal sinus rhythm

84. **Rate:** 68 beats/min
    Rhythm: Irregular
    P Waves: Present; precede the first and third QRS complexes
    PRI: About 0.08 sec
    QRS: 0.08 sec (first and third QS complex); 0.18 sec (second and fourth QRS complex)
    Interp: Atrial rhythm with premature ventricular complexes (ventricular bigeminy)

85. **Rate:** 68 beats/min
    Rhythm: Irregular
    P Waves: Present; precede each QRS complex. The first and third P waves are positive; the second and fourth P waves are negative.
    PRI: 0.20 sec
    QRS: 0.12 sec
    Interp: Sinus rhythm with first-degree atrioventricular (AV) block, and premature atrial complexes (atrial bigeminy)

86. **Rate:** 34 beats/min (atrial rate: 163 beats/min)
    Rhythm: Undeterminable
    P Waves: Present, but the negative P waves have no set relation to the QRS complexes.
    PRI: None
    QRS: 0.16 sec
    Interp: Third-degree atrioventricular (AV) block with wide QRS complexes

87. **Rate:** 75 beats/min
    Rhythm: Irregular
    P Waves: None; fine atrial fibrillation waves are present.
    PRI: None
    QRS: 0.16 sec
    Interp: Atrial fibrillation (fine)

88. **Rate:** 107 beats/min
    Rhythm: Irregular
    P Waves: Present; precede each QRS complex
    PRI: 0.14 sec
    QRS: 0.16 sec
    Interp: Sinus tachycardia with first-degree atrioventricular (AV) block, bundle-branch block, and an isolated premature junctional complex (fourth QRS complex)

89. **Rate:** 230 beats/min
    Rhythm: Slightly irregular
    P Waves: None
    PRI: None
    QRS: 0.20 sec
    Interp: Ventricular tachycardia

90. **Rate:** 170 beats/min
    Rhythm: Irregular
    P Waves: None; fine atrial fibrillation waves are present.
    PRI: None
    QRS: 0.08 sec
    Interp: Atrial fibrillation (fine)

91. **Rate:** 80 beats/min
    Rhythm: Irregular
    P Waves: Present; precede the first and third QRS complexes
    PRI: 0.14 sec
    QRS: 0.12 sec
    Interp: Sinus rhythm with bundle-branch block and premature junctional complexes (bigeminy)

92. **Rate:** 115 beats/min
    Rhythm: Irregular
    P Waves: None; atrial flutter waves are present.
    PRI: None
    QRS: 0.12 sec
    Interp: Atrial flutter with variable conduction ratio

93. **Rate:** Unmeasurable
    Rhythm: Irregular
    P Waves: None; coarse ventricular fibrillation waves are present.
    PRI: None
    QRS: None
    Interp: Ventricular fibrillation (coarse)

94. **Rate:** 46 beats/min
    Rhythm: Irregular
    P Waves: Present; the first, second, and fourth P waves are followed by QRS complexes.
    PRI: 0.20–0.32 sec. The PR intervals progressively increase until a QRS complex fails to follow the P wave.
    QRS: 0.10 sec
    Interp: Sinus rhythm with second-degree type I atrioventricular (AV) block (Wenckebach)

95. **Rate:** 82 beats/min
    Rhythm: Regular
    P Waves: None; atrial and ventricular pacemaker spikes are present.
    PRI: None
    QRS: 0.16 sec
    Interp: Pacemaker rhythm (atrioventricular [AV] sequential pacemaker)

96. **Rate:** 61 beats/min
    Rhythm: Irregular
    P Waves: Present; precede the first, second, and fourth QRS complexes
    PRI: 0.22 sec
    QRS: 0.11 sec

Interp: Normal sinus rhythm with first-degree atrioventricular (AV) block and isolated premature ventricular complex (third QRS complex)

97. Rate: 224 beats/min
Rhythm: Regular
P Waves: None
PRI: None
QRS: 0.06 sec
Interp: Supraventricular tachycardia

98. Rate: 98 beats/min
Rhythm: Irregular
P Waves: Present; precede the first, second, third, and sixth QRS complexes
PRI: 0.16 sec
QRS: 0.16–0.18 sec
Interp: Normal sinus rhythm with bundle-branch block and premature junctional complexes (group beats)

99. Rate: 136 beats/min
Rhythm: Regular
P Waves: Present; negative P waves follow each QRS complex.
PRI: None
QRS: 0.06 sec
Interp: Junctional tachycardia

100. Rate: 63 beats/min
Rhythm: None
P Waves: None; positive wide artifacts are present.
PRI: None
QRS: None
Interp: Ventricular asystole with artifacts (chest compressions)

101. Rate: 184 beats/min
Rhythm: Regular
P Waves: None
PRI: None
QRS: 0.10 sec
Interp: Supraventricular tachycardia

102. Rate: 102 beats/min
Rhythm: Regular
P Waves: Present; precede each QRS complex
PRI: 0.16 sec
QRS: 0.06 sec
Interp: Sinus tachycardia. Abnormally tall T waves characteristic of hyperkalemia are present.

103. Rate: 68 beats/min
Rhythm: Regular
P Waves: None
PRI: None
QRS: About 0.22 sec
Interp: Accelerated idioventricular rhythm

104. Rate: 164 beats/min
Rhythm: Regular
P Waves: Present; precede each QRS complex
PRI: 0.12 sec

QRS: 0.08 sec
Interp: Atrial tachycardia

105. Rate: 123 beats/min
Rhythm: Regular
P Waves: Present; precede each QRS complex
PRI: 0.12 sec
QRS: 0.16 sec
Interp: Sinus tachycardia with bundle-branch block

106. Rate: 76 beats/min
Rhythm: Irregular
P Waves: Present; precede the second and fourth QRS complex. The fifth QRS complex is superimposed on a P wave.
PRI: 0.16 sec
QRS: 0.08 sec (third and fifth QRS complexes); 0.12 sec (first, second, and fourth QRS complexes)
Interp: Normal sinus rhythm with bundle-branch block and premature junctional complexes

107. Rate: 61 beats/min
Rhythm: Irregular
P Waves: Present; precede the first, second, and fourth QRS complexes.
PRI: 0.24 sec
QRS: 0.10 sec
Interp: Sinus rhythm with first-degree atrioventricular (AV) block and an isolated premature junctional complex

108. Rate: 41 beats/min
Rhythm: Regular
P Waves: Present; precede each QRS complex
PRI: About 0.14 sec
QRS: 0.08 sec
Interp: Sinus bradycardia

109. Rate: 69 beats/min
Rhythm: Regular
P Waves: Present; precede each QRS complex
PRI: About 0.24 sec
QRS: 0.16 sec
Interp: Sinus rhythm with first-degree atrioventricular (AV) block and bundle-branch block

110. Rate: 48 beats/min (atrial rate: 125 beats/min)
Rhythm: Regular
P Waves: Present, but have no set relation to the QRS complexes
PRI: None
QRS: 0.10 sec
Interp: Third-degree atrioventricular (AV) block

111. Rate: 41 beats/min
Rhythm: Irregular
P Waves: Present; the first, fourth, and sixth P waves are followed by QRS complexes. Atrioventricular (AV) conduction ratios are 2:1 and 3:1.
PRI: 0.20 sec
QRS: 0.12 sec

Interp: Sinus rhythm with second-degree, 2:1, and advanced AV block

112. **Rate:** 92 beats/min
Rhythm: Regular
P Waves: Present; precede each QRS complex
PRI: 0.14 sec
QRS: About 0.08 sec
Interp: Normal sinus rhythm

113. **Rate:** 161 beats/min
Rhythm: Regular
P Waves: None
PRI: None
QRS: 0.08 sec
Interp: Supraventricular tachycardia

114. **Rate:** 320 beats/min
Rhythm: Slightly irregular
P Waves: None
PRI: None
QRS: 0.14–0.20 sec
Interp: Torsades de pointes

115. **Rate:** 50 beats/min
Rhythm: Regular
P Waves: Present; precede each QRS complex
PRI: 0.16 sec
QRS: 0.08 sec
Interp: Junctional escape rhythm

116. **Rate:** 60 beats/min
Rhythm: Irregular
P Waves: None; fine atrial fibrillation waves are present.
PRI: None
QRS: 0.08 sec
Interp: Atrial fibrillation (fine)

117. **Rate:** 97 beats/min
Rhythm: Regular
P Waves: Present; precede each QRS complex
PRI: 0.16 sec
QRS: 0.20 sec
Interp: Normal sinus rhythm with bundle-branch block

118. **Rate:** Unmeasurable
Rhythm: Irregular
P Waves: None; coarse ventricular fibrillation waves present
PRI: None
QRS: None
Interp: Ventricular fibrillation (coarse)

119. **Rate:** 48 beats/min
Rhythm: Regular
P Waves: Present; follow each QRS complex
PRI: None
QRS: About 0.16 sec
Interp: Junctional escape rhythm with bundle-branch block or accelerated idioventricular rhythm

120. **Rate:** 73 beats/min
Rhythm: Irregular
P Waves: Present; precede the first, second, and fourth QRS complexes
PRI: 0.18 sec
QRS: 0.08 sec (first, second, and fourth QRS complexes); 0.16 sec (third QRS complex)
Interp: Normal sinus rhythm with an isolated premature ventricular complex (interpolated)

121. **Rate:** 62 beats/min
Rhythm: Regular
P Waves: Present; precede each QRS complex
PRI: 0.20 sec
QRS: About 0.08 sec
Interp: Normal sinus rhythm

122. **Rate:** 78 beats/min
Rhythm: Irregular
P Waves: None; fine atrial fibrillation waves are present.
PRI: None
QRS: 0.08 sec
Interp: Atrial fibrillation (fine)

123. **Rate:** 87 beats/min
Rhythm: Irregular
P Waves: Present; precede the first and fourth QRS complexes
PRI: 0.16 sec
QRS: 0.10 sec (first and fourth QRS complexes); about 0.16–0.18 sec (second, third, and fifth QRS complexes)
Interp: Normal sinus rhythm with uniform premature ventricular complexes (group beats)

124. **Rate:** 80 beats/min
Rhythm: Regular
P Waves: None; ventricular pacemaker spikes are present.
PRI: None
QRS: 0.16 sec
Interp: Pacemaker rhythm (ventricular pacemaker)

125. **Rate:** 31 beats/min (atrial rate: 97 beats/min)
Rhythm: Undeterminable
P Waves: Present, but have no set relation to the QRS complexes
PRI: None
QRS: 0.12–0.14 sec
Interp: Third-degree atrioventricular (AV) block with wide QRS complexes

126. **Rate:** 57 beats/min
Rhythm: Regular
P Waves: None
PRI: None
QRS: About 0.16 sec
Interp: Junctional escape rhythm with bundle-branch block

127. **Rate:** 47 beats/min
Rhythm: Regular
P Waves: Present; precede each QRS complex

PRI: 0.48 sec
QRS: 0.08 sec
Interp: Sinus bradycardia with first-degree atrioventricular (AV) block

128. **Rate:**   149 beats/min
    Rhythm: Regular
    P Waves: Present; precede each QRS complex
    PRI: Unmeasurable
    QRS: 0.08 sec
    Interp: Atrial tachycardia

129. **Rate:**   160 beats/min
    Rhythm: Irregular
    P Waves: Undeterminable
    PRI: Undeterminable
    QRS: 0.12 sec (first QRS complex); $\geq$0.16 sec (rest of the QRS complexes)
    Interp: A wide QRS complex followed by ventricular tachycardia

130. **Rate:**   160 beats/min
    Rhythm: Regular
    P Waves: None
    PRI: None
    QRS: 0.16 sec
    Interp: Supraventricular tachycardia

131. **Rate:**   150 beats/min
    Rhythm: Regular
    P Waves: Present; follow each QRS complex
    PRI: None
    QRS: 0.10 sec
    Interp: Junctional tachycardia

132. **Rate:**   Ventricular rate 31 beats/min; atrial rate 100 beats/min.
    Rhythm: Undeterminable
    P Waves: Present, but have no set relation to the QRS complexes
    PRI: None
    QRS: About 0.15 sec
    Interp: Third-degree atrioventricular (AV) block with wide QRS complexes

133. **Rate:**   31 beats/min
    Rhythm: Undeterminable
    P Waves: Present; precede each QRS complex
    PRI: 0.14 sec
    QRS: 0.08 sec
    Interp: Sinus bradycardia

134. **Rate:**   59 beats/min
    Rhythm: Regular
    P Waves: None; atrial flutter waves are present.
    PRI: None
    QRS: 0.16 sec
    Interp: Atrial flutter with bundle-branch block

135. **Rate:**   178 beats/min
    Rhythm: Regular
    P Waves: None
    PRI: None
    QRS: 0.08 sec
    Interp: Supraventricular tachycardia

136. **Rate:**   91 beats/min
    Rhythm: Regular
    P Waves: Present; precede each QRS complex
    PRI: 0.28 sec
    QRS: 0.12 sec
    Interp: Sinus rhythm with first-degree atrioventricular (AV) block and bundle-branch block

137. **Rate:**   47 beats/min
    Rhythm: Regular
    P Waves: Present; the first, third, and fifth P waves are followed by QRS complexes.
    PRI: 0.28 sec
    QRS: 0.12 sec
    Interp: Sinus rhythm with second-degree 2:1 atrioventricular (AV) block and bundle-branch block

138. **Rate:**   78 beats/min
    Rhythm: Irregular
    P Waves: Present; precede each QRS complex. The second and fourth P waves are abnormal, each in a different way.
    PRI: About 0.22 sec (first and third PR intervals); about 0.16 second (second and fourth PR intervals)
    QRS: About 0.10 sec
    Interp: Sinus rhythm with multifocal premature atrial complexes

139. **Rate:**   64 beats/min
    Rhythm: Regular
    P Waves: None
    PRI: None
    QRS: About 0.10 sec
    Interp: Accelerated junctional rhythm

140. **Rate:**   222 beats/min
    Rhythm: Regular
    P Waves: None
    PRI: None
    QRS: 0.12 sec
    Interp: Supraventricular tachycardia with wide QRS complexes or ventricular tachycardia

141. **Rate:**   None (pacemaker spikes: 63 beats/min)
    Rhythm: Regular
    P Waves: None; pacemaker spikes are present
    PRI: None
    QRS: None
    Interp: Asystole with pacemaker spikes without capture

142. **Rate:**   99 beats/min
    Rhythm: Irregular
    P Waves: Present; precede the first, second, and fifth QRS complexes
    PRI: 0.28 sec
    QRS: 0.10 sec (first, second, and fifth QRS complexes); 0.12–0.16 second (third and fourth QRS complexes)
    Interp: Sinus rhythm with first-degree atrioventricular (AV) block and multifocal premature ventricular complexes (group beats)

143. **Rate:** 61 beats/min
     Rhythm: Regular
     P Waves: Present: precede each QRS complex. P waves are abnormally tall (P pulmonale).
     PRI: 0.26 sec
     QRS: 0.10 sec
     Interp: Sinus rhythm with first-degree atrioventricular (AV) block
144. **Rate:** 114 beats/min
     Rhythm: Regular
     P Waves: Present; precede each QRS complex
     PRI: 0.16 sec
     QRS: 0.08 sec
     Interp: Sinus tachycardia
145. **Rate:** 100 beats/min
     Rhythm: Regular
     P Waves: Present; retrograde P waves follow each QRS complex.
     PRI: None
     QRS: 0.10 sec
     Interp: Junctional tachycardia
146. **Rate:** Unmeasurable
     Rhythm: Irregular
     P Waves: None; coarse ventricular fibrillation waves are present.
     PRI: None
     QRS: None
     Interp: Ventricular fibrillation (coarse)
147. **Rate:** 21 beats/min
     Rhythm: Undeterminable
     P Waves: None
     PRI: None
     QRS: 0.20 sec
     Interp: Ventricular escape rhythm
148. **Rate:** 68 beats/min
     Rhythm: Irregular
     P Waves: None; fine atrial fibrillation waves are present.
     PRI: None
     QRS: 0.10 sec
     Interp: Atrial fibrillation (fine)
149. **Rate:** 65 beats/min (atrial rate: 113 beats/min)
     Rhythm: Regular
     P Waves: Present, but have no set relation to the QRS complexes
     PRI: None
     QRS: Undeterminable
     Interp: Third-degree atrioventricular (AV) block
150. **Rate:** 88 beats/min
     Rhythm: Irregular
     P Waves: Present; precede each QRS complex. Third wave is negative.
     PRI: About 0.14 sec
     QRS: About 0.08 sec
     Interp: Normal sinus rhythm with an isolated premature junctional complex
151. **Rate:** 55 beats/min
     Rhythm: Regular
     P Waves: Present; abnormally wide, positive P waves precede each QRS complex.
     PRI: About 0.40 sec
     QRS: About 0.10 sec
     Interp: Sinus rhythm with first-degree atrioventricular (AV) block. Possible 2:1 AV block.
152. **Rate:** 148 beats/min
     Rhythm: Regular
     P Waves: Present; precede each QRS complex
     PRI: Undeterminable; P waves are buried in the preceding QRS complexes.
     QRS: 0.10 sec
     Interp: Sinus tachycardia
153. **Rate:** 118 beats/min
     Rhythm: Irregular
     P Waves: None; fine atrial fibrillation waves are present.
     PRI: None
     QRS: 0.08 sec
     Interp: Atrial fibrillation (fine)
154. **Rate:** 36 beats/min
     Rhythm: Undeterminable
     P Waves: None
     PRI: None
     QRS: About 0.16 sec
     Interp: Ventricular escape rhythm
155. **Rate:** 50 beats/min
     Rhythm: Regular
     P Waves: None; atrial flutter waves are present.
     PRI: None
     QRS: 0.16 sec
     Interp: Atrial flutter with bundle-branch block
156. **Rate:** 163 beats/min
     Rhythm: Regular
     P Waves: None
     PRI: None
     QRS: 0.16 sec
     Interp: Ventricular tachycardia
157. **Rate:** 63 beats/min
     Rhythm: Regular
     P Waves: Present; negative P waves follow each QRS complex.
     PRI: None
     QRS: About 0.08 sec
     Interp: Accelerated junctional rhythm
158. **Rate:** 103 beats/min
     Rhythm: Regular
     P Waves: Present: P waves precede each QRS complex. The P waves are abnormally tall (P pulmonale).
     PRI: 0.19 sec
     QRS: About 0.15 sec
     Interp: Sinus tachycardia with bundle-branch block
159. **Rate:** 312 beats/min
     Rhythm: Slightly irregular
     P Waves: None
     PRI: None
     QRS: 0.12–0.14 sec
     Interp: Ventricular tachycardia (multiform)

160. **Rate:** 101 beats/min
     Rhythm: Regular
     P Waves: None
     PRI: None
     QRS: 0.14 sec
     Interp: Junctional tachycardia with wide QRS complexes or ventricular tachycardia

161. **Rate:** 92 beats/min
     Rhythm: Irregular
     P Waves: Present; precede the first, second fourth, and fifth QRS complexes
     PRI: 0.14 sec
     QRS: 0.16 sec
     Interp: Normal sinus rhythm with bundle-branch block and an isolated premature ventricular complex (interpolated)

162. **Rate:** 70 beats/min
     Rhythm: Regular
     P Waves: Present; precede each QRS complex
     PRI: About 0.12 sec
     QRS: 0.12 sec
     Interp: Normal sinus rhythm

163. **Rate:** 72 beats/min
     Rhythm: Regular
     P Waves: None
     PRI: None
     QRS: 0.12–0.16 sec
     Interp: Accelerated idioventricular rhythm

164. **Rate:** Unmeasurable
     Rhythm: Irregular
     P Waves: None; fine ventricular waves are present.
     PRI: None
     QRS: None
     Interp: Ventricular fibrillation (fine)

165. **Rate:** 57 beats/min
     Rhythm: Regular
     P Waves: Present; precede each QRS complex
     PRI: 0.24 sec
     QRS: About 0.10 sec
     Interp: Sinus bradycardia with first-degree atrioventricular (AV) block

166. **Rate:** 43 beats/min
     Rhythm: Regular
     P Waves: Present; positive P waves precede each QRS complex.
     PRI: 0.10 sec
     QRS: About 0.10 sec
     Interp: Sinus bradycardia with atrio–His pre-excitation.

167. **Rate:** 57 beats/min
     Rhythm: Regular
     P Waves: None
     PRI: None
     QRS: About 0.16 sec
     Interp: Accelerated idioventricular rhythm

168. **Rate:** None
     Rhythm: None
     P Waves: None
     PRI: None
     QRS: None
     Interp: Asystole

169. **Rate:** 43 beats/min
     Rhythm: Regular
     P Waves: Present; negative P waves follow each QRS complex.
     PRI: None
     QRS: About 0.10 sec
     Interp: Junctional escape rhythm

170. **Rate:** Unmeasurable
     Rhythm: Irregular
     P Waves: None; coarse ventricular fibrillation waves are present.
     PRI: None
     QRS: None
     Interp: Ventricular fibrillation (coarse)

171. **Rate:** 25 beats/min
     Rhythm: Undeterminable
     P Waves: None
     PRI: None
     QRS: 0.16 sec
     Interp: Junctional escape rhythm with wide QRS complexes

172. **Rate:** 213 beats/min
     Rhythm: Regular
     P Waves: None
     PRI: None
     QRS: 0.12 sec
     Interp: Supraventricular tachycardia with wide QRS complexes or ventricular tachycardia

173. **Rate:** 70 beats/min
     Rhythm: Irregular
     P Waves: None; fine atrial fibrillation waves are present.
     PRI: None
     QRS: 0.10 sec
     Interp: Atrial fibrillation (fine)

174. **Rate:** 89 beats/min
     Rhythm: Regular
     P Waves: Present; precede each QRS complex
     PRI: About 0.18 sec
     QRS: 0.12 sec
     Interp: Normal sinus rhythm with bundle-branch block

175. **Rate:** 165 beats/min
     Rhythm: Regular
     P Waves: None
     PRI: None
     QRS: 0.10 sec
     Interp: Supraventricular tachycardia

176. **Rate:** 48 beats/min
     Rhythm: Regular

P Waves: Present; appear to precede each QRS complex
PRI: 0.08 sec
QRS: 0.08 sec
Interp: Sinus bradycardia with atrio–His pre-excitation

177. **Rate:** 79 beats/min
Rhythm: Irregular
P Waves: Present; positive P waves precede the first, second, fourth, and fifth QRS complexes. A negative P wave precedes the third QRS complex.
PRI: 0.12 sec (first, second, fourth, and fifth QRS complexes); 0.09 sec (third QRS complex)
QRS: 0.10 sec
Interp: Normal sinus rhythm with an isolated premature junctional complex

178. **Rate:** 33 beats/min (atrial rate: 39 beats/min)
Rhythm: Undeterminable
P Waves: Present; the first and fifth P waves are followed by QRS complexes. Atrioventricular (AV) conduction ratio is 4:1.
PRI: Variable
QRS: 0.14 sec
Interp: Third-degree heart block

179. **Rate:** 59 beats/min
Rhythm: Irregular
P Waves: Present; the first, third, and fourth P waves are followed by QRS complexes.
PRI: 0.20–0.28 sec
QRS: About 0.05 sec
Interp: Sinus rhythm with second-degree atrioventricular (AV) block (probably type I [Wenckebach])

180. **Rate:** 96 beats/min
Rhythm: Irregular. An incomplete compensatory pause follows the fourth QRS complex.
P Waves: Present; precede the second, third, fifth, and sixth QRS complexes
PRI: 0.18 sec
QRS: 0.10 sec
Interp: Normal sinus rhythm with an isolated premature junctional complex

181. **Rate:** 60 beats/min
Rhythm: Regular
P Waves: Present; precede each QRS complex
PRI: 0.15 sec
QRS: 0.07 sec
Interp: Normal sinus rhythm

182. **Rate:** Unmeasurable
Rhythm: Irregular
P Waves: None
PRI: None
QRS: None
Interp: Asystole

183. **Rate:** 98 beats/min
Rhythm: Regular

P Waves: Present; precede each QRS complex
PRI: About 0.20 sec
QRS: About 0.16 sec
Interp: Normal sinus rhythm with bundle-branch block

184. **Rate:** 64 beats/min
Rhythm: Regular
P Waves: None
PRI: None
QRS: About 0.16 sec
Interp: Accelerated idioventricular rhythm

185. **Rate:** 35 beats/min (atrial rate: 167 beats/min)
Rhythm: Undeterminable
P Waves: Present, but have no set relation to the QRS complexes
PRI: None
QRS: 0.12 sec
Interp: Third-degree atrioventricular (AV) block with wide QRS complexes

186. **Rate:** 79 beats/min
Rhythm: Regular
P Waves: Present; precede each QRS complex
PRI: 0.15 sec
QRS: 0.08 sec
Interp: Normal sinus rhythm

187. **Rate:** 87 beats/min
Rhythm: Irregular
P Waves: None; atrial flutter waves are present. The atrioventricular (AV) conduction ratios vary.
PRI: None
QRS: 0.12 sec
Interp: Atrial flutter

188. **Rate:** 181 beats/min
Rhythm: Regular
P Waves: None
PRI: None
QRS: About 0.22 sec
Interp: Supraventricular tachycardia with wide QRS complexes or ventricular tachycardia.

189. **Rate:** 103 beats/min
Rhythm: Regular
P Waves: None; atrial flutter waves are present
PRI: None
QRS: 0.06 sec
Interp: Atrial flutter

190. **Rate:** 161 beats/min
Rhythm: Regular
P Waves: Present; precede each QRS complex
PRI: 0.12 sec
QRS: 0.08 sec
Interp: Sinus tachycardia

191. **Rate:** 130 beats/min
Rhythm: Regular
P Waves: None
PRI: None

QRS: About 0.10 sec
Interp: Supraventricular tachycardia

192. **Rate:** Ventricular rate: none (atrial rate: 70 beats/min)
    Rhythm: Regular
    P Waves: Present
    PRI: None
    QRS: None
    Interp: Asystole (ventricular standstill)

193. **Rate:** 31 beats/min (atrial rate 106 beats/min)
    Rhythm: Undeterminable
    P Waves: Present, but have no set relation to the QRS complexes
    PRI: None
    QRS: About 0.16 sec
    Interp: Third-degree atrioventricular (AV) block with wide QRS complexes

194. **Rate:** 36 beats/min
    Rhythm: Undeterminable
    P Waves: None
    PRI: None
    QRS: 0.16 sec
    Interp: Ventricular escape rhythm

195. **Rate:** 59 beats/min
    Rhythm: Regular
    P Waves: Inverted prior to each QRS
    PRI: 0.05–0.06 sec
    QRS: About 0.12 sec
    Interp: Junctional escape rhythm

196. **Rate:** 71 beats/min
    Rhythm: Irregular. A complete compensatory pause follows the third QRS complex.
    P Waves: Present; precede each QRS complex
    PRI: 0.16 sec
    QRS: 0.08 sec
    Interp: Normal sinus rhythm with an isolated premature atrial complex

197. **Rate:** 122 beats/min
    Rhythm: Regular
    P Waves: None
    PRI: None
    QRS: 0.12 sec
    Interp: Junctional tachycardia

198. **Rate:** None
    Rhythm: None
    P Waves: None
    PRI: None
    QRS: 0.16 sec
    Interp: A single wide QRS complex, probably ventricular in origin, followed by asystole

199. **Rate:** 169 beats/min
    Rhythm: Irregular
    P Waves: None; atrial flutter waves are present. The atrioventricular (AV) conduction ratios vary.
    PRI: None
    QRS: 0.08 sec

    Interp: Atrial flutter with rapid ventricular response

200. **Rate:** 128 beats/min
    Rhythm: Regular
    P Waves: Present; precede each QRS complex. The P waves are abnormally tall (P pulmonale).
    PRI: 0.24 sec
    QRS: About 0.12 sec
    Interp: Sinus tachycardia with first-degree atrioventricular (AV) block and bundle-branch block

201. **Rate:** 63 beats/min
    Rhythm: Regular
    P Waves: None
    PRI: None
    QRS: About 0.16 sec
    Interp: Accelerated junctional rhythm with wide QRS complexes or accelerated idioventricular rhythm

202. **Rate:** 60 beats/min
    Rhythm: Regular
    P Waves: Present; precede each QRS complex
    PRI: 0.16 sec
    QRS: 0.07 sec
    Interp: Normal sinus rhythm

203. **Rate:** Unmeasurable
    Rhythm: None
    P Waves: None
    PRI: None
    QRS: None
    Interp: Asystole

204. **Rate:** 238 beats/min
    Rhythm: Regular
    P Waves: None
    PRI: None
    QRS: About 0.10 sec
    Interp: Supraventricular tachycardia

205. **Rate:** 165 beats/min
    Rhythm: Regular
    P Waves: None
    PRI: None
    QRS: About 0.24 sec
    Interp: Ventricular tachycardia

206. **Rate:** 72 beats/min
    Rhythm: Regular
    P Waves: None; atrial flutter waves are present.
    PRI: None
    QRS: 0.08 sec
    Interp: Atrial flutter

207. **Rate:** 33 beats/min
    Rhythm: Undeterminable
    P Waves: None
    PRI: None
    QRS: Unmeasurable; greater than 0.12 sec
    Interp: Ventricular escape rhythm

208. **Rate:** 126 beats/min
    Rhythm: Regular

P Waves: None
PRI: None
QRS: 0.11 sec
Interp: Sinus tachycardia with first-degree atrioventricular (AV) block

209. **Rate:** 81 beats/min
Rhythm: Irregular
P Waves: Present; precede each QRS complex. The shape and direction of the fourth P wave differs from the others.
PRI: 0.13 sec (first, second, third, and fifth PR intervals); 0.18 sec (fourth PR interval)
QRS: 0.10 sec (first, second, third, and fifth QRS complex)
Interp: Normal sinus rhythm with an isolated premature atrial complex

210. **Rate:** 31 beats/min (atrial rate: 83 beats/min)
Rhythm: Undeterminable
P Waves: Present, but have no set relation to the QRS complexes
PRI: None
QRS: About 0.14 sec
Interp: Third-degree atrioventricular (AV) block with wide QRS complexes

211. **Rate:** 180 beats/min
Rhythm: Regular
P Waves: Present; precede each QRS complex
PRI: 0.08 sec
QRS: 0.12 sec
Interp: Atrial tachycardia with atrio–His preexcitation and bundle-branch block

212. **Rate:** 45 beats/min (atrial rate 111 beats/min)
Rhythm: Regular
P Waves: Present, but have no set relation to the QRS complexes
PRI: None
QRS: 0.12 sec
Interp: Third-degree atrioventricular (AV) block

213. **Rate:** 52 beats/min
Rhythm: Regular
P Waves: Present; the first, third, and fifth P waves are followed by QRS complexes. The atrioventricular (AV) conduction ratio is 2:1.
PRI: 0.20 sec
QRS: 0.14 sec
Interp: Sinus rhythm with second-degree 2:1 AV block and bundle-branch block

214. **Rate:** 44 beats/min
Rhythm: Irregular
P Waves: None; atrial flutter waves are present. The atrioventricular (AV) conduction ratios vary.
PRI: None
QRS: About 0.14 sec
Interp: Atrial flutter with wide QRS complexes

215. **Rate:** 71 beats/min
Rhythm: Regular
P Waves: Present; precede each QRS complex
PRI: 0.26 sec
QRS: 0.10 sec
Interp: Sinus rhythm with first-degree atrioventricular (AV) block

216. **Rate:** 103 beats/min
Rhythm: Regular
P Waves: Present; precede each QRS complex
PRI: 0.12 sec
QRS: 0.14 sec
Interp: Sinus tachycardia with bundle-branch block

217. **Rate:** 104 beats/min
Rhythm: Regular
P Waves: None
PRI: None
QRS: 0.14 sec
Interp: Junctional tachycardia with wide QRS complexes

218. **Rate:** 109 beats/min
Rhythm: Irregular
P Waves: Present; precede the first, second, third, fourth, and fifth QRS complexes
PRI: 0.14 sec
QRS: 0.09 sec (first, second, third, fourth, and fifth QRS complexes); 0.11 sec (sixth QRS complex)
Interp: Normal sinus rhythm with premature ventricular complexes and a fusion beat (third QRS complex)

219. **Rate:** None
Rhythm: None
P Waves: None
PRI: None
QRS: None
Interp: Asystole

220. **Rate:** 81 beats/min
Rhythm: Regular
P Waves: None
PRI: None
QRS: 0.10 sec
Interp: Accelerated junctional rhythm with possible Osborn waves

221. **Rate:** 109 beats/min
Rhythm: Irregular
P Waves: Present; precede the first, second, fourth, and fifth QRS complexes
PRI: About 0.14 sec
QRS: 0.09 sec (first, second, fourth, and fifth QRS complexes); 0.11 sec (third and sixth QRS complexes)
Interp: Normal sinus rhythm with unifocal (uniform) premature ventricular complexes (trigeminy)

222. **Rate:** 37 beats/min
Rhythm: Undeterminable

P Waves: Present; the second and fifth P waves are followed by QRS complexes. The third and sixth P waves are buried in the preceding T waves. The atrioventricular (AV) conduction ratio is 3:1.
PRI: 0.16 sec
QRS: 0.14 sec
Interp: Sinus rhythm with second-degree advanced AV block and bundle-branch block

223. **Rate:** 128 beats/min
Rhythm: Irregular
P Waves: None; final atrial fibrillation waves are present
PRI: None
QRS: 0.12–0.16 sec
Interp: Atrial fibrillation (fine) with bundle-branch block

224. **Rate:** 108 beats/min
Rhythm: Regular
P Waves: None
PRI: None
QRS: 0.16 sec
Interp: Supraventricular tachycardia

II. BUNDLE-BRANCH AND FASCICULAR BLOCKS

225. Left bundle-branch block
226. Left posterior fascicular block
227. Right bundle-branch block
228. Right bundle-branch block with an intact interventricular septum
229. Left anterior fascicular block

III. MYOCARDIAL INFARCTIONS

230. Anterolateral myocardial infarction
231. Septal myocardial infarction
232. Extensive anterior myocardial infarction
233. Anterior myocardial infarction
234. Lateral myocardial infarction
235. Inferior myocardial infarction
236. Anteroseptal myocardial infarction
237. Posterior myocardial infarction
238. Right ventricular myocardial infarction

IV. QRS AXES

239. QRS axis: +150°
240. QRS axis: −30° to −90°
241. QRS axis: +90°
242. QRS axis: +90° to +150°
243. QRS axis: 0° to +30°
244. QRS axis: 0° to −30°

V. ECG CHANGES: DRUG AND ELECTROLYTE

245. Hypercalcemia
246. Procainamide/quinidine toxicity
247. Hyperkalemia
248. Digitalis effect
249. Hypocalcemia
250. Hypokalemia

VI. ECG CHANGES: MISCELLANEOUS

251. Left ventricular hypertrophy
252. Chronic obstructive pulmonary disease (COPD)
253. Right ventricular hypertrophy/cor pulmonale
254. Pericarditis
255. Acute pulmonary embolism
256. Early repolarization
257. Hypothermia
258. Ventricular preexcitation
259. Atrio–His preexcitation
260. Nodoventricular/fasciculoventricular preexcitation

VII. SCENARIOS

Scenario 1

261. (A) The rhythm is regular, with P waves preceding each QRS complex. All P waves are identical. The rate is between 60 and 100 and therefore is a **normal sinus rhythm.**
262. (B) The T waves in the precordial leads are **tall and peaked.** Although the ST segment appears to be slightly elevated in V₂ and V₃, the ST segment is "upsloping," which is not characteristic of ischemia. The QT interval is normal at 352 ms.
263. (B) Peaked T waves are caused by **hyperkalemia.** Coronary artery occlusion results in ST elevation. Hypocalcemia causes QT interval prolongation. Hypothermia is manifested by prolonged PR and QT intervals, QRS complexes, and the presence of Osborn waves.

Scenario 2

264. (C) Although it is true that atrial tachycardia and atrial flutter with 1:1 conduction are supraventricular tachycardias, this patient reports a sudden onset of the dysrhythmia, which places it in the special category of **paroxysmal supraventricular tachycardia (PSVT).** There are no P waves; therefore sinus tachycardia is unlikely.
265. (A) A wide QRS complex tachycardia may be either supraventricular tachycardia with aberrant conduction or

ventricular tachycardia. If the patient is stable, a **12-lead ECG** may be used to determine the axis of the QRS and assist in the differentiation. Performing vagal maneuvers will not assist in the differentiation. Administration of adenosine in ventricular tachycardia is contraindicated and can result in asystole. Amiodarone will treat either dysrhythmia but will not aid in differentiating the two.

266. (D) The electrophysiologic mechanism responsible for PSVT is a **reentry mechanism involving the atrioventricular (AV) node alone or the AV node in conjunction with an accessory conduction pathway.**

Scenario 3

267. (D) **Third-degree atrioventricular (AV) heart block** is characterized by total dissociation between the P waves and the QRS complexes. Examination of the rhythm strip—marking the P waves and attempting to correlate them with any QRS complex—makes it clear that no association exists. The wide QRS complex and rate are consistent with a ventricular escape rhythm or junctional escape rhythm with aberrant conduction.

268. (A) It is more probable that the **AV-node** pacemaker has assumed the escape rhythm with aberrant conduction because ventricular escape rhythms are more often slower than 40.

269. (D) Although the patient's blood pressure is slightly low, she is awake and conscious. Therefore she is tolerating the relative bradycardia well. Initial care would include **placing her in a supine position, administering oxygen, and obtaining vascular access.** It would be prudent to apply a transcutaneous pacemaker on the patient so as to be prepared in the event her rate slowed. If she continues to tolerate this rate, she can await a cardiology consultation for pacemaker placement. In the event she was to deteriorate, sedation and transcutaneous pacing would be appropriate.

Scenario 4

270. (A) The rhythm is totally irregular, there are no discernable P waves, and the baseline in the R-R interval appears to contain f waves and F waves. The QRS complex rate is 128, which is fast. This meets the criteria of **atrial fibrillation/flutter with rapid ventricular response.**

271. (D) The R-R intervals vary across the strip without a pattern. This is called *grossly or irregularly irregular.*

272. (B) The patient admits to taking cold medication containing decongestants. These agents contain antihistamine and other adrenergic-stimulating chemicals. This, combined with fatigue and mild dehydration, results in **increased adrenergic stimulation of the atria,** which can precipitate atrial fibrillation.

Scenario 5

273. (C) There are no P waves. The QRS complex is wide and bizarre at a rate of 40. This is consistent with a **ventricular escape rhythm,** which is common following defibrillation.

Pulseless electrical activity (PEA) is not a rhythm but is instead a condition.

274. (C) Because there is no pulse, cardiopulmonary resuscitation (CPR) must be continued. The goal now is to encourage the rate to increase and produce a sustainable pulse. This is accomplished by **administering 40 units of vasopressin,** which is a potent vasoconstrictor. Vasopressin will additionally stimulate the heart's pacemakers to fire. It is too early to consider termination of resuscitation. Only ventricular fibrillation (VF) and ventricular tachycardia (VT) are susceptible to defibrillation. The administration of too many agents this early in the resuscitation is not warranted, and until the heart's pacemaker is above the atrioventricular (AV) node, the administration of amiodarone or lidocaine could extinguish the ventricular escape rhythm, resulting in asystole.

275. (D) When the heart is defibrillated, the entire myocardium is **depolarized** simultaneously. This results in asystole and the **termination of VF/VT.** At this point, if quality CPR has been performed and the heart is perfused, the goal is for one of the pacemaker sites to "awaken" and begin an organized rhythm, which produces a pulse.

Scenario 6

276. (C) The most notable finding on this 12-lead ECG is the marked ST elevation in leads II, III, and aVF, which is consistent with an acute inferior wall myocardial infarction. However, looking at the lateral precordial leads V_5 and V_6 reveals ST-segment elevation as well. Examination of V_1 to V_3 reveals marked ST-segment depression. Together, this indicates a myocardial infarction involving the inferior, lateral, and posterior walls of the left ventricle.

277. (A) The majority of inferior wall myocardial infarctions are caused by occlusion of the right coronary artery because 80% to 90% of hearts are "right artery" dominant. However, the lateral and posterior walls of the left ventricle are perfused by the left circumflex artery. Therefore this heart is "left artery" dominant, and the **occlusion is in the distal left circumflex.**

278. (A) The primary goal for patients suffering acute myocardial infarction is to limit ischemic time. Therefore the goal is to rapidly assess the patient for **candidacy for either percutaneous coronary intervention (PCI) or fibrinolytic therapy.** Oxygen, aspirin, and nitrates are the only medications included in the initial therapy of all acute coronary syndromes. The decision to administer the other agents listed is case dependent.

Scenario 7

279. (B) The rhythm is patterned irregularity. There are more P waves than QRS complexes; therefore an atrioventricular block (AVB) is present. The PR interval is 0.20 second in complex 2 and 0.24 second in complex 3. There is no QRS following the next P wave. The progressive lengthening of the PR interval and "dropped" QRS complex are characteristic of second-degree **AVB type I (Wenckebach).**

280. (D) The conduction ratio is always the number of P waves to the number of QRS complexes. In this case there are three P waves to every two QRS complexes. Therefore the ratio is **3:2.**

281. (A) More than likely, this is the **patient's underlying cardiac rhythm**. The rate is normal and would not be expected to result in hemodynamic compromise. This is common dysrhythmia in the elderly and does not require treatment.

Scenario 8

282. (D) Although it is possible that a wide QRS complex tachycardia could be supraventricular tachycardia in the emergent situation, it **is prudent to assume the rhythm is ventricular tachycardia until proven otherwise.** The QRS complexes are uniform "monomorphic" and therefore do not meet the criteria for torsades de pointes. Ventricular fibrillation would not produce a pulse and would appear totally chaotic on the monitor.

283. (D) Despite the presence of a pulse, the dysrhythmia has resulted in shock and must be terminated immediately. This is accomplished by administering **synchronized cardioversion at 100 joules.** Defibrillation would be effective in terminating the dysrhythmia, but the higher energy and lack of synchronized delivery are more likely to result in producing ventricular fibrillation.

284. (D) The presence of inverted T waves in leads V_1 to V_6 is consistent with extensive myocardial ischemia. The ST segments in V_1 to V_3 are upsloping, which is characteristic of ischemia. These are common findings after defibrillation or could represent an underlying acute coronary syndrome, which precipitated the dysrhythmia.

Scenario 9

285. (A) The rhythm is regular. P and P′ waves are present. The PR interval varies as a result of the varying location of the P waves. The QRS complex is less than 0.12 second. The conduction ratio is 1:1. The rate is 70. This is characteristic of **junctional tachycardia.** A junctional escape rhythm would have a rate between 40 and 60. Multiatrial tachycardia would have a rate greater than 100. A wandering atrial pacemaker requires the identification of three or more ectopic P waves.

286. (B) Damage to the atrioventricular (AV) node, which occurs during an **inferior wall myocardial infarction,** is a common cause of this dysrhythmia. Although it can occur in rheumatic heart disease, the patient's history is consistent with acute coronary syndrome. Adrenergic agents and pericarditis are not associated with junctional tachycardia.

287. (A) Junctional tachycardia results from **disruption of normal conduction through the AV node.**

Scenario 10

288. (B) This is a dual-chamber pacemaker that senses and paces both the atria and ventricles and is inhibited by electrical activity from both sites. Therefore it is referred to as *D (dual-chamber sense), D (dual-chamber pace), I (inhibited).* The AAI pacemaker only senses and paces the atria. VDD pacemakers sense the ventricles, pace both atria and ventricles, and are demand pacemakers. VVI pacemakers only sense and pace the ventricle.

289. (C) There are pacer spikes without corresponding P′ and QRS complexes. This indicates that the pacemaker is firing but the electrical discharge is not, resulting in depolarization of the myocardium. **This condition is referred to as *failure to capture* because the pacemaker is not "capturing" the myocardium.**

290. (C) The patient has a history of congestive heart failure; therefore **a large-volume fluid resuscitation would be contraindicated.** Although the patient's blood pressure is low, the patient is conscious, and therefore cautious therapy would include supplemental oxygen, institution of transcutaneous pacing once the patient is sedated, and a cardiology consultation for evaluation of the malfunctioning pacemaker.

GLOSSARY

2:1 AV BLOCK An atrioventricular (AV) block with a 2:1 AV conduction ratio. Also referred to as an *advanced AV block*.

12-LEAD ELECTROCARDIOGRAM (ECG): The routine (or conventional) ECG consisting of three standard (bipolar) limb leads (leads I, II, and III), three augmented (unipolar) leads (leads aVR, aVL, and aVF), and six precordial (unipolar) leads (leads V_1, V_2, V_3, V_4, V_5, and V_6).

A

ABERRANCY See *Aberrant ventricular conduction (aberrancy).*

ABERRANT VENTRICULAR CONDUCTION (ABERRANCY) An electrical impulse originating in the sinoatrial (SA) node, atria, or atrioventricular (AV) junction that is temporarily conducted abnormally through the bundle branches, resulting in a bundle-branch block. This is usually caused by the appearance of the electrical impulse at the bundle branches prematurely, before the bundle branches have been sufficiently repolarized. Aberrancy may occur with atrial fibrillation; atrial flutter; premature atrial and junctional complexes; and sinus, atrial, and junctional tachycardias. Also referred to simply as *ventricular aberrancy.*

ABSOLUTE REFRACTORY PERIOD The period of ventricular depolarization and most of ventricular repolarization during which the ventricles cannot be stimulated to depolarize. It begins with the onset of the QRS complex and ends at about the peak of the T wave.

ACCELERATED IDIOVENTRICULAR RHYTHM (AIVR) A dysrhythmia originating in an ectopic pacemaker in the ventricles with a rate between 40 and 100 beats per minute. Also referred to as *accelerated ventricular rhythm, idioventricular tachycardia,* and *slow ventricular tachycardia.*

ACCELERATED JUNCTIONAL RHYTHM A dysrhythmia originating in an ectopic pacemaker in the atrioventricular (AV) junction, with a rate between 60 and 100 beats per minute.

ACCELERATED RHYTHM Three or more consecutive beats originating in an ectopic pacemaker with a rate faster than the inherent rate of the escape pacemaker but less than 100 beats per minute. Examples are accelerated junctional rhythm and accelerated idioventricular rhythm (AIVR).

ACCELERATED VENTRICULAR RHYTHM See *Accelerated idioventricular rhythm (AIVR).*

ACCESSORY ATRIOVENTRICULAR (AV) PATHWAYS (BUNDLES OF KENT) Abnormal accessory conduction pathways located between the atria and the ventricles that bypass the AV junction, resulting in the so-called Wolff–Parkinson–White (WPW) conduction. The result is an abnormally wide QRS complex with a delta wave and an abnormally short PR interval, the classic form of ventricular preexcitation. When this type of AV conduction is associated with a paroxysmal supraventricular tachycardia with normal QRS complexes, it is known as *WPW syndrome.* Three separate accessory AV pathways have been found:

type A WPW conduction pathway, type B WPW conduction pathway, and posteroseptal WPW conduction pathway.

ACCESSORY AV PATHWAY CONDUCTION See *Accessory atrioventricular (AV) pathways (bundles of Kent).*

ACCESSORY CONDUCTION PATHWAYS Several distinct abnormal electrical conduction pathways within the heart that bypass the atrioventricular (AV) node, the bundle of His, or both, thus allowing the electrical impulses to travel from the atria to the ventricles more rapidly than usual. They include the accessory AV pathways (the bundles of Kent), the atrio–His fibers, and the nodoventricular/fasciculoventricular fibers.

ACIDOSIS A disturbance in the acid–base balance of the body caused by excessive amounts of carbon dioxide (respiratory acidosis), lactic acid (metabolic acidosis), or both.

ACTION POTENTIAL See *Cardiac action potential.*

ACUTE CORONARY SYNDROMES Include silent ischemia, stable and unstable angina, acute myocardial infarction (MI), and sudden cardiac death.

ACUTE MYOCARDIAL INFARCTION (ACUTE MI, AMI) A condition that is present when necrosis of the myocardium occurs because of prolonged and complete interruption of blood flow to the area. The area of the myocardium involved identifies the acute myocardial infarction: anterior MI, septal MI, lateral MI, anterior (localized) MI, anterolateral MI, anteroseptal MI, extensive anterior MI, inferior (diaphragmatic) MI, inferolateral MI, posterior MI, or right ventricular MI.

ADENOSINE DIPHOSPHATE (ADP) A substance released from platelets when the platelets are activated after damage to the blood vessel walls. ADP promotes thrombus formation by stimulating platelet aggregation. Other substances released on platelet activation are serotonin and thromboxane A2.

ADP See *Adenosine diphosphate (ADP).*

ADRENERGIC Having the characteristics of the sympathetic nervous system; sympathomimetic.

ADVANCED AV BLOCK An atrioventricular (AV) block with a 3:1 or higher conduction ratio.

AFTERDEPOLARIZATION An abnormal condition of latent pacemaker and myocardial cells (nonpacemaker cells) in which spontaneous depolarization occurs because of a spontaneous and rhythmic increase in the level of the phase 4 membrane action potential after a normal depolarization. If afterdepolarization occurs early in phase 4, it is called *early afterdepolarization;* if late in phase 4, it is called *delayed afterdepolarization.* This abnormal condition is also referred to as *triggered activity.*

AGONAL Occurring at the moment of or just before death.

AGONAL RHYTHM Cardiac dysrhythmia present in a dying heart. Ventricular escape rhythm.

AMPLITUDE (VOLTAGE) With respect to ECGs, the height or depth of a wave or complex measured in millimeters (mm).

ANEURYSM Dilation of an artery (such as the aorta) or a chamber of the heart (such as the ventricle).

ANGINAL EQUIVALENTS Presence of associated symptoms in the absence of typical angina.

ANION An ion with a negative charge (for example, Cl^-, PO_4^{---}, SO_4^{--})

ANOXIA Absence or lack of oxygen.

ANTEGRADE (OR ANTEROGRADE) CONDUCTION Conduction of the electrical impulse in a forward direction, that is, from the sinoatrial (SA) node or atria to the ventricles or from the atrioventricular (AV) junction to the ventricles.

ANTERIOR LEADS Leads I, aVL, and V_1 to V_6.

ANTERIOR (LOCALIZED) MI A myocardial infarction (MI) commonly caused by occlusion of the diagonal arteries of the left anterior descending (LAD) coronary artery and characterized by early changes in the ST segments and T waves (that is, ST elevation and tall, peaked T waves) and the later appearance of abnormal Q waves in leads V_3 to V_4.

ANTERIOR MI A myocardial infarction (MI) caused by the occlusion of the left anterior descending (LAD) coronary artery or the left circumflex coronary artery or any of their branches, singly or in combination. Anterior MI includes septal, anterior (localized), anteroseptal, lateral, anterolateral, and extensive anterior myocardial infarctions and is characterized by early changes in the ST segments and T waves (that is, ST elevation and tall, peaked T waves) and the appearance early or later of abnormal Q waves in two or all of leads I, aVL, and V_1 to V_6, depending on the site of the infarction.

ANTEROLATERAL MI A myocardial infarction (MI) commonly caused by occlusion of the diagonal arteries of the left anterior descending (LAD) coronary artery alone or in conjunction with the anterolateral marginal artery of the left circumflex coronary artery and characterized by early changes in the ST segments and T waves (that is, ST elevation and tall, peaked T waves) and the appearance later of abnormal Q waves in leads I, aVL, and V_3 to V_6.

ANTEROSEPTAL MI A myocardial infarction (MI) commonly caused by occlusion of the left anterior descending (LAD) coronary artery involving both the septal perforator and diagonal arteries and characterized by early changes in the ST segments and T waves (that is, ST elevation and tall, peaked T waves) in leads V_1 to V_4 and the appearance early of abnormal Q waves in leads V_1 to V_2 and then later in leads V_3 to V_4.

AORTA The main trunk of the arterial system of the body, consisting of the ascending aorta, the aortic arch, and the descending aorta. The descending aorta is further divided into the thoracic and abdominal aorta.

AORTIC DISSECTION Splitting of the media layer of the aorta, leading to the formation of a dissecting aneurysm.

AORTIC VALVE The one-way valve located between the left ventricle and the ascending aorta.

APEX OF THE HEART The pointed lower end of the heart formed by the pointed lower ends of the right and left ventricles.

ARTIFACTS Abnormal waves and spikes in an ECG that result from sources other than the electrical activity of the heart and interfere with or distort the components of the ECG. Common causes of artifacts are muscle tremor, alternating current (AC) interference, loose electrodes, interference related to biotelemetry, and external chest compression. Artifacts are also referred to as *electrical interference* or *noise*.

ARTIFICIAL PACEMAKER An electronic device used to stimulate the heart to beat when the electrical conduction system of the heart malfunctions, causing bradycardia or ventricular asystole. An artificial pacemaker consists of an electronic pulse generator, a battery, and a wire lead that senses the electrical activity of the heart and delivers electrical impulses to the atria or ventricles or both when the pacemaker senses an absence of electrical activity.

ASYMPTOMATIC BRADYCARDIA A bradycardia with a systolic blood pressure greater than 90 to 100 mm Hg and stable, with the absence of congestive heart failure, chest pain, dyspnea, signs and symptoms of decreased cardiac output, and premature ventricular complexes. Treatment may not be indicated even if the heart rate falls below 50 beats per minute.

ASYSTOLE Absence of electrical activity in the heart, evidenced by a lack of QRS complexes.

ATHEROSCLEROTIC PLAQUE A lesion in the arterial wall that varies in size and composition from a well-demarcated, yellowish, raised area or swelling on the intimal surface of an artery, produced by subintimal fatty deposits (atheroma), to a large, protruding, dull, white, fibrous plaque filled with pools of gruel-like lipid and foam cells filled with lipid, surrounded by fibrous tissue, necrotic debris, various amounts of blood, and calcium, all covered by a fibrous cap.

ATRIAL AND VENTRICULAR DEMAND PACEMAKER An artificial pacemaker that paces either the atria or ventricles when there is no appropriate spontaneous underlying atrial or ventricular rhythm.

ATRIAL DEMAND PACEMAKER (AAI) An artificial pacemaker that senses spontaneously occurring P waves and paces the atria when they do not appear.

ATRIAL DEPOLARIZATION The electrical process of discharging the resting (polarized) myocardial cells producing the P, P′, F, and f waves and causing the atria to contract.

ATRIAL DIASTOLE The interval or period during which the atria are relaxed and filling with blood. The period between atrial complexes.

ATRIAL DILATATION Distention of the atria because of increased pressure and/or volume within the atria; it may be acute or chronic.

ATRIAL DYSRHYTHMIA Dysrhythmia originating in the atria, such as wandering atrial pacemaker (WAP), premature atrial complexes (PACs), atrial tachycardia (ectopic atrial tachycardia, multifocal atrial tachycardia), atrial flutter, and atrial fibrillation.

ATRIAL ENLARGEMENT Includes atrial dilatation and hypertrophy. Common causes include heart failure, ventricular hypertrophy from whatever cause, pulmonary diseases, pulmonary or systemic hypertension, heart valve stenosis or insufficiency, and acute myocardial infarction. See *Left atrial enlargement (left atrial dilatation and hypertrophy)* and *Right atrial enlargement (right atrial dilatation and hypertrophy)*.

ATRIAL FIB-FLUTTER Occurs when the rhythm may exhibit atrial fibrillation with an irregularly irregular rhythm.

ATRIAL FIBRILLATION A dysrhythmia arising in numerous ectopic pacemakers in the atria characterized by very rapid atrial fibrillation (f) waves and an irregular, often rapid, ventricular response. Atrial fibrillation is "fast" if the ventricular rate is greater than 100 per minute and "slow" if it is less than 60. When fast, atrial fibrillation is considered uncontrolled (untreated) atrial fibrillation; when slow, it is controlled (treated) atrial fibrillation.

ATRIAL FIBRILLATION (f) WAVES: Irregularly shaped, rounded (or pointed), and dissimilar atrial waves originating in multiple ectopic pacemakers in the atria at a rate between 350 and 600 (average 400) beats per minute. May be "fine" (less than 1 mm in height) or "coarse" (1 mm or greater in height).

ATRIAL FLUTTER A dysrhythmia arising in an ectopic pacemaker in the atria, characterized by abnormal atrial flutter waves with a sawtooth appearance and usually a regular ventricular response after every other or every fourth F wave. If the QRS complexes occur irregularly at varying ratios of F waves to QRS complexes, a variable atrioventricular (AV) block is present. Atrial flutter may be transient (paroxysmal) or chronic (persistent). When fast, atrial flutter is considered uncontrolled (untreated) atrial flutter; when slow, it is controlled (treated) atrial flutter.

ATRIAL FLUTTER-FIBRILLATION A dysrhythmia arising in the atria alternating between atrial flutter and atrial fibrillation.

ATRIAL FLUTTER (F) WAVES Regularly shaped, usually pointed, atrial waves with a sawtooth appearance originating in an ectopic pacemaker in the atria at a rate between 240 and 360 (average 300) beats per minute.

ATRIAL HYPERTROPHY Increase in the thickness of the atrial wall because of chronic increase in pressure and/or volume within the atria.

"ATRIAL KICK": Refers to the complete filling of the ventricles brought on by the contraction of the atria during the last part of ventricular diastole just before the ventricles contract.

ATRIAL OVERLOAD Refers to increased pressure and/or volume within the atria.

ATRIAL REPOLARIZATION The electrical process by which the depolarized atria return to their polarized, resting state. Atrial repolarization produces the atrial T (Ta) wave.

ATRIAL STANDSTILL Absence of electrical activity of the atria.

ATRIAL SYNCHRONOUS VENTRICULAR PACEMAKER (VDD) An artificial pacemaker that is synchronized with the patient's atrial rhythm and paces the ventricles when an AV block occurs.

ATRIAL SYSTOLE The interval or period during which the atria are contracting and emptying of blood.

ATRIAL TACHYCARDIA A dysrhythmia originating in an ectopic pacemaker in the atria with a rate between 160 and 240 beats per minute. It includes ectopic atrial tachycardia and multifocal atrial tachycardia (MAT). Atrial tachycardia may occur with or without an atrioventricular (AV) block, which may be constant or variable. It may occur with narrow QRS complexes or abnormally wide QRS complexes because of a preexisting bundle-branch block, aberrant ventricular conduction, or ventricular preexcitation. When abnormal QRS complexes occur with the tachycardia because of aberrant ventricular conduction, the tachycardia is called *atrial tachycardia with aberrant ventricular conduction (aberrancy)*.

ATRIAL TACHYCARDIA WITH ABERRANCY A dysrhythmia with abnormal QRS complexes only during tachycardia. See *Aberrant ventricular conduction (aberrancy)*.

ATRIAL TACHYCARDIA WITH BLOCK When the atrioventricular (AV) block occurs only during tachycardia.

ATRIAL T WAVE (Ta): Represents atrial repolarization; often buried in the following QRS complex.

ATRIO–HIS FIBERS (JAMES FIBERS) Abnormal accessory conduction pathways connecting the atria with the lower part of the atrioventricular (AV) node at its junction with the bundle of His. See *Atrio–His preexcitation*.

ATRIO–HIS PREEXCITATION Abnormal conduction of the electrical impulses from the atria to the bundle of His via the atrio–His fibers (James fibers), bypassing the atrioventricular (AV) node and resulting in PR intervals that are usually shortened to less than 0.12 second and normal QRS complexes.

ATRIOVENTRICULAR (AV) BLOCK See *AV block* and specific AV blocks.

ATRIOVENTRICULAR (AV) DISSOCIATION Occurs when the atria and ventricles beat independently.

ATRIOVENTRICULAR (AV) JUNCTION The part of the electrical conduction system that normally conducts the electrical impulse from the atria to the ventricles. It consists of the AV node and the bundle of His.

ATRIOVENTRICULAR (AV) NODE The part of the electrical conduction system located in the posterior floor of the right atrium near the interatrial septum, through which the electrical impulses are normally conducted from the atria to the bundle of His.

ATRIOVENTRICULAR NODAL REENTRY TACHYCARDIA (AVNRT) A dysrhythmia when the reentry mechanism involves only the atrioventricular (AV) node.

ATRIOVENTRICULAR VALVES Tricuspid and mitral valves.

ATRIUM The thin-walled chamber into which venous blood flows before reaching the ventricle. The two atria, the right and left atria, form the upper part of the heart, or the base, and are separated from the ventricles by the mitral and tricuspid valves.

AUGMENTED (UNIPOLAR) LEADS Leads aVR, aVL, and aVF; each is obtained using a positive electrode attached to one extremity and a negative electrode to a central terminal:

Lead aVR. The positive electrode attached to the right arm and the negative electrode attached to the central terminal.

Lead aVL. The positive electrode attached to the left arm and the negative electrode attached to the central terminal.

Lead aVF. The positive electrode attached to the left leg and the negative electrode attached to the central terminal.

AUTOMATICITY, PROPERTY OF The property of a cell to reach a threshold potential and generate electrical impulses spontaneously. Also referred to as the *property of self-excitation*.

AUTONOMIC NERVOUS SYSTEM Part of the nervous system that is involved in the constant control of involuntary bodily functions, including the control of cardiac output (by regulating the heart rate and stroke volume) and blood pressure (by regulating blood vessel activity). It includes the sympathetic (adrenergic) and parasympathetic (cholinergic or vagal) nervous systems, each producing opposite effects when stimulated.

AV Abbreviation for *atrioventricular*.

AV BLOCK: Delay or failure of conduction of electrical impulses through the atrioventricular (AV) junction.

AV BLOCK, FIRST-DEGREE A dysrhythmia in which there is a constant delay in the conduction of electrical impulses through the atrioventricular (AV) node. It is characterized by abnormally prolonged PR intervals (longer than 0.20 second).

AV BLOCK, SECOND-DEGREE, 2:1 AND ADVANCED A dysrhythmia caused by defective conduction of electrical impulses through the atrioventricular (AV) node or bundle branches or both. It is characterized by regularly or irregularly absent QRS complexes (commonly producing an AV conduction ratio of 2:1 or greater), with or without a bundle-branch block.

AV BLOCK, SECOND-DEGREE, TYPE I (WENCKEBACH) A dysrhythmia in which progressive prolongation of the conduction of electrical impulses through the atrioventricular (AV) node occurs until conduction is completely blocked. It is characterized by progressive lengthening of the PR interval until a QRS complex fails to appear after a P wave. This phenomenon is cyclical.

AV BLOCK, SECOND-DEGREE, TYPE II A dysrhythmia in which a complete block of conduction of the electrical impulses occurs in one bundle branch and an intermittent block in the other. It is characterized by regularly or irregularly absent QRS complexes (producing, commonly, an atrioventricular [AV] conduction ratio of 4:3 or 3:2) and a bundle-branch block.

AV BLOCKS WITH WIDE QRS COMPLEXES Second-degree atrioventricular (AV) block, type II and 2:1 and advanced AV block, and third-degree AV block with wide QRS complexes require a temporary transcutaneous pacemaker immediately, regardless of whether not the bradycardia is symptomatic.

AV BLOCK, THIRD-DEGREE (COMPLETE AV BLOCK) A dysrhythmia in which there is a complete block of the conduction of electrical impulses through the atrioventricular (AV) node, bundle of His, or bundle branches. It is characterized by independent beating of the atria and ventricles. Third-degree AV block may be transient and reversible or permanent (chronic).

AV CONDUCTION RATIO The ratio of P, P′, F, or f waves to QRS complexes. For example, an atrioventricular (AV) conduction ratio of 4:3 indicates that for every four P waves, three are followed by QRS complexes.

AV DISSOCIATION Occurs when the atria and ventricles beat independently. Occurs when QRS complexes occur totally unrelated to the P, P′, or F waves.

AV JUNCTION See *Atrioventricular (AV) junction.*

AV NODE See *Atrioventricular (AV) node.*

AV REENTRY TACHYCARDIA (AVRT) A dysrhythmia when both the atrioventricular (AV) node and an accessory conduction pathway are involved in the reentry mechanism.

AV SEQUENTIAL PACEMAKER (DVI) An artificial pacemaker that paces either the atria or ventricles or both sequentially when spontaneous ventricular activity is absent.

AXIS Used alone, usually refers to the QRS axis—the single large vector representing the mean (or average) of all the ventricular vectors. It is usually graphically displayed as an arrow. See *P axis, ST axis,* and *T axis.*

AXIS OF A LEAD (LEAD AXIS) A hypothetical line joining the poles of a lead. A lead axis has a direction and a polarity.

B

BACHMANN'S BUNDLE A branch of the internodal atrial conduction tracts that extends across the atria, conducting the electrical impulses from the sinoatrial (SA) node to the left atrium.

BASELINE The part of the ECG during which electrical activity of the heart is absent. Commonly the interval between the end of the T wave and the onset of the P wave (the TP segment) is considered the baseline and is used as the reference for the measurement of the amplitude of the ECG waves and complexes.

BASE OF THE HEART The upper part of the heart formed by the right and left atria.

BIDIRECTIONAL VENTRICULAR TACHYCARDIA Ventricular tachycardia characterized by two distinctly different forms of QRS complexes alternating with each other, indicating the presence of two ventricular ectopic pacemakers.

BIGEMINY A dysrhythmia in which every other beat is a premature complex. The premature beat may be atrial, junctional, or ventricular in origin (that is, atrial bigeminy, junctional bigeminy, or ventricular bigeminy).

BIPHASIC DEFLECTION A deflection with both a positive and a negative component (for example, a biphasic P wave, a biphasic T wave).

BIPOLAR LEAD A lead that has both a positive and negative electrode that measures the electrical potential between the electrodes.

BIPOLAR LIMB LEADS Leads I, II, and III.

BLOCK Delay or failure of conduction of an electrical impulse through the electrical conduction system because of tissue damage or increased parasympathetic (vagal) tone.

BLOCKED PAC A P′ wave not followed by a QRS complex.

BRADYCARDIA A dysrhythmia with rates of less than 60 beats per minute (for example, sinus bradycardia; sinus arrest and sinoatrial [SA] exit block; junctional escape rhythm; ventricular escape rhythm; second-degree type I AV block [Wenckebach]; second-degree type II AV block; second-degree, 2:1, and advanced atrioventricular [AV] block; and third-degree AV block).

BRUGADA SYNDROME Sudden cardiac arrest from ST-segment elevation in the right precordial leads, right bundle-branch block, susceptibility to ventricular tachydysrhythmias, and structurally normal hearts.

BUNDLE-BRANCH BLOCK (BBB) Defective conduction of electrical impulses through the right or left bundle branch from the bundle of His to the Purkinje network, causing a right or left bundle-branch block. It may be complete or incomplete (partial) or permanent (chronic) or intermittent (transient). It may be present with or without an intact interventricular septum.

BUNDLE BRANCHES The part of the electrical conduction system in the ventricles consisting of the right and left bundle branches that conducts the electrical impulses from the bundle of His to the Purkinje network of the myocardium.

BUNDLE OF HIS The part of the electrical conduction system located in the upper part of the interventricular septum that conducts the electrical impulses from the atrioventricular (AV) node to the right and left bundle branches. The bundle of His and the AV node form the AV junction.

BUNDLES OF KENT See *Accessory atrioventricular (AV) pathways (bundles of Kent).*

BURIED P WAVE Refers to a P wave partially or completely hidden in a preceding T wave. This occurs when a sinus, atrial, or junctional P wave occurs during the repolarization of a previous beat, as in a sinus, atrial, or junctional tachycardia or a premature atrial or junctional premature beat.

BURSTS (OR SALVOS) Refers to the occurrence of two or more consecutive premature atrial, junctional, or ventricular complexes.

C

CALIBRATION (OR STANDARDIZATION) Accomplished by inserting a standard 1-millivolt (mV) electrical signal to produce a 10-mm deflection (two large squares) on the ECG.

CAMEL'S HUMP Descriptive term referring to the distinctive narrow, positive wave—the Osborn wave—that occurs at the junction of the QRS complex and the ST segment in patients with hypothermia with a core body temperature of 95°F. Also referred to as the *J wave* or the *J deflection.*

CAPTURE Refers to the ability of a pacemaker's electrical impulse to depolarize the atria or ventricles or both.

CAPTURE BEAT A normally conducted QRS complex of the underlying rhythm occurring within a ventricular tachycardia.

CARDIAC ACTION POTENTIAL Refers to the membrane potential of a myocardial cell and the changes it undergoes during depolarization and repolarization. The phases of the cardiac action potential include the following:

Phase 0—depolarization phase

Phase 1—early rapid repolarization phase

Phase 2—plateau phase of slow repolarization

Phase 3—terminal phase of rapid repolarization

Phase 4—period between action potentials

CARDIAC ARREST The sudden and unexpected cessation of an adequate circulation to maintain life in a patient who was not expected to die.

CARDIAC CELLS Cells of the heart, consisting of the myocardial (or "working") cells and the specialized cells of the electrical conduction system of the heart.

CARDIAC CYCLE The interval from the beginning of one heartbeat to the beginning of the next one. The cardiac cycle normally consists of a P wave, a QRS complex, and a T wave. It represents a sequence of atrial contraction and relaxation and ventricular contraction and relaxation, in that order.

CARDIAC OUTPUT The amount of blood circulated by the heart in 1 minute, in liters per minute. Obtained by multiplying the amount of blood expelled by the left ventricle with each contraction (stroke volume) by the heart rate per minute.

CARDIAC PACEMAKER An artificial pacemaker. See *Artificial pacemaker.*

CARDIAC STANDSTILL Absence of atrial and ventricular complexes. This term is used interchangeably with *ventricular asystole.*

CARDIAC TAMPONADE: Acute compression of the heart because of effusion of fluid into the pericardial cavity (as occurs in pericarditis) or accumulation of blood in the pericardium from rupture of the heart or penetrating trauma.

CARDIAC VECTOR A graphic presentation, using an arrow, representing the moment-to-moment electric current generated by depolarization or repolarization of a small segment of the atrial or ventricular wall.

CARDIOACCELERATOR CENTER One of the nerve centers of the sympathetic nervous system located in the medulla oblongata, a part of the brainstem. Impulses from the cardioaccelerator center reach the electrical conduction system of the heart and the atria and ventricles by way of the sympathetic nerves.

CARDIOGENIC Originating in the heart.

CARDIOGENIC SHOCK A life-threatening complication of acute myocardial infarction caused by the inability of the damaged ventricles to maintain adequate systemic circulation. One of the consequences of pump failure.

CARDIOINHIBITOR CENTER One of the nerve centers of the parasympathetic nervous system located in the medulla oblongata, a part of the brainstem. Impulses from the cardioinhibitor center, by way of the right and left vagus nerves, innervate the atria, sinoatrial (SA) node, and atrioventricular (AV) junction and, to a small extent, the ventricles.

CARDIOMYOPATHY A primary disease of the myocardium affecting the bundle branches, causing bundle-branch and fascicular blocks, often of unknown etiology.

CARDIOVERSION Application of a synchronized countershock to convert certain dysrhythmias—atrial flutter, atrial fibrillation, paroxysmal supraventricular tachycardia (PSVT), wide-QRS-complex tachycardia of unknown origin with pulse, and ventricular tachycardia with pulse—to an organized supraventricular rhythm.

CAROTID ARTERY DISEASE Primarily atherosclerotic in nature, with progressive formation of lumen-narrowing (stenotic) atheromatous plaques. A carotid occlusive disease.

CAROTID BRUIT An abnormal sound or murmur heard by auscultation over a stenotic (narrowed) carotid artery, usually a sign of an atheromatous plaque.

CAROTID SINUS A slightly dilated section of the common carotid artery at the point where it bifurcates, containing sensory nerve endings involved in the nervous reflexes regulating blood pressure and heart rate.

CAROTID SINUS MASSAGE Application of pressure to one of the carotid sinuses with the fingertips to convert paroxysmal supraventricular tachycardia (PSVT) and narrow-QRS-complex tachycardia of unknown origin (with pulse).

CATECHOLAMINES Hormonelike substances, such as epinephrine and norepinephrine, that have a strong sympathetic action on the heart and peripheral blood vessels, increasing the cardiac output and blood pressure.

CATION An ion with a positive charge (for example, K^+, Na^+).

cc: Abbreviation for cubic centimeter. It is often substituted for mL (milliliter).

CELL MEMBRANE POTENTIAL The difference in electrical potential across the cell membrane (that is, the difference between the electrical potential within the cell and a reference potential in the extracellular fluid surrounding the cell).

CENTRAL TERMINAL The central terminal, in the case of the augmented ECG leads, consists of connecting together two of the three electrodes used (the right and left arm electrodes and the left leg electrode) other than the positive electrode. In the case of the precordial leads, the central terminal consists of connecting all three extremity electrodes—the right and left arm electrodes and the left leg electrode. The central terminal is considered to be an indifferent, zero reference point.

CEREBROVASCULAR ACCIDENT (CVA) Cerebral ischemia caused by a decrease in blood flow resulting from obstruction of a blood vessel by an embolus or a thrombus or from cerebrovascular hemorrhage. Cerebral stroke.

CEREBROVASCULAR DISEASE General term for a brain dysfunction caused by an inadequacy of the cerebral blood supply.

CHAMBERS OF THE HEART Consists of the two thin-walled atria (the right and left atrium) and the two thick-walled ventricles (the right and left ventricle).

CHEST DISCOMFORT Described as a crushing, viselike constriction, a feeling equivalent to an "elephant sitting on the chest," or heartburn.

CHIEF COMPLAINT Short statement of the patient's major symptoms requiring emergency medical care.

CHRONIC OBSTRUCTIVE PULMONARY DISEASE (COPD) A chronic disease of the lungs characterized by a chronic productive cough and dyspnea. The typical ECG pattern is poor R-wave progression in the precordial leads V_1 to V_5 or V_1 to V_6.

CIRCULATORY SYSTEM The blood vessels in the body, including the systemic and pulmonary circulatory systems.

COAGULATION CLOTTING The process of changing from a liquid to a solid (that is, changing from liquid blood to a solid blood clot or thrombus).

COARSE ATRIAL FIBRILLATION Atrial fibrillation with large fibrillatory waves—1 mm or greater in height.

COARSE FIBRILLATORY WAVES When the f waves are greater than 1 mm high.

COARSE VENTRICULAR FIBRILLATION Ventricular fibrillation with large fibrillatory waves—greater than 3 mm in height.

COLLAGEN FIBERS The white protein fibers present in the connective tissue within the intima of the arterial wall that, when exposed to blood after an injury, immediately bind to the platelets directly (via glycoprotein [GP] Ia receptors) and indirectly through von Willebrand factor (vWF; via GP Ib and GP IIb/IIIa receptors). This action adheres the platelets to the arterial wall and activates them.

COMPENSATORY PAUSE The R-R interval after a premature complex. It may be full or incomplete, depending on whether the sinoatrial (SA) node, for example, is depolarized by the premature complex. If the SA node is not depolarized by the premature complex, the compensatory pause is called "full"; the sum of a "full" compensatory pause and the preceding R-R interval is equal to the sum of two R-R intervals of the underlying rhythm. If the SA node is depolarized by the premature complex, resetting the timing of the SA node, the compensatory pause is called *incomplete;* the sum of an incomplete compensatory pause and the preceding R-R interval is less than the sum of two R-R intervals of the underlying rhythm.

COMPLETE ATRIOVENTRICULAR (AV) BLOCK See *AV block, third-degree (complete AV block).*

COMPLETE BUNDLE-BRANCH BLOCK (RIGHT, LEFT) Complete disruption of the conduction of electrical impulses through the right or left bundle branch. The duration of the QRS complex is 0.12 second or greater.

COMPONENTS OF THE ELECTROCARDIOGRAM Includes the P wave, PR interval, PR segment, QRS complex, ST segment, T wave, U wave, QT interval, TP segment, and R-R interval.

CONDUCTED PAC A positive P′ wave (in lead II) followed by a QRS complex.

CONDUCTED PJC A negative P′ wave (in lead II) followed by a QRS complex.

CONDUCTIVITY, PROPERTY OF The property of cardiac cells to conduct electrical impulses.

CONGESTIVE HEART FAILURE (CHF) Excessive blood or tissue fluid in the lungs or body or both caused by the inefficient pumping of the ventricles. One of the consequences of pump failure. May be of recent origin (acute) or of prolonged duration (chronic).

CONTRACTILE FILAMENT See *Myofibril.*

CONTRACTILITY, PROPERTY OF The property of cardiac cells to contract when they are depolarized by an electrical impulse.

CONTROLLED ATRIAL FIBRILLATION When fewer than 100 QRS complexes per minute are conducted.

CONTROLLED ATRIAL FLUTTER A "treated" atrial flutter with a slow ventricular rate of about 60 to 75 beats per minute.

COPD See *Chronic obstructive pulmonary disease (COPD).*

CORONARY ARTERY CIRCULATION The coronary artery circulation consists of the left coronary artery (LCA) and the right coronary artery (RCA). The left coronary artery has a short main stem—the left main coronary artery—that branches into the left anterior descending (LAD) coronary artery and the left circumflex coronary artery. The arteries that commonly arise from the LAD coronary artery, the left circumflex coronary artery, and the right coronary artery are as follows:

Left anterior descending coronary artery	Right coronary artery
Diagonal arteries	Conus artery
Septal perforator arteries	Sinoatrial node artery
Right ventricular arteries	Anterior right ventricular artery
Left circumflex coronary artery	Right atrial artery
Left atrial circumflex arteries	Acute marginal artery
Anterolateral marginal artery	Posterior descending coronary artery
Posterolateral marginal arteries	AV node artery
Distal left circumflex artery	Posterior left ventricular arteries

CORONARY ARTERY DISEASE Progressive narrowing and eventual obstruction of the coronary arteries by atherosclerosis.

CORONARY CIRCULATION Passage of blood through the coronary arteries and their branches and the capillaries in the heart and then back to the right atrium via the coronary venules and veins and the coronary sinus.

CORONARY OCCLUSION (OR OBSTRUCTION) Obstruction of a coronary artery, usually by a blood clot (coronary thrombus); the major cause of acute myocardial infarction.

CORONARY SINUS The outlet in the right atrium draining the coronary venous system.

CORONARY THROMBOSIS The formation of a blood clot (thrombus) within a coronary artery, resulting in coronary artery obstruction; the major cause of acute myocardial infarction.

CORONARY VASOSPASM Coronary artery spasm. One of the causes of coronary artery obstruction.

COR PULMONALE Right heart disease with right ventricular hypertrophy and right atrial dilatation caused by pulmonary hypertension secondary to chronic lung disease.

CORRECTED QT INTERVAL (QTc): The average duration of the QT interval normally expected at a given heart rate.

COUNTERSHOCK See *Synchronized countershock.*

COUPLED BEATS Atrial or ventricular ectopic beats occurring in groups of two. Also called *paired beats* or *couplet.*

COUPLET Two consecutive premature complexes. Also referred to as *coupled beats* or *paired beats.*

COUPLING Ventricular bigeminy with the premature ventricular complexes following the QRS complexes of the underlying rhythm at equal coupling intervals.

COUPLING INTERVAL The R-R interval between a premature complex and the preceding QRS complex of the underlying rhythm.

C-REACTIVE PROTEIN A plasma protein that becomes abnormally elevated in many acute inflammatory conditions and in tissue necrosis, as occurs in acute myocardial infarction (MI). It becomes elevated in about 24 hours after acute MI.

CURRENT OF INJURY The theoretical cause of ST-segment elevation in acute myocardial infarction; an electrical manifestation of the inability of cardiac cells "injured" by severe ischemia to maintain a normal resting membrane potential during diastole.

CVA See *Cerebrovascular accident (CVA).*

CYANOSIS Slightly bluish, grayish, slatelike, or purplish discoloration of the skin caused by the presence of unoxygenated blood.

D

DEFIBRILLATION SHOCK An unsynchronized direct-current (DC) shock used to terminate pulseless ventricular tachycardia and ventricular fibrillation.

DEFLECTION Refers to the waves in the ECG. A deflection may be positive (upright), negative (inverted), biphasic (both positive and negative), or equiphasic (equally positive and negative). When a series of waves, such as a QRS complex, is composed of positive and negative deflections, it may be (1) predominantly positive (the sum total of the positive and negative deflections is positive, no matter by how much), (2) predominantly negative (the sum total of the positive and negative deflections is negative, no matter by how much), or (3) equiphasic (the positive deflections are equal to the negative deflections).

DELAYED AFTERDEPOLARIZATION See *Afterdepolarization.*

DELTA WAVE The slurring of the onset of the QRS complex—the fusion of the depolarization wave of a prematurely activated ventricle, the result of premature ventricular excitation, and the depolarization wave of the other, normally activated ventricle. Present in ventricular preexcitation and nodoventricular/fasciculoventricular preexcitation.

DEMAND PACEMAKERS Artificial pacemakers that have a sensing device that senses the heart's electrical activity and fires at a preset rate when the heart's electrical activity drops below a predetermined rate level.

DEMAND PACING Refers to a mode of pacing by an artificial pacemaker in which the pacemaker is turned on when an appropriate underlying spontaneous atrial or ventricular rhythm fails to occur.

DEPOLARIZATION The electrical process by which the resting potential of a polarized, resting cell of the atria, ventricles, or electrical conduction system is reduced to a less negative value.

DEPOLARIZATION WAVES The parts of the ECG representing the depolarization of the atria and ventricles—the P wave (atrial depolarization) and the QRS complex (ventricular depolarization).

DEPOLARIZED STATE The condition of the cell when it has been completely depolarized.

DIABETIC HEMORRHAGIC RETINOPATHY A disorder of the retinal blood vessels characterized by degeneration of the blood vessels and hemorrhage within the eye, the result of long-standing, poorly controlled diabetes.

DIAGONAL CORONARY ARTERY Arises from the left main coronary artery instead of from the left anterior descending coronary artery.

DIASTOLE (ELECTRICAL) Phase 4 of the action potential.

DIASTOLE (MECHANICAL) The period of atrial or ventricular relaxation.

DIAZEPAM An antianxiety agent used to produce amnesia in conscious patients before cardioversion of certain dysrhythmias. A drug that relieves apprehension and anxiety. Trade name: Valium.

DIGITALIS A cardiac glycoside obtained from the leaves of *Digitalis lanata,* used to decrease rapid ventricular rate in atrial flutter, atrial fibrillation, and paroxysmal supraventricular tachycardia (PSVT) and to improve ventricular contraction in congestive heart failure.

DIGITALIS EFFECT The changes in the ECG caused by the administration of digitalis. They include prolongation of the PR interval over 0.2 second; depression of the ST segment by 1 mm or more in many of the leads, with a characteristic "scooped-out" appearance; alteration of the T waves so that they appear flattened, inverted, or biphasic; and shortening of the QT interval to less than normal for the heart rate.

DIGITALIS OVERDOSE Excessive administration of digitalis, often accompanied by signs and symptoms of digitalis toxicity, which includes the appearance of dysrhythmias, such as sinus dysrhythmia and bradycardia; premature atrial, junctional, and ventricular complexes; atrial, junctional, and ventricular tachycardias; accelerated idioventricular rhythm (AIVR); ventricular fibrillation; and atrioventricular (AV) blocks. In fact, almost any dysrhythmia may be caused by excess digitalis.

DIGITALIS TOXICITY Digitalis overdose.

DIGITALIZATION The process of administering an adequate amount of digitalis over a period of time in the treatment of certain dysrhythmias. See *Digoxin.*

DILATATION AND HYPERTROPHY Refers to the two kinds of enlargement of the atria and ventricles. Distention of an individual heart chamber; it may be acute or chronic.

DIRECT-CURRENT (DC) SHOCK Used as defibrillation shock, synchronized countershock, and unsynchronized shock to terminate various dysrhythmias. See *Defibrillation shock, Synchronized countershock,* and *Unsynchronized shock.*

DIRECTIONAL CORONARY ATHERECTOMY (DCA) The mechanical removal of a noncalcified thrombus through a catheter inserted in the occluded or narrowed coronary artery.

DIURETIC A drug used in congestive heart failure to decrease excess body fluid by increasing the secretion of urine by the kidney.

DIVING REFLEX The technique of immersing the patient's face in ice water to elicit the parasympathetic reflex in an attempt to terminate paroxysmal supraventricular tachycardia (PSVT) and narrow-QRS-complex tachycardia of unknown origin (with pulse). It should only be tried if other vagal maneuvers are not effective and ischemic heart disease is not present or suspected.

DOMINANT CORONARY ARTERY (RIGHT, LEFT) Refers to the coronary artery, right or left, that gives rise to both the posterior left ventricular arteries and the posterior descending coronary artery.

DOMINANT (OR PRIMARY) PACEMAKER OF THE HEART The sinoatrial (SA) node.

DOPAMINE HYDROCHLORIDE A sympathomimetic that increases blood pressure; used in the treatment of hypotension and shock.

DOWNSLOPING ST-SEGMENT DEPRESSION A type of ST-segment depression that is most specific for myocardial ischemia, including that present in acute subendocardial non–Q-wave myocardial infarction (MI).

DROPPED BEATS Nonconducted P waves in atrioventricular (AV) blocks.

DROPPED P WAVES Absent P waves in sinus arrest and sinoatrial (SA) exit block.

DUAL-CHAMBER PACEMAKER An artificial pacemaker that paces the atria, ventricles, or both when appropriate.

DYING HEART A heart with feeble, ineffectual ventricular contractions and an ECG showing markedly abnormal QRS complexes, usually a ventricular escape rhythm.

DYSRHYTHMIA A rhythm other than a normal sinus rhythm when (1) the heart rate is less than 60 or greater than 100 beats per minute, (2) the rhythm is irregular, (3) premature complexes occur, or (4) the normal progression of the electrical impulse through the electrical conduction system is blocked. A term more correct than *arrhythmia* but used less frequently.

E

EARLY AFTERDEPOLARIZATION See *Afterdepolarization.*

EARLY REPOLARIZATION A normal variant of myocardial repolarization in which the ST segment is elevated or depressed 1 to 3 mm above or below the baseline, respectively. Most commonly elevated in leads I, II, and aVF and the precordial leads V_2 to V_6.

ECG Abbreviation for *electrocardiogram.*

ECG ARTIFACTS: See *Artifacts.*

ECG CALIPERS A device used to measure distances and intervals on an ECG tracing as an aid in determining the heart rate and rhythm.

ECG GRID The grid on the ECG paper is formed by dark and light horizontal and vertical lines. It is used to measure the time in seconds (sec) and distance in millimeters (mm) along the horizontal lines and voltage (amplitude) in millimeters (mm) along the vertical lines. The dark vertical lines are 0.20 second (5 mm) apart; the light vertical lines 0.04 second (1 mm) apart. The dark horizontal lines are 5 mm apart; the light horizontal lines are 1 mm apart.

ECG LEAD An ECG lead measures the difference in electrical potential generated by the heart, obtained by using a positive and a negative electrode—the positive electrode attached to an extremity or the anterior chest wall and the negative electrode to an extremity or a central terminal. Includes leads I, II, III, aVR, aVL, aVF, and V_1 to V_6.

ECG LEAD V_4 R: A precordial lead obtained by placing the positive electrode in the right midclavicular line in the right fifth intercostal space. Used primarily to rule out a right ventricular myocardial infarction after the initial finding of an inferior myocardial infarction.

ECG MONITOR The screen of an oscilloscope used in viewing the ECG.

ECTOPIC ATRIAL TACHYCARDIA An atrial tachycardia that originates in a single atrial ectopic pacemaker site, characterized by P′ waves that are usually identical.

ECTOPIC BEATS Premature beats originating in ectopic pacemakers in the atria, atrioventricular (AV) junction, and ventricles (for example, premature atrial complexes [PACs], premature junctional complexes [PJCs], and premature ventricular complexes [PVCs]).

ECTOPIC FOCUS A pacemaker other than the sinoatrial (SA) node.

ECTOPIC PACEMAKERS Abnormal pacemakers in the atria, atrioventricular (AV) junction, bundle branches, Purkinje network, and ventricular myocardium.

ECTOPIC P WAVE (P′ WAVE) A P wave produced by the depolarization of the atria in an abnormal direction, initiated by an electrical impulse arising in an ectopic pacemaker in the atria, atrioventricular (AV) junction, or ventricles. The ectopic P wave may be either positive (upright) or negative (inverted) in lead II and may precede or follow the QRS complex.

ECTOPIC RHYTHMS Dysrhythmias originating in ectopic pacemakers in the atria, atrioventricular (AV) junction, and ventricles, as follows:

Atrial. Wandering atrial pacemaker (WAP), premature atrial complexes (PACs), atrial tachycardia (ectopic atrial tachycardia, multifocal atrial tachycardia), atrial flutter, atrial fibrillation

Junctional. Premature junctional complexes (PJCs), nonparoxysmal junctional tachycardia (accelerated junctional rhythm, junctional tachycardia), paroxysmal supraventricular tachycardia (PSVT)

Ventricular. Accelerated idioventricular rhythm (AIVR), premature ventricular complexes (PVCs), ventricular tachycardia (VT), ventricular fibrillation (VF)

ECTOPIC TACHYCARDIAS Abnormal rhythms originating in ectopic pacemakers with a rate of over 100 beats per minute, such as atrial tachycardia (ectopic atrial tachycardia, multifocal atrial tachycardia), atrial flutter, atrial fibrillation, junctional tachycardia, paroxysmal supraventricular tachycardia (PSVT), and ventricular tachycardia (VT).

ECTOPIC VENTRICULAR DYSRHYTHMIAS Abnormal rhythms originating in ectopic pacemakers in the ventricles, such as accelerated idioventricular rhythm (AIVR), premature ventricular complexes (PVCs), ventricular tachycardia, and ventricular fibrillation.

ECTOPY A condition signifying the presence of ectopic beats and rhythms (for example, ventricular ectopy).

EDEMA A condition in which the body tissues have accumulated excessive tissue fluid or exudate (as in congestive heart failure).

EINTHOVEN'S EQUILATERAL TRIANGLE An equilateral triangle depicted in the frontal plane using the lead axes of the three limb leads as the sides with the heart and its zero reference point in the center.

EINTHOVEN'S LAW The sum of the electrical currents recorded in leads I and III equals the sum of the electrical currents recorded in lead II.

ELECTRICAL ACTIVITY OF THE HEART The electric current generated by the depolarization and repolarization of the atria and ventricles, which can be graphically displayed on the ECG.

ELECTRICAL ALTERNANS Periodic alternation in the size of the QRS complexes between normal and small, coincident with respiration; typically present in cardiac tamponade.

ELECTRICAL AXIS AND VECTOR A graphic presentation, using an arrow, of the electric current generated by the depolarization and repolarization of the atria and ventricles.

ELECTRICAL CONDUCTION SYSTEM OF THE HEART Includes the sinoatrial (SA) node, internodal atrial conduction tracts, interatrial conduction tract (Bachmann's bundle), atrioventricular (AV) node, bundle of His, right and left bundle branches, and Purkinje network.

ELECTRICAL CONDUCTION SYSTEM OF THE VENTRICLES The His–Purkinje system, which includes the bundle of His, the right and left bundle branches, and the Purkinje network.

ELECTRICAL IMPULSE The tiny electric current that normally originates in the sinoatrial (SA) node automatically and is conducted through the electrical conduction system to the atria and ventricles, causing them to depolarize and contract.

ELECTRICAL NONUNIFORMITY A condition of the ventricles during the vulnerable period of ventricular repolarization (that is, the relative refractory period of the ventricles coincident with the peak of the T wave) when the ventricular muscle fibers may be completely repolarized, partially repolarized, or completely refractory. Stimulation of the ventricles at this point by an intrinsic electrical impulse, such as that generated by a premature ventricular complex (PVC) or by an extrinsic impulse from a cardiac pacemaker or an electrical countershock, may result in nonuniform conduction of the electrical impulse through the muscle fibers, setting up a reentry mechanism that may precipitate repetitive ventricular complexes and result in ventricular tachycardia or fibrillation. Responsible for the "R-on-T phenomenon."

ELECTRICAL POTENTIAL Refers to the amount of electric current generated by the depolarization and repolarization of the heart and expressed as millivolts (mV). It ranges between 0 and 620 mV or more.

ELECTRIC CURRENT The flow of electricity along a conductor in a closed circuit.

ELECTROCARDIOGRAM (ECG): The graphic display of the electrical activity of the heart generated by the depolarization and repolarization of the atria and ventricles. The ECG includes the QRS complex; the P, T, and U waves; the PR, ST, and TP segments; and the PR, QT, and R-R intervals.

ELECTRODE A sensing device that detects electrical activity, such as that of the heart. May be positive or negative.

ELECTROLYTE A substance that, when in solution, dissociates into cations and anions, thus becoming capable of conducting electricity.

ELECTROLYTE IMBALANCE Abnormal concentrations of serum electrolytes within the body caused by excessive intake or loss of such electrolytes as calcium, chloride, potassium, and sodium.

ELECTROMECHANICAL DISSOCIATION (EMD) A term no longer used that referred to a condition in which the electrical activity of the heart is present and can be recorded on the ECG, but effective ventricular contractions, blood pressure, and pulse are absent. See *Pulseless electrical activity.*

EMBOLISM Obstruction of a blood vessel by an embolus that reduces or stops blood flow, resulting in ischemia or necrosis of the tissue supplied by the blood vessel.

EMBOLUS A mass of solid, liquid, or gaseous material carried from one part of the circulatory system to another.

ENDOCARDIUM The thin membrane lining the inside of the heart.

ENHANCED AUTOMATICITY An abnormal condition of latent pacemaker cells in which their firing rate is increased beyond their inherent rate because of a spontaneous increase in the slope of phase 4 depolarization. See *Slope of phase 4 depolarization.*

EPICARDIAL SURFACE The outside surface of the heart.

EPICARDIUM The thin connective tissue lining the outside of the heart.

EPINEPHRINE (ADRENALIN) A hormone produced by the adrenal gland and other tissues of the body. It is an alpha- and beta-stimulator causing an increase in blood pressure by means of peripheral artery vasoconstriction and an increase in cardiac output by increasing the heart rate and force of ventricular contraction. Used in the treatment of bronchial asthma, acute allergic disorders, bradycardia from whatever cause, ventricular fibrillation/pulseless ventricular tachycardia, ventricular asystole, and pulseless electrical activity.

EQUIPHASIC DEFLECTION A biphasic deflection in which the sum of the positive (upright) deflection or deflections in an ECG is equal to that of the negative (inverted) deflection or deflections.

EROSION Occurs when the endothelial cover of the plaque is torn away, exposing the plaque itself.

ESCAPE BEAT OR COMPLEX A QRS complex arising in an escape (or secondary pacemaker) in the atrioventricular (AV) junction or ventricles when the underlying rhythm slows to less than the escape or secondary pacemaker's inherent firing rate. Such rhythms are called *junctional or ventricular escape beats or complexes.*

ESCAPE (OR SECONDARY) PACEMAKER A latent pacemaker in the atrioventricular (AV) junction or ventricles that takes over pacing the heart when the pacemaker of the underlying rhythm slows to less than the latent pacemaker's inherent firing rate or stops functioning altogether.

ESCAPE PACEMAKER CELLS The pacemaker cells in the rest of the electrical conduction system that hold the property of automaticity in reserve should the sinoatrial (SA) node fail to function properly or electrical impulses fail to reach them for any reason, such as disruption in the electrical conduction system.

ESCAPE RHYTHM Three or more consecutive QRS complexes that result when the underlying rhythm slows to less than the escape or secondary pacemaker's inherent firing rate or stops altogether and the escape pacemaker takes over. Examples of escape rhythms are junctional escape rhythm and ventricular escape rhythm.

ESSENTIALLY REGULAR RHYTHM A rhythm in which the shortest and longest R-R interval varies by less than 0.08 second (two small squares) in an ECG tracing.

EVOLVING MI Necrosis progresses from the endocardium to the epicardium.

EXCITABILITY, PROPERTY OF The ability of a cell to respond to stimulation.

EXTENSIVE ANTERIOR MI A myocardial infarction commonly caused by occlusion of the left anterior descending (LAD) coronary artery alone or in conjunction with the anterolateral marginal artery of the left circumflex coronary artery and characterized by early changes in the ST segments and T waves (that is, ST elevation and tall, peaked T waves) in leads I, aVL, and V_1 to V_6 and the appearance early of abnormal Q waves in leads V_1 to V_2 and then later in leads I, aVL, and V_3 to V_6.

EXTERNAL CARDIAC PACING Transcutaneous pacing (TCP, TC pacing). A technique to treat bradycardias from whatever cause, ventricular asystole, and pulseless electrical activity using an external artificial pacemaker.

EXTRASYSTOLE A premature beat or complex independent of the underlying rhythm caused by an electrical impulse originating in an ectopic focus in the atria, atrioventricular (AV) junction, or ventricles. Examples of extrasystoles are premature atrial complexes (PACs), premature junctional complexes (PJCs), and premature ventricular complexes (PVCs).

EXTREME RAD When a QRS axis falls between −90° and ±180°. Also called an *indeterminate axis (IND)*.

F

FACING ECG LEADS Leads that view specific surfaces of the heart (for example, leads V_1–V_4 are facing leads viewing the anterior of the heart).

FASCICLE A band or bundle of muscle or nerve fibers. The left anterior fascicle and the left posterior fascicle form the two major divisions of the left bundle branch before it divides into the Purkinje fibers, forming the Purkinje network. See *Left bundle branch (LBB)*.

FASCICULAR BLOCK Absent conduction of electrical impulses through one of the fascicles of the left bundle branch (that is, left anterior fascicular block, left posterior fascicular block).

FASCICULOVENTRICULAR FIBERS (MAHAIM FIBERS) An accessory conduction pathway located between the bundle of His and the ventricles, resulting in fasciculoventricular preexcitation.

FASCICULOVENTRICULAR PREEXCITATION Abnormal conduction of the electrical impulses through the fasciculoventricular fibers, resulting in abnormally wide QRS complexes of greater than 0.10 second in duration and of abnormal shape, with a delta wave. PR intervals are normal.

FAST SODIUM CHANNELS Structures in the cell membrane called *pores* that facilitate the rapid flow of sodium ions into the cell during depolarization, rapidly changing the electrical potential within the cell from negative to positive. Fast sodium channels are typically found in the myocardial cells and the cells of the electrical conduction system other than those of the sinoatrial (SA) and atrioventricular (AV) nodes.

FIBRILLATION Chaotic, disorganized beating of the myocardium in which each myofibril contracts and relaxes independently, producing rapid, tremulous, and ineffectual contractions. Fibrillation may occur in both the atria and ventricles.

FIBRILLATION (f) WAVES: On the ECG, these waves appear as numerous irregularly shaped, rounded (or pointed), and dissimilar waves originating in multiple ectopic foci in the atria or ventricles.

FIBRIN An elastic threadlike filament that binds the platelets firmly together to form the thrombus after being converted from fibrinogen.

FIBRINOGEN A plasma protein that converts to fibrin, an elastic threadlike filament, when exposed to thrombin.

FIBRINOLYSIS The process of dissolving the fibrin strands binding the platelets together within a thrombus, initiating the breakup of the thrombus (thrombolysis).

FIBROUS PERICARDIUM The outer tough layer of the pericardium that comes in contact with the lung.

FINE ATRIAL FIBRILLATION Atrial fibrillation with fine fibrillatory waves—less than 1 mm in height.

FINE FIBRILLATORY WAVES When the f waves are less than 1 mm high.

FINE VENTRICULAR FIBRILLATION Ventricular fibrillation with small fibrillatory waves—less than 3 mm in height.

FIRING RATE The rate at which electrical impulses are generated in a pacemaker, whether it is the sinoatrial (SA) node or an ectopic or escape pacemaker.

FIRST-DEGREE AV BLOCK A dysrhythmia in which there is a constant delay in the conduction of electrical impulses through the atrioventricular (AV) node. It is characterized by abnormally prolonged PR intervals (longer than 0.20 second).

FIXED COUPLING Equal intervals of time between each premature beat and the preceding QRS complex of the underlying rhythm (that is, equal [constant] coupling intervals).

FIXED-RATE PACEMAKERS Artificial pacemakers designed to fire constantly at a preset rate without regard to the patient's own heart's electrical activity.

FLUTTER Rapid, regular, repetitive beating of the atria or ventricles.

FLUTTER-FIBRILLATION Refers to the simultaneous occurrence of flutter and fibrillation, as in atrial flutter-fibrillation.

FLUTTER (F) WAVES On the ECG, these waves appear as numerous repetitive, similar, usually pointed waves originating in an ectopic pacemaker in the atria or ventricles.

FREQUENT PVCs: Five or more premature ventricular complexes (PVCs) per minute.

FRONTAL PLANE A flat surface passing through the body at right angles to a plane passing through the body from front to back in the midline (sagittal plane), as viewed from the front of the body.

FULL (FULLY) COMPENSATORY PAUSE See *Compensatory pause.*

FUSION BEAT A ventricular complex unlike the QRS complexes of the underlying rhythm and those of the ventricular dysrhythmia in a given ECG lead, having features of both. This results from the stimulation of the ventricles by two electrical impulses, one originating in the sinoatrial (SA) node or an ectopic focus in the atria or atrioventricular (AV) junction and the other in an ectopic focus in the ventricles. A fusion beat can occur in accelerated idioventricular rhythm (AIVR), pacemaker rhythm, premature ventricular complexes (PVCs), and ventricular tachycardia.

f WAVES: See *Atrial fibrillation (f) waves.*

F WAVES See *Atrial flutter (F) waves.*

G

GAP JUNCTION A structure within the intercalated disks located at the junctions of the branches of myocardial cells, permitting very rapid conduction of electrical impulses from one cell to another.

GLYCOPROTEIN (GP) RECEPTORS Adhesive GPs located on platelet surfaces that bind with various components of connective tissue and blood to form thrombi. The major receptors and their function include the following:

GP Ia binds the platelets directly to collagen fibers present in connective tissue.

GP Ib binds the platelets to von Willebrand factor (vWF).

GP IIb/IIIa binds the platelets to vWF and, after the platelets are activated, to fibrinogen.

GOALS IN THE MANAGEMENT OF AN ACUTE MI The three major goals in the management of acute MI are as follows:
- Prevent the further expansion of the original thrombus and/or prevent the formation of a new thrombus.
- Dissolve or lyse the existing thrombus (thrombolysis).
- Enlarge the lumen of the occluded section of the affected coronary artery.

GP Ia RECEPTOR: The platelet receptor that binds the platelets directly to collagen fibers present in connective tissue.

GP Ib RECEPTOR: The platelet receptor that binds the platelets to von Willebrand factor (vWF).

GP IIb/IIIa RECEPTOR: The platelet receptor that binds the platelets to von Willebrand factor (vWF) and, after the platelets are activated, to fibrinogen.

GP IIb/IIIa RECEPTOR INHIBITOR: Inhibits platelet adhesion and aggregation by blocking the platelets' glycoprotein (GP) IIb/IIIa receptors. Examples include abciximab and eptifibatide.

GRID, ECG See *ECG grid.*

GROSSLY IRREGULAR RHYTHM When there appears to be no fixed pattern or ratio of the R-R intervals on an ECG.

GROUND ELECTRODE The ECG lead other than the positive and negative leads that grounds the input to prevent extraneous noise from entering the amplifier circuit.

GROUP BEATING Repetitive sequence of two or more consecutive beats followed by a dropped beat, as seen in second-degree atrioventricular (AV) block.

GROUP BEATS Occurrence of two or more consecutive atrial, junctional, or ventricular premature complexes preceded and followed by the underlying rhythm.

H

HEART RATE The number of heartbeats, QRS complexes, or R-R intervals per minute.

HEART-RATE CALCULATOR RULER A rulerlike device used to calculate the heart rate.

HEMIBLOCK Blockage to the conduction of electrical impulses in one of the fascicles (anterior or posterior) of the left bundle branch. See *Left anterior fascicular block (LAFB), Left posterior fascicular block (LPFB).*

HEMODYNAMICALLY STABLE (OR UNSTABLE) Refers to a patient who is normotensive, without chest pain or congestive heart failure, and not having an acute myocardial infarction or ischemic episode. A patient who is hemodynamically unstable, on the other hand, is hypotensive with evidence of poor peripheral perfusion, has chest pain or congestive heart failure, or is having an acute myocardial infarction or ischemic episode.

HEMORRHAGIC DIATHESIS Any tendency for spontaneous bleeding or bleeding from minor trauma caused by a defect in clotting or a defect in the structure of blood vessels.

HEMOSTATIC DEFECTS Abnormal conditions that stop the flow of blood within the vessels.

HEXAXIAL REFERENCE FIGURE A guide for determining the direction of the QRS axis in the frontal plane, formed by the lead axes of the three limb leads and three augmented leads, spaced 30° apart around a zero reference point.

HIS–PURKINJE SYSTEM (OF THE VENTRICLES) The part of the electrical system consisting of the bundle of His, bundle branches, and Purkinje network.

"HOCKEY STICK" PATTERN: The ventricular "strain" pattern in the QRS-ST-T complex produced by a downsloping ST-segment depression and T-wave inversion; characteristic of long-standing right or left ventricular hypertrophy. Synonymous with *left* or *right ventricular strain pattern.*

HORIZONTAL PLANE: A flat surface passing through the body at right angles to the sagittal and frontal planes and, in the case of electrocardiography, dividing the chest into an upper and a lower half at the level of the heart.

HYPERCALCEMIA Elevated levels of serum calcium in the blood.

HYPERCAPNIA Excessive amount of carbon dioxide in the blood, defined as a blood gas carbon dioxide level over 45 mm Hg.

HYPERCARBIA Hypercapnia.

HYPERKALEMIA Excessive amount of serum potassium in the blood. Normal is 3.5 to 5.0 mEq/L.

HYPERTENSION Blood pressure over 140/90 mm Hg.

HYPERTROPHY Chronic condition of the heart characterized by an increase in the thickness of a chamber's myocardial wall secondary to the increase in the size of the muscle fibers.

HYPERVENTILATION Increased ventilation of the alveoli caused by abnormally rapid, deep, and prolonged respirations; the result is a loss of carbon dioxide from the body and eventually alkalosis.

HYPOCALCEMIA Low amount of serum calcium in the blood.

HYPOCAPNIA Low amount of carbon dioxide in the blood.

HYPOCARBIA Hypocapnia. Low amount of carbon dioxide in the blood.

HYPOKALEMIA Low amount of serum potassium in the blood.

HYPOTENSION Low blood pressure; generally considered to be a systolic blood pressure of 80 to 90 mm Hg or less.

HYPOTHERMIA A state of low body temperature. When the core body temperature drops to 95°F, a distinctive narrow, positive wave—the Osborn wave—appears in the ECG. See *Osborn wave.*

HYPOVENTILATION Decreased ventilation of the alveoli.

HYPOVOLEMIA Decreased amount of blood in the body's cardiovascular system.

HYPOXEMIA Reduced oxygenation of the blood.

HYPOXIA Reduced amount of oxygen.

I

IDIOVENTRICULAR Pertaining to the ventricles.

IDIOVENTRICULAR RHYTHM See *Ventricular escape rhythm.*

IDIOVENTRICULAR TACHYCARDIA See *Accelerated idioventricular rhythm (AIVR).*

IM Abbreviation for *intramuscular.*

IMPLANTABLE CARDIOVERTER-DEFIBRILLATOR (ICD): Internal placement of a device capable of delivering electrical shocks to the heart to interrupt a life-threatening run of ventricular tachycardia or ventricular fibrillation. Prevents syncope or sudden death.

IMPLANTED CARDIAC PACEMAKER-INDUCED QRS COMPLEX Generally 0.12 second or greater in width and appears bizarre.

INCOMPLETE AV BLOCK (SECOND-DEGREE AV BLOCK) A dysrhythmia in which one or more P waves are not conducted to the ventricles. See *Second-degree type I AV block (Wenckebach); Second-degree type II AV block; Second-degree, 2:1, and advanced AV block.*

INCOMPLETE BUNDLE-BRANCH BLOCK (RIGHT, LEFT) Defective conduction of electrical impulses through the right or left bundle branch from the bundle of His to the Purkinje network in the myocardium, resulting in a slightly widened QRS complex (that is, greater than 0.10 second but less than 0.12 second).

INCOMPLETE COMPENSATORY PAUSE The R-R interval following a premature complex that, if added to the R-R interval preceding the premature complex, would result in a sum less than the sum of two R-R intervals of the underlying rhythm. See *Compensatory pause*.

INDETERMINATE AXIS A QRS axis between 90° and 180° (that is, extreme right axis deviation).

INDIFFERENT, ZERO REFERENCE POINT See *Central terminal*.

INFARCTION Death (necrosis) of tissue caused by interruption of the blood supply to the affected tissue.

INFERIOR (DIAPHRAGMATIC) MI A myocardial infarction commonly caused by occlusion of the posterior left ventricular arteries of the right coronary artery or, less commonly, of the left circumflex coronary artery of the left coronary artery and characterized by early changes in the ST segments and T waves (that is, ST elevation and tall, peaked T waves) and the appearance later of abnormal Q waves in leads II, III, and aVF.

INFERIOR VENA CAVA One of the two largest veins in the body that empty venous blood into the right atrium.

INFEROLATERAL MI A myocardial infarction that may be caused by (1) occlusion of (a) the laterally located diagonal arteries of the left anterior descending (LAD) coronary artery and/or the anterolateral marginal artery of the left circumflex coronary artery, and (b) the posterior left ventricular arteries of the right coronary artery, or, less commonly, of the left circumflex coronary artery of the left coronary artery; or (2) occlusion of the left circumflex artery of a dominant left coronary artery. The infarct is characterized by early changes in the ST segments and T waves (that is, ST elevation and tall, peaked T waves) and the later appearance of abnormal Q waves in leads I, II, III, aVL, aVF, and V_5 or V_6.

INFRANODAL Below the atrioventricular (AV) node.

INFREQUENT PVCs: Fewer than five premature ventricular complexes (PVCs) per minute.

INHERENT FIRING RATE The rate at which a given pacemaker of the heart normally generates electrical impulses.

INSTANTANEOUS ELECTRICAL OR CARDIAC AXIS OR VECTOR A graphic presentation, using an arrow, of the electric current generated by the depolarization or repolarization of the atria and ventricles at any given moment.

INTERATRIAL CONDUCTION TRACT See *Bachmann's bundle*.

INTERATRIAL SEPTUM The membranous wall separating the right and left atria.

INTERCALATED DISKS Specialized structures located at the junctions of the branches of myocardial cells that permit very rapid conduction of electrical impulses from one cell to another.

INTERNODAL ATRIAL CONDUCTION TRACTS Part of the electrical conduction system of the heart consisting of three pathways of specialized conducting tissue located in the walls of the right atrium between the sinoatrial (SA) node and atrioventricular (AV) node.

INTERPOLATED PVC A premature ventricular complex (PVC) that occurs between two normally conducted QRS complexes without greatly disturbing the underlying rhythm. A full compensatory pause, commonly present with PVCs, is absent.

INTERVALS The sections of the ECG between waves and complexes. Includes waves, complexes, and segments. See *P-P interval, PR interval, QT interval,* and *R-R interval.*

INTERVENTRICULAR SEPTUM The membranous, muscular wall separating the right and left ventricles. The anterior portion of the interventricular septum is supplied by the left anterior descending (LAD) coronary artery; the posterior portion is supplied by the posterior descending coronary artery.

INTIMA The innermost layer lining a blood vessel.

INTRACARDIAC Within the heart.

INTRAVENTRICULAR CONDUCTION DISTURBANCE Defective conduction of electrical impulses from the atrioventricular (AV) junction to the myocardium via the bundle branches and Purkinje fibers, resulting in an abnormally wide QRS complex. It occurs most commonly as a right or left bundle-branch block and, to a lesser extent, as a nonspecific, diffuse intraventricular conduction defect (IVCD) seen in myocardial infarction, fibrosis, and hypertrophy; electrolyte imbalance; and excessive administration of certain cardiac drugs.

INTRINSICOID DEFLECTION The downstroke of the R wave; the part of the QRS complex that begins at the peak of the last R wave and ends at the J point or tip of the following S wave. Follows the ventricular activation time (VAT; or preintrinsicoid deflection).

INTRINSICOID DEFLECTION TIME (IDT) The downstroke of the R wave, which begins at the peak of the R wave and ends at the J point or tip of the following S wave.

ION An atom or group of atoms with a positive charge (cation) or a negative one (anion).

IRREGULARLY IRREGULAR RHYTHM See *Grossly irregular rhythm.*

ISCHEMIA Reduced blood flow to tissue caused by narrowing or occlusion of the artery supplying blood to it. Ischemia results in tissue anoxia. Ischemia may be localized under the endocardium (subendocardial ischemia) or under the epicardium (subepicardial ischemia).

ISCHEMIC HEART DISEASE Heart disease caused by a deficiency of the blood supply to the heart (the myocardium, the electrical conduction system, and other structures), caused by obstruction or constriction of the coronary arteries. Manifestations of ischemic heart disease include acute myocardial infarction (MI), angina pectoris, bundle-branch and fascicular blocks, right and left heart failure, and arrhythmias.

ISCHEMIC T WAVES Symmetrically positive and abnormally tall, peaked T waves or symmetrically and deeply inverted T waves that appear over an ischemic myocardium. Generally, the ischemic T waves are upright over subendocardial ischemia and inverted over subepicardial ischemia.

ISOELECTRIC LINE The flat (sometimes wavy) line in an ECG during which electrical activity is absent. Synonymous with *baseline*.

ISOLATED BEAT: A premature complex occurring singly.

J

JAMES FIBERS The other name for atrio–His fibers, the abnormal accessory conduction pathway connecting the atria with the lower part of the atrioventricular (AV) node at its junction with the bundle of His.

J DEFLECTION See *Osborn wave*.

JOULES Unit of electrical energy delivered for 1 second by an electrical source, such as a defibrillator. Used interchangeably with the term *watt-seconds*.

J POINT See *Junction (or "J") point*.

JUNCTION Between the QRS complex and the ST segment.

JUNCTIONAL DYSRHYTHMIA A dysrhythmia arising in an ectopic or escape pacemaker in the atrioventricular (AV) junction, such as premature junctional complexes, junctional escape rhythm, nonparoxysmal junctional tachycardia (accelerated junctional rhythm, junctional tachycardia), and paroxysmal supraventricular tachycardia (PSVT).

JUNCTIONAL ESCAPE BEATS (COMPLEXES) AND RHYTHMS Beats (or complexes) and rhythms originating in an escape pacemaker in the atrioventricular (AV) junction that occur when the rate of the underlying supraventricular rhythm drops to less than 40 to 60 beats per minute.

JUNCTIONAL ESCAPE RHYTHM A dysrhythmia originating in an escape pacemaker in the atrioventricular (AV) junction with a rate of 40 to 60 beats per minute.

JUNCTIONAL TACHYCARDIA A dysrhythmia originating in an ectopic pacemaker in the atrioventricular (AV) junction with a rate greater than 100 beats per minute. When abnormal QRS complexes occur with tachycardia because of aberrant ventricular conduction, the tachycardia is called *junctional tachycardia with aberrant ventricular conduction (aberrancy)*.

JUNCTIONAL TACHYCARDIA WITH ABERRANCY See *Aberrant ventricular conduction (aberrancy)*.

JUNCTION (AV) See *Atrioventricular (AV) junction*.

JUNCTION (OR "J") POINT The point where the QRS complex becomes the ST segment or the ST-T wave.

J WAVE See *Osborn wave*.

K

K⁺ Symbol for potassium.

L

LAD Left anterior descending coronary artery. See *Coronary circulation*.

LARGE SQUARES The areas on ECG paper enclosed by the dark horizontal and vertical lines of the grid.

LATENT (OR SUBSIDIARY) PACEMAKER CELLS Cells in the electrical conduction system with the property of automaticity, located below the sinoatrial (SA) node. These cells hold the property of automaticity in reserve should the SA node fail to function properly or electrical impulses fail to reach them for any reason, such as a disruption in the electrical conduction system.

LATERAL LEADS Leads V_5 and V_6. The left precordial leads.

LATERAL MI A myocardial infarction commonly caused by occlusion of the laterally located diagonal arteries of the left anterior descending (LAD) coronary artery and/or the anterolateral marginal artery of the left circumflex coronary artery and characterized by early changes in the ST segments and T waves (that is, ST elevation and tall, peaked T waves) and the appearance later of abnormal Q waves in leads I, aVL, and V_5 or V_6.

LBB See *Left bundle branch (LBB)*.

LBBB See *Left bundle-branch block (LBBB)*.

LEAD A lead of the ECG. See *ECG lead*.

LEAD AXIS See *Axis of a lead (lead axis)*.

LEAD I, MONITORING LEAD See *Monitoring lead I*.

LEAD II, MONITORING LEAD See *Monitoring lead II*.

LEAD III, MONITORING LEAD See *Monitoring lead III*.

LEAD MCL1, MONITORING LEAD See *Monitoring lead MCL1*.

LEAD MCL6, MONITORING LEAD See *Monitoring lead MCL6*.

LEFT ANTERIOR DESCENDING CORONARY ARTERY Travels anteriorly and downward within the interventricular groove over the interventricular septum and circles the apex of the heart to end behind it.

LEFT ANTERIOR FASCICULAR BLOCK (LAFB) Absent conduction of electrical impulses through the left anterior fascicle of the left bundle branch. Typical ECG pattern: q1r3 pattern. Also referred to as *left anterior hemiblock*.

LEFT ATRIAL ENLARGEMENT (LEFT ATRIAL DILATATION AND HYPERTROPHY) Usually caused by increased pressure and/or volume in the left atrium. It is found in mitral valve stenosis and insufficiency, acute myocardial infarction, left heart failure, and left ventricular hypertrophy from various causes, such as aortic stenosis or insufficiency, systemic hypertension, and hypertrophic cardiomyopathy.

LEFT AXIS DEVIATION (LAD) A QRS axis greater than 230° (230°–290°).

LEFT BUNDLE BRANCH (LBB) Part of the electrical conduction system of the heart that conducts electrical impulses into the left ventricle. It consists of the left common bundle branch (or main stem), which divides into two bundles of fibers, the left anterior fascicle (LAF) and the left posterior fascicle (LPF).

LEFT BUNDLE-BRANCH BLOCK (LBBB) Defective conduction of electrical impulses through the left bundle branch. LBBB may be complete or incomplete and be present with or without an intact interventricular septum.

LEFT CIRCUMFLEX CORONARY ARTERY Courses over the anterior and lateral surface of the left ventricle between the left anterior descending coronary artery and the anterolateral marginal branch of the left circumflex coronary artery.

LEFT CORONARY ARTERY Arises from the base of the aorta just above the left coronary cusp of the aortic valve.

LEFT HEART Left side of the heart consisting of the left atrium and left ventricle.

LEFT MAIN CORONARY ARTERY Short main stem of about 2 to 10 mm in length that divides into two equal major branches: the left anterior descending coronary artery (LAD) and the left circumflex coronary artery (LCx).

LEFT POSTERIOR FASCICULAR BLOCK (LPFB) Absent conduction of electrical impulses through the left posterior fascicle of the left bundle branch. Typical ECG pattern: q3r1 pattern. Also referred to as *left posterior hemiblock*.

LEFT PRECORDIAL (OR LATERAL) LEADS Leads V_5 and V_6.

LEFT VENTRICULAR FAILURE Inadequacy of the left ventricle to maintain normal circulation of blood. This results in pulmonary congestion and edema.

LEFT VENTRICULAR HYPERTROPHY (LVH) Increase in the thickness of the left ventricular wall because of a chronic increase in pressure and/or volume within the ventricle. Common causes include mitral insufficiency, aortic stenosis or insufficiency, and systemic hypertension.

LENÈGRE'S DISEASE/LEV'S DISEASE Idiopathic degenerative disease of the electrical conduction system with fibrosis and/or sclerosis and disruption of the conduction fibers. A cause of bundle-branch and fascicular blocks.

LEUKOCYTES White blood cells.

LIFE-THREATENING DYSRHYTHMIAS Include ventricular fibrillation, pulseless ventricular tachycardia, ventricular asystole, and pulseless electrical activity.

LIMB OR EXTREMITY LEADS The three standard (bipolar) limb leads (leads I, II, and III) and the three augmented (unipolar) leads (leads aVR, aVL, and aVF).

LOWERCASE LETTERS Lowercase letters, such as *q, r,* and *s,* are used to designate small deflections of the ECG.

LOWN–GANONG–LEVINE (LGL) SYNDROME Atrio–His preexcitation typified by an abnormally short PR interval.

LPFB See *Left posterior fascicular block (LPFB)*.

LVH See *Left ventricular hypertrophy (LVH)*.

LYSE To break up, to disintegrate (for example, to lyse a thrombus).

LYSIS The process of breaking up or disintegrating (for example, thrombolysis).

M

MAHAIM FIBERS See *Nodoventricular fibers; Fasciculoventricular fibers*.

MARKED BRADYCARDIA A bradycardia with a heart rate between 30 and 45 beats per minute or less accompanied by hypotension and signs and symptoms of decreased perfusion of the brain and other organs.

MARKED SINUS BRADYCARDIA See *Marked bradycardia.*

MAT See *Multifocal atrial tachycardia (MAT).*

MCL1
See *Monitoring lead MCL1.*

MEAN QRS AXIS The average of all the ventricular vectors; also called the *QRS axis* or, simply, the *axis.*

MEAN VECTOR: An average of one or more vectors.

MEDIASTINUM Tissues and organs separating the sternum in front and the vertebral column behind, containing the heart and its large vessels, trachea, esophagus, thymus, and lymph nodes.

MEDULLA OBLONGATA Part of the brainstem connecting the cerebral hemispheres with the spinal cord; it contains specialized nerve centers for special senses, respiration, and circulation, including the sympathetic and parasympathetic nervous systems and their respective cardioaccelerator and cardioinhibitor centers.

MEMBRANE POTENTIAL The electrical potential measuring the difference between the interior of a cell and the surrounding extracellular fluid.

MIDCLAVICULAR LINE An imaginary line beginning in the middle of the left clavicle and running parallel to the sternum slightly inside the left nipple.

MIDPRECORDIAL (OR ANTERIOR) LEADS Leads V_3 and V_4.

MILD BRADYCARDIA A bradycardia with a heart rate between 50 and 59 beats per minute and the absence of hypotension and signs and symptoms of decreased perfusion of the brain or other organs.

MILD SINUS BRADYCARDIA See *Mild bradycardia.*

MILLIVOLT (mV): A unit of electrical energy. One thousand millivolts equal 1 volt.

MITRAL STENOSIS Pathologic narrowing of the orifice of the mitral valve, commonly the result of rheumatic fever or age-related calcification of the valve leaflets. One of the causes of left atrial enlargement.

MITRAL VALVE The one-way valve located between the left atrium and the left ventricle.

MOBITZ TYPE I AV BLOCK Type I atrioventricular (AV) block. A form of second-degree AV heart block characterized by progressively lengthening PR intervals until a QRS complex fails to occur.

MOBITZ TYPE II AV BLOCK Type II atrioventricular (AV) block. A form of second-degree AV heart block characterized by constant PR intervals. There are more P waves than QRS complexes, usually in a fixed ratio (2:1, 3:2, etc.).

MONITORED CARDIAC ARREST Cardiac arrest in a patient who is being monitored.

MONITORING LEAD I The single ECG lead used for monitoring the heart for dysrhythmias. Lead I is obtained by attaching the negative electrode to the right arm or the upper-right anterior chest wall and the positive electrode to the left arm or the upper-left anterior chest wall.

MONITORING LEAD II The single ECG lead commonly used for monitoring the heart solely for dysrhythmias. Lead II is obtained by attaching the negative electrode to the right arm or the upper-right anterior chest wall and the positive electrode to the left leg or the lower-left anterior chest wall at the intersection of the left fifth intercostal space and the midclavicular line.

MONITORING LEAD III The single ECG lead used for monitoring the heart for dysrhythmias. Lead III is obtained by attaching the negative electrode to the left arm or the upper-left anterior chest wall and the positive electrode to the left leg or the lower-left anterior chest wall at the intersection of the fifth intercostal space and the midclavicular line.

MONITORING LEAD MCL1 An ECG lead commonly used in the monitoring of dysrhythmias in the hospital, particularly in differentiating supraventricular dysrhythmias with aberrant ventricular conduction (aberrancy) from ventricular dysrhythmias. Lead MCL1 is obtained by attaching the positive electrode to the right side of the anterior chest in the fourth intercostal space just right of the sternum. The negative electrode is attached to the left chest in the midclavicular line below the clavicle.

MONITORING LEAD MCL6 The single ECG lead commonly used for monitoring the heart solely for dysrhythmias. Lead MCL6 is obtained by attaching the negative electrode to the upper-left anterior chest wall and the positive electrode to the lower-left anterior chest wall at the intersection of the sixth intercostal space and the midaxillary line.

MONOMORPHIC V-TACH V-tach with QRS complexes that are of the same or almost the same shape, size, and direction.

MORPHINE SULFATE A narcotic analgesic and sedative used to produce amnesia in conscious patients before cardioversion of certain dysrhythmias. Also used as a vasodilator to relieve congestive heart failure secondary to left-heart failure.

"M" (OR RABBIT-EARS) PATTERN: Refers to the rSR′ pattern of the QRS complex in V_1, representative of a right bundle-branch block.

MULTIFOCAL Indicates a dysrhythmia originating in different pacemaker sites (for example, a ventricular dysrhythmia with QRS complexes that differ in size, shape, and direction).

MULTIFOCAL ATRIAL TACHYCARDIA (MAT) An atrial tachycardia that originates in three or more different ectopic pacemaker sites, characterized by P′ waves that usually vary in size, shape, and direction in each given lead.

MULTIFOCAL PREMATURE VENTRICULAR COMPLEXES (PVCs): Different-appearing PVCs in the same tracing that originate from different ectopic pacemaker sites in the ventricles.

MULTIFORM Applies to a ventricular dysrhythmia with QRS complexes that differ in size, shape, and direction, originating in single or multiple pacemaker sites.

MULTIFORM PREMATURE VENTRICULAR COMPLEXES (PVCs): Different-appearing PVCs in the same tracing that originate in one or more ectopic pacemaker sites in the ventricles.

MULTIFORM VENTRICULAR TACHYCARDIA Ventricular tachycardia with QRS complexes that differ markedly from beat to beat.

MUSCLE TREMOR The cause of extraneous spikes and waves in the ECG brought on by voluntary or involuntary muscle movement or shivering; often seen in elderly persons or in a cold environment.

mV: Abbreviation for *millivolt.*

MYOCARDIAL: Pertaining to the muscular part of the heart.

MYOCARDIAL INFARCTION (MI) See *Acute myocardial infarction (acute MI, AMI).*

MYOCARDIAL INJURY Reversible changes in the myocardial cells from prolonged lack of oxygen. ECG manifestations include ST elevation or depression over injured myocardial cells.

MYOCARDIAL ISCHEMIA Reversible changes in myocardial cells from a temporary lack of oxygen. ECG manifestations include symmetrical T-wave elevation or inversion over ischemic myocardial cells.

MYOCARDIAL NECROSIS (INFARCTION) Irreversible damage to myocardial cells, causing their death; the result of prolonged lack of oxygen. ECG manifestations include abnormal Q waves over necrotic myocardial cells.

MYOCARDIAL (OR "WORKING") CELLS Myocardial cells other than those in the electrical conduction system of the ventricles.

MYOCARDIAL RUPTURE Rupture of the myocardial wall, usually occurring in the left ventricle in the area of necrosis after an acute transmural myocardial infarction.

MYOCARDIUM Middle layer of heart tissue that contains the muscle cells.

MYOFIBRIL Tiny structure within a muscle cell that contracts when stimulated. Contains the contractile protein filaments actin and myosin.

MYOSIN One of the contractile protein filaments in myofibrils that give the myocardial cells the property of contractility. The other is actin.

N

Na$^+$: Symbol for sodium ion.

NECROSIS Death of tissue.

NEGATIVE DEFLECTION Occurs when an electric current flows away from the positive electrode.

NERVOUS CONTROL OF THE HEART Emanates from the autonomic nervous system, which includes the sympathetic (adrenergic) and parasympathetic (cholinergic or vagal) nervous systems, each producing opposite effects when stimulated.

NODOVENTRICULAR FIBERS (MAHAIM FIBERS) An accessory conduction pathway located between the lower part of the atrioventricular (AV) node and the ventricles, resulting in nodoventricular preexcitation.

NODOVENTRICULAR PREEXCITATION Abnormal conduction of the electrical impulses through the nodoventricular fibers, resulting in abnormally wide QRS complexes of greater than 0.10 second in duration and of abnormal shape, with a delta wave. PR intervals are normal.

NOISE Extraneous spikes, waves, and complexes in the ECG signal caused by muscle tremor; 60-cycle alternating-current (AC) interference; improperly attached electrodes; and biomedical telemetry-related events, such as out-of-range ECG transmission and weak transmitter batteries. See *Artifact*.

NONCOMPENSATORY PAUSE The R-R interval after a premature complex that, if added to the R-R interval preceding the premature complex, would result in a sum that is less than the sum of two R-R intervals of the underlying rhythm. Synonymous with *incomplete compensatory pause*. See *Compensatory pause*.

NONCONDUCTED PAC A positive P′ wave (in lead II) not followed by a QRS complex. A blocked premature atrial complex (PAC).

NONCONDUCTED PJC A negative P′ wave (in lead II) not followed by a QRS complex. A blocked premature junctional complex (PJC).

NONCONDUCTED P WAVE A P wave not followed by a QRS complex. A dropped beat.

NONPACEMAKER CELL A cardiac cell without the property of automaticity.

NONPAROXYSMAL ATRIAL TACHYCARDIA When atrial tachycardia starts and ends gradually.

NONPAROXYSMAL JUNCTIONAL TACHYCARDIA A dysrhythmia originating in an ectopic pacemaker in the atrioventricular (AV) junction with a rate between 60 and 150 beats per minute. It includes accelerated junctional rhythm (60–100 beats per minute) and junctional tachycardia (100–150 beats per minute). It may occur with narrow QRS complexes or abnormally wide QRS complexes because of a preexisting bundle-branch block or aberrant ventricular conduction. When abnormal QRS complexes occur with the tachycardia because of aberrant ventricular conduction, the tachycardia is called *junctional tachycardia with aberrant ventricular conduction (aberrancy)*.

NONPITTING EDEMA Results from swelling caused by trauma or inflammation.

NON–Q-WAVE MI A myocardial infarction (MI) where abnormal Q waves are absent in the ECG. In the majority of such MIs, a nontransmural MI is present; in the rest, it is transmural.

NONSUSTAINED VENTRICULAR TACHYCARDIA Paroxysms of three or more premature ventricular complexes (PVCs) separated by the underlying rhythm. Paroxysmal ventricular tachycardia.

NONTRANSMURAL Not extending from the endocardium to the epicardium (that is, partial involvement of the myocardial wall, either in the subendocardial area or the midportion of the myocardium).

NONTRANSMURAL MYOCARDIAL INFARCTION A myocardial infarction in which the ventricular wall is only partially involved with the infarction.

NORMAL QRS AXIS A QRS axis between −30° and 190°.

NORMAL SINUS RHYTHM (NSR) Normal rhythm of the heart, originating in the sinoatrial (SA) node, with a rate of 60 to 100 beats per minute.

NOTCH A sharply pointed upright or downward wave in the QRS complex or T wave that does not go below or above the baseline, respectively.

O

OCCASIONALLY IRREGULAR RHYTHM Occurs when premature complexes occur in an otherwise regular rhythm. Seen in premature atrial complexes and premature ventricular complexes.

OPPOSITE (OR RECIPROCAL) ECG LEADS See "Reciprocal" ECG changes.

OPTIMAL SEQUENTIAL PACEMAKER (DDD) An artificial pacemaker that paces the atria or ventricles or both when spontaneous atrial or ventricular activity is absent.

ORTHOPNEA Severe dyspnea that is relieved only by the patient assuming a sitting or semireclining position or standing up.

OSBORN WAVE The distinctive narrow, positive wave that occurs at the junction of the QRS complex and the ST segment—the QRS-ST junction—in hypothermic patients with a core body temperature of 95°F. Also referred to as the *J wave*, the *J deflection*, or the *camel's* hump. Associated ECG changes include prolonged PR and QT intervals and widening of the QRS complex.

OVERDRIVE SUPPRESSION The suppression of spontaneous depolarization of the sinoatrial (SA) node or an escape or ectopic pacemaker by a series of electrical impulses (from whatever source) that depolarize the pacemaker cells prematurely. After termination of the electrical impulses, there may be a slight delay in the appearance of the next expected spontaneous depolarization of the affected pacemaker cells because of a depressing effect that premature depolarization has on their automaticity.

OVERLOAD Refers to increased pressure, volume, or both within a chamber of the heart from various causes, resulting in chamber enlargement from dilatation, hypertrophy, or both. Examples are right atrial enlargement, left atrial enlargement, right ventricular hypertrophy, and left ventricular hypertrophy.

P

PAC Abbreviation for *premature atrial complex*.

PACEMAKER, ARTIFICIAL: An electronic device used to stimulate the heart to beat when the electrical conduction system of the heart malfunctions, causing bradycardia or ventricular asystole. An artificial pacemaker consists of an electronic pulse generator, a battery, and a wire lead that senses the electrical activity of the heart and delivers electrical impulses to the atria or ventricles or both when the pacemaker senses an absence of electrical activity.

PACEMAKER CELL A myocardial cell with the property of automaticity.

PACEMAKER OF THE HEART The sinoatrial (SA) node or an escape or ectopic pacemaker in the electrical system of the heart or in the myocardium. May be sinus nodal, atrial, atrioventricular (AV) junctional, or ventricular.

PACEMAKER RHYTHM A cardiac rhythm produced by an artificial pacemaker.

PACEMAKER SITE The site of the origin of an electrical impulse. It can be the sinoatrial (SA) node or an escape or ectopic pacemaker in any part of the electrical system of the heart or in the myocardium.

PACEMAKER'S INHERENT FIRING RATE The rate at which the sinoatrial (SA) node or an escape pacemaker normally generates electrical impulses.

PACEMAKER SPIKE The narrow, sharp deflection in the ECG caused by the electrical impulse generated by an artificial pacemaker.

PAIRED BEATS Atrial or ventricular ectopic beats occurring in groups of two. Also called *coupled beats* or a *couplet.*

PAIRED PVCs: Two consecutive premature ventricular complexes (PVCs).

PARASYMPATHETIC (CHOLINERGIC OR VAGAL) ACTIVITY The inhibitory action on the heart, blood vessels, and other organs brought on by the stimulation of the parasympathetic nervous system. The effect on the heart and blood vessels results in a decrease in heart rate, cardiac output, and blood pressure and, sometimes, an atrioventricular (AV) block.

PARASYMPATHETIC (CHOLINERGIC OR VAGAL) NERVOUS SYSTEM Part of the autonomic nervous system involved in the control of involuntary bodily functions, including the control of cardiac and blood vessel activity. Activation of this system depresses cardiac activity and produces effects opposite those of the sympathetic nervous system. Some effects of parasympathetic stimulation are slowing of the heart rate, decreased cardiac output, drop in blood pressure, nausea, vomiting, bronchial spasm, sweating, faintness, and hypersalivation.

PARASYMPATHETIC (CHOLINERGIC OR VAGAL) TONE Pertains to the degree of parasympathetic activity.

PAROXYSM Sudden unexpected occurrence.

PAROXYSMAL NOCTURNAL DYSPNEA (PND) Sudden attacks of dyspnea, occurring at night, in a patient who may be asymptomatic during the day.

PAROXYSMAL SUPRAVENTRICULAR TACHYCARDIA (PSVT) A dysrhythmia with a rate between 160 and 240 beats per minute and usually an abrupt onset and termination. It originates in the atrioventricular (AV) junction as a reentry mechanism involving the AV node alone (AV nodal reentry tachycardia [AVNRT]) or the AV node and an accessory conduction pathway (AV reentry tachycardia [AVRT]). It may occur with narrow QRS complexes or abnormally wide QRS complexes because of a preexisting bundle-branch block or aberrant ventricular conduction. When abnormal QRS complexes occur only with paroxysmal supraventricular tachycardia (PSVT) because of aberrant ventricular conduction, the tachycardia is called *PSVT with aberrant ventricular conduction (aberrancy).*

PAROXYSMAL SUPRAVENTRICULAR TACHYCARDIA WITH ABERRANCY See *Aberrant ventricular conduction (aberrancy).*

PAROXYSMAL VENTRICULAR TACHYCARDIA A short burst of ventricular tachycardia consisting of three or more QRS complexes.

PAROXYSMS OF BEATS Bursts of three or more beats. A burst of three or more beats is considered a tachycardia.

PAST CARDIAC HISTORY Brief review of previous cardiovascular disease and its treatment.

PATTERNED IRREGULARITY Occurs when there is an ECG pattern seen between the measured R-R intervals.

P AXIS The mean of all the vectors generated during the depolarization of the atria.

PEA See *Pulseless electrical activity.*

PCI See *Percutaneous coronary intervention (PCI).*

PEAK OF THE T WAVE Coincident with the vulnerable period of ventricular repolarization, during which a premature ventricular complex (PVC) can initiate ventricular tachycardia or ventricular fibrillation.

PERCUTANEOUS CORONARY INTERVENTION (PCI) Catheter-based technique to enlarge the lumen of the occluded section of the affected coronary artery mechanically by means of one or more of the following:
- Percutaneous transluminal coronary angioplasty (PTCA)
- Coronary artery stenting
- Directional coronary atherectomy (DCA)
- Rotational atherectomy

PERFUSION Passage of a fluid such as blood through the vessels of a tissue or organ.

PERICARDIAL EFFUSION Fluid within the pericardial cavity or sac.

PERICARDIAL FLUID Helps lubricate the movements of the heart within the pericardium.

PERICARDIAL SPACE OR CAVITY Located between the visceral pericardium and the pericardial sac. It contains up to 50 mL of pericardial fluid.

PERICARDIAL TAMPONADE Accumulation of fluid under pressure within the pericardial cavity.

PERICARDITIS Inflammation of the pericardium accompanied by chest pain somewhat resembling that of acute myocardial infarction. The ECG in acute pericarditis mimics that of acute myocardial infarction because of marked ST-segment elevation.

PERICARDIUM The tough fibrous sac containing the heart and origins of the superior vena cava, inferior vena cava, aorta, and pulmonary artery. The pericardium consists of an inner, two-layered, fluid-secreting membrane (serous pericardium) and an outer, tough fibrous sac (fibrous pericardium). The inner layer of the serous pericardium, the visceral pericardium—or, as it is more commonly known, *the epicardium*—covers the heart itself; the outer layer, the parietal pericardium, lines the fibrous pericardium. Between the two layers of the serous pericardium is the pericardial space or cavity (or sac), which contains the pericardial fluid.

PERIPHERAL VASCULAR RESISTANCE The resistance to blood flow in the systemic circulation that depends on the degree of constriction or dilation of the small arteries, arterioles, venules, and small veins making up the peripheral vascular system.

PERIPHERAL VASOCONSTRICTION Constriction of blood vessels, especially the small arteries, arterioles, venules, and small veins, causing an increase in blood pressure and a decrease in the circulation of blood beyond the point of vasoconstriction.

PERIPHERAL VASODILATATION Dilation of blood vessels, especially the small arteries, arterioles, venules, and small veins, causing a decrease in blood pressure.

PERPENDICULAR OF A LEAD AXIS (PERPENDICULAR AXIS) A line intersecting or connecting with the lead axis at 90° (or a right angle), at its electrically "zero" point. Also referred to simply as the *perpendicular.*

pH: Symbol for the concentration of hydrogen ions (H^+) in a solution.

PHASES OF ACUTE MI
Phase 1: 0 to 2 hours
Phase 2: 2 to 24 hours
Phase 3: 24 to 72 hours
Phase 4: 2 to 8 weeks

PHASES OF DEPOLARIZATION AND REPOLARIZATION See *Cardiac action potential.*

PHASES OF THROMBOLYSIS (1) Release of tissue plasminogen activator (tPA) from the endothelium of the blood vessel wall into the plasma; (2) plasmin formation by conversion of plasminogen attached to the fibrin strands within the thrombus through the action of tPA; (3) fibrinolysis by the breakdown of fibrin through the action of plasmin, causing the platelets to separate from each other and the thrombus to break apart.

PHYSIOLOGIC AV BLOCK An atrioventricular (AV) block that occurs only when a rapid atrial dysrhythmia, such as atrial fibrillation, atrial flutter, and atrial tachycardia, is present.

PITTING EDEMA When pressure is applied with a finger, a dent appears in the edematous tissue that does not disappear immediately upon withdrawal of pressure. Sign of peripheral edema.

PJC Abbreviation for *premature junctional complex.*

PLASMIN: An enzyme that dissolves fibrin within the thrombus, helping to break the thrombus apart (thrombolysis). See *Plasminogen.*

PLASMINOGEN A plasma glycoprotein that converts to an enzyme, plasmin, when activated by tissue plasminogen activator (tPA). Plasmin, in turn, dissolves the fibrin strands (fibrinolysis) binding the platelets together within a thrombus, initiating thrombolysis.

PLATELET ACTIVATION The second phase of thrombus formation that occurs after the platelets become bound to the collagen fibers. The platelets become activated and change their shape from smooth ovals to tiny spheres while releasing adenosine diphosphate (ADP), serotonin, and thromboxane A2 (TxA2), substances that stimulate platelet aggregation. Platelet activation is also stimulated by the lipid-rich gruel within the atherosclerotic plaque. At the same time, the glycoprotein (GP) IIb/IIIa receptor is turned on to bind with fibrinogen. While this is happening, tissue factor is being released from the tissue and platelets.

PLATELET ADHESION The first phase of thrombus formation. After the denudation or rupture of an atherosclerotic plaque, the platelets are exposed to collagen fibers and von Willebrand factor (vWF). The platelets' receptor glycoprotein (GP) Ia binds with the collagen fibers and GP Ib and GP IIb/IIIa with vWF, which in turn also binds with collagen fibers. The result is the adhesion of platelets to the collagen fibers within the plaque, forming a layer of platelets overlying the damaged plaque.

PLATELET AGGREGATION The third phase of thrombus formation. Once activated, the platelets bind to each other by means of fibrinogen, which binds to the platelets' glycoprotein (GP) IIb/IIIa receptors. Stimulated by adenosine diphosphate (ADP) and thromboxane A2 (TxA2), the binding of fibrinogen to the GP IIb/IIIa receptors is greatly enhanced, resulting in rapid growth of the platelet plug. By this time, the prothrombin has been converted to thrombin by the tissue factor.

PLATELETS Small cells present in the blood that are necessary for coagulation of blood and maintenance of hemostasis. Contain adhesive glycoprotein (GP) receptors that bind with various components of connective tissue and blood to form thrombi. The major receptors are GP Ia, GP Ib, and GP IIb/IIIa. Platelets also contain several substances that, when released upon platelet activation, promote thrombus formation by stimulating platelet aggregation. These include adenosine diphosphate (ADP), serotonin, and thromboxane A2 (TxA2).

PLEURA The serous membrane enveloping the lungs and lining the thoracic cavity, completely enclosing a space filled with fluid, the pleural cavity.

P MITRALE A wide, notched P wave occurring in the presence of left atrial dilatation and hypertrophy. Typically associated with severe mitral stenosis.

PNEUMOTHORAX, TENSION Accumulation of air under positive pressure within the pleural cavity.

POLARITY The condition of being positive or negative.

POLARIZED (OR RESTING) STATE OF THE CELL The condition of the cell after repolarization, when the interior of the cell is negative and the outside is positive.

POLYMORPHIC V-TACH Ventricular tachycardia (V-tach) in which the QRS complexes differ markedly in shape, size, and direction from beat to beat.

POOR R-WAVE PROGRESSION Refers to the presence of small R waves in the precordial leads V_1 to V_6, characteristic of chronic obstructive pulmonary disease (COPD). Also seen after an anterior myocardial infarction.

POSITIVE DEFLECTION Occurs when an electric current flows toward the positive electrode of a lead.

POSTDEFIBRILLATION DYSRHYTHMIA A dysrhythmia occurring after defibrillatory shocks (for example, premature beats, bradycardias, and tachycardias).

POSTERIOR MI A myocardial infarction (MI) commonly caused by occlusion of the distal left circumflex artery and/or posterolateral marginal artery of the left circumflex artery and characterized by early changes in the ST segments and T waves (that is, ST depression in V_1 to V_4, inverted T waves in V_1 to V_2).

POTENTIAL (ELECTRICAL) The difference in the concentration of ions across a cell membrane, for instance, measured in millivolts.

P-P INTERVAL The section of the ECG between the onset of one P wave and the onset of the following P wave.

P PRIME (P′) WAVE An abnormal P wave originating in an ectopic pacemaker in the atria or atrioventricular (AV) junction or, rarely, in the ventricles. Usually negative in lead II.

P PULMONALE A wide, tall P wave (greater than 2.5 mm in height) occurring in the presence of right atrial dilatation and hypertrophy. Typically associated with pulmonary disease, such as chronic obstructive pulmonary disease (COPD), pulmonary embolism, and cor pulmonale.

PRECORDIAL Pertaining to the precordium.

PRECORDIAL REFERENCE FIGURE An outline of the chest wall in the horizontal plane superimposed by the six precordial lead axes and their angles of reference in degrees, radiating out from the heart's zero reference point.

PRECORDIAL THUMP A sharp, brisk blow delivered to the midportion of the sternum with a clenched fist in an initial attempt to terminate ventricular fibrillation or pulseless ventricular tachycardia.

PRECORDIAL (UNIPOLAR) LEADS Leads V_1, V_2, V_3, V_4, V_5, and V_6; each is obtained using a positive electrode attached to a specific area of the anterior chest wall and a central terminal. The positive electrode for each precordial lead is attached as follows:
V_1: Right side of the sternum in the fourth intercostal space.
V_2: Left side of the sternum in the fourth intercostal space.
V_3: Midway between V_2 and V_4.
V_4: Left midclavicular line in the fifth intercostal space.
V_5: Left anterior axillary line at the same level as V_4.
V_6: Left midaxillary line at the same level as V_4.

V_1 and V_2: The right precordial (or septal) leads overlie the right ventricle.

V_3 and V_4: The midprecordial (or anterior) leads overlie the interventricular septum and part of the left ventricle.

V_5 and V_6: The left precordial (or lateral) leads overlie the left ventricle.

PRECORDIUM The region of the thorax over the heart, the midportion of the sternum.

PREEXCITATION SYNDROME An abnormal ECG pattern consisting of an abnormally short PR interval or an abnormally wide QRS complex with a delta wave, or both, that results when electrical impulses travel from the atria or atrioventricular (AV) junction into the ventricles through accessory conduction pathways, causing the ventricles to depolarize earlier than they normally would. Accessory conduction pathways are abnormal strands of myocardial fibers that conduct electrical impulses (1) from the atria to the ventricles (accessory AV pathways), (2) from the atria to the AV junction (atrio–His fibers), or (3) from the AV junction to the ventricles (nodoventricular/fasciculoventricular fibers), bypassing various parts of the normal electrical conduction system. Preexcitation syndromes include ventricular preexcitation, atrio–His preexcitation, and nodoventricular/fasciculoventricular preexcitation.

PREINTRINSICOID DEFLECTION The part of the QRS complex measured from its onset to the peak of the R wave or, if there is more than one R wave, to the peak of the last R wave. See *Ventricular activation time (VAT)*.

PREMATURE ATRIAL COMPLEX (PAC) An extra beat consisting of an abnormal P wave originating in an ectopic pacemaker in the atria followed by a normal or abnormal QRS complex. PACs with abnormal QRS complexes that occur only with the PACs are called *PACs with aberrancy*; such PACs resemble PVCs. Also called *premature atrial beats (PABs) or complexes*.

PREMATURE ATRIAL COMPLEX WITH ABERRANCY See *Aberrant ventricular conduction (aberrancy)*.

PREMATURE COMPLEX QRS complex that occurs unexpectedly at some point in the P-QRS-T cycle or between cycles.

PREMATURE ECTOPIC BEAT (COMPLEX) An extra beat or complex originating in the atria, atrioventricular (AV) junction, or ventricles, such as a premature atrial complex (PAC), premature junctional complex (PJC), or premature ventricular complex (PVC).

PREMATURE JUNCTIONAL COMPLEX (PJC) An extra beat that originates in an ectopic pacemaker in the atrioventricular (AV) junction, consisting of a normal or abnormal QRS complex, with or without an abnormal P wave. If a P wave is present, the PR interval is shorter than normal. PJCs with abnormal QRS complexes that occur only with the PJCs are called *PJCs with aberrancy*. Such PJCs resemble premature ventricular complexes (PVCs).

PREMATURE JUNCTIONAL COMPLEX WITH ABERRANCY See *Aberrant ventricular conduction (aberrancy)*.

PREMATURE VENTRICULAR COMPLEX (PVC) An extra beat consisting of an abnormally wide and bizarre QRS complex originating in an ectopic pacemaker in the ventricles.

PRINZMETAL ANGINA A severe form of angina pectoris occurring at rest, caused by coronary artery spasm.

PROCAINAMIDE TOXICITY Excessive administration of procainamide, manifested by wide QRS complexes, low and wide T waves, U waves, prolonged PR intervals, depressed ST segments, and prolonged QT intervals.

PRODUCTIVE COUGH Cough accompanied by sputum.

PROPERTY OF AUTOMATICITY When pacemaker cells are capable of generating electrical impulses simultaneously.

PROPERTY OF CONDUCTIVITY The ability of cardiac cells to conduct electrical impulses.

PROPERTY OF CONTRACTILITY The ability of myocardial cells to shorten and return to their original length when stimulated by an electrical impulse.

PROTHROMBIN A plasma protein that, when activated by exposure of the blood-to-tissue factor released from damaged arterial wall tissue, converts to thrombin. Thrombin, in turn, converts fibrinogen to fibrin.

PR (P′R) INTERVAL The section of the ECG between the onset of the P (or P′) wave and the onset of the QRS complex. The normal PR interval is 0.12 to 2.0 seconds.

PR SEGMENT The section of the ECG between the end of the P wave and the onset of the QRS complex.

PSEUDOELECTROMECHANICAL DISSOCIATION A life-threatening condition in which the ventricular contractions are too weak to produce a detectable pulse and blood pressure because of the failure of the myocardium or electrical conduction system or both from a variety of causes. A form of pulseless electrical activity.

PULMONARY CIRCULATION Passage of blood from the right ventricle through the pulmonary artery, all of its branches, and capillaries in the lungs and then to the left atrium through the pulmonary venules and veins. The blood vessels within the lungs and those carrying blood to and from the lungs.

PULMONARY EMBOLISM Obstruction (occlusion) of pulmonary arteries by small amounts of solid, liquid, or gaseous material carried to the lungs through the veins. Typical ECG pattern: S1Q3T3 pattern.

PULMONARY INFARCTION Localized necrosis of lung tissue caused by obstruction of the arterial blood supply, commonly caused by pulmonary embolism.

PULMONIC VALVE The one-way valve located between the right ventricle and the pulmonary artery.

PULSE DEFICIT Occurs when some cardiac contractions are weak and cannot produce a strong enough pulse wave to reach the radial artery.

PULSELESS ELECTRICAL ACTIVITY The absence of a detectable pulse and blood pressure in the presence of electrical activity of the heart, as evidenced by some type of an ECG rhythm other than ventricular fibrillation or ventricular tachycardia.

PULSELESS VENTRICULAR TACHYCARDIA A life-threatening dysrhythmia equivalent to ventricular fibrillation and treated the same way, by immediate defibrillation.

PULSE OXIMETRY The continuous measurement of the oxygen saturation of hemoglobin and the pulse.

PUMP FAILURE Partial or total failure of the heart to pump blood forward effectively, causing congestive heart failure and cardiogenic shock. It is a complication of acute myocardial infarction, occurring more frequently in the presence of a bundle-branch block.

PURKINJE FIBERS Tiny, immature muscle fibers forming an intricate web, the Purkinje network, spread widely throughout the subendocardial tissue of the ventricles, whose ends finally terminate at the myocardial cells.

PURKINJE NETWORK OF THE VENTRICLES The part of the electrical conduction system between the bundle branches and the ventricular myocardium consisting of the Purkinje fibers and their terminal branches.

PVC Abbreviation for *premature ventricular complex*.

P WAVE: Normally, the first wave of the P-QRS-T complex, representing the depolarization of the atria. The P wave may be positive (upright), symmetrically tall and peaked, or wide and notched; negative (inverted); biphasic (partially upright, partially inverted); or flat.

Q

q1r3 PATTERN: Typical ECG pattern of an initial small q wave in lead I and an initial small r wave in lead III indicative of a left anterior fascicular block.

q3r1 PATTERN: Typical ECG pattern of an initial small q wave in lead III and an initial small r wave in lead I indicative of a left posterior fascicular block.

QRS AXIS The single large vector representing the mean (or average) of all the ventricular vectors.

QRS COMPLEX Normally, the wave following the P wave; consisting of the Q, R, and S waves; and representing ventricular depolarization. May be normal (narrow), 0.10 second or less, or abnormal (wide), greater than 0.10 second.

QRS PATTERN The QRS pattern present in leads V_5 to V_6 typical of a right bundle-branch block with an intact interventricular septum. An example of a QRS complex with a "terminal S" wave.

QRS-ST-T PATTERN Refers to the abnormally wide "sine-wave"–appearing QRS-ST-T complex that occurs in hyperkalemia.

qSR PATTERN: The QRS pattern present in leads V_1 to V_2 typical of a right bundle-branch block with a damaged interventricular septum.

QS WAVE A QRS complex that consists entirely of a single, large negative deflection.

QTc: See *Corrected QT interval (QTc)*.

QT INTERVAL The section of the ECG between the onset of the QRS complex and the end of the T wave, representing ventricular depolarization and repolarization.

QUADRANTS Refers to the four quadrants of the hexaxial reference figure—quadrants I, II, III, and IV.

QUADRIGEMINY A series of groups of four beats, usually consisting of three normally conducted QRS complexes followed by a premature complex that may be atrial, junctional, or ventricular in origin (that is, atrial quadrigeminy, junctional quadrigeminy, or ventricular quadrigeminy).

QUINIDINE TOXICITY Excessive administration of quinidine, manifested electrocardiographically by wide, often notched, P waves; wide QRS complexes; low, wide T waves; U waves; prolonged PR intervals; depressed ST segments; and prolonged QT intervals.

Q WAVE The first negative deflection of the QRS complex not preceded by an R wave.

Q-WAVE MYOCARDIAL INFARCTION (MI) An MI in which abnormal Q waves are present in the ECG. In the majority of the Q-wave MIs, a transmural MI is present; in the rest, the infarction involves only the subendocardium or midportion of the myocardium.

R

RABBIT-EARS PATTERN See *rSR′ pattern*.

RATE CONVERSION TABLE A table converting the number of small squares between two adjacent R waves into the heart rate per minute.

RATE OF IMPULSE FORMATION (THE FIRING RATE) See *Slope of phase 4 depolarization*.

R DOUBLE PRIME (R″) The third R wave in a QRS complex.

"RECIPROCAL" ECG CHANGES: ECG changes of evolving acute myocardial infarction present in opposite ECG leads, being, for the most part, opposite in direction to those in the facing ECG leads (that is, a mirror image). For example, an elevated ST segment and a symmetrically tall, peaked T wave in a facing ECG lead are mirrored as a depressed ST segment and a deeply inverted T wave in an opposite ECG lead.

REENTRY A condition in which the progression of an electrical impulse is delayed or blocked in one or more segments of the electrical conduction system while being conducted normally through the rest of the conduction system.

REENTRY MECHANISM A mechanism by which an electrical impulse repeatedly exits and reenters an area of the heart, causing one or more ectopic beats.

REFRACTORY Inability to respond to a stimulus.

REFRACTORY PERIOD The time during which a cell or fiber may or may not be depolarized by an electrical stimulus, depending on the strength of the electrical impulse. It extends from phase 0 to the end of phase 3 and is divided into the absolute refractory period (ARP) and relative refractory period (RRP). The ARP extends from phase 0 to about midway through phase 3. The RRP extends from about midway through phase 3 to the end of phase 3.

REGULARLY IRREGULAR RHYTHM See *Patterned irregularity*.

RELATIVE BRADYCARDIA The heart rate is too slow relative to the existing metabolic needs.

RELATIVE REFRACTORY PERIOD The period of ventricular repolarization during which the ventricles can be stimulated to depolarize by an electrical impulse that is stronger than usual. It begins at about the peak of the T wave and ends with the end of the T wave.

REPOLARIZATION The electrical process by which a depolarized cell returns to its polarized, resting state.

REPOLARIZATION WAVE The progression of the repolarization process through the atria and ventricles that appears on the ECG as the atrial and ventricular T waves.

REPOLARIZED STATE The condition of the cell when it has been completely repolarized.

RESTING MEMBRANE POTENTIAL Electrical measurement of the difference between the electrical potential of the interior of a fully repolarized, resting cell and that of the extracellular fluid surrounding it.

RESTING STATE OF A CELL The condition of a cell when a layer of positive ions surrounds the cell membrane and an equal number of negative ions lines the inside of the cell membrane directly opposite each positive ion. A cell in such a condition is called a *polarized cell*.

RESUSCITATION The restoration of life by artificial respiration and external chest compression.

RETROGRADE Movement in the opposite direction compared with normal.

RETROGRADE ATRIAL DEPOLARIZATION Abnormal depolarization of the atria that begins near the atrioventricular (AV) junction, producing a negative P′ wave in lead II; typically associated with junctional dysrhythmias.

RETROGRADE AV BLOCK Delay or failure of backward conduction through the atrioventricular (AV) junction into the atria of electrical impulses originating in the bundle of His or ventricles.

RETROGRADE CONDUCTION Conduction of an electrical impulse in a direction opposite to normal (that is, from the atrioventricular [AV] junction or ventricles [through the AV junction] to the atria or sinoatrial [SA] node). Same as retrograde AV conduction.

RIGHT AND LEFT ATRIA Two upper chambers of the heart; are thin walled.

RIGHT AND LEFT VENTRICLES The lower two chambers of the heart; are thick walled and muscular.

RIGHT ATRIAL ENLARGEMENT (RIGHT ATRIAL DILATATION AND HYPERTROPHY) Usually caused by increased pressure and/or volume in the right atrium. It is found in pulmonary valve stenosis, tricuspid valve stenosis and insufficiency (relatively rare), and pulmonary hypertension and right ventricular hypertrophy from various causes. These include chronic obstructive pulmonary disease (COPD), cor pulmonale, status asthmaticus, pulmonary embolism, pulmonary edema, mitral valve stenosis or insufficiency, and congenital heart disease.

RIGHT ATRIAL OVERLOAD Increased pressure and/or volume in the right atrium.

RIGHT AXIS DEVIATION (RAD) A QRS axis greater than 90°. Extreme right axis deviation – a QRS axis between −180° and −90°.

RIGHT BUNDLE BRANCH (RBB) Part of the electrical conduction system of the heart that conducts electrical impulses into the right ventricle.

RIGHT BUNDLE-BRANCH BLOCK (RBBB) Defective conduction of electrical impulses through the right bundle branch. It may be complete or incomplete and be present with or without an intact interventricular septum. Typical ECG patterns:

- rSR′ pattern in lead V1, the so-called "M" (or rabbit-ears) pattern
- Tall "terminal" R waves in leads aVR and V_1 to V_2
- Deep and slurred "terminal" S waves in leads I, aVL, and V_5 to V_6
- qRS pattern in leads V_5 to V_6—typical of a right bundle-branch block with an intact interventricular septum
- QSR pattern in leads V_1 to V_2—typical of a right bundle-branch block without an intact interventricular septum

RIGHT CORONARY ARTERY Arises from the aorta just above the right aortic coronary cusp.

RIGHT HEART The right half of the heart, consisting of the right atrium and right ventricle.

RIGHT-HEART FAILURE Inadequacy of the right ventricle to maintain the normal circulation of blood. This results in distended veins of the body, especially the jugular veins; body tissue edema; and congestion and distention of the liver and spleen. The lungs are typically clear.

RIGHT PRECORDIAL (OR SEPTAL) LEADS Leads V_1 to V_2.

RIGHT PRECORDIAL (UNIPOLAR) LEADS Leads V_2 R, V_3 R, V_4 R, V_5 R, and V_6 R; each is obtained using a positive electrode attached to a specific area of the right anterior chest wall and a central terminal. The right precordial leads overlie the right ventricle. The positive electrode for each right precordial lead is attached as follows:

V_2 R: Right side of the sternum in the fourth intercostal space

V_3 R: Midway between V_2 R and V_4 R

V_4 R: Right midclavicular line in the right fifth intercostal space

V_5 R: Right anterior axillary line at the same level as V_4 R

V_6 R: Right midaxillary line at the same level as V_4 R

RIGHT VENTRICULAR HYPERTROPHY (RVH) Increase in the thickness of the right ventricular wall because of a chronic increase in pressure and/or volume within the ventricle. It is found in pulmonary valve stenosis and other congenital heart defects (for example, atrial and ventricular septal defects), tricuspid valve insufficiency (relatively rare), and pulmonary hypertension from various causes. These include chronic obstructive pulmonary disease (COPD), status asthmaticus, pulmonary embolism, pulmonary edema, and mitral valve stenosis or insufficiency.

RIGHT VENTRICULAR MI A myocardial infarction (MI) caused by the occlusion of the right coronary artery and characterized by early changes in the ST segments and T waves (that is, ST elevation and tall, peaked T waves) and taller-than-normal R waves in leads II, III, and aVF; ST-segment elevation in V_4 R; and the later appearance of abnormal QS waves or complexes with T-wave inversion in leads II, III, and aVF and T-wave inversion in V_4 R.

RIGHT VENTRICULAR OVERLOAD Increased pressure and/or volume in the right ventricle.

R-ON-T PHENOMENON An ominous type of premature ventricular complex (PVC) that falls on the T wave of the preceding QRS-T

complex. This can cause ventricular tachycardia or ventricular fibrillation.

RP′ INTERVAL The section of the ECG between the onset of the QRS complex and the onset of the P′ wave following it. This is present in junctional dysrhythmias and occasionally in ventricular dysrhythmias.

R PRIME (R′) The second R wave in a QRS complex.

R-R INTERVAL The section of the ECG between the onset of one QRS complex and the onset of an adjacent QRS complex or between the peaks of two adjacent R waves.

RS PATTERN Refers to the appearance of a QRS complex in which there is an initial tall R wave followed by a deep S wave.

rSR′ PATTERN: A typical QRS complex pattern in V_1 present in a right bundle-branch block. Also referred to as the *M* or *rabbit-ears pattern*.

RUPTURE (DISRUPTION) OF THE FIBROUS CAP An abrupt tear in the leading edge of atheromatous plaque. Most likely to occur at its leading edge, the area of the cap where it connects with the normal arterial wall.

R WAVE The positive wave or deflection in the QRS complex. An uppercase "R" indicates a large R wave; a lowercase "r," a small R wave. May be tall or small, narrow or wide, slurred, or notched.

S

SALVOS Refers to two or more consecutive premature complexes. Bursts.

SA NODE The dominant pacemaker of the heart located in the wall of the right atrium near the inlet of the superior vena cava.

SAWTOOTH APPEARANCE Description given to atrial flutter waves.

SCOOPED-OUT APPEARANCE Description given to the depression of the ST segment caused by digitalis. Also referred to as the *digitalis effect*.

S DOUBLE PRIME (S″) The third S wave in the QRS complex.

SECONDARY PACEMAKER OF THE HEART A pacemaker in the electrical system of the heart other than the sinoatrial (SA) node; an escape or ectopic pacemaker.

SECOND-DEGREE AV BLOCK A dysrhythmia in which one or more P waves are not conducted to the ventricles. Incomplete atrioventricular (AV) block. See *AV block, second-degree, type I (Wenckebach); AV block, second-degree, type II;* and *AV block, second-degree, 2:1 and advanced.*

SECOND-DEGREE, 2:1, AND ADVANCED AV BLOCK A dysrhythmia caused by defective conduction of the electrical impulses through the atrioventricular (AV) node or the bundle branches or both. It is characterized by regularly or irregularly absent QRS complexes (producing, commonly, an AV conduction ratio of 2:1 or greater). The QRS complexes may be narrow (0.10 second or less) or abnormally wide (longer than 0.12 second in duration).

SECOND-DEGREE TYPE I AV BLOCK (WENCKEBACH) A dysrhythmia in which progressive prolongation of the conduction of electrical impulses through the atrioventricular (AV) node occurs until conduction is completely blocked. It is characterized by progressive lengthening of the PR interval until a QRS complex fails to appear after a P wave. This phenomenon is cyclical. See *Mobitz type I AV block.*

SECOND-DEGREE TYPE II AV BLOCK A dysrhythmia in which a complete block of conduction of the electrical impulses occurs in one bundle branch and an intermittent block in the other. It is characterized by regularly or irregularly absent QRS complexes (producing, commonly, an atrioventricular [AV] conduction ratio of 4:3 or 3:2). The QRS complexes typically are abnormally wide (greater than 0.12 second in duration). See *Mobitz type II AV block.*

SEGMENT A section of the ECG between two waves (for example, PR segment, ST segment, and TP segment). A segment does not include waves or intervals.

SELF-EXCITATION, PROPERTY OF The property of a cell to reach a threshold potential and generate electrical impulses spontaneously without being externally stimulated. Also referred to as the *property of automaticity.*

SEPTAL DEPOLARIZATION Refers to the depolarization of the interventricular septum early in ventricular depolarization, producing the septal q and r waves.

SEPTAL LEADS Leads V_1 to V_2. The right precordial leads.

SEPTAL MI A myocardial infarction (MI) commonly caused by occlusion of the left anterior descending (LAD) coronary artery beyond the first diagonal branch, involving the septal perforator arteries and characterized by early changes in the ST segments and T waves (that is, ST elevation and tall, peaked T waves) and the early appearance of abnormal Q waves in leads V_1 to V_2.

SEPTAL q WAVES: The small q waves produced by the normal left-to-right depolarization of the interventricular septum early in ventricular depolarization. Present in one or more of leads I, II, III, aVL, aVF, and V_5 to V_6.

SEPTAL r WAVES: The small r waves produced by the normal left-to-right depolarization of the interventricular septum early in ventricular depolarization. Present in the right precordial leads V_1 and V_2.

SEPTUM A wall separating two cavities.

SEROTONIN A substance released from platelets after the platelets are activated after damage to the blood vessel walls. Serotonin is a potent vasoconstrictor and promotes thrombus formation by stimulating platelet aggregation. Other substances released on platelet activation are adenosine diphosphate (ADP) and thromboxane A2 (TxA2).

SEROUS PERICARDIUM The inner layer of the pericardium.

SERUM CARDIAC MARKERS Proteins and enzymes released from damaged or necrotic myocardial tissue into the blood. These serum markers include myoglobin, creatinine kinase MB isoenzyme (CK-MB), and troponin T and I (cTnT, cTnI).

SHOCK A state of cardiovascular collapse caused by numerous factors, such as severe acute myocardial infarction (AMI), hemorrhage, anaphylactic reaction, severe trauma, pain, strong emotions, drug toxicity, or other causes. A patient in decompensated shock typically has dulled senses and staring eyes, a pale and cyanotic color, cold and clammy skin, systolic blood pressure of 80 to 90 mm Hg or less, a feeble rapid pulse (over 110 beats per minute), and a urinary output of less than 20 mL per hour.

SHORT VERTICAL LINES The vertical lines inscribed at every 3-second interval along the top of the ECG paper.

SICK SINUS SYNDROME A clinical entity manifested by syncope or near-syncope, dizziness, increased congestive heart failure, angina, and/or palpitations as a result of a dysfunctioning sinus node, especially in the elderly. The ECG may show marked sinus bradycardia, sinus arrest, sinoatrial (SA) block, chronic atrial fibrillation or flutter, atrioventricular (AV) junctional escape rhythm, or tachydysrhythmias interspersing with the bradycardias (sinus-tachydysrhythmia syndrome).

SIGNS Physical findings seen in the patient's body structure and function that are detected by initial inspection of the patient and by the physical examination.

SINGLE-CHAMBER PACEMAKER Artificial pacemaker that paces either the atria or the ventricles when appropriate.

SINOATRIAL (SA) EXIT BLOCK A dysrhythmia caused by a block in the conduction of the electrical impulse from the SA node to the atria, resulting in bradycardia, episodes of asystole, or both.

SINOATRIAL (SA) NODE See *SA node.*

SINUS ARREST A dysrhythmia caused by a decrease in the automaticity of the sinoatrial (SA) node, resulting in bradycardia, episodes of asystole, or both.

SINUS ARRHYTHMIA Irregularity of the heart rate caused by fluctuations of parasympathetic activity on the sinoatrial (SA) node during breathing.

SINUS BRADYCARDIA A dysrhythmia originating in the sinoatrial (SA) node with a rate of less than 60 beats per minute.

SINUS NODE DYSRHYTHMIAS Dysrhythmias arising in the sinus node include sinus dysrhythmia, sinus bradycardia, sinus arrest and sinoatrial (SA) exit block, and sinus tachycardia.

SINUS P WAVE A P wave produced by the depolarization of the atria initiated by an electrical impulse arising in the sinoatrial (SA) node.

SINUS TACHYCARDIA A dysrhythmia originating in the sinoatrial (SA) node with a rate of over 100 beats per minute.

SITE OF ORIGIN Pacemaker site.

SIX-SECOND COUNT METHOD A method of determining the heart rate by counting the number of QRS complexes within a 6-second interval and multiplying this number by 10 to get the heart rate per minute.

SIX-SECOND INTERVALS The period between every third 3-second interval mark.

SLIGHTLY IRREGULAR RHYTHM Over the length of the ECG, the amount of R-R interval variation is rarely more than 0.08 second.

SLOPE OF PHASE 4 DEPOLARIZATION Refers to the rate at which a cell membrane depolarizes spontaneously, becoming progressively less negative, during phase 4—the period between action potentials. As soon as the threshold potential is reached, rapid depolarization of the cell (phase 0) occurs. The rate of spontaneous depolarization is dependent on the degree of sloping of phase 4 depolarization. The steeper the slope of phase 4 depolarization, the faster the rate of spontaneous depolarization and the rate of impulse formation (the firing rate). The flatter the slope, the slower the firing rate.

SLOW CALCIUM-SODIUM CHANNELS A mechanism in the membrane of certain cardiac cells, predominantly those of the sinoatrial (SA) and atrioventricular (AV) nodes, by which positively charged calcium and sodium ions enter the cells slowly during depolarization, changing the potential within these cells from negative to positive. The result is a slower rate of depolarization compared with the depolarization of cardiac cells with fast sodium channels.

SLOW VENTRICULAR TACHYCARDIA See *Accelerated idioventricular rhythm (AIVR).*

SLURRING OF THE QRS COMPLEX The delta wave.

SMALL SQUARES The areas on ECG paper enclosed by the light horizontal and vertical lines of the grid.

SODIUM–POTASSIUM PUMP A mechanism in the cell membrane, activated during phase 4—the period between action potentials—that transports excess sodium out of the cell and potassium back in to help maintain a stable membrane potential between action potentials.

SPECIALIZED CELLS OF THE ELECTRICAL CONDUCTION SYSTEM OF THE HEART One of two kinds of cardiac cells in the heart, the other being the myocardial (or "working") cells. The specialized cells conduct electrical impulses extremely rapidly (six times faster than do the myocardial cells) but do not contract. Some of these cells, the pacemaker cells, are also capable of generating electrical impulses spontaneously, having the property of automaticity.

SPIKES Artifacts in the ECG. If numerous and occurring randomly, they are most likely caused by muscle tremor, alternating-current (AC) interference, loose electrodes, or biotelemetry-related interference.

If they are regular, occurring at a rate of about 60 to 80/minute, they are most likely caused by an artificial pacemaker.

SPONTANEOUS DEPOLARIZATION Property possessed by pacemaker cells, allowing them to achieve threshold potential and depolarize without external stimulation.

S PRIME (S′) The second S wave in the QRS complex.

S1Q3T3 PATTERN Typical ECG changes in lead I and lead III that occur in acute pulmonary embolism (that is, large S wave in lead I and a Q wave and inverted T wave in lead III).

STANDARD (BIPOLAR) LIMB LEADS Standard limb leads I, II, and III; each is obtained using a positive electrode attached to one extremity and a negative electrode to another extremity, as follows:
Lead I: The positive electrode attached to the left arm and the negative electrode attached to the right arm.
Lead II: The positive electrode attached to the left leg and the negative electrode attached to the right arm. Commonly used as a monitoring lead in prehospital emergency cardiac care.
Lead III: The positive electrode attached to the left leg and the negative electrode attached to the left arm.

STANDARDIZATION OF THE ECG TRACING A means of standardizing the amplitude of the waves and complexes of the ECG using a 1-mV/10-mm standardization impulse.

STANDARD LEADS Usually refers to the 12 ECG leads—leads I, II, III, aVR, aVL, aVF, and V₁ to V₆.

STANDARD LIMB LEADS Leads I, II, and III.

STANDARD PAPER SPEED A rate of 25 mm per second.

ST AXIS The mean of all the vectors generated during the ST segment.

STENT A cylindrical coil or wire mesh. See *Coronary artery stenting*.

STRAIN PATTERN Refers to the combination of a downsloping ST-segment depression and a T-wave inversion, characteristic of long-standing right or left ventricular hypertrophy. Along with the R wave, gives the so-called "hockey stick" appearance to the QRS-ST-T complex.

ST SEGMENT The section of the ECG between the end of the QRS complex, the J point, and onset of the T wave. May be flat (horizontal), downsloping, or upsloping.

ST-SEGMENT DEPRESSION An ECG sign of severe myocardial ischemia, appearing in the leads facing the ischemia. An ST segment is considered to be depressed when it is 1 mm (0.1 mV) below the baseline, measured 0.04 second (1 small square) after the J point of the QRS complex. It may be flat, upsloping, or downsloping. ST depression is also seen in the leads opposite those with ST elevation.

ST-SEGMENT ELEVATION An ECG sign of severe, extensive myocardial ischemia and injury in the evolution of an acute Q-wave myocardial infarction (MI), usually indicating transmural involvement. Less frequently, it may be seen in an acute non–Q-wave MI. An ST segment is considered to be elevated when it is 1 mm (0.1 mV) above the baseline, measured 0.04 second (1 small square) after the J point of the QRS complex. ST elevation usually occurs in the leads facing the myocardial ischemia and injury. ST elevation is also present in pericarditis and early repolarization.

ST-T WAVE The section of the ECG between the end of the QRS complex and the end of the T wave that includes the ST segment and T wave.

SUBENDOCARDIAL Located under the endocardium.

SUBENDOCARDIAL AREA The inner half of the myocardium.

SUBENDOCARDIAL, NON–Q-WAVE MI A myocardial infarction (MI) localized in the subendocardial area of the myocardium with absent Q waves in the ECG most of the time. See *Non–Q-wave MI*.

SUBEPICARDIAL Located under the epicardium.

SUBEPICARDIAL AREA The outer half of the myocardium.

SUBSTERNAL Under the sternum (retrosternal).

SUDDEN CARDIAC DEATH Sudden and unexpected death, usually from coronary heart disease, in patients with relatively minor or vague premonitory symptoms who appear well. Usual cause: a life-threatening dysrhythmia.

SUPERIOR VENA CAVA One of the two largest veins in the body that empty venous blood into the right atrium.

SUPERNORMAL PERIOD The short terminal phase of repolarization (phase 3) of cardiac cells near the end of the T wave, just before the cells return to their resting potential, during which a stimulus weaker than is normally required can depolarize the cardiac cells.

SUPERNORMAL PERIOD OF VENTRICULAR REPOLARIZATION The last phase of repolarization, during which the cell can be stimulated to depolarize by an electrical stimulus weaker than usual (that is, a subthreshold stimulus).

SUPRAVENTRICULAR Refers to the part of the heart above the bundle branches; includes the sinoatrial (SA) node, atria, and atrioventricular (AV) junction.

SUPRAVENTRICULAR DYSRHYTHMIA A dysrhythmia originating above the bifurcation of the bundle of His.

SUPRAVENTRICULAR TACHYCARDIA A dysrhythmia originating above the bifurcation of the bundle of His in the sinoatrial (SA) node, atria, or atrioventricular (AV) junction, with a rate of over 100 beats per minute.

SUSTAINED VENTRICULAR TACHYCARDIA Prolonged ventricular tachycardia.

S WAVE The first negative or downward wave of deflection of the QRS complex that is preceded by an R wave. An uppercase "S" indicates a large S wave; a lowercase "s" indicates a small S wave. May be deep and narrow or wide and slurred.

SYMPATHETIC (ADRENERGIC) ACTIVITY The excitatory action on the heart, blood vessels, and other organs brought on by the stimulation of the sympathetic nervous system. The effect on the heart and blood vessels results in an increase in heart rate, cardiac output, and blood pressure.

SYMPATHETIC (ADRENERGIC) NERVOUS SYSTEM Part of the autonomic nervous system involved in the control of involuntary bodily functions, including the control of cardiac and blood vessel activity. This system stimulates cardiac activity and produces effects opposite those of the parasympathetic nervous system, which depresses cardiac activity. Some effects of sympathetic stimulation are an increase in heart rate, cardiac output, and blood pressure.

SYMPATHETIC TONE Pertains to the degree of sympathetic activity.

SYMPATHOMIMETIC DRUGS Drugs that mimic the effects of stimulation of the sympathetic nervous system (for example, epinephrine and norepinephrine).

SYMPTOM An abnormal feeling of distress or an awareness of disturbances in bodily function experienced by the patient.

SYMPTOMATIC BRADYCARDIA A bradycardia with one or more of the following signs or symptoms: (1) hypotension (systolic blood pressure less than 90 mm Hg), (2) congestive heart failure, (3) chest pain, (4) dyspnea, (5) signs and symptoms of decreased cardiac output, or (6) premature ventricular complexes. Requires treatment immediately.

SYMPTOMATIC "RELATIVE" BRADYCARDIA Normal sinus rhythm or a dysrhythmia with a heart rate somewhat above 60 beats per minute with signs or symptoms associated with a symptomatic bradycardia because of the heart rate being too slow relative to the existing metabolic needs. Requires treatment immediately.

SYNCHRONIZED COUNTERSHOCK A direct-current (DC) shock synchronized with the QRS complex used to terminate the following:
- Atrial flutter/atrial fibrillation
- Paroxysmal supraventricular tachycardia (PSVT) with narrow QRS complexes
- Wide-QRS-complex tachycardia of unknown origin (with pulse)
- Ventricular tachycardia, monomorphic (with pulse)
- Ventricular tachycardia, polymorphic, with normal QT interval (with pulse)

SYNCYTIUM A branching and anastomosing network of cells, such as that formed by the interconnection of the cardiac cells to form the myocardium.

SYSTEMIC CIRCULATION Passage of blood from the left ventricle through the aorta, all its branches, and capillaries in the tissue of the body and then to the right atrium through the venules, veins, and vena cava. The blood vessels in the body (except those in the lungs) and those carrying blood to and from the body.

SYSTOLE (ELECTRICAL) The period of time from phase 0 to the end of phase 3 of the cardiac action potential.

SYSTOLE (MECHANICAL) The period of atrial or ventricular contraction.

T

TACHYCARDIA Considered to be three or more beats occurring at a rate exceeding 100 beats per minute.

Ta WAVE: Atrial T wave; usually buried in the following QRS complex.

T AXIS The mean of all the vectors generated during the repolarization of the ventricles (that is, during the T wave).

TEMPORARY TRANSVENOUS PACEMAKER Delivery of electrical impulses generated by an external artificial pacemaker through a catheter threaded through a vein and positioned in the right ventricle.

TERMINAL The final wave of the QRS complex.

TERMINAL R AND S WAVES Typical ECG findings in a right bundle-branch block—tall "terminal" R waves in leads aVR and V_1 to V_2; deep and slurred "terminal" S waves in leads I, aVL, and V_5 to V_6.

THIRD-DEGREE AV BLOCK (COMPLETE AV BLOCK) Complete absence of conduction of electrical impulses from the atria to the ventricles through the atrioventricular (AV) junction. May be transient and reversible or permanent (chronic). Usually associated with abnormally wide QRS complexes, but the QRS complexes may be narrow. See *AV block, third-degree (complete AV block)*.

THREE-SECOND INTERVAL The period between two adjacent 3-second interval lines.

THRESHOLD POTENTIAL The value of intracellular negativity that a cardiac cell must reach before the cell will depolarize.

THROMBIN An enzyme formed from prothrombin when prothrombin is exposed to tissue factor released from damaged arterial wall tissue. Thrombin, in turn, converts fibrinogen to fibrin.

THROMBOLYSIS The breakdown (lysis) of a thrombus (blood clot) by thrombolytic agents such as the normally occurring tissue plasminogen activator (tPA), which converts plasminogen attached to the fibrin strands within the thrombus to plasmin (an enzyme). Plasmin, in turn, breaks down the fibrin into soluble fragments (fibrinolysis), causing the platelets to separate from each other and the thrombus to break apart. Drugs used for thrombolysis include alteplase (t-PA; Activase), reteplase (r-PA; Retavase), and tenecteplase (TNK-tPA; TNKase).

THROMBOLYTIC AGENTS A tissue plasminogen activator that converts plasminogen, normally present in the blood, to plasmin, an enzyme that dissolves fibrin (fibrinolysis) within the thrombus, helping to break the thrombus apart (thrombolysis). The following

are thrombolytic agents: alteplase (t-PA), reteplase (r-PA), and tenecteplase (TNK-tPA).

THROMBOXANE A2 (TxA2): A substance released from platelets after the platelets are activated after damage to the blood vessel walls. Thromboxane A2 promotes thrombus formation by stimulating platelet aggregation. Other substances released on platelet activation are adenosine diphosphate (ADP) and serotonin. Aspirin inhibits thromboxane A2 (TxA2) formation and its release from the platelets, thus partially impeding platelet aggregation.

THROMBUS (BLOOD CLOT) An aggregation of platelets, fibrin, clotting agents, and red and white blood cells attached to a blood vessel wall.

THROMBUS FORMATION The formation of a blood clot (coagulation) involving a complex interaction between certain blood components (that is, platelets, prothrombin, and fibrinogen) and von Willebrand factor (vWF), collagen fibers, and tissue factor present in the endothelium and intima lining the blood vessel walls. The four phases of thrombus formation are as follows:

Phase I: Platelet adhesion. See *Platelet adhesion*.

Phase II: Platelet activation. See *Platelet activation*.

Phase III: Platelet aggregation. See *Platelet aggregation*.

Phase IV: Thrombus formation.

Also refers to the fourth phase of thrombus formation when the fibrinogen between the platelets is converted into stronger strands of fibrin by the action of thrombin, itself converted from prothrombin by tissue factor. Plasminogen usually becomes attached to the fibrin during its formation. As the thrombus grows, red blood cells and leukocytes (white blood cells) become entrapped in the platelet–fibrin mesh.

TISSUE FACTOR A substance present in tissue, platelets, and leukocytes that, when released after injury, initiates the conversion of prothrombin to thrombin.

TORSADES DE POINTES A form of ventricular tachycardia characterized by QRS complexes that gradually change back and forth from one shape and direction to another over a series of beats. A French expression meaning "twisting around a point."

TOTALLY IRREGULAR RHYTHM See *Grossly irregular rhythm*.

TP SEGMENT The section of the ECG between the end of the T wave and the onset of the P wave. Used as the baseline reference for the measurement of the amplitude of the ECG waves and complexes.

T/P WAVE When the following P wave is embedded or hidden in the preceding T wave.

TRANSCUTANEOUS OVERDRIVE PACING The use of a transcutaneous pacemaker to terminate certain dysrhythmias, such as polymorphic ventricular tachycardia with a prolonged QT interval (with pulse) and torsades de pointes (with pulse). This is done by adjusting the pacemaker's rate to one that is greater than that of the dysrhythmia.

TRANSCUTANEOUS PACING (TCP, TC PACING) The delivery of electrical impulses through the skin to treat bradycardia from whatever cause, ventricular asystole, and pulseless electrical activity using an external artificial pacemaker. External cardiac pacing.

TRANSMURAL Extending from the endocardium to the epicardium.

TRANSMURAL INFARCTION When the zone of infarction involves the entire or almost entire thickness of the ventricular wall, including both the subendocardial and subepicardial areas of the myocardium.

TRANSMURAL, Q-WAVE MI An infarction in which the zone of infarction involves the entire full thickness of the ventricular wall, from the endocardium to the epicardial surface. Abnormal Q waves are usually present.

TRENDELENBURG POSITION One in which the patient is supine on the backboard, the head of which is tilted downward 30 to 40 degrees, and the patient's knees are bent.

TRIAXIAL REFERENCE FIGURE A guide for determining the direction of the QRS axis in the frontal plane, formed by the lead axes of the three limb leads or the three augmented leads, spaced 60° apart around a zero reference point. The two triaxial reference figures, one formed by the standard limb leads and the other by the augmented leads, superimposed, form the hexaxial reference figure.

TRICUSPID VALVE The one-way valve located between the right atrium and the right ventricle.

TRIGEMINY A series of groups of three beats, usually consisting of two normally conducted QRS complexes followed by a premature complex. The premature complex may be atrial, junctional, or ventricular in origin (that is, atrial trigeminy, junctional trigeminy, or ventricular trigeminy).

TRIGGERED ACTIVITY See *Afterdepolarization.*

TRIPHASIC rSR′ PATTERN OF RBBB: See *"M"* (or rabbit-ears) pattern.

TRIPLICATE METHOD A method used to determine the heart rate.

T WAVE The part of the ECG representing repolarization of the ventricles that follows the QRS complex from which it is separated by the ST segment if it is present. It may be positive (symmetrically tall and peaked) or negative (deeply inverted).

T-WAVE ELEVATION/INVERSION See *Ischemic T waves.*

TxA2: Thromboxane A2 (TxA2).

U

UNCONTROLLED Refers to dysrhythmias such as atrial flutter and atrial fibrillation that are untreated and, consequently, have rapid ventricular rates.

UNCONTROLLED ATRIAL FIBRILLATION When more than 100 QRS complexes per minute are conducted in the presence of atrial fibrillation.

UNDERLYING RHYTHM The basic rhythm upon which certain dysrhythmias are superimposed, such as sinus arrest and sinoatrial (SA) exit block; atrioventricular (AV) blocks; pacemaker rhythm; and premature atrial, junctional, and ventricular complexes.

UNIFOCAL Pertains to a single ectopic pacemaker.

UNIFOCAL PVCs: Premature ventricular complexes (PVCs) that originate in the same ventricular ectopic pacemaker site, usually appearing identical.

UNIPOLAR CHEST ("V") LEADS Leads V_1 to V_6.

UNIPOLAR LEADS A lead that has only one electrode, which is positive.

UNIPOLAR LIMB LEADS Leads aVR, aVL, and aVF.

UNMONITORED CARDIAC ARREST Cardiac arrest that is witnessed by the resuscitation team or that has occurred before the arrival of the team and the patient is not being monitored.

UNSYNCHRONIZED SHOCK A direct-current (DC) shock not synchronized with the QRS complex, used to treat the following:
- Ventricular tachycardia, polymorphic, with prolonged QT interval (with pulse)
- Torsades de pointes (with pulse)
- Pulseless ventricular tachycardia
- Ventricular fibrillation

UPPERCASE LETTERS Uppercase letters, such as *Q, R,* and *S,* are used to designate large deflections of the ECG.

U WAVE The positive wave superimposed on or following the T wave. Possibly represents the final phase of repolarization of the ventricles.

V

VAGAL MANEUVERS Methods to increase the vagal (parasympathetic) tone to convert paroxysmal supraventricular tachycardia. See *Valsalva maneuver.*

VAGAL (PARASYMPATHETIC) TONE See *Parasympathetic (cholinergic or vagal) tone.*

VAGUS NERVE The parasympathetic nerve. Consists of the right and left vagus nerves.

VALSALVA MANEUVER Forceful act of expiration against a closed glottis (nose and mouth), producing a bearing down and subsequent rise in intrathoracic pressure. Also accomplished by gentle massage of the carotid bodies on the side of the neck. Used to increase the parasympathetic tone to convert paroxysmal supraventricular tachycardia.

VARIABLE AV BLOCK Refers to an atrioventricular (AV) block with varying AV conduction ratios (that is, the ratio of P, P′, F, or f waves to QRS complexes varies).

VASOCONSTRICTION Narrowing of the lumen of blood vessels.

VASOVAGAL Pertaining to a vascular and neurogenic cause.

VAT See *Ventricular activation time (VAT).*

VECTOR A graphic presentation, using an arrow, of the electric current generated by the depolarization or repolarization of the atria and ventricles at any one moment of time.

VENTRICLE The thick-walled muscular chamber that receives blood from the atrium and pumps it into the pulmonary or systemic circulation. The two ventricles form the larger lower part of the heart and the apex. They are separated from the atria by the mitral and tricuspid valves.

VENTRICULAR ACTIVATION TIME (VAT) The time it takes for depolarization of the interventricular septum, the right ventricle, and most of the left ventricle, up to and including the endocardial to epicardial depolarization of the left ventricular wall under the facing lead. Also called the *preintrinsicoid deflection* or *intrinsicoid deflection time (IDT).*

VENTRICULAR ASYSTOLE (CARDIAC STANDSTILL) Cessation of ventricular complexes. See *Asystole.*

VENTRICULAR BIGEMINY When premature ventricular complexes (PVCs) alternate with the QRS complexes of the underlying rhythm.

VENTRICULAR DEMAND PACEMAKER (VVI) A pacemaker that senses spontaneously occurring QRS complexes and paces the ventricles when they do not appear.

VENTRICULAR DIASTOLE The interval or period during which the ventricles are relaxed and filling with blood. The period between ventricular contractions.

VENTRICULAR DILATATION Distention of the ventricle because of increased pressure and/or volume within the ventricle; it may be acute or chronic.

VENTRICULAR DYSRHYTHMIA A dysrhythmia originating in an ectopic pacemaker in the ventricles. Also referred to as *ventricular ectopy.*

VENTRICULAR ECTOPY Occurrence of ventricular ectopic beats or rhythms.

VENTRICULAR ENLARGEMENT Ventricular enlargement includes ventricular dilatation and hypertrophy. Common causes include heart failure, pulmonary diseases, pulmonary or systemic hypertension, heart valve stenosis or insufficiency, congenital heart defects, and acute myocardial infarction. See *Left ventricular hypertrophy (LVH); Right ventricular hypertrophy (RVH).*

VENTRICULAR ESCAPE RHYTHM A dysrhythmia arising in an escape pacemaker in the ventricles with a rate of less than 40 beats per minute.

VENTRICULAR FIBRILLATION/PULSELESS VENTRICULAR TACHYCARDIA Two life-threatening ventricular dysrhythmias that result in cardiac arrest. Treatment is immediate defibrillation.

VENTRICULAR FIBRILLATION (VF, V-FIB) A dysrhythmia originating in multiple ectopic pacemakers in the ventricles and characterized by numerous ventricular fibrillatory waves and no QRS complexes.

VENTRICULAR FIBRILLATION (VF) WAVES Bizarre, irregularly shaped, rounded or pointed, and markedly dissimilar waves originating in multiple ectopic pacemakers in the ventricles.

VENTRICULAR HYPERTROPHY Enlargement of the ventricular myocardium, the result of an increase in the size of the muscle fibers because of a chronic increase in pressure and/or volume within the ventricle. Common causes include heart failure, pulmonary diseases, pulmonary or systemic hypertension, heart valve stenosis or insufficiency, and congenital heart defects. See *Left ventricular hypertrophy (LVH); Right ventricular hypertrophy (RVH).*

VENTRICULAR OVERLOAD Refers to increased pressure and/or volume within the ventricles.

VENTRICULAR PREEXCITATION The premature depolarization of the ventricles associated with an abnormal accessory conduction pathway, such as the accessory atrioventricular (AV) pathways or nodoventricular/fasciculoventricular fibers that bypass the AV junction or bundle of His, respectively, allowing the electrical impulses to initiate depolarization of the ventricles earlier than usual. This results in an abnormally wide QRS complex of greater than 0.10 second that characteristically has an abnormal slurring and sometimes notching at its onset—the delta wave. The PR interval is usually less than 0.10 second when ventricular preexcitation is the result of an accessory AV pathway and usually normal when nodoventricular/fasciculoventricular fibers are the cause. The term *ventricular preexcitation* is most commonly used to indicate ventricular preexcitation associated with accessory AV pathway conduction.

VENTRICULAR REPOLARIZATION The electrical process by which the depolarized ventricles return to their polarized, resting state. Ventricular depolarization is represented by the T wave on the ECG.

VENTRICULAR "STRAIN" PATTERN The changes in the QRS-ST-T complex produced by a downsloping ST-segment depression and T-wave inversion, characteristic of long-standing right or left ventricular hypertrophy. Also known as the "hockey stick" pattern.

VENTRICULAR SYSTOLE The interval or period during which the ventricles are contracting and emptying of blood.

VENTRICULAR TACHYCARDIA (VT, V-TACH) A dysrhythmia originating in an ectopic pacemaker in the ventricles with a rate between 100 and 250 beats per minute.

VENTRICULAR TRIGEMINY Occurs when there is one premature ventricular complex (PVC) for every two QRS complexes of the underlying rhythm, or one QRS complex of the underlying rhythm for every two PVCs.

VENTRICULAR T WAVE (T WAVE) Represents ventricular repolarization.

VERAPAMIL An antiarrhythmic used to treat paroxysmal atrial and junctional tachycardias.

VISCERAL PERICARDIUM See *Epicardium.*

V LEADS Leads V_1, V_2, V_3, V_4, V_5, and V_6. See *Precordial (unipolar) leads.*

VOLTAGE (AMPLITUDE) See *Amplitude (voltage).*

VON WILLEBRAND FACTOR (vWF): A protein stored in the endothelium of blood vessels that, when exposed to blood, binds to the platelets' glycoprotein (GP) Ib and GP IIb/GP IIIa receptors, adhering the platelets to the collagen fibers in the blood vessel wall.

VULNERABLE PERIOD OF VENTRICULAR REPOLARIZATION The part of the last phase of repolarization during which the ventricles can be stimulated to depolarize prematurely by a greater-than-normal electrical stimulus. This corresponds to the downslope of the T wave.

vWF: See *von Willebrand factor (vWF).*

W

WANDERING ATRIAL PACEMAKER (WAP) A dysrhythmia originating in pacemakers that shifts back and forth between the sinoatrial (SA) node and an ectopic pacemaker in the atria or atrioventricular (AV) junction. It is characterized by P waves varying in size, shape, and direction in any given lead.

WARNING DYSRHYTHMIAS Premature ventricular complexes (PVCs) that are more prone than others to initiate life-threatening dysrhythmias, particularly after an acute myocardial infarction or ischemic episode:

- PVCs falling on the T wave (the R-on-T phenomenon)
- Multiform and multifocal PVCs
- Frequent PVCs of more than five or six per minute
- Ventricular group beats with bursts or salvos of two, three, or more

WAVES Refers to various components of the ECG—the P, Q, R, S, T, and U waves. Waves may be large or small.

WENCKEBACH BLOCK See *Second-degree type I AV block (Wenckebach).*

WENCKEBACH PHENOMENON A progressive prolongation of the conduction of electrical impulses through the atrioventricular (AV) node, most commonly until conduction is completely blocked, occurring in cycles. A conduction block may also occur infranodally.

WIDE-QRS-COMPLEX TACHYCARDIA A tachycardia with abnormally wide QRS complexes (greater than 0.12 second) that may be ventricular tachycardia or a supraventricular tachycardia with wide QRS complexes resulting from a preexisting bundle-branch block, aberrant ventricular conduction, or ventricular preexcitation.

WINDOW THEORY Refers to the popular theory of why Q waves occur over infarcted myocardium. According to this theory, the facing leads over electrically inert infarcted myocardium (or "window") view the endocardium of the opposite noninfarcted ventricular wall and detect the R waves generated by the opposite wall as large Q waves.

WOLFF–PARKINSON–WHITE (WPW) CONDUCTION Accessory atrioventricular (AV) pathway conduction, resulting in abnormally wide QRS complexes.

WOLFF–PARKINSON–WHITE (WPW) SYNDROME When Wolff–Parkinson–White conduction is associated with paroxysmal supraventricular tachycardia with normal QRS complexes.

Z

ZERO CENTER OF THE HEART Refers to the hypothetical reference point with an electrical potential of zero, located in the electrical center of the heart—left of the interventricular septum and below the atrioventricular (AV) junction. Formed by connecting the extremity electrodes together, the "indifferent" zero reference point is used as the central terminal for the unipolar leads. It also represents the central point for the hexaxial reference figure.

ZONE OF INJURY Layer of injured myocardial tissue.

ZONE OF ISCHEMIA Outer layer of ischemic tissue.

ZONES OF INFARCTION (NECROSIS), INJURY, AND ISCHEMIA A myocardial infarction at its height typically consists of a central area of dead, necrotic tissue known as the *zone of infarction* (or *necrosis*); surrounded immediately by a layer of injured myocardial tissue, the *zone of injury*; and, last, by an outer layer of ischemic tissue, the *zone of ischemia*.

INDEX

Note: Page numbers followed by *f* indicate figures, *t* indicate tables, and *b* indicate boxes.